Instructor's Resource Manual

to accompany

Medical Language

Susan Turley, MA(Educ), BSN, RN, RHIT, CMT

Adjunct Professor; School of Health Professions,
Wellness, and Physical Education
Anne Arundel Community College
Arnold, Maryland

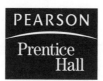

PEARSON

Prentice
Hall

Upper Saddle River, New Jersey 07458

Pearson Prentice Hall™ is a trademark of Pearson Education, Inc.
Pearson® is a registered trademark of Pearson plc.
Prentice Hall® is a registered trademark of Pearson Education, Inc.

Pearson Education Ltd., *London*
Pearson Education Australia Pty. Limited, *Sydney*
Pearson Education Singapore, Pte. Ltd.
Pearson Education North Asia Ltd., *Hong Kong*
Pearson Education Canada, Ltd., *Toronto*

Pearson Educación de Mexico, S.A. de C.V.
Pearson Education—Japan, *Tokyo*
Pearson Education Malaysia, Pte. Ltd.
Pearson Education, Upper Saddle River, New Jersey

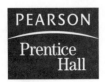

10 9 8 7 6 5 4 3 2 1
ISBN 0-13-094000-3

CONTENTS

PREFACE

Thank you for adopting *Medical Language*! The goal of this book is to immerse your students in the real world of medicine. I propose to do this by way of various visual, auditory, and pedagogical features throughout the textbook and the student and instructor's resources. Combined with your instructional expertise and guidance, this textbook and these resources will help your students discover the way to become fluent in medical language. By taking full advantage of what this textbook and these resources have to offer, you and your students will discover a system of learning medical language that is simple and yet challenging.

By selecting *Medical Language* as your textbook you have given yourself access to a wide variety of excellent text-specific instructional tools. In the pages of this preface that follow, I will introduce you to the most advanced instructor resources of any medical terminology textbook on the market today.

Instructor's Resource Manual

The goal of this manual is to help you synthesize all of the resources you now have at your disposal in connection with your adoption of *Medical Language*. The manual is designed not only to aid your course preparation, but also to help you truly shine in the classroom. I have taken a novel approach to designing this manual. Each chapter follows a consistent format:

- Instructor Activity for the Beginning of Class begins each chapter. These are "conversation starters" that you can use to infuse interest, stimulate discussion, and help get each class session off on the right foot.
- Teaching Strategies and Content Abstracts are organized according to the learning objectives in each chapter. The Teaching Strategy gives the overall goal for teaching that section, while the Content Abstract is a short summary of the essential content covered within the chapter.
- Instructor Activities provide a wealth of fascinating facts, authentic medical stories, and thought-provoking current events that you can share with your students as well as ideas for novel ways to spice up the classroom experience.
- Classroom Activities present a treasure chest of ideas for bringing your classroom alive. From games to group activities to videos to tips for guest speakers, these sections will give you many valuable resources.
- Experience Multimedia boxes refer you to appropriate presentation opportunities within Prentice Hall's robust instructional media program. These media assets are found on the Instructor's Media Library. The Instructor's Media Library (0-13-112380-7) is available upon adoption of *Medical Language*.
- Homework Activities provide you with a comprehensive list of unique assignment options directly correlated to the chapter content. Included are a broad range of activities that run the gamut from Internet research to the creation of crossword puzzles to writing a paper about the experience of donating blood.

Other components of this manual include:

- Test questions that measure student mastery of pertinent objectives are provided in a variety of formats for use in quizzes and examinations. An electronic version of the test bank can be found in the Instructor's Media Library.
- The Art and Craft of Teaching discusses various teaching techniques to ensure that students learn the material effectively. This section also highlights classroom management techniques that help to make learning enjoyable.
- *Medical Terminology Pearls of Wisdom.* Dozens of highly successful medical terminology instructors from around the United States (see page PW-6 for a list of their names) shared their "pearls of wisdom" for teaching medical terminology. These tips from master instructors have been compiled and arranged in their own section at the beginning of this manual. Refer to this section often when you are looking for good ideas. You may also wish to share your own ideas with Prentice Hall by sending them to Medical Terminology Pearls, Prentice Hall Health Editorial, 1 Lake St., Upper Saddle River, NJ 07458.

Instructor's Media Library

The Instructor's Media Library (0-13-112380-7) is available upon adoption and gives you access to a number of powerful tools in electronic format.

- A 3,436-question test bank allows instructors to design customized quizzes and exams using our award-winning TestGen 7.0 test building engine. You will find the test bank by clicking on Assessment Resources from the main dashboard screen of the CD-ROM. The TestGen wizard steps you through the creation of a simple test with drag-and-drop or point-and-click transfer. You can select test questions either manually or randomly and use online spellchecking and other tools to quickly polish your test content and presentation. The question formats include multiple-choice, fill-in-the-blank, true/false, and essay. You can save your test in a variety of formats both locally and on a network, print up to 25 variations of a single test, and publish your tests in an online course. For more information go to www.prenhall.com/testgen.
- A PowerPoint lecture package contains key discussion points, along with color images, animations, and videos for each chapter. You will find the PowerPoint lectures by clicking on Presentation Resources from the main dashboard screen of the CD-ROM. This feature provides dynamic, fully designed, integrated lectures that are ready to use and allow instructors to customize the materials to meet their specific course needs. These ready-made lectures will save you time and ease the transition into your use of *Medical Language*.
- A library of 453 medical images is also available to you. You will find the image library by clicking on Presentation Resources from the main dashboard screen of the CD-ROM. You are free to copy and paste these images into your PowerPoint lectures, printed documents, and Web site, as long as you are using *Medical Language* as your course textbook. If you do not have access to a video projector, you may still make use of these slides by printing them out on acetate film and presenting them by using an overhead projector.
- *Real People, Real Medicine* videos are short segments in which we have profiled 22 different health professionals doing their daily jobs. You will find the video collection by clicking on Presentation Resources from the main dashboard screen of the CD-ROM. These videos were produced during the development of *Medical Language*, and they are tied directly to the Career Focus boxes toward the end of each chapter. We encourage you to use the Career Focus boxes with your students and then explain that you have a bonus video to show them that directly correlates to these boxes. These will provide you with an extra resource to help you pre-

sent a seamless lecture and also help your students draw the connection between this textbook and real-life experiences of healthcare professionals on the job.

- An electronic version of this Instructor's Resource Manual in PDF format can be accessed by clicking on Instructor's Resources from the main dashboard screen of the CD-ROM.

Other Components of the Teaching and Learning Package

- An interactive student CD-ROM is packaged in the back of the textbook and contains a host of interactive study aids. This CD-ROM is self-loading. It runs as soon as it is placed in the CD-ROM drive of any computer, and therefore requires no installation or downloading. The CD-ROM includes a custom flashcard generator that allows the students to create flashcards designed for their personal study needs. The videos and animations help the students to visualize the content they are learning. Interactive exercises, games, and activities provide students with extra practice to master the chapter content. There are also listening/typing exercises that have real physicians dictating excerpts from real medical reports. You may wish to assign the CD-ROM activities as homework and ask students to use the Print function to print their answers and turn them in to you at the start of class.

- A companion Web site is available at www.prenhall.com/turley. This is an open-access online "home base" for the book. Here you will find two bonus chapters, Dietetics and Dentistry. Additionally, students may access a daily health news update service and an audio pronunciation glossary.

- OneKey is Prentice Hall's online course system. Those instructors wishing to facilitate on-line courses will be able to access a premium on-line course management option, which is available in WebCT, Blackboard, or CourseCompass formats. OneKey is an integrated online resource that brings a wide array of supplemental resources together in one convenient place for both students and faculty. OneKey features everything you and your students need for out-of-class work, conveniently organized to match your syllabus. OneKey's online course management solution features interactive modules, text and image PowerPoints, animations, videos, and more. OneKey also provides course management tools so faculty can customize course content, build online tests, create assignments, enter grades, post announcements, communicate with students, and much more. Testing materials, gradebooks, and other instructor resources are available in a separate section that can be accessed by instructors only. OneKey content is available in three different platforms. A nationally hosted version is available in the reliable, easy-to-use CourseCompass platform. The same content is also available for download to locally hosted versions of BlackBoard and WebCT. Please contact your Prentice Hall Sales Representative for a demonstration or go online to **www.prenhall.com/onekey.**

CONTRIBUTORS

Instructor's Resource Manual

Toni Cade, MBA, RHIA, CCS, FAHIMA
Associate Professor, Health Information Management
University of Louisiana at Lafayette
Lafayette, Louisiana

Test Bank

Toni Cade, MBA, RHIA, CCS, FAHIMA
Associate Professor, Health Information Management
University of Louisiana at Lafayette
Lafayette, Louisiana

Anne Loochtan, MEd
Assistant Dean, Health and Public Safety
Columbus State Community College
Cincinnati, Ohio

Patricia McLane, RHIA, MA
Instructor, Health Information Technology
Henry Ford Community College
Dearborn, Michigan

Donna Jeanne Pugh, BSN, RN
Department Chair, Medical Programs
Florida Metropolitan University
Jacksonville, Florida

PowerPoint™ Lectures

Kathy Stau, CPhT
Program Director, Pharmacy Technician
Medix School
Smyrna, Georgia

Classroom Response System

Beulah Hofmann, RN, MSN, CMA
Assistant Professor/Director, Nursing
Ivy Tech Community College
Greencastle, Indiana

Student CD-ROM

Alice Noblin, MBA, RHIA, LHRM
Instructor, Health Information Management
University of Central Florida
Orlando, Florida

Kim Webb, RN, MN
Chair, Nursing Program
Northern Oklahoma College
Tonkawa, Oklahoma

REVIEWERS

Instructor's Resource Manual

Karen Myers, CPC
Instructor, Office Technology
Pierce College—Puyallup
Puyallup, Washington

Alice Noblin, MBA, RHIA, LHRM
Instructor, Health Information Management
University of Central Florida
Orlando, Florida

Mary Jane Tremethick, PhD, RN, CHES
Instructor, Health/Physical Education and Recreation
Northern Michigan University
Marquette, Michigan

Scott Zimmer, MS
Instructor, Biology
Metropolitan Community College
Omaha, Nebraska

Test Bank

Judy Anderson, MEd
Instructor, Medical Office Administration
Coastal Carolina Community College
Jacksonville, North Carolina

Valentina Spencer Holder, MA Ed, RHIA
Instructor, Medical Office Administration
Pitt Community College
Winterville, North Carolina

Marsha Lalley, BSM, MSM
Instructor, Medical Assisting
Minneapolis Community and Technical College
Minneapolis, Minnesota

Mary Rahr, MS, RN, CMA
Instructor, Health Sciences
Northeast Wisconsin Technical College
Madison, Wisconsin

Mary Sayles, RN, MSN, PHN
Instructor, Health Sciences
Sierra College—Nevada County Campus
Rocklin, California

Donna Sue Shellman, CMA, CPC
Instructor, Office Systems Technology
Gaston College
Dallas, North Carolina

Carolyn Stariha, BS, RHIA
Clinical Coordinator, Health Sciences
Houston Community College—Coleman Campus
Houston, Texas

Jay W. Wilborn, MEd, MT(ASCP)
Program Director, Medical Laboratory Technology
National Park Community College
Hot Springs, Arkansas

Tammy Wilder, RN, MSN, CMSRN
Assistant Professor, Nursing
Ivy Tech Community College
Evansville, Indiana

PowerPoint™ Lectures

Darla Sparacino, MEd, RHIA
Associate Professor, Health Information Management
Arkansas Tech University
Russellville, Arkansas

Classroom Response System

Alice Noblin, MBA, RHIA, LHRM
Instructor, Health Information Management
University of Central Florida
Orlando, Florida

Sheila G. Rockoff, EdD, MSN, BSN, ADN, RN
Professor and Chairperson, Medical Assisting
Santa Ana College
Santa Ana, California

Timothy J. Skaife, RT(R), MA
Director, Radiography Program
National Park Community College
Hot Springs, Arkansas

THE ART AND CRAFT OF TEACHING

George Bernard Shaw once said, "He who can, does; he who cannot, teaches." This tongue-in-cheek comment on poor teachers compels us to strive to be better. We may start out not knowing a lot about teaching techniques, but that doesn't mean we should continue in that state. It is the responsibility of each teacher to continually improve and refine his or her teaching techniques.

Please take some time to read the following material on the art and craft of teaching and allow it to influence your teaching.

Teaching Styles

This list shows the natural progression from beginning teaching techniques to a more mature and effective teaching style.

1. **Subject-centered teaching.** This teaching style places the subject matter on a pedestal. If there are 30 chapters in the book, then all 30 must be covered before the end of the course. If one chapter is especially long, it still must be covered in the same amount of time given to other, smaller chapters. The order of the chapters can never be varied from what is found in the Table of Contents.

2. **Teacher-centered teaching.** This teaching style places the teacher on a pedestal. Each chapter covered must be presented by the teacher who is the sole source of information. The teacher knows all aspects of the subject; the students know nothing. Lecture is the preferred method of presenting material and students cannot be expected to learn in any other way. The lecture is always about telling students something, and there is very little dialogue coming from the students to the teacher. The teacher feels the role of the teacher is to initiate and the role of the student is to respond, because discovering knowledge is beyond the power of the average student. The teacher asks few questions and views spontaneous questions from students as an interruption to the flow of the lecture. The teacher's authority is the final word and student's questions are viewed as a challenge to her authority rather than an opportunity for further study.

    Beginning and experienced teachers can become trapped in either of the two teaching styles described above. Fortunately, enthusiasm and caring in the classroom cover a multitude of teaching sins! Students can still learn a lot about medical language even when the teacher uses either of these teaching styles. However, the teacher should always be striving to embrace the third teaching style described below.

3. **Student-centered teaching.** This teaching style places the student on a pedestal. The teacher actively considers the students' needs in planning the course material. The teacher consciously follows Maslow's Hierachy of Needs (as described in the next section) to direct course activities. Students are encouraged to ask questions, do research projects, form study groups, etc. The teacher should provide opportunities to help students realize that they can give intelligent answers based on life experience and general fund of knowledge. For example: What is it called when your tonsils are red and inflamed? [tonsillitis]. What is the surgical procedure to remove your tonsils? [tonsillectomy].

Use group participation to "piece together" answers to questions. Keep rewording the question to stimulate thinking and show there is more than one way to look at things.

Ask "why" questions and then provide the answer to show connections and relationships in the course material.

Maslow's Hierarchy of Needs

This adaptation of Maslow's Hierarchy of Needs is a graphic representation that depicts the full spectrum from students' most basic needs to the highest need, self-actualization. Needs are met from the bottom of the pyramid to the top, and a need higher on the pyramid cannot be met until all of the needs below it have been fulfilled. This section describes how a teacher can best meet these needs.

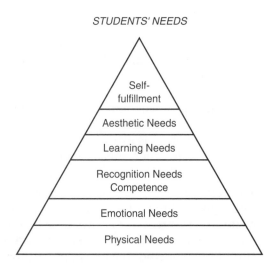

STUDENTS' NEEDS

Self-fulfillment
Aesthetic Needs
Learning Needs
Recognition Needs Competence
Emotional Needs
Physical Needs

Physical Needs

Learning stops when the physical needs of the student have not been met. Make sure the temperature and lighting in the room are conducive to learning. Take one or more breaks during a long session. Inform students where the restrooms are on the first day of class. If the class continues during lunch or dinner hours and food is not allowed in the classroom, discuss ways that students can work around this.

Emotional Needs

Learning stops when the emotional needs of the student have not been met. On the first day of class, allay fears about the course. Teach students specific ways they can assure their success (flashcard review, designated study time in small segments, involve family members, etc.). Do not allow any student to belittle another student. Do not have students grade each others' test papers. Encourage group activities to break the ice with students who do not know each other, but discourage cliques.

Recognition Needs and Competence

Keep an open atmosphere that allows student questions of any type. All questions are an opportunity for learning. Inspire student self-confidence by taking each question seriously and complimenting the student who thought to ask it ("Oh, that was a very good point!"). Allow students who are familiar with a medical condition to share their point of view about it.

Learning Needs

When the physical needs, emotional needs, and recognition/competence needs of students are being met, then, and only then, will the learning needs be met. Students need to learn the course materials in a way that they can recall that information and apply it to real life situations in the medical field. In many cases, students need to be taught how to learn before they can begin to learn.

Aesthetic Needs

Above the need for learning is the need to have an aesthetic experience. This relates to feeling connected and responding to the beauty and emotion of the world around us as opposed to having a purely intellectual connection. The aesthetic needs of the student are not difficult to meet because the human body is full of wondrous things and the field of medicine is compelling in the emotions of life and death that it deals with every day. The textbook includes the famous painting *The Starry Night* by Vincent van Gogh to illustrate the possible side effects of the cardiac drug digitalis in Chapter 5, Cardiology. It also includes the famous drawing of the skeleton by Andreas Vesalius in Chapter 8, Orthopedics (Skeletal). Other paintings can be obtained from art history books and shown to the class when teaching the following chapters:

Chapter 5, Cardiology
The Doctor's Wife, by Frans van Mieris
Shows a doctor feeling the patient's pulse. It was not until the invention of watches with second hands around 1700 that that pulse rate could be accurately measured.

The Dropsical Woman, by Gerard Dou
Shows the same type of scene as *The Village Doctor.* Dropsy is an old word for congestive heart failure.

Chapter 10, Urology
The Village Doctor, by David Teniers
Shows the doctor examining a urine specimen. It was not unusual for the doctor to also taste the urine as part of the examination.

Chapter 16, Otolaryngology
Portrait of an Old Man and a Young Boy, by Domenico Ghirlandaio
Shows the medical condition of rhinophyma on the old man.

Chapter 18, Oncology
Painting of the first successful demonstration of surgical anesthesia at Massachusetts General Hospital by Robert Hinckley.
Shows a young man (Gilbert Abbott) unconscious after ether anesthesia. He is seated in a chair while a tumor is being removed from his jaw.

Self-Fulfillment

The final step of Maslow's Hierarchy of Needs is self-fulfillment. The empowered student has fulfilled his or her own learning needs and implemented that knowledge in the practice of a career and success in life.

Poor Teaching Techniques

Aristotle said, "All men, by nature, desire to know." But poor teachers can thwart the efforts of even the most dedicated students. During her long career as a student and an educator, the author has encountered the following poor teaching techniques. Read this section to make sure these DO NOT describe your teaching! If they do, follow the *Solution* given.

Boring

The teacher lacks enthusiasm, does not change the inflection of his or her voice, and stands behind a podium without moving.

Solution: Be passionate! Get excited about the material and how it applies to a career in the healthcare field. Let your voice reflect this! Move around the class as you teach, from side to side, and even teach from the back of the classroom occasionally. Even if you have taught this medical terminology course 10 times and it seems boring to you, this is the first time your students will have heard it. Good teaching involves a little bit of acting. Sometimes you have to act like you are interested even when you are not! Be sure to get a good night's sleep and come to class with plenty of energy because good teaching is active and demands energy. Inject humor into your lectures and include classroom activities as described in this instructor's manual.

Insecure

The teacher stands in front of the students and reads from the textbook, offering few additional comments or insights.

Solution: Learn the material well enough that you are not reading from the textbook but only glancing at it to keep your place. Collect interesting medical facts to share during class or use some of the ones presented in this instructor's manual for each chapter.

Technically challenged

The teacher has not kept up with the latest technology advances in the classroom. Not only does the teacher not know how to operate PowerPoint slides, but he or she does not know how to use the overhead projector and create overheads and may not be computer literate and cannot create the course syllabus, handouts, and tests.

Solution: Pick one area of technology at a time and master it. It's your job to do that and do it right!

Not relevant

The teacher does not make a strong connection between what is being learned in class and the real world.

Solution: Bring in newspaper articles and report what you hear on the news or relevent TV shows. Bring in medical reports. Do your own research on the Internet to find out what's new in medicine. These Internet sites are particularly helpful:

www.webmd.com

www.sciencentral.com

www.nlm.nih.gov (National Library of Medicine and Medline Plus)

www.news-medical.net

www.medicineNet.com

www.cbsnews.com/sections/health.html (CBSHealthWatch)

http:/pubs.ama-assn.org (*Journal of the American Medical Assoc.*)

www.nejm.org (*New England Journal of Medicine*)

www.eurekalert.org (Comprehensive web site of new advances in medicine and health)

www.personalmd.com

Digressive	The teacher presents little course material but always seems to have time to talk about personal concerns and a myriad of other subjects.
	Solution: Make the majority of what you present to be course material and sprinkle anecdotes and activities in sparingly. Remember, students are paying you to provide them with a comprehensive experience in medical terminology.
Careless	The teacher feels that presentation of the material is the equivalent of learning. This mirrors the expression, "If you build it, they will come" by saying "If you teach it, they will learn."
	Solution: It is the teacher's responsibility to make sure students learn the material by using good teaching techniques. It is also the teacher's responsibility to administer tests to make sure students have retained the material.

The Teacher's Role

"My job as a teacher is to empower my students, to demystify a subject for them, and so to give up my power over them. If I am doing my job, by the end of the semester my students are independent of me. I strive every semester to give my students power, even though when I succeed I inevitably disempower myself. I hate that feeling of powerlessness at the end of the semester. And I love it!"

Source: Peter G. Beidler, *Distinguished Teachers on Effective Teaching.* San Francisco: Jossey-Bass Publishers, 1986.

The teacher's role has many facets:

Gardener	One who tills and cultivates the fertile soil of students' minds, plants the seeds of knowledge, and then watches as understanding blossoms
Potter	One who shapes and molds students' thoughts and opinions
Dietitian	One who feeds students' minds with good information and then poses critical questions to help students digest that information
Builder	One who lays a foundation of knowledge in the subject and then helps students build on it throughout the course
Electrician	One who connects all the vital links of knowledge and then turns on the switch and watches for that "ah-ha" moment when the light bulb goes on to illuminate students' minds

"Teaching is a craft, and as with any craft, one's performance can be bettered by careful attention to detail. Choosing textbooks, assigning papers, preparing for class, testing, grading, learning to improvise despite the best-laid plans—these are all important skills well worth your continuing attention. Yet the center of all teaching and learning is the interaction between the teacher and the learner. Developing as a teacher can be described as becoming wiser and less judgmental, more generous, less arrogant and yet more confident; being more honest with oneself and students and subject matter; taking more risks; showing forth without showing off; being impatient with ignorance but not appalled by it."

Source: Kenneth Eble, *The Craft of Teaching.* Jossey-Bass Publishers, pp. xvii, 212.

Great Beginnings: What to Do on the First Day of Class

For most teachers, the longest, loneliest minute of life occurs in facing a class for the first time, when students quiet down and look up expectantly. Where to begin and what to do on the first day of class can seem both overwhelming and perplexing, particularly to an inexperienced teacher. The tips below can help you provide a smooth introduction to a medical terminology course for all of your students. Your efforts will produce students who can work confidently and productively in the weeks ahead.

1. **Provide a relaxed atmosphere.** Begin by assessing your classroom, its equipment, lighting, temperature, and so on, to assure that they are conducive to learning. A modified version of Maslow's hierarchy of needs is presented here to clarify the point that physical comfort must be established before the student can progress to the next level. Fear and anxiety caused by unclear expectations for performance can prevent students from reaching the level where learning takes place.

   Get acquainted. Rather than immediately plunging into course content and requirements, take a few minutes to allow students to become acquainted with each other. Ask them to stand and introduce themselves and state what they hope to gain from the course. A slightly longer version of this involves having students take out a blank piece of paper and write down the following things: name, why they are taking the course, something interesting about themselves (like their hobbies), and their greatest fear about the course. Then collect these papers. Call out the name on each paper and have the student raise his or her hand. That way you can put a face with the student's name. Take some notes on each paper to help you remember who is who. Students often sit in the same spot in the classroom each time and by the third week, you should be calling each student by his or her correct name. If the student has an interesting hobby, share it with the class and make a brief comment. Finally, take a moment to review all of the papers to identify the students' greatest fears. Then summarize them for the entire class and tell how you will help them overcome these fears. By developing a cooperative atmosphere in which students feel a part of the group and not isolated, you can help allay fears. Research has shown that a strongly supportive peer group in a learning situation helps students to cope successfully with the frustrations inherent in learning a new subject.

   Slow and steady. As a new teacher, I remember that my only thoughts on the first day of class dealt with how much material needed to be covered and the short time that I had to do it. I wrongly felt that if I didn't plunge right in to work on the first day that I would fall so far behind in presenting the material that I could never catch up for the rest of the course. That was a misperception on my part, but I am sure it caused quite a few anxious moments for my overwhelmed students.

   When you do begin to present course material, proceed at a slower-than-normal pace. When every part of an instructional process is new, students need extra time to understand detailed instructions. Speak slowly and allow pauses during which students can digest what you have presented. There is nothing more frustrating than having a teacher present course requirements so quickly that they become impossible to remember. Your students will not be able to immediately see patterns of learning in your course and will not be able to initiate their own learning/studying process if your presentation is hurried and pressured.

   Address student anxiety. Every learner, regardless of age, has feelings of anxiety when confronted with a new learning situation, particularly if the learning involves being graded or evaluated in any way. It is important for the teacher to acknowledge this anxiety and discuss it with the group in order to help defuse it. Humorous sayings on the chalkboard (such as "Does medical terminology give you cephalalgia?") can provide a release of tension for students. One simple exercise that acknowledges the difficulty of learning a new skill is to ask students to fold their arms across their chests in the usual way that is comfortable for them. Then ask them to fold their arms with the other arm on the top. This usually provokes laughter and strange arm movements as the difficulty of this seemingly simple task becomes apparent. The teacher should then remind students that learning medical terminology is a mental skill that takes some time to properly coordinate and that they should not feel frightened or frustrated if their efforts do not immediately produce perfect results. Share this Khmer proverb with them: "A journey of 1,000 miles begins with a single step."

2. **Provide general, then specific, information.** First, present the big picture (the entire course) before you discuss the details. This will give students a framework on which to hang the details you discuss later. Go over the information in the course syllabus and weekly reading assignments very slowly, reading it aloud while students follow along. Read through at least three weeks to show the repeating structure of the course objectives and assignments. This helps students get a sense of continuity within the course.

Explore the textbook and CD-ROM. Display and discuss the required textbook. Students will then know if they have purchased the correct textbook, and your positive comments about why this textbook was selected will generate confidence.

Some students are so worried about a course that it prevents them from doing anything but what the instructor specifically says for them to do. On their own, they may fail to explore the textbook and enjoy what it has to offer. For all students, however, it is also helpful to go through the textbook chapter names and sections so that they do not feel intimidated and, when you give them their first assignment, they have the tools they need to do it and can confidently say, "Oh, I know where that section is in the textbook!" Go from cover to cover in the textbook, pointing out sections that the student will need to use during the course (brief table of contents, index, answer key, glossary of word parts, etc.). Ask students to look up the meaning of several word parts in the Glossary and look in the Index to find on what page "appendectomy" and "rhinorrhea" are located in the text. Be sure to point out special features of the textbook that make learning easier or more interesting (Word Alert boxes, A Closer Look, cartoons, etc.). You can do this by going through "Dive Into Something Different" on pp. vi–viii that elaborate on these special features. A number of teachers follow up this in-depth review with a brief quiz on the syllabus and parts of the textbook the following week. They have found that this approach has lowered their attrition rate dramatically.

If possible, run the CD-ROM during class and show how easy it is to navigate through it to allay the fears of some students who are technophobic. Also demonstrate some of its features and games to entice students to make it an integral part of their learning experience. Mention that Prentice Hall's CD-ROM technology is advanced and much richer than that of any other medical terminology book publisher on the market, and how fortunate the students are for their school to have picked this textbook that contains this CD-ROM. Tell students who are not computer savvy to find a child, family member, or friend who can quickly tell them how to use this CD-ROM.

3. **Be enthusiastic.** A major airline advertises, "We love to fly, and it shows!" Like that airline, an instructor who loves to teach will show it, and one who has a love for the subject will not be able to hide it. Nothing is more important to teaching than an enthusiasm for the subject. That enthusiasm will be contagious. This is especially important in medical language because learning word parts and vocabulary is often associated with boring repetition and mind-numbing drill.

4. **Introduce the concepts of good study habits.**

Take advantage of small blocks of time. Have students explore the Web site http://www.exploratorium.edu/memory/index.html. "The Memory Exhibition" Web site contains activities to test your memory—and some things you can try to help you remember things better.

Urge students to keep their flashcards with them and study them while they wait to pick up their children from an activity, stop at a red light, or sit in a doctor's waiting room. Emphasize the importance of using every available moment. The successful student is the one who is best able to identify a study moment and seize it. Tiny study moments add up and contribute more to long-term retention than does a single, memorize-until-you-drop study session.

Involve family; urge students to get family members involved in what they are learning. Even small children can enjoy helping as they hold up a flashcard printed from the CD-ROM that accompanies the textbook. Use water-soluble markers to label body parts on family members.

Summary

In short, make the first day of class a relaxed, confidence-building memorable experience for your students. "We tend to forget how difficult it is for [students] . . . Our grasp of our subject matter is apt to become automatic . . . It is our duty to assume nothing and explain everything."

This material was adapted from the following articles:

Susan Turley, "Great Beginnings: What to Do on the First Day," *Perspectives on the Medical Transcription Profession,* Fall 1991, pp. 4–5.

Ellen Drake, "Teaching Medical Terminology," *Perspectives on the Medical Transcription Profession,* Fall 1992, pp. 12–15.

Classroom Management Techniques

Chapter Questions and Exercises

Give extra credit to every student who can show that they completed all the chapter exercises. This includes the anatomy-labeling exercises or word-building exercises in the middle of the chapter as well as the final section of Chapter Review Exercises. You do not need to check for correct or incorrect answers (that is the student's job). You are just rewarding diligent study habits that pay off in better test scores and more knowledge retained at the end of the course. Some students may want to resell their textbook and may not want to write in it. Stress to them that doing the exercises right in the textbook is a very helpful learning tool and that many students want to keep their textbook as a very useful reference book as they finish their other studies and later during their careers.

Weekly Spelling Practice

Select one of the following techniques to reinforce spelling each week for the chapter being studied.

Beanbag Spelling Toss.   The members of the class stand in a circle. The first player, who is holding the beanbag, pronounces a medical word from the chapter while tossing the beanbag to another student. The student catching the beanbag must quickly spell the word. If the student spells the word correctly, then he/she thinks of and pronounces a new medical word while tossing the beanbag to another student, and so on. If the student cannot spell the word correctly, the student is eliminated, gives the beanbag to the instructor, and sits down. The instructor then pronounces a medical word while tossing the beanbag to another student and the game continues. The game is over when only one player remains standing.

Scrabble.   Bring in a standard Scrabble game board set. The rules of the game are modified in that only medical words are allowed. Players work together in groups of two or three. Players may use a medical dictionary or the textbook to verify the correct spelling (but only half of the points are awarded). Option: Players can be required to define the words as they play them.

Spelling Bee.   Divide the class into three or four equal groups. Have each group line up at the whiteboard at the front of the class. At the same time, give each of four students at the head of each group a different word to spell. They should write it on the whiteboard. If the word is spelled correctly, the student stays standing with his/her group but goes to the end of the group. If the word is spelled incorrectly, the student must sit down. The group with the last person left standing wins the spelling bee and a few points can be given to each member of that group.

Gridlock.   Use this grid to review chapter terminology. Draw two identical grids on the board. Divide the class into two groups. Each group should stand at the board and collectively think of and write words from the chapter that begin with the initial letters on the grid. The team that thinks of the most words wins, but misspelled words do not count.

M	
E	
D	
I	
C	
A	
L	
W	
O	
R	
D	

Hangman.   This game reinforces spelling but also pronunciation and the definitions of medical words. Pick one student to be the hangman. He/she mentally picks a medical word that is at least eight letters in length, goes to the board and draws a scaffold and a noose and a series of blanks indicating the number of letters in the word. Going around the room, each student calls out a letter. If the letter is present in the word, the hangman writes it in the appropriate blank. If the letter is not present, the hangman draws a body part. As the game progresses, the body should be drawn in six steps (head, torso, left leg, right leg, left arm, right arm). The student who guesses the word before the hangman picture is completed is declared the winner, but only if he/she can also correctly pronounce the word and define it. If so, then that student becomes the hangman for the next round.

Weekly Pronunciation Practice

Select one of the following techniques to reinforce pronunciation each week for the chapter being studied.

Parroting.   Using the comprehensive "see and say" pronunciation guide in the Pronunciation Checklist, say each word and then have the students as a group repeat the pronunciation to you. This promotes active listening and helps them to develop competence in their pronunciation of medical words aside from the standard times of practice that occur as they study the chapter or use the CD-ROM. Alternatively, give the pronunciation of one word and then have the students as a group give the pronunciation of the next word.

Hieroglyphics.   Randomly pick and write a few of the "see and say" pronunciations on the board and see if students can pronounce the medical word.

Beach Ball Blast.   If students seem to be tired and unable to concentrate on the lecture, stop the class and surprise them with this activity. Have each of them quickly pick out four medical words from the chapter. Specify that at least one should be a long medical word. Have them quickly review the pronunciations of the words they picked (they can say them out loud to practice the pronunciations). It is okay if some students pick some of the same words. As they are doing this, quickly blow up an inflatable beach ball. Tell them each time the beach ball comes to them they are to punch or hit it to another student (or pick it up and punch it if it falls to the floor) and, at the same time, they are to correctly pronounce one of the vocabulary words they have picked. They are not to catch the ball, just react to it and punch or hit it away. The next time the ball comes to them, they are to punch or hit the ball while pronouncing their second vocabulary word. Continue this until most students have pronounced at least three of their words. Start the activity by hitting the ball high in the air toward the back row of students while you say the word for the medical specialty of the chapter you are currently studying. If the activity is done correctly, the ball should be moving quickly around the room and there should be lots of medical words being pronounced.

Weekly Chapter Test

Each week, the class should cover one chapter of material and take a test on that material the following week at the beginning of class. This keeps the learning segments at a size that is manageable and prevents students from falling behind and doing poorly (which can happen when the course only has one large midterm test and one large final test). The test should be taken in the first 30 minutes of class, and then the answers quickly reviewed. I often allow students to skip one weekly test that does not count toward their grade to allow for unforeseen events like illness and family emergencies.

Weekly Spelling Test

For each chapter, provide students with a list of 20 spelling words to study. Then, next week, at the conclusion of the weekly chapter test, have students turn their test paper over and number the back for the spelling test. Pronounce each spelling word and use it in a sentence. Include at least 10 of the spelling words.

Weekly Pronunciation Test

Assign 20 words from the Pronunciation Checklist. Any time before the next weekly test, tell each student to call your office or home and leave a message on your answering machine in which they give their name and then pronounce the list of words.

Take-Home Test

If you don't have time to cover every chapter, consider using a take-home test to be completed during mid-semester break or over the course of several class sessions. This would be an open-book test.

Comprehensive Review before the Final Examination

Some colleges require that a comprehensive final examination be given. This is a good strategy to make sure students review and relearn material from the entire course. This leads to better retention of course material for the future when the student is on the job. However, a final examination can cause students great anxiety. Devote some of your final class time to helping students prepare for the final examination by using this fun exercise.

Have each student make up 10 *Jeopardy*-like questions the week before the final review. The questions can be based on anything and everything studied during the whole course. Have students write the answer on one side and the question on the other side of an index card. Questions are always phrased as an answer and the answer is then always given in the form of a question.

> Answer: Ren/o- and nephr/o- [on the front of the index card]
>
> Question: What are the two combining forms that both mean *kidney?*

For the final review class, collect all the index cards and shuffle them. Divide the students into two or three teams and have them remain standing. Read an index card "answer" to each group. The group members can help each other come up with the answer in a form of a question and write it on the board. If they are correct, give them another "answer" to work on. The first group to write 10 correct questions on the board wins.

Interesting Quotations to Use During Class

The beginnings of all things are small. —Cicero

A journey of 1,000 miles begins with one step. —Khmer proverb

The distance is nothing; it is only the first step that is difficult. —Marquise Du Deffand (1697–1780)

Learning is a continuous process of combining the familiar with the new. —Stanford C. Ericksen (1974)

If we succeed in giving the love of learning, the learning itself is sure to follow. —Sir John Lubbock

Perfection is the child of time. —Joseph Hall (1574–1656)

Knowledge is power. —Francis Bacon (1500s)

Learn from the mistakes of others—you can't live long enough to make them all yourself. —Anonymous

Examinations are formidable even to the best prepared, for the greatest fool may ask more than the wisest man can answer. —Charles Colton (1888–1965)

Intelligent thinking is the basis of all great endeavors. —Anonymous

Genius is one percent inspiration and ninety-nine percent perspiration. —Thomas Alva Edison (1874–1931)

Whatever is worth doing at all is worth doing well. —Philip Chesterfield (1694–1773)

Nothing great was every achieved without enthusiasm. —Ralph Waldo Emerson (1803–1882)

If you're going to do it, do it RIGHT. —Lee Iacocca

I have not failed; I have discovered 50,000 things that will not work. —Thomas Alva Edison (1874–1931)

Getting an idea should be like sitting on a tack; it should make you get up and do something about it. —Herbert Prochnow

If you would hit the mark, you must aim a little above it. —Henry Wadsworth Longfellow (1807-1882)

He who aims at nothing will likely hit it. —Anonymous

The secret of success is constancy of purpose. —Benjamin Disraeli

Ambition, energy, and perseverance are the levers that move obstacles in our path. —Ida Scott Taylor (1894)

The best way to escape from a problem is to solve it. —Brendan Frances

Life is a daring adventure, or it is nothing. —Helen Keller

The most important thing in life is to love what you're doing, because it's the only way you'll ever really be good at it. —Donald Trump

"Mnifty" Mnemonic Devices

Many of us are familiar with the term *mnemonic device* (pronounced "ne-MAWN-ik"). Certainly we have all used mnemonic devices in one way or another throughout our lifetimes. Do you remember learning these mnemonic devices?

"Roy G. Biv" (red, orange, yellow, green, blue, indigo, violet) to remember the colors of the rainbow

There are two *s*'s in "dessert" because you always want two helpings of dessert. This mnemonic helps you differentiate between the spelling of "dessert" and "desert."

"**M**y very excellent **m**other **j**ust **s**erved **u**s **n**ine **p**izzas" to remember the names of the planets (Mercury, Venus, Earth, Mars, Jupiter, Saturn, Uranus, Neptune, Pluto)

A mnemonic device is simply a memory aid that helps link the unfamiliar with the familiar, so that we can retrieve information from our brains more quickly. Using mnemonic devices and learning how to construct them helps students remember the spellings of the many new words they have to learn in medical terminology.

1. **First-letter cues.** To spell difficult words or to remember long lists, use the letters of the word or the first letters of each of the words in the phrase to construct a sentence. For example, the spelling of "rhythm" is difficult to remember, but constructing the sentence, "Ruby had yams; Tommy had muffins" can help you remember. Anatomy students use "Every child must nap" to remember the four major types of body tissues (epithelial, connective, muscle, nerve).

2. **Imagery link.** Linking medical words to mental images makes them easier to remember. "Dysphagia" and "dyspasia" are frequently confused, and are more easily remembered by llnking "dysphagia" with "gag" and "dysphasia" with "speech."

3. **Associate spelling with "logical order."** To remember the difference between "perineal" and "peroneal," associate the word with its order of appearance in the body from head to toe: the perineal area (external genital area) comes before the peroneal area (leg area). Also, the "i" (in perineal) comes before the "o" (in peroneal) alphabetically.

4. The CD-ROM of the textbook contains several good mnemonic devices for each chapter. Encourage students to develop their own as well!

This textbook's CD-ROM shares many mnemonic devices for each chapter, but the ones that students make up themselves are the ones they often remember best. Give two extra credit points for each good mnemonic that a student submits (limit 10 points throughout the course). Share the best ones with the rest of the class. Mnemonic devices can be in the form of an abbreviation where each letter stands for something, or in the form of a riddle, a poem, or a song.

Source: Adapted from Linda Campbell, "Using Mnemonic Devices," *Perspectives on the Medical Transcription Profession,* Fall 1991.

All of the Above

Test questions:
    a. are not easy to construct.
    b. can mean different things to the teacher and student.
    c. may inaccurately test students' knowledge.
    d. can give away the correct answer.
    e. All of the above.
[The correct answer is "e. All of the above."]

When I first began teaching, my immediate priorities were to quickly develop a course syllabus, select an appropriate textbook, and research additional lecture material for each class. Sometimes in the week-to-week busyness of class preparation, I would have to construct a test. Often I found myself doing this hurriedly and late at night. Some last-minute preparation is certainly unavoidable for a new teacher or even for an experienced teacher developing and presenting a course for the first time. However, last-minute test preparation is not conducive to thoroughness and may inaccurately test students' knowledge.

It is important to recognize some of the finer points of test construction. As in all areas of teaching, we grow in our ability to teach as well as to evaluate students' learning. The writing of test questions is something of an art, the perfection of which depends on two factors: knowledge of the mechanics/techniques of proper test construction, and the time to practice and refine those techniques.

1. **Draw from course objectives.** No course syllabus is complete without a list of course objectives. Chapter objectives can be found at the beginning of every chapter in the textbook. The test must be drawn from these same objectives. Consider the following example in which the test questions do *not* correlate with the chapter objectives.

   Chapter Objectives
   List the main structures of the cardiovascular system.
   Identify common diseases of the cardiovascular system.

   Test Questions
   Give a brief history of the discovery of the circulatory system.
   Identify five common radiology procedures performed on the circulatory system.

2. **Consider time and scope.** Consider the length of the testing time period and the scope of the material that is to be tested. It is common to include too many questions for the time allowed. It is also common to pick questions that focus too much attention on one area of content. It may be helpful to keep a chart as you prepare a test and check off each subject area when you finish its test questions.

3. **Vary the types of questions used.** There are several test question formats that can be used to approach the material in different ways. These formats include multiple choice, true-false, matching, fill in the blank, short answer, sequencing, selection, and case studies. Not every question format is suitable to each testing situation. However, the use of several different test question formats is preferred.

Multiple-Choice Questions

This format is widely used but can be inaccurate if a question is not constructed properly. All of the answers must be plausible and constructed in such a way that the sentence structure does not give a clue as to the correct answer. Consider the following example in which the sentence structure is faulty, making it easy to determine the correct answer.

A ronguer is an _____ instrument.
   a. neurological
   b. cardiovascular
   c. orthopedic
   d. gastrointestinal
[Answer: c. The use of "an" clues the student that the correct answer must begin with a vowel.]

Because multiple-choice formats allow the student to guess the right answer, it is best to include five answers rather than four to reduce the probability of a correct guess from 25 percent to 20 percent.

Beginning test writers tend to shy away from the first alternative [a] being the correct answer. In fact, the third position [c] tends to be the correct answer a disproportionate number of times. The goal should be to have the correct answer appear in each position an equal number of times. The position of the correct answer should be selected randomly. No pattern of the correct answer position should appear in the test.

True/False Questions

This format is also widely used, but is more restricted in the scope of information it can test. It is best to avoid test questions that contain the words *always, never,* or *none,* as this provides a clue that the answer is probably false. True/false questions also provide an opportunity for students to guess at the answer with a 50 percent chance of being correct. Therefore, this type of question should be used sparingly.

Matching Questions

This format can test relationships and the ability to classify. It is best not to provide an exact match between the number of items in Column A and those in Column B. An uneven match makes students evaluate each item based on its own merits rather than just matching it to whatever is left over. Never continue the matching columns from the bottom of one page to the top of another. Make sure that the entire matching question is on the same page.

One twist on the matching question is to use this format (answers provided):

Column A		Column B
1. A is caused by B	3, 4	femur: bone
2. A is a source of B	5	MI: elevated CPK-MB
3. A is made of B	2	pancreas: insulin
4. A is a type of B	1	stroke: blood clot
5. A is proven by B	1, 5	syphilis: Treponema

This format requires a bit of thinking on the part of the student. It is very important that the teacher review and explain this type of question and how to employ thinking strategies to answer it correctly BEFORE presenting it in a testing situation.

Fill-in-the-Blank Questions

This format effectively measures memorization of specific facts but cannot measure understanding or relationships. If the question is not well constructed, students may have a difficult time trying to guess what should go in the blank. The teacher may also inadvertently give a clue to the correct answer by making a long or short blank line.

Short-Answer Questions

This format is similar to that of fill-in-the-blank questions but differs in that there is no line drawn to write in the answer.

Sequencing Questions

This format is particularly useful in testing anatomy in which there is a well defined sequence of structures. Example:

Arrange the structures of the urinary tract in the correct anatomical order, beginning with the flow of blood in the renal artery and ending with the production of urine. Pick from these structures to complete the sequence.

Renal artery   ureter   glomerulus   renal pelvis [etc.]

Renal artery   →   _____   →   _____   →   _____ [etc.]

Selection Questions

In this format, students are asked to select only those answers that correspond to a particular category, disease condition, etc.

Circle those drugs used to treat cardiac arrhythmias.

Nexium   Procan-SR   Corgard
Lasix   Lipitor   Avodart

Case Studies

This format presents the opportunity to test not only students' knowledge of facts but their understanding of relationships. Case studies should be used sparingly on tests because they are time consuming. Case studies should be presented in class to allow students to develop the skills needed to correctly answer questions associated with a case study.

A final thought on test construction. Just as there is no perfect student and no perfect teacher, there is also no perfect test question. A question that seems perfectly clear to the teacher may be confusing to a student. Teachers should make every effort to word questions clearly and to use only terminology that has been presented in class or in the textbook. The wise teacher will listen to the student who has a logical explanation for a "wrong" answer. It is not heresy to admit that there might be more than one correct interpretation of the wording of a question.

Source: Adapted from Turley, Susan, "All of the Above," *Perspectives on the Medical Transcription Profession,* Fall 1990, pp. 8-10.

When is an Adult an Adult?

Students in a medical terminology course can range in age from 18 to 55 years of age or more. This is a wide span and it behooves the teacher to be aware of the differences and similarities of these students and the practical challenges this presents when teaching adult learners.

Traditional educational research has extensively addressed the question of what constitutes an adult learner, what personal characteristics are common to adult learners, and what basic characteristics can be attributed to them. Two schools of thought attempt to describe the adult learner.

The first school of thought views adult learners as a generic group with similar characteristics based on their sharing of adulthood. Malcolm S. Knowles, an educational researcher, is one of the main proponents for this group. According to Knowles, the foundation of modern adult learning theory is based on several key assumptions which ascribe particular attributes to all adult learners. In general, these assumptions state that all adults are motivated, inquiring, mature, self-directed, experienced, and have attained a formal operational level of thought processes.

- **Motivated.** Adult learners are more motivated to learn. They often have a sense of urgency and are more willing to make sacrifices in their pursuit of learning.
- **Inquiring.** Adult learners are less willing to accept the authority of the teacher as the final and sole source of knowledge. Adult learners demand that teachers be accountable and that course work be meaningful.
- **Mature.** Adult learners are more mature in the behavior and attitudes they bring to the learning experience. Their goals are more clearly defined, and they take their studies seriously. Adult learners have a strong self-concept and confidence gained from coping with the responsibilities of adult life.
- **Self-directed.** Adult learners are self-directed in their pursuit of knowledge. They value the right to make independent decisions about their own learning needs.
- **Experienced.** Adult learners bring to the classroom a rich background of varied experiences. This past learning becomes a touchstone for relating to new learning. In contrast to younger learners, adult learners possess sophisticated insights springing from their knowledge of the world of work and from the skills they have acquired there.
- **Formal operational.** Adult learners function at the level of formal operational thinking and are able to deal with abstract concepts as well as concrete (hands-on) learning.

There is considerable uncertainty from other authors (from the second school of thought) as to whether all adult learners can be so categorically labeled and whether this labeling accurately reflects a true picture of *any* individual adult learner. Stephen D. Brookfield, a professor and author in the field of adult education, notes that individual learning behaviors are so idiosyncratic as to cast considerable doubt on any general assertions about adults as learners. Although some adult learners may be highly self-directed, many adults regress in a classroom situation to relive their role as passive childhood learners. Some are even visibly intimidated, and it is unrealistic to claim that self-directed learning is a commonality across the spectrum of adult learners. Brookfield cautions not to assume that all adults will enter a course as self-directed learners or will even want to become so with the assistance of the teacher.

While some adult learners possess a wide range of learning experiences, some minority, poor, and disadvantaged adult learners come from an environment that did not foster critical thinking and a self-directed attitude toward learning.

For those adult learners who do possess a rich variety of experiences, it still cannot be said that this is a positive resource to learning. Life experiences can enrich and enlarge an individual's perception of self and society, but they can also result in mental habits and biases that tend to close the mind to new ideas and alternative ways of thinking.

While some adult learners have a strong self-concept and confidence, other adult learners are hesitant and lack confidence in their ability to learn. While some adult learners have clear goals and take their studies seriously, others have goals and priorities that are poorly defined.

Some adult learners may actively participate in the learning process, while others may sit back and expect to be spoon fed by the instructor. This calls to mind the title of the infant nutrition book *Feed Me, I'm Yours.*

So when is an adult an adult? For some students, maybe never. We must, then, acknowledge the flaw of attempting to put the same labels on all adult learners. We must remember that adult learners come with all different levels of motivation, curiosity, maturity, and independence. Our job as teachers is to recognize each student as an individual with distinct strengths and weaknesses, to praise their strengths, correct their weaknesses, and help them on their journey to become an adult learner.

Source: Adapted from Susan Turley, "When is an Adult an Adult?," *Perspectives on the Medical Transcription Profession,* Winter 1990–91, pp. 25–27.

SAMPLE COURSE SYLLABUS

Instructor: (Teacher's name here)
E-mail: (Teacher's e-mail address here)
Course Text: Turley, Susan. *Medical Language* (Prentice Hall, 2007).

Course Goals

1. Give the medical meaning of prefixes, suffixes, and combining forms for each body system.
2. Demonstrate the ability to use word parts to build medical words.
3. Analyze the meaning of medical words for each body system.
4. Correctly make plural and adjective forms of medical words.
5. Demonstrate the ability to interpret medical words in the context of medical reports.
6. Pronounce and spell medical words correctly for each body system.
7. Translate common abbreviations, acronyms, and slang terms for each body system.
8. Make a personal commitment to learning medical terminology.
9. Describe methods of time management and good study habits and apply them to this course.

Course Outline and Weekly Learning Objectives

Week 1: Introduction to Medical Language/Chapter 1

1. Describe tips on how to manage your time and develop good study habits.
2. Describe the origins of medical words.
3. Analyze the component parts of a medical word: prefixes, suffixes and combining forms.
4. Identify medical words you already know from real life.
5. Describe how to build medical words.
6. Practice dictionary skills.
7. List the 5 language skills needed to communicate medical language.
8. Practice correctly pronouncing and spelling medical words.
9. Differentiate between sound-alike words.

Week 2: The Body in Health and Disease/Chapter 2

1. Define anatomy and physiology.
2. Use medical words to identify body positions, planes, directions, and cavities.
3. Identify the component organs of various body systems.
4. Correctly form plurals and adjectives of medical words.
5. List several types of disease categories.
6. List several sites where health care is provided.

Note: The following weeks correlate to specific body systems and medical specialties. The weekly learning objectives are the same for each of these weeks.

Weekly Learning Objectives for Weeks 3-15

1. Name the organs and structures of this body system.
2. Build medical words using combining forms from this body system.
3. Describe common symptoms and diseases related to this body system.
4. Describe common diagnostic tests related to this body system.
5. Describe common surgeries related to this body system.
6. Define common abbreviations related to this body system.
7. Correctly spell and pronounce medical words related to this body system.
8. Apply your knowledge by analyzing medical reports related to this body system.

Week 3: Gastroenterology/Gastrointestinal System   Chapter 3
Week 4: Pulmonology/Respiratory System   Chapter 4
Week 5: Cardiology/Cardiovascular System   Chapter 5
Week 6: Hematology and Immunology/Blood and the Lymphatic System   Chapter 6
Week 7: Dermatology/Integumentary System   Chapter 7
Week 8: Orthopedics/Skeletal System   Chapter 8
Week 9: Orthopedics/Muscular System   Chapter 9
Week 10: Neurology/Nervous System   Chapter 10
Week 11: Urology/Urinary System   Chapter 11
Week 12: Reproductive Medicine/Male Genitourinary System   Chapter 12
Week 13: Obstetrics and Gynecology/Female Reproductive System   Chapter 13
Week 14: Endocrinology/Endocrine System   Chapter 14
Week 15: Ophthalmology and Otolaryngology/Eyes, Ears, Nose, and Throat   Chapters 15 and 16
Independent Study Chapters throughout the Course
  Psychiatry   Chapter 17
  Oncology   Chapter 18
  Radiology   Chapter 19
Final Examination

Course Management

Attendance

Students are expected to be present for all class sessions. We all, on occasion, have times when illness or family situations prevent us from attending class. You need not provide the instructor with an explanation or a note or a reason for your absence. No points are deducted for missing a class lecture. However, regular attendance promotes success, and absenteeism may adversely affect your overall grade.

If you are absent from a class, it is YOUR responsibility to find out what you missed, to copy notes from another student, and to ask the instructor for the handouts. Being absent does not excuse you from being responsible for learning any subject matter that was presented or discussed, whether in the textbook or during class time.

Basis for a Final Grade

Weekly Quiz.   A quiz will be given weekly (beginning on the third week). Each weekly quiz will cover the material presented in class or assigned in the textbook during the previous week(s). There are no make up quizzes under any circumstances. In calculating your final grade for the course, your one lowest weekly quiz grade will be automatically dropped. In addition to that, if you are absent and miss one quiz (or circumstances left you unprepared and you elect not to take one quiz), that one quiz will be omitted from your grade and will not count against you.

Take-Home Quizzes.   Occasionally a chapter quiz will be a take-home quiz that you complete at home over 1-2 weeks and then turn in. These are open-book quizzes.

Homework.   Occasional homework assignments may be given. Late homework assignments are not accepted unless you were absent from class on the day that the assignment was due.

Optional Extra Credit Work.   If you complete all the chapter review exercises by writing directly in the textbook, you can receive 3 extra points per chapter. Show your textbook to your instructor to receive credit.

During the course, you may submit mnemonic devices (memory aids) that you think of yourself to help you remember the course material (like the sequence of body structures in the GI system, etc.). Each is worth 2 points, and you may submit up to 5 during the course for a possible total of 10 points.

Comprehensive Final Examination.   This is a college requirement for passing this course. If you have a scheduling conflict at the time the Final Examination is scheduled, you must make prior arrangements with your instructor for a copy of the Final Examination to be sent to the college Testing and Tutoring Center, and the Final Examination must always be taken before the regularly scheduled classroom Final Examination.

Grading Scale

89.5 to 100%	A
79.5 to 89.4%	B
69.5 to 79.4%	C
Below 69.4%	F

Let's Keep in Touch

The instructor will inform you of your midterm grade before it is turned into the Records and Registration Office. Students with a low C or below at midterm will be referred by the instructor to the Counseling Center.

You may ask the instructor what your current grade is at any time during the course.

Don't be afraid to ask your instructor for help in clarifying the expectations of the course and/or how to improve your grade. It is your responsibility to do this.

IMPORTANT: If you feel confused, anxious, not "on track," or concerned about anything about the course, immediately contact your instructor by e-mail, before class, or during class break. Believe it or not, every student feels that way from time to time! It's a normal response to the stress of learning something new!

Drop/Withdraw

Your instructor has given you a dates sheet that gives the last date to withdraw from the course. If you decide to drop/withdraw from this course, it is your responsibility to notify the Records and Registration Office at the college and complete paperwork to formally drop/withdraw. If you do this before the Final Drop Date for the semester, the course will be taken off your transcript. If you drop/withdraw after that, you will receive a "W" on your transcript for this course. If you do not complete the paperwork at the Records and Registration Office, you will receive an F on your transcript for this course.

Medical Terminology Pearls of Wisdom

Lynette M. Veach, MA, MLT(ASCP)

Marsha M. Holtsberry, CMA, RMA/AMT

Prentice Hall is committed to creating tools to help instructors and students succeed in the classroom and beyond. Along these lines, *Medical Terminology Pearls of Wisdom* is a treasure chest of ideas to help infuse a new spark into your classroom. This manual is organized topically and provides a collection of best practices from a nationwide panel of master teachers who agreed to share tips and ideas for teaching medical terminology. We hope that this serves as a valuable resource and helps you and your students to shine brightly.

Medical Terminology Pearls of Wisdom

Lynette M. Veach, MA, MLT(ASCP)

Former Instructor, Medical Assisting Department
Columbus State Community College and Ohio Institute of Health Careers
Columbus, Ohio

Marsha M. Holtsberry, CMA, RMA/AMT

Program Manager, Healthcare Office Technology
Ohio Institute of Health Careers
Columbus, Ohio

Contents

Contributors

Ellen Anderson, RHIA, CCS
Instructor, Health Information Technology
College of Lake County
Grayslake, Illinois

Judy Anderson, MEd
Instructor, Medical Office Administration
Coastal Carolina Community College
Jacksonville, North Carolina

Lorraine Baskin, BSc
Instructor, Medical Assisting
Heald College
Concord, California

Mary Elizabeth Browder, CMA
Assistant Professor, Office Information Technology
Raymond Walters College
Cincinnati, Ohio

Patricia Burkhard, RN, MSN
Professor, Nursing
Moorpark College
Moorpark, California

Marilyn R. Davidian, MA, RHIA
Chair and Assistant Professor, Health Information
    Management
Loma Linda University
Loma Linda, California

Sherry Gamble, RN, MSN, CNS, CNOR
Director and Associate Professor, Surgical
    Technology
The University of Akron
Akron, Ohio

Mary Garcia, BA, AD, RN
Instructor, Allied Health
Northwestern Business College
Chicago, Illinois

Michele Heller, CMA, RMA
Program Director, Medical Assisting
Ohio Institute of Health Careers
Columbus, Ohio

Janice C. Hess, MA
Program Coordinator, Health Information
    Management Systems
Metropolitan Community College
Omaha, Nebraska

Sherry L. Jones, RN, ASN
Instructor, Medical Assisting
Western School of Health and Business
Community College of Allegheny County
Pittsburgh, Pennsylvania

Trudi James-Parks, BS
Instructor, Radiologic Technology
Lorain County Community College
Elyria, Ohio

Michael Murphy, AAS, CMA, CLP
Instructor, Allied Health
Berdan Institute
Union, New Jersey

Pamela J. Posey, CMT
Program Coordinator, Health and Legal Studies
El Centro College
Dallas, Texas

Sheila D. Rockoff, EdD, MSN, BSN, AS, RN
Professor and Chair, Medical Assisting
Santa Ana College
Santa Ana, California

Marilyn Turner, RN, CMA
Program Advisor, Medical Assisting
Ogeechee Technical College
Statesboro, Georgia

**Gail S. Williams, PhD, MT(ASCP)SBB,
    CLS(NCA)**
Assistant Professor, Clinical Laboratory Science
Northern Illinois University
DeKalb, Illinois

1

General Teaching Ideas Related to Medical Terminology

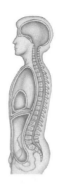

INTRODUCTION

In this section of the book, various ideas for teaching medical terminology will be introduced. Varying teaching styles help keep the attention and involvement of the students. By keeping them actively involved, the instructor will be able to ascertain their level of understanding. It will follow that the more completely a student understands, the more smoothly the learning process will proceed.

Language, by its definition, is fluid and always changing. English dictionaries must constantly be updated to reflect the changes in the manner in which we express ourselves. New words evolve from many sources—technology to street lingo. That evolution allows our language to keep pace with changes in society. Medical terminology is the same. If you were to take a look at an older version of a medical dictionary, many words used today would be missing. For example, Human Immunodeficiency Virus, Acquired Immunodeficiency Syndrome, Magnetic Resonance Imaging, Computed Tomography and many more are not in the dictionaries that were used 30 years ago. Either the technology had not been invented or the disease had not yet been discovered. This keeps medical language as flexible and ever changing as any other language. The instructor must keep up with those changes.

Successful teaching of medical terminology should include understanding the rules of building a term, memorization (for word elements), and, finally, a connection between the term and its relationship to anatomy and physiology.

The authors hope that by using the ideas in this guide instructors will find that they can add enthusiasm and eagerness to the classroom teaching process.

SECTION 1: STUDENT MOTIVATION ISSUES

Each student will enter the class with his/her own purpose for taking the course. Each will have a personal perspective on what they intend to achieve by learning medical terminology. In addition, the instructor may have a combination of continuing learners and new adult learners. This adds another dimension to the classroom.

For some students, it may be a mandatory course for further studies. Others may be just returning to the classroom and consider medical terminology a good place to start. These adult students may be wondering if they can learn after being out of school for many years. Still others may have had a basic understanding of medical terms from previous experience but have decided to take that learning a step further. Motivation for each will be different. Meeting the needs of each student can be daunting but are possible. Let's start out by looking at the specific needs of each of these students.

Terminology as a Prerequisite Course

The student interested in nursing, medical assisting, radiology, or any other clinical aspect of medicine will need a good basic understanding of medical terminology early in their program. In these cases, further, more intensive studies of anatomy and physiology will be needed.

However, giving the student an early connection with the terminology and anatomy and physiology will allow the student to get a jump start on those courses. The motivation of this student may be to get through the course and on to more "exciting" classes. The instructor must be able to help the student understand that terminology is a necessity for additional learning. To accomplish this, an instructor must use teaching skills that emphasize the connection between terminology and clinical medicine. Keeping the attention of this particular student can be difficult. That is why varying one's style of instruction becomes critical. Imagination plays a major role in keeping the interest of the student.

A student who is pursuing a clinical medical education may have a long road of learning ahead. The task may even be somewhat intimidating at first. Since terminology is usually taken early in a program, the student may also need to polish study skills. The instructor who understands this and makes room for it in their curriculum will have a far better chance of reaching the student. If the student recognizes the correlation between the terminology course and further learning, he/she will be more interested in truly acquiring a strong knowledge of the language of medicine.

Nonclinical students who need medical terminology may have a stronger interest in the course. Their hope is to use terminology in a more immediate way, such as for transcription or medical coding. This student will need to be more aware of the need for accurate spelling and correct usage in context. It is somewhat easier to keep this type of student involved in class participation.

The Adult Student

Returning to the classroom environment can be stressful and intimidating for adult learners. They may feel insecure and doubt their ability to understand and retain what they have learned. Up front, let them know they bring a great deal of knowledge to the class, whether or not they recognize it. Emphasize the value of lifelong learning. This will lessen the anxiety and give the student a much needed boost. If the class is primarily comprised of adult returning students (and even if it isn't), begin the course with a list of general study tips. Let the students know that everyone can continue to learn throughout their lifetimes. Dedication to study is paramount to learning. Older, returning students generally have a strong desire to learn. They are attempting to carve out a new direction for their lives. As a result, they generally ask more questions than the younger students. Instructors can use this to the advantage of all the students. Students without any interruption in their education may feel that they should know more about how to study, what to study, etc. By emphasizing the structure of the class early on, the instructor can help both types of students.

Students with Some Medical Background

This last category may be the most difficult student with which to work. Some students may arrive in class with the attitude that they all ready know everything and just need the course to continue. These students may have learned on the job, be self-taught, taken a correspondence (or online) class, or learned in some other manner. The key to this student is for the instructor to recognize the potential of this knowledge and use it to the advantage of all the students. This has to be well controlled. A student with a strong medical background can easily overwhelm and take over a class. The instructor needs to be able to continue to be the leader of the class and keep classroom disruption to a minimum.

In summary, the motivation of each student will be different. How to keep the interest of the whole class depends on using humor and imagination, while recognizing the need to keep structure in the classroom. A seasoned instructor will recognize the desire to learn and use methods that enhance that process. Ways in which to accomplish that will be presented in following sections.

SECTION 2: GAMES AND ACTIVITIES

Games and activities can be created by the instructor and the class. Some forms of *Jeopardy, Bingo, Family Feud* and other TV game shows can be modified to work with medical terms in the classroom.

SECTION 3: CLASSROOM MANAGEMENT

The instructor's approach to managing the classroom environment is paramount for effective learning to take place. Just as there are various learning styles, so are there different teaching styles.

One of the most important aspects of the class is that the students should feel welcomed and relaxed. The instructor should make it clear that no question will go unanswered. The instructor should know the names of the students and call them by name.

Let's begin with the physical layout of the classroom. If the classroom is a large room with standard lecture chairs, little can be done to change this configuration. The mere size of the class can intimidate even the most experienced instructor. However, there are ways to overcome the vastness of this style classroom. Using presentation software or overheads can bring the material closer to the students; using video or audio supplements can add a new dimension to the lecture. Keeping eye contact with the class will also offer the students a connection with the instructor.

A smaller space can often be awkward to work in. The physical closeness of the students can work to the instructor's advantage if managed well. If the room has lecture chairs, the instructor might want to arrange them in a "U" shape to allow the students to see each other. This creates a more intimate setting where the students feel they can more easily offer and receive assistance to and from each other. Activities are also easier to implement with this configuration. If the room has tables, a similar arrangement can be achieved by placing the table in a square with the instructor on one side. This gives the instructor the ability to work within in the group.

Both of these arrangements offer the instructor a good view of the students' faces. Looking at them while teaching has a two-fold value. It is easier to assess whether learning is occurring when the instructor is able to "read" the expressions of the students. Confusion or lack of understanding can be seen and the instructor has the opportunity to restate or reiterate the material. Catching this kind of problem early prevents students from becoming "lost" or frustrated. In addition, the physical accessibility of each student allows the instructor to give more one on one attention to the class.

Other physical aspects of the classroom must be controlled as well. Distractions such as outside noise should be kept to a minimum; the room should be a comfortable temperature, and lighting should be sufficient.

Next, the teaching style of the instructor should make learning interesting and enjoyable. Instructors should make clear at the beginning of the course that medical terminology cannot be learned by memorization alone. Using the terms in context will increase a student's complete understanding of the language. Just as students can not learn English strictly from reading a dictionary, neither can they learn medical terms just by seeing them on a page with a definition.

The instructor needs to make sure that every student has access to a medical dictionary from the start of the class. These may be purchased by the student or made available in the library and classroom. Regular use of the dictionary during class and lecture will help the students recognize the value of looking up definitions. Not all terms can easily be broken down and defined. A dictionary clarifies the meaning, gives the etymology of the word and may list synonyms and antonyms.

The instructor should introduce terms in context by having the students decipher a medical record such as a radiology report, discharge summary or pathology report. This exercise requires the student to show not only knowledge of the terms but an understanding of the manner in which terms are incorporated into the English language. Grammar, punctuation, and spelling must be understood in order for a report to make sense. The student who struggles with this exercise may need some tutoring in basic English.

In addition to using the printed word, students should use their other senses to help them understand. Verbally pronouncing the word, both in context and by itself; writing the term and its definition many times as an exercise; seeing the word used on the blackboard; using visual images relating to the term; and listening to the other students say the term all add dimension to the learning process.

Activities should be included that bring the class together, either as teams or groups. Games can be played that entertain as well as teach. Working together in small groups can bring out the reticent student who may not be as willing to participate in larger discussions. The student who learns more quickly may be able to coach slower students. Interaction between the students can be as valuable as any other study technique.

An instructor should strive to make a class enjoyable, informative and relatively painless. Learning should be a pleasant task, not tedious. The more interest the instructor shows in the subject being taught, the more the students will want to learn.

SECTION 4: TESTING/QUIZZING/HOMEWORK/ GRADING POLICIES

Each institution will have its own grading policy but the instructor will most likely have flexibility in how and when to test and evaluate students. Achieving fairness and yet making sure that the students are not just memorizing but also truly understanding the concepts presented can be bewildering for an instructor.

Homework should be assigned on a regular basis. Worksheets, review sections of the textbook, written reports, and Internet research projects all make great homework. Some instructors assign a poster to be designed. Grading of homework may be on a completion basis or be checked according to the instructor and/or the policy of the school. Using the homework as a review is helpful to the student. Give the students constant input and feedback. Be involved with them.

Quizzes should be given no less than once per chapter or system. They can include matching, multiple choice, fill-in-the-blank and deconstructing terms. Combining several of these styles of questions keeps the student interested in the test. If he/she does poorly on one style of question, they may do well on another.

Spelling tests may also be given. The instructor can dictate the terms or a list of correctly spelled or misspelled words can be used on a written test.

Tests at mid-term and a final exam are valuable to evaluate how well a student has assimilated the material. The above-mentioned styles of questions can be used along with a medical report to be reviewed and "translated."

Keeping tabs on the level of learning that students are achieving is important, as is feedback to them. If they are not evaluated regularly, students can become frustrated or not sure of their skill level. Students like to find out how well they are doing. They may not be thrilled with the grade received but they know where they stand.

Students will look to the instructor to tell them if they are excelling or failing. Quizzes and tests are effective ways to assess them.

SECTION 5: TEACHING ONLINE

Online classes are a fairly new concept. Some instructors have not had any experience with this form of teaching. There are definite advantages and disadvantages to online classes.

One of the obvious advantages is to make the course accessible to students who might otherwise be unable to attend a regular class. In addition, the students can work on the course at their own convenience.

The disadvantages are lack of test security, lack of personal connections and the inability to control the level of study. These can be overcome by using the technology available. Unfortunately, the instructor can never know whether the student is getting more "help" than they should.

It is important for the instructor of a distance learning course be actively involved with the students. Having regular chat sessions, email feedback and offering assistance to those who ask for it are ways to stay actively involved.

Teaching correct pronunciation is of particular concern when teaching an online course. The software should have audio so that the student can hear the words pronounced. Encourage the students to say the words out loud regularly. You may want to have the students send a tape or other media with examples of them pronouncing the words.

Keep up with the newest technology available. Network with other seasoned instructors of online courses. Connect with publishers to see if they have materials that would adapt well to distance learning classes. Keep in touch with the students! Don't ever let them feel they are out in cyberspace alone.

SECTION 6: USING PRESENTATION SOFTWARE (POWERPOINT™)

Slide presentation software is becoming increasingly more available. Most textbooks will now come with these presentations already created for the instructor. These materials are great ways of showing new information to the students. They allow information to be seen as well as heard and it will reinforce the information that the instructor is trying to get across.

All instructors will find their own comfort level with this software. Some will be very comfortable and will want to create their own presentations. Others will be new to the technology and will tend to rely more on prepared material. Either way works if the instructor uses it efficiently.

For those instructors that would like to create their own presentations there are some guidelines that should be kept in mind. For those that are new to creating their own slides, there are some pitfalls that are easily fallen into.

The first thing to watch for is including too much information on a slide. There is a general rule that states that you should not have more than seven words on a line and no more than seven lines on a page. This will help not to overwhelm the student when looking at the slide. The information also becomes very difficult to read when there are too many lines on a slide.

The next guideline that should be kept in mind is to keep the slides simple. Do not go overboard with pictures and sound effects. They are fun but only in moderation. Too much will become distracting to the students. On the same note, it is important to keep the presentations interesting. It is possible to have too little on the slides. Give them some motion and pictures to draw their attention to the information being presented. In particular, when teaching medical terminology, pictures and diagrams can really help to create a connection for the students.

One last note to keep in mind is that the presentation should be unified. Keep the same background or theme throughout. Be careful not to change every slide. The best slide shows will have smooth transitions throughout.

Once you have your presentation, whether you created it yourself or are using one from a publisher, how you present it becomes key. Slide presentations can be very boring if not used correctly. They are meant to interactive. Too many believe that all they need to do is stand there and read the slides, but that will have your students asleep in no time. The best instructors will understand that you must work with the presentation, and even have the students work with the material to create a learning environment.

2

Teaching Word Structure and Word Parts

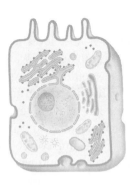

GENERAL TIPS FOR TEACHING

Medical terminology can be quite an intimidating language for students who are being introduced to it for the first time. It is the "new" language that must be mastered to communicate successfully with other health care professionals. By first laying a solid foundation, the instructor can take students through this learning process more easily. Approach this task as if constructing a building. Begin first by laying that solid foundation and building each level on top of the previous one.

First of all, you might ask the students to suggest some learning methods that have been successful in the past. Allow them to tell you how they would like to begin learning word parts and word building. Ask them to relate both their life and employment experiences, as these may often help with the learning process.

Begin by reviewing basic language skills go over nouns, verbs, pronouns, adverbs, and adjectives. Inform the students that many medical terms are constructed from word parts. Introduce the word parts (prefixes, suffixes, roots, and combining forms) and explain how each is used. Since students often struggle with which word part to use and when, strongly stress the rules of word building. Understanding the rules is as important as memorizing the terminology. Other suggestions for approaching word building follow.

- Go over basic study skills, especially with adult students who have been out of the learning arena for some time.
- Write the four word parts as headings on the board. Under each heading, make a list of the most common word parts in that category. Stress the definition of the word part, as well as the correct pronunciation.
- Stress the importance of learning by memorization and repetition.
- Use different colors for each word part. For example, use red for prefixes, blue for suffixes, green for word roots, and black for combining forms. Each time the student sees a color; they will associate that color with a particular word part.
- Demonstrate how to use all the resources found in a medical dictionary.

TEACHING USING DIFFERENT FORMATS

To keep the learning process interesting, teach using different formats. Catch the students by surprise! Do something different, something they are not accustomed to.

- Use visual images like PowerPoint™ presentations, overheads, and three-dimensional props. Often, a visual image will stick with the students more than a verbal one.
- Share real-life scenarios that you have experienced as a teacher and in the work force. Try to relate to the students by sharing similar experiences you have been involved in during procedures. Talk about any situations that were connected to a particular disease they may be studying. Students often find the material more relevant when it can be related to a real situation.

- Approach word building from as many directions as possible. Ask the students to sound out and pronounce the terms before you give them the correct pronunciation. Have the students write the definitions as they are explained.
- Stress correct spelling of the word parts and make sure the students are using the correct spelling.
- Face-to-face teaching can be coupled with online courses. This format gives the students a chance to review in-class material and to obtain the lecture when they can't attend class.
- An independent study format can allow students to learn at their own rate. Continue to lecture, but allow the students to advance through the lessons at their own individual level of ability. With this type of format, the students must end their independent study at the same time as the lectures.
- Case studies and actual medical records are a great way to expose students to terminology. Have the students find the terms within the document and break them down into their individual components.
- Once different word parts are on the way to being mastered, instruct the students to choose one root and add prefixes and suffixes to make as many different words as possible. Stress how the parts can be mixed and matched.

It is the opinion of some instructors that A&P and terminology should be taught during the same time period. Because a different instructor will probably teach each course, this would require the instructors to work together very closely to cover the same body system at the same time.

The atmosphere in which terminology is taught can also make a difference. Different seating arrangements may be more conducive to learning depending on the students' needs. However, some students may feel as if they are in the spotlight if seated in a circle or other less conventional method.

A structured, yet relaxed and somewhat informal atmosphere can be very valuable. Many students are intimidated if the atmosphere is too structured and formal.

Testing is almost always a source of anxiety for students. A variety of practice tests and quizzes can help the student feel confident about taking the "big" test, which counts for a grade. Depending on how often your class meets, the following suggestions for testing formats may be considered.

- Give several small quizzes throughout the unit or chapter instead of one large test.
- Give the definition and have the students create the term.
- Use case studies and ask the students to pick out the terms and divide them into their parts.
- Multiple choice and matching formats give the students a chance to pick from a group of words rather than having to come up with the correct answer on their own.
- Give just spelling tests.
- Give the students a paragraph and have them proofread it for terms and correct any that are incorrect.
- Give one large test at the end of each chapter.

GROUP ACTIVITY SUGGESTIONS FOR TEACHING

Most students, especially the introverted ones, benefit by taking part in group activities. Let your imagination and creativity guide you. There are endless possibilities. Suggestions for group activities follow.

- Of course, flash cards containing the different word parts are always a great way to facilitate word building. Students can use the cards for mix and match exercises to construct as many words as possible.

- Break the class up into groups and set a time limit. Have each group use the same word parts, and build the longest word they can come up with. Offer bonus points to the group with the largest word.

- Use worksheets with one word root on them and have the students build as many words as possible by adding prefixes and suffixes.

- Using the class as a whole, write a short root on the board and have the students build a long word, maybe even one that stretches all the way across the board. Stress to the students how they can define even the longest word by breaking it down and defining each part.

- Divide the class into groups and give each group a list of terms. Have the students dissect the terms into prefixes, suffixes, roots, and combining forms, and define each part. Allow the students to make this activity a group effort.

- Break down words and construct a list of prefixes, suffixes, and roots and create new words from the lists without repeating the original terms.

Activities are a great way to stimulate the students and to keep word building from becoming routine and boring.

GAME SUGGESTIONS FOR TEACHING

The use of games in teaching has become very popular. A fast paced, fun game can make word building exciting and interesting instead of boring and repetitious. A game can stimulate a student who is having problems learning the new language of medical terminology. Most terminology books include a student CD-ROM with great activities and games that the student can use outside of class time. The CD-ROM can also be implemented within the classroom. Set aside some time during every class period, perhaps at the end, for games. This activity can be used to recap the lecture material and review material from previous chapters.

Some additional suggestions for games are:

- A game similar to *Jeopardy,* in which the definition is given and the student must answer with the category and word part. For example, the game facilitator will say "inflammation," and the student will answer, "What is the suffix -itis?"

- Create a *Wheel of Fortune* type game, in which letters are filled in one at a time until the word part or term is guessed or totally revealed.

- Crossword puzzles can be created using word parts.

- Create a game like *Family Feud* and divide the class into two opposing teams to play against one another.

- Have the students create their on "bingo" cards with different prefixes, suffixes, and roots listed beneath the letters B-I-N-G-O. Call out the word parts and have the students locate them on their cards until someone has a "bingo" vertically, horizontally, or diagonally.

Establishing a routine and guidelines from the start will help to maintain structure in your class. Learning the rules of word building is essential from the beginning to eliminate problems later on. The foundation must be strong to support the different levels of medical terminology as the students work their way through each body system. Keep it fun and stimulating and enjoy teaching word building and watching a whole new language open up for your students.

3

Teaching the Terminology of the Whole Body

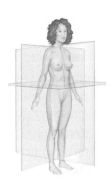

After the students have been introduced to the concept of prefixes, suffixes and word roots, they will begin the anatomy and physiology portion of the course. How much depth anatomy and physiology will be taught is dependent on the overall purpose of the terminology course. This topic is discussed in the general tips section.

Bringing together all of the word parts into logical medical terms can be daunting to the student. The idea of which word parts to use and the order to use them can confuse students. Also, learning anatomy and physiology may seem unnecessary to some students. Reinforce the point that even administrative employees need to understand how the body works. Medical coding and billing accuracy relies on the knowledge of the structures of the body and how they all work together.

The best way to begin this part of the course is to start at the beginning. The cell is the simplest form of life that should be discussed; then move on to the bio-organization of life, i.e., cells, tissues, organs, systems. Using diagrams, photos, and models on an overhead projector or presentation software, the students will be able to understand how all of these structures work together to form a functioning human body.

Usually anatomical planes, quadrants, positions and directions are taught in this section. Make sure the students are aware that two-dimensional drawings are reversed on the page so that the right side of the body will look like the left side on a page. They might imagine their body lying on the page to understand this concept. If they don't "get it," they will tend to label diagrams backwards.

The students will appreciate being able to actively participate in the class at this point. They have been in class long enough to feel more comfortable with open discussions and interactive opportunities.

GROUP ACTIVITIES

- Make of model of a cell using household items. This allows the creativity of students to be brought out. Explain that they shouldn't go out and purchase items. Instead, have them look at home for things like buttons, pasta, paper clips, etc. Discuss what cellular component each item resembles. The more they use their imaginations, the more fun this assignment becomes. The truly artistic students will be able to use the concepts that will encourage others to look for ways to express their thoughts about the structures of the body and their relationships. Have the students label each item with the proper term for that cellular component. Again, let them use imagination for the labels. The idea is to make this introduction to anatomy fun and draw in the more reticent students.

- There are excellent videos and slide presentations available to illustrate the functions of the body systems. Students could check out Internet sites such as WebMD, PBS (NOVA), Discovery Health and report on appropriate shows. The students should take note of whether the shows use layman's terms or the correct medical terminology. Why would the terminology make a show less understandable to the general population?

- On the Internet, by searching for images, the students will find unusual images particularly ideas of how the body worked in ancient times. Have them do research on how science has progressed in its understanding of anatomy and physiology.
- Team up students and have them do a presentation showing the manner in which body systems coordinate with each other. It could be done in the form of a skit, posters, or slide show presentation. The point is to show that various systems depend on each other to function correctly.

GAMES

See the list of games and descriptions of each in the general section. Any game can be adapted to correlate to a specific body system or specialty.

4

Teaching the Terminology of Gastroenterology/ Gastrointestinal System

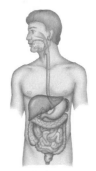

Gastroenterology is the study of the entire digestive system and metabolism of nutrients. Nutrition is usually included as a portion of this chapter.

A good place to begin teaching any body system is to differentiate between the specialists that treat the structures related to the system. For instance, gastroenterology is a general specialty that treats all organs. That can be seen by deconstructing the term: "gastr" means stomach, "enter" means intestine, and "ology" means the study of. Beginning with the suffix "-ology," the student can readily define the term as study of the stomach and intestines. Obviously, this a broad definition of a complex specialty.

Subspecialties include proctology, bariatrics, and colorectal surgeons. Dentistry can also be considered a specialty for the digestive system, since the alimentary canal begins with the mouth and teeth. Descriptions of each of these specialties will introduce the student to the basic terminology of this system.

Diagnostic techniques for the gastrointestinal system involve the use of contrast materials, radiology, scopes, MRI and CT scans. The terminology of such methods should be begin by emphasizing the differences between such suffixes as -scope and -scopy, -stomy and -tomy, and ectomy.

Another area to discuss is the accessory organs that are not naturally thought of as part of the digestive system. The alimentary canal is only part of the system. The liver, gallbladder and pancreas are organs that secrete enzymes to assist in digestion and absorption of nutrients.

The digestive system is also a system of elimination. Sometimes students will enter the course with little to no knowledge of anatomy. They may not realize that the human body has two systems by which it gets rid of waste products. A brief introduction into the difference between solid waste and liquid waste elimination can help. Explain that the body eliminates liquid waste through the urinary system and solid waste through the intestinal system.

Needless to say, spelling should be of major concern to the instructor and students. Recognition of the terms used in context can be accomplished by having the students read operative reports, imaging reports, and scope reports. These reports can be complex but do offer excellent opportunities for learning spelling and contextual use of terms.

GROUP ACTIVITIES

As with all group activities, insist that the students use the correct medical terminology and avoid the use of layman's terms. Verbal discussion, along with written reports, provides the instructor with a way to evaluate the pronunciation and true understanding of the terms.

- An interesting way to illustrate the manner in which saliva begins the breakdown of carbohydrates is the "saltine" test. Chew on a saltine cracker. At first, the taste is one of salt and starch. The longer one chews, the sweeter the flavor. This is due to the enzymes in saliva starting to change the complex carbohydrates into simple sugars.
- Discuss the innovations in abdominal surgery such as laparoscopic appendectomies, cholecystectomies and exploratory surgeries. Surgery no longer needs to be invasive and is often done on an outpatient basis.
- Use of anatomical models, diagrams and pictures help the students see in three dimensions, which makes the system easier to understand.
- If students are comfortable and willing, ask them about surgeries they, or someone they know, have undergone.
- Obtain information from the American Cancer Society regarding cancers that affect the gastrointestinal organs such as colon cancer, stomach cancer and pancreatic cancer.

5

Teaching the Terminology of Pulmonology/ Respiratory System

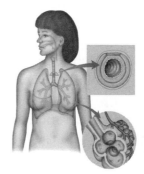

The function of the respiratory system is to provide the body with oxygen and eliminate carbon dioxide. It is a rather straightforward system to teach. The terminology consists of basic word roots, suffixes and prefixes.

Begin this chapter by describing the flow of air through the nose, sinuses and trachea into the lungs using medical language instead of layman's terms. This provides a quick introduction to the terminology and helps make it real to the student. Since the respiratory system is generally one with which most people are familiar, it is not as intimidating and the class may be more willing to openly participate. It is a good idea to present this system early in the course.

The recent emphasis on stopping/preventing smoking is an excellent way to capture the interest of the students. The public is constantly made aware of the environmental issues that relate to the respiratory system. Some are controllable (stop smoking) while others are not (smog). Students may not realize that there can be unseen pollutants in the air we breathe. Damage to the respiratory system is not a rare occurrence. Research the recent increase in tuberculosis and the dramatic changes in treatment since the 1920s. Asthma, emphysema, and COPD are other relatively common disorders that can be researched by students. Encourage the use of the proper medical terms when having discussions regarding the above issues.

Presentations can include models, diagrams, and anatomical drawings. The instructor should make sure that the students are able to recognize the structures and the correct pronunciation of the medical name. One may find regional and dialectic differences in pronunciation of terms.

Explain the disparities in language itself. Using the potato/tomato analogy will help assure the students that sometimes neither is wrong.

Describe the various diagnostic and imaging techniques used in the treatment of pulmonary diseases. Use an operative report along with a pre-op imaging report. This will illustrate the need for accurate reports. Ask what would have happened if the typist had inadvertently typed "right" instead of "left" lung.

GROUP ACTIVITIES

As with all group activities, insist that the students use the correct medical terminology and avoid the use of layman's terms. Verbal discussion, along with written reports, provides the instructor with a way to evaluate the pronunciation and true understanding of the terms.

- The simple act of blowing up a balloon can explain the act of exhalation. The concept of atmospheric pressure can also be illustrated using this approach.
- Have the students build a "lung" using a two-liter soda bottle, a regular balloon, a section of thick balloon material and a couple of rubber bands. Cut the bottom off of the bottle. Place the regular balloon inside the top of the bottle wrapped around the lip of the opening. Place the thick rubber on the cut-off bottom of the bottle and attach it with a rubber band. When you pull down on the rubber on the bottom, it acts as the diaphragm does in the body. The balloon inside the bottle will inflate due to the atmospheric pressure change.
- Use materials from the American Cancer Society that show the effect that smoking has on the lungs. Research recent statistics and compare them with numbers from years ago.
- Relate the difference between living and working in an urban vs. rural environment, again comparing the agricultural vs. industrial ages.
- If available, show the students how lung volume can vary by using a basic spirometer.
- Use a large bunch of grapes to demonstrate how the alveoli can have a large surface area within a smaller structure.
- Have the students use a stethoscope to listen to lung sounds or use an audio CD that allows the students to hear normal and abnormal breath sounds such as rales, rhonchi, and wheezing.
- If appropriate for the course, introduce the mechanics of CPR.

6

Teaching the Terminology of Cardiology/ Cardiovascular System

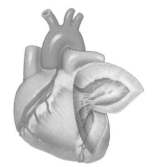

Begin this section with a discussion of the importance of the heart's function in circulating the blood throughout the body. This circulation of blood delivers oxygen to the cells and transports carbon dioxide away from the cells.

Use an anatomy and physiology model or diagram to explain the structure of the heart, including the chambers and valves. Check with a local butcher shop to see if a beef heart can be obtained and dissect it to reveal a cross section, which will allow the students to actually see the appearance of the structures they are learning the terminology for. Other teaching suggestions include:

- Create a list of the different vessels in the circulatory system and the word roots and combining forms for each. Stress the importance of the aorta as the largest artery in the body. Show the students a rubber hose that is 1 in. in diameter, the same diameter as the aorta. This type of visual aid will impress upon the students how large 1 in. really is.
- Trace a drop of blood through the entire system. Stress the difference between arteries and veins and point out which type of blood each vessel carries. Name the branches of the veins and arteries.
- Review the conduction system of the heart.
- Explain that the meaning of a prefix or suffix usually will not change. It is by combining them with a root or combining form that the meanings of the terms are created.
- Create a list on the board of the new combining forms and roots that pertain to the heart and vessels and allow the students to construct and define the new terms of the cardiovascular system.
- List some prefixes that can be used by more than one system, like epi-, peri-, myo-, and endo-.
- Have a discussion about the different subspecialists that are involved in treating the cardiovascular system: cardiologist, cardiac surgeon, vascular surgeon.
- Illustrate the connection between the anatomy and physiology terms and the medical terms.
- Give examples of terms that are not built using roots, prefixes, and suffixes.
- List the abbreviations for the cardiovascular system and their definitions.
- With the students' help, build a list of abbreviations of the cardiovascular system that could have two meanings.
- Discuss diseases and disorders of the cardiovascular system along with special medications used and other treatment options.
- Use visual images. Whenever possible, obtain actual photos of disorders and diseases of the vessels. Obtain a photo of the inside of a normal artery and one that is occluded with plaque.
- Show a video of an open-heart surgery or cardiac catheterization and ask the students to list the related terms in the video.
- Write a list of terms on the board that are related to a cardiovascular surgery or diagnostic procedure. Have the students dissect the words into their parts: for example, *aneurysmectomy.*
- Invite a health care provider who is currently working in a cardiology practice to speak to the class about different diseases and disorders of the system that they have worked with directly.
- Ask an EKG technician to speak to the class and show tracings of abnormal heart rhythms. Have the students make a list of the terms and then divide them into their parts: for example, *ventricular tachycardia.*
- Ask a cardiac stress test technician to speak to the class and explain the mechanisms related to a stress test and the use of the correct terminology.
- Obtain a page from the medical record of a hospital patient in the CCU. Ask the students to read the record and translate it into lay terms.
- Explain the connection between certain dental procedures and how the heart can be affected following the procedure or because of a dental abscess.

GROUP/INDIVIDUAL ACTIVITIES

- Give the students a blank diagram of the major arteries and veins and ask them to label it.
- Ask the students to relate common cardiovascular terms to the correct medical term. For example, heart attack = myocardial infarction, high blood pressure = hypertension, clot = embolus, or stroke = CVA.
- Divide the students into two groups. Have one group research arteriosclerosis and the other atherosclerosis, and then have a discussion to compare and contrast the two.
- Have the class compare the differences and similarities between an EKG and a Holter monitor.
- Ask the students to surf the Internet and create a list of different health care professions that relate to cardiology.
- Ask the students to visit the American Heart Association's Web site and gather the latest statistics on heart disease and cardiac deaths in the United States.
- Give the students an enjoyable assignment like watching a medical documentary or television episode of a medical drama and list any procedures performed that relate to the cardiovascular system.
- Ask the students to write a patient education scenario in lay terms with the medical terms in parentheses.
- Give the students a case study in lay terms and have them translate it into medical terms.
- Have a class discussion about the differences between echocardiography, electrocardiography, and Doppler ultrasound.
- With the students' help, make a list on the board of factors that can and cannot be changed to help prevent heart disease.

7

Teaching the Terminology of Hematology and Immunology/Blood, Lymphatic, and Immune Systems

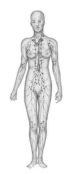

The students may find it odd to see these systems grouped together. An explanation of the connection between them is essential. Explain that blood and lymph are both body fluids, which have a function within the immune system. A discussion of the different elements found in the blood and the function of each element as part of the immune response can come alive with actual pictures of the different types of blood cells.

Use anatomy and physiology diagrams and visual aids to review the placement and location of lymph nodes and the circulation of the lymph fluid. Keep the anatomy basic, as some students may not have had anatomy and physiology or are taking it simultaneously with terminology.

Once the foundation of the blood and lymphatic systems has been laid, a presentation of the prefixes, suffixes, and roots that relate to them can be introduced. When the word parts have been presented, give a pretest to see how many terms the students know by simply defining the different parts. Assuring the students that this pretest will not count for a grade will help them to perform better. Students can prove to themselves how much they know from the basics and then see how much they have improved when a post-test is given. Other suggestions for teaching the system are as follows:

- An audio glossary or PowerPoint™ presentation of the correct pronunciation of related terms may be used if available. It is very helpful for the students to hear the correct pronunciation repeatedly.
- Have the students repeat the word parts as you pronounce them to ensure that they are pronouncing them correctly.
- Discuss some of the more common disorders of these systems and the terminology related to each.
- List and discuss the diagnostic and laboratory tests associated with these systems.
- Review an actual lab report, such as a CBC, and have the students identify and define the terms and abbreviations listed on the report form.
- Explain the different medical specialists associated with these body systems, such as hematologist, allergist, and immunologist.
- Use a video with related subject matter and have students list terms and break them down into parts.
- Spend 5-10 minutes reviewing terms from previous chapters to help refresh the terms the students already know.
- Stress correct spelling and pronunciation.
- If students are learning online, be sure they have access to support and automatic feedback of their progress.
- Have students make a list of new words at home and give bonus or extra credit points for the funniest, longest, most creative, etc.
- Relate the word parts to an anatomical drawing or to photos of some diseases and disorders associated with these systems.

GROUP/INDIVIDUAL ACTIVITIES

Use or create activities that directly relate to these body systems.

- Invite a laboratory technician to speak to the class about hematology and immunology tests or take the class on a field trip to these departments within the lab.
- Encourage the students to surf the Web for articles or papers on blood disorders and to circle the medical terms within the article.
- Have each student pick a type of blood or immunological disorder and prepare a short paper to present to the class. During the presentation, have the other students jot down the terms related to these systems.
- Introduce drugs used to treat disorders of the blood or immune system.
- Find a magazine article and give the students a copy and ask them to circle the medical terms.
- Give the students a diagnostic test report and have them translate the results into "plain English."

- Have the students complete and turn in any worksheets included in the text.
- Allow the students to suggest any activities or to create original games.
- Have the students research procedures or surgeries related to the blood or the lymphatic or immune systems.
- Introduce the term "immunosuppressed" and ask the students to list the types of patients who may fall into this category. Ask the students to come up with situations in which the physician would want to suppress a patient's immune system.

8

Teaching the Terminology of Dermatology/ Integumentary System

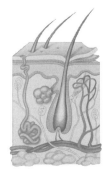

Dermatology is the study of the skin and its diseases. The name of the system that includes the skin is the integumentary system. The term comes from the Latin word integument, which means covering. In addition to the skin, this system includes the hair, nails, and the underlying subcutaneous tissues and glands.

The primary practitioner for the skin is the dermatologist. There are several subspecialties within this group such as reconstructive surgeons, burn specialists and oncologists.

The integumentary system is usually taught at the beginning of the course. Most of the word roots involved are basic to terminology and will be used in other body systems. The study of the skin and the medical terms is made easier by the fact that the system can actually be seen. It isn't hidden like the heart or nervous system. We are able to feel and touch the skin. Students can relate the terms directly to themselves.

Begin by explaining that the skin and its structure is the largest organ in the body. This helps build the concept of skin as a system in and of itself, not just a covering to keep the rest of the body intact. The skin has physiological functions such as temperature control, protection against invading organisms, and elimination of waste. It is the organ for our sense of touch, pressure, pain and temperature. The body needs the skin to remain intact to allow it to function completely.

Students should be made aware that skin cancers have been on the rise for many years. This may be due to several factors. One of these factors is that people live longer. Some scientists also believe that there is a correlation between the increase of skin cancers and the depletion of the earth's ozone layer. Regardless of the cause, the effect is that physicians who specialize in dermatology have to be on the lookout for suspicious lesions that may or may not be malignant. Much research involving skin cancers is being done to improve that outcome of such a diagnosis.

The science and practice of plastic surgery is always changing and improving as it relates to the aging of the skin. With surgeries and less invasive techniques such as laser, the condition of the skin can be improved to avoid the tell-tale signs of age such as wrinkles, sagging, thinning and discolorations.

Relate the integumentary system to the other body systems that affect or may be affected by its injury or disease, such as the nervous system and the immune system. Give the students an opportunity to look ahead to learning these other systems and their terms by introducing them in the chapter.

Relate the pertinent word parts to anatomical structures via presentation software, handouts and overheads to allow the student to recognize the structures of the skin. Emphasize correct pronunciation early, so that the student doesn't acquire any bad habits by mispronouncing a term.

GROUP ACTIVITIES

The advantage of this particular body system is its availability to be studied visually. As with all group activities, insist that the students use the correct medical terminology and avoid the use of layman's terms. Verbal discussion, along with written reports, provides the instructor with a way to evaluate the pronunciation and true understanding of the terms.

- Have the students visually examine their own skin to recognize the structure on the surface such as pores, hair, and visible blood vessels.
- Have the students do research on the prevalence of skin cancers in their geographical area and compare this to other areas of the world.
- Discuss the practice of plastic surgery and the evolving techniques for preventing or repair of the aging of the skin.
- Have students research the local "spas" and other businesses that relate to skin care. Compare the promises to the actual outcome of a particular procedure. Are the ads reliable?
- Have a cosmetologist do a demonstration explaining hair and nail care.

9

Teaching the Terminology of Orthopedics/Skeletal System

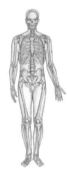

Tackling the terminology related to the 206 bones in the adult skeleton can be an insurmountable task to many students. Reassurance that words for this system are built in the same manner as all other body systems will help most students to relax. Start by explaining the term orthopedics, review the parts of a long bone, and on an anatomy and physiology model or diagram, point out some of the *major* bones of the skeleton.

Allow the students to relate their own experiences with orthopedics, such as broken bones or sports injuries. Explain to the class about the belief that many disease states of the body can be caused by a misalignment of the spinal column. The practice of chiropractics was founded on this belief.

After reviewing the bones, again lay the foundation by introducing the prefixes, suffixes, roots, and combining forms that relate to the bones. Have the students write the word parts on flash cards. Stress the importance of correct pronunciation of the word parts and ask the students to repeat them after you pronounce them. Explain that sometimes terms related to the bones/skeleton can have two different combining forms, one from Greek and one from Latin.

Divide the skeleton into the two parts, appendicular and axial, and review the bones in each part. Other teaching suggestions include:

- Relate English words to medical terms. For example, thigh bone = femur, funny bone = humerus.

- Conduct a class discussion about sports or other types of exercise and have the students talk about the movements involved in each and the possible injuries that could occur. List the correct terminology for those injuries.

- Once the terminology of the bones has been introduced, use visual aids to explain the different types of fractures and diseases.

- Discuss different diagnostic procedures like MRIs, scans, scopes, and x-rays. If possible, obtain an arthroscope to show the class or an x-ray film that clearly shows a fracture.

- Include the pharmaceutical terms related to the treatment of skeletal disorders and diseases.

- Use large flash cards, which have a bone on each card and ask the students to list the related terms.

- Use word association when possible to make learning the terms easier.

- Give practice word sheets with fill-in-the-blank sentences and several terms from which to choose.

- Introduce current surgical and therapeutic procedures used for the treatment of injuries, birth defects, and diseases.

GROUP/INDIVIDUAL ACTIVITIES

Activities, whether individual or group, are fun and a stimulating method of teaching. An activity produces a more relaxed atmosphere than a graded test. Once the students appear to have a solid grasp on the terminology of the bones, integrate some fun activities.

- Divide the class into two groups and assign each group a division of the skeleton, appendicular or axial. As a group, have the students identify the bones on a diagram.

- Visit an orthopedics office and arrange for the office manager or one of the other office assistants to give a presentation about the practice and to show the different instruments and scopes used. Ask the presenter to explain the different types of casting materials, splints, and any other immobilization devices.

- Talk about osteoarthritis and how common it is. Ask the students to go online and research the latest information about joint replacement surgery.

- Instead of a spelling bee, have a pronunciation bee. Show the term or word part on a flash card, and have the students pronounce it. If is not pronounced correctly, the player is eliminated.

- Have the students read an actual ER report of an injury to the skeletal system and circle and translate the medical terms.

- Divide the class into two groups and assign the topic of rheumatoid arthritis to one group and the topic of osteoarthritis to the other. Ask them to research the disorders and then have a discussion to compare and contrast the two.

10

Teaching the Terminology of Orthopedics/Muscular System

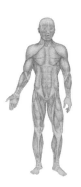

With 700+ muscles in the human body, deciding which ones to teach can be daunting. A review of the major muscles on an anatomical diagram may be the best way to begin. The difference among tendons, ligaments, and cartilage should also be explained.

The next step might be to divide the body into sections, like the head, chest, arms, legs, etc., and review or introduce the muscles in each body part. Once a good anatomy and physiology review has been completed, introduce the terms relative to the muscles. Divide the terms into their word parts, and define each part. Some instructors prefer to introduce roots and combining forms first and then add the prefixes and suffixes. Other methods include:

- If possible, allow students to observe in an anatomy lab that uses cadavers or animals so they can actually see the muscles, tendons, ligaments, and cartilage.
- Explain how many muscles get their names.

  Size = maximus, medius
  Where they originate
  Where they are inserted
  By their action = flexor, extensor
  Location = latissimus dorsi

- Discuss the relationship between the bones and muscles and the rehabilitation required to strengthen muscles following an injury or surgery. Students should have a basic understanding of why strengthening the muscles helps with the support and function of the bones. Explain terms related to rehabilitation.
- Have an open discussion with the class about the difference between a strain and a sprain. Have the students talk about their own experiences with the two and list the terminology for both.
- Introduce the laboratory and diagnostic tests related to the muscles and have the students build a list of the abbreviations for each. Discuss why x-rays cannot be used to view muscles as they can be for viewing bones.
- Discuss the difference between the treatment options for muscle injuries and bone injuries. Discuss physical therapy vs. surgical intervention.
- When the students are comfortable with the terms related to the muscles, introduce the terminology of movement, like, abduction, adduction, flexion, extension, etc. While reviewing these terms, have the students perform each movement.
- Discuss the difference between muscle relaxants and muscle stimulants. The students could also list the brand or generic names under the correct heading.
- Bring in a newspaper/magazine article related to the muscles, such as one on injuries, any new neuromuscular disorders, or other related diseases. Ask the students to make a list of the medical terms contained in the article and to define each.

- Review a lab or diagnostic report and have a discussion about the implication of the results. Ask the students to identify the medical terms contained within.
- Encourage the students to form study groups to help each other learn and review.
- Point out the exercises and games related to the muscles on the student CD-ROM. Assign some pages from the CD-ROM for homework and bonus points.

GROUP/INDIVIDUAL ACTIVITIES

- Take the class to a rehabilitation facility. Ask the physical therapist to explain the different equipment and modalities used in physical therapy. Relate the movement terms to certain injuries and rehabilitation and stress the importance of range of motion (ROM) exercises.
- Ask the students to do some research and find the smallest and largest muscle in the body and the shortest and longest.
- Divide the class into two groups and ask the students to research the diseases muscular dystrophy and myasthenia gravis. Students should compare and contrast the information found and make a list of the medical terms related to each disease. Have the students research the different types of paralysis: hemiplegia, paraplegia, and quadraplegia.
- Ask the students to look up information about work-related injuries such as repetitive motion disorders, like carpal tunnel syndrome, and include any statistics about the frequency and commonality of certain work-related injuries.
- Encourage the students to make a list of those words they are having problems spelling and to write each word 15 times.
- Ask the students to list the medical terms related to the common terms for disorders like tennis elbow, golf elbow, tennis shoulder, pitcher's shoulder, etc.

11

Teaching the Terminology of Neurology/Nervous System

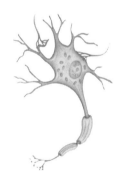

Neurology is the study of the nervous system and related diseases and disorders. It includes the central nervous system and the peripheral nervous system.

It is important to begin this subject with a discussion of the relationships of all body function to the nervous system. Without an intact nervous system, the body will not be able to function normally. The brain and spinal cord are the primary structures that permit the actions of all of the peripheral nerves.

The brain is the principal organ of the nervous system. If it cannot function, neither will any other system. Without sufficient oxygenation, brain tissue will quickly die; this death is irreversible. Therefore, the proper function of the body is dependent on the brain working correctly.

Unfortunately, brain damage can affect the physical and/or mental capabilities of a person. The study of neurology should closely relate to the study of mental impairment. Some medical terminology textbooks do not cover the psychology issues of injury to the nervous system. It may be up to the instructor to include information regarding the mental processes and how they relate to the nervous system.

Most terminology courses aren't long enough to devote time to understanding the nervous system in detail. It is a complicated, involved process to explain. Therefore, the instructor should emphasize the terms that are basic to the workings of the nervous system.

Physicians who specialize in neurology usually have a subspecialty such as surgery, physical therapy (including physiatrists), reconstruction (plastic surgery for reattachment of an amputated body part), and neurobiology (study of the chemical aspect of the nervous system).

Recent studies have shown the close relationship between neurotransmitters and mental health, particularly regarding depression, obsessive-compulsive disorders, and bipolar illness. The nervous system relies on these chemicals to maintain a balance among the neurons. New medications affect these neurotransmitters, allowing a more normal reaction.

Discussion of the effects that a spinal cord injury can have and how dependent the outcome is on the level of injury should address the current studies of stem cell research. Be careful not to allow this to become a political issue; stay on the science. Students may have very strong feelings regarding stem cell research.

Neurological oncology is the study of malignancies that attack structures of the nervous system. Surgery, chemotherapy, and radiology are the methods most commonly used to treat cancers of the nervous system.

GROUP ACTIVITIES

As with all group activities, insist that the students use the correct medical terminology and avoid the use of layman's terms. Verbal discussion, along with written reports, provides the instructor with a way to evaluate the pronunciation and true understanding of the terms.

- Research the most recent advances in the treatment of spinal cord injuries.
- Have students compare the differences between paraplegia and quadriplegia.
- Have the students research the increase in late effects of poliomyelitis and the effect it is having on victims.
- Have a wheelchair-bound person speak with the students regarding the stigma that society has placed on the disabled.
- Discuss the American Disabilities Act and the positive effect it has had for disabled persons.
- Research the recent improvements in microsurgery that allow the reattachment and full use of an amputated limb.

12

Teaching the Terminology of Endocrinology/ Endocrine System

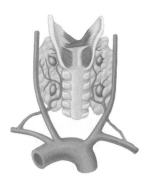

The endocrine system is a system of ductless glands and glands that secrete internally. One way to describe the endocrine system to your students is to describe it as being similar to the nervous system. The nervous system is used to transport messages throughout the body to control function. The endocrine system is similar in that it also sends messages throughout the body to control functions, just with different means. The nervous system uses electric impulses, and the endocrine system uses chemicals.

The reason why your students are taking medical terminology will have an effect on how you teach the terminology of the endocrine system. This system is very complicated and intricate. It can be very intimidating to your students. Try taking it slow in this system if your program allows.

One of the first things that you will want to explain to students is the difference between exocrine and endocrine. The terms are very similar, so it will be easy for students to confuse them. Talk about the idea that the prefix exo- means outside; exocrine glands secrete to the outside of the body. The prefix endo- means within; the endocrine glands secrete within the body. With this initial confusion out of the way it will help to start asking the students about different glands they already know. Then follow that by having them determine whether or not those glands are endocrine or exocrine.

Now that the students have a good idea what the system includes you can begin introducing the different organs. The students will need to have an understanding of each gland and which hormones are secreted. Many students will just try to memorize this information. However, it is much better if connections are made. For example, the location of the parathyroid gland can be revealed just by breaking down the word. The same approach will help with hormones. Breaking down the word antidiuretic makes it easier to understand what job it performs.

The concept of feedback as it relates to the endocrine system may help the students understand how the hormones actually need each other in order to perform correctly. The pituitary gland secretes many hormones that act on other endocrine glands such as the thyroid, ovaries, and testes. It acts as a "master gland" controlling functions of the body. Using diagrams and tables explaining these connections will simplify this system for the students.

GROUP ACTIVITIES

You may find that this is one of the more difficult systems to create group activities. Here are a few to get you started.

- Create cards with the different glands and the different hormones. Have the students match up the hormones to the glands. This will work with large groups—or split the students into teams—and make a game out of it.
- Have a class discussion regarding diabetes. What are common beliefs and myths surrounding this disease? Many will know someone that suffers from the disease. Have students look up new medications and technology updates such as insulin pumps.
- Have students research the controversy surrounding HRT. What did we believe before about HRT? What do we know now and how has it changed the use of HRT?

13

Teaching the Terminology of Urology/Urinary System

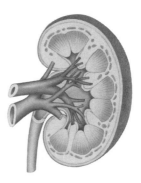

Personal preference will often dictate how an instructor begins to teach the terminology of each body system. Some prefer to introduce the anatomy first and then proceed to the word parts and word building, or vice versa.

Visual aids are very important and make learning easier and make the language come alive. For instance, a picture of a polycystic kidney makes a much larger impact than just the term itself. Other teaching suggestions follow.

- Relate to the students the history of urinalysis.
- Introduce the terminology of the urinary tract and urinalysis and ask the students to repeat the pronunciation of each term.
- Explain the composition of urine and discuss how much information can be gained about a patient's state of health by performing a simple urinalysis.
- Explain that an urologist treats both the male and female urinary tract and the male reproductive system.
- Demonstrate how many of the urinary tract terms are constructed from word parts.
- Introduce abbreviations related to the urinary system and the abbreviations of the diagnostic and laboratory tests. Stress the importance of learning the full meaning of the abbreviations.
- Start with a blank diagram and relate the terms to the structures.
- Create a word scramble game.
- When introducing the diseases and disorders of this system, read an actual medical record or case study to the class and ask them to listen for the medical terms.
- When discussing the anatomy and physiology of the urinary system, try to obtain a beef kidney to dissect so the internal structures can be revealed and studied.
- Explain how the kidneys not only filter the blood and create urine, but secrete a hormone—erythropoeitin—which signals the bone marrow to make more red blood cells when their level becomes low.
- Explain the difference between the male and female urinary system. Explain how the male shares structures with both the reproductive system and the urinary tract. In the male the system is referred to as the *genitourinary* system or the *urogenital* system.
- Introduce the different medications of the urinary system: diuretics, antibiotics, drugs that improve bladder function, and urinary tract analgesics.
- Since visual aids really reinforce the learning process, when discussing kidney stones or renal calculi, show an actual x-ray film, which clearly shows a stone. A KUB would be interesting to show the outline of the kidneys, ureters, and bladder.

    Try to obtain an actual kidney stone and pass it around for the students to examine. Point out the sharp edges and the shape, which is what causes the pain as it is being passed.

- Another interesting visual aid would be a video of an actual cystoscopy or transurethral prostate surgery.
- Discuss the two laboratory tests, urinalysis and culture and sensitivity.
- Talk about renal failure, dialysis, and transplant.
- Invite a dialysis nurse to speak to the class about hemodialysis and peritoneal dialysis or take the class to a dialysis center to see the process in person.

GROUP/INDIVIDUAL ACTIVITIES

- Give the students lists of word parts related to the urinary system and have them create new terms.
- Ask the students to choose two words that have the same meaning.
- Ask for volunteers to research a disease of the urinary system and any current or new treatment options.
- Give the students an IVP report and have them circle the medical terms contained in the report and translate them into lay terms.
- Have the students research the process of lithotripsy and then have a class discussion on the subject.
- Obtain a urinalysis report and ask the students to interpret and define the results.
- Give the students a list of misspelled words and have them correctly spell the terms.
- Ask the students to create a concentration game from urinary system terms and abbreviations.
- Assign the students to give a presentation with visual aids.
- Alter a page from a medical record, and ask the students to correct it.
- Divide the students into two groups and assign one group the topic of hemodialysis and the other group peritoneal dialysis.

14

Teaching the Terminology of Gynecology and Obstetrics/Female Reproductive System

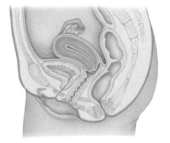

When teaching the terminology of OB-GYN and the female reproductive system, the structures of the system may be a good place to begin, since they are all involved in both branches of the specialty.

Introducing the terminology of the anatomy and physiology first—before tackling the subjects of pregnancy, labor and delivery, and diseases and disorders of the system—is a logical way to approach the subject. Relay the terminology related to each suggestion below.

- Use anatomy and physiology models and diagrams and review the structures of the system.
- Introduce the roots and combining forms to be coupled with prefixes and suffixes to create the terminology of obstetrics and gynecology.
- Divide terms into the separate categories of obstetrics and gynecology. Place each term under the correct heading. Relate the terms to anatomical structures, diagnostic and laboratory tests, medications for treating gynecological patients, medications for treating obstetrical patients, surgical procedures, diseases, and disorders.
- When teaching the GYN section, invite a speaker from the local health department to talk about STDs and AIDS. Have the students note any terms they are familiar with.
- Explain the different stages of breast cancer.
- Introduce the terminology for different surgical procedures of the breast.
- Invite a cytotechnologist to talk about PAP smears and how they are graded. Also ask the tech to explain the special training they are required to have in order to read the PAP slides and the fact that they are limited to reading a certain number of slides per shift.
- Obtain a video of a pelvic laparoscopy and point out the uterus, ovaries, and tubes. While pointing out the structures, discuss the function of each.
- Review the menstrual cycle, along with the terminology associated with each phase.
- Discuss the relationship between problems like endometriosis and some autoimmune diseases like lupus.
- Explain the development of the fetus using anatomy and physiology diagrams, videos, or actual photos.
- Explain the trimesters of pregnancy and the complications that may arise.
- Obtain a sonogram of a fetus and point out the visible structures.
- Discuss the use of ultrasound in obstetrics and gynecology.
- Using visual aids, introduce and define the terms zygote, embryo, fetus, neonate, and newborn.
- Show a video of a vaginal delivery and a C-section delivery.
- Invite a labor and delivery nurse to speak to the class and to compare and contrast the difference between assisting with each type of delivery.
- When teaching the medications and laboratory and diagnostic tests, it may be easier to separate the terms into two categories.

GROUP/INDIVIDUAL ACTIVITIES

- Divide the class into two groups and have each group create their own words and then quiz each other by giving a definition and guessing the term.
- Have the students watch a TV show such as *Maternity Ward* and make a list of all OB-GYN terms used in the episode.
- Instead of a spelling bee, have an abbreviation bee.
- Divide the class into two groups. Give one group an actual hospital report of a C-section delivery and the other group a hospital report of a vaginal delivery. Have the students circle the medical terms and then compare the differences and similarities between the two deliveries.
- Ask the students to break down and explain the terms *hysterectomy, salpingectomy, oophorectomy,* and *hysterosalpingo-oophorectomy.*
- Ask the students to do research on amniocentesis and list the information that can be gained from analyzing the amniotic fluid.

- Ask for volunteers to do a short presentation on in-vitro and assisted fertilization. Ask the rest of the class to write down any OB-GYN terms included in the presentation.
- Divide the class into the appropriate number of groups and have each group do a report on one of the stages of breast cancer and the treatment options for each.
- Have one or two students prepare a short presentation on the pros and cons of HRT.

15

Teaching the Terminology of Male Reproductive Medicine/Male Reproductive System

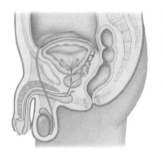

Urology and andrology are the two specialties for diseases and disorders of the male reproductive system. Urology studies the structure and function of the testes and penis along with related organs. Andrology is the study of male hormones and their effect on aging, body structure, psychology and sexual behavior.

The study of the urinary system should precede this subject since they are integral. The male reproductive system should be studied as an adjunct to the urinary system and female reproductive system. It is necessary to teach in this order so that the correlations between the systems can be understood. In addition, students should have a basic understanding of the endocrine system to be able to understand the male hormones and how they work in the body.

Many of the prefixes and suffixes of this system will be the same as in most other chapters. Also, if the student has already studied the process of reproduction, many of the word roots will be recognized.

Begin teaching the chapter by discussing the connection to the urinary system and the structures that both systems have in common. As a result of this introduction, the students will realize that he/she has already learned a great deal about the subject within the study of other chapters. Much of the terminology for this system will be redundant. That should be looked upon as a positive aspect since it allows for the review of familiar terms.

Use presentation software, anatomical models and drawings to explain the manner in which sperm are developed, mature, and fertilize an ovum. There are several excellent videos available that show the physiological action of the male and female reproductive systems. Care should be used in their use since they are graphic in nature. However, the instructor shouldn't shy away from discussion of the subject. As a matter of fact, the more comfortable the instructor is, the more comfortable the students will be.

Due to the evolution of infertility treatments, the science has changed our way of thinking about reproduction. Sterility and erective disorders are openly discussed and treated. Society has become more open regarding sexuality in general. This should make it easier for the instructor to keep the students on task.

GROUP ACTIVITIES

As with all group activities, insist that the students use the correct medical terminology and avoid the use of layman's terms. Verbal discussion, along with written reports, provides the instructor with a way to evaluate the pronunciation and true understanding of the terms. Because the subject may make some students uncomfortable, emphasize the use of medical terms instead of euphemisms and slang.

- Research new treatments for infertility and sterility.
- Discuss the difference between female menopause and male andropause.
- Discuss genetic issues and how they relate to the reproductive systems of both males and females.
- Research the issue of erectile dysfunction and the pharmaceutical industry's approach to it.

16

Teaching the Terminology of Ophthalmology/Eyes

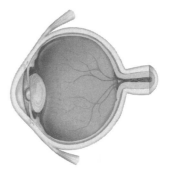

Ophthalmology is the study of the eye structures and the sense of sight. When teaching this section, there are several areas in particular to emphasize.

There are three primary specialists in this field of medicine: ophthalmologists, optometrists, and opticians. There are also subspecialties such as cosmetic, reconstructive plastic, refractive (LASIK), glaucoma, and cataract surgeons. The instructor should start out with defining each and describing the differences between each discipline. In addition, stress the differences in spelling. In this instance, pronunciation is key to the correct spelling. There should be no regional differences in pronunciation of these specialties.

The students should be able to relate the terminology to the structures of the eye, sense of vision, and related nervous system connections. Begin by listing pertinent word parts, and then relate them to anatomical drawings. This can be done via presentation software, handouts, and overheads. Do not rely on the student to understand the drawings in their textbook without input from the instructor. Move on to adding prefixes and suffixes that relate to procedures that are performed on the eye.

Correct spelling cannot be emphasized enough. Since many terms are similar but have very different meanings in the field of ophthalmology, the accurate spelling may make a difference within the context of the material.

Make known that constant improvements and new procedures are being developed but, in general, the terminology will contain the same basic word parts. Since surgical procedures are quite often acronyms or eponyms, giving a background explanation will help the students understand. Explain the particular procedures that may be eponyms and the process through which they were named. Understanding the basis for a term enables the student to have a different viewpoint from which to grasp the concept.

GROUP ACTIVITIES

Ophthalmology is one of the less common specialties. As a result, students are likely to have less knowledge of the specialty. Introducing them to the activities of this type of practice will help reinforce the terminology. As with all group activities, insist that the students use the correct medical terminology and avoid the use of layman's terms. Verbal discussion, along with written reports, provides the instructor with a way to evaluate the pronunciation and true understanding of the terms.

- Have students relate their own experiences with ophthalmologists, optometrists, and opticians. Have them discuss the training and the limitations of each practice.

- Have the students do "eye exams" on each other. These should be as simple as noting the difference of the iris color, PERRLA, eye movement. These are noninvasive and do not invade the privacy of the person. Have the students use the correct terms as they discuss the exam. This will also allow the student to involve him/herself with the hands-on concept of the exam.

- Have students do research on various practices in the area that perform refractive surgeries. This can be done with television and radio advertisements, telephone book listings and Web pages for practices in their geographical area. Have them compare these to information on practices outside their general area. Discuss the various types of advertising and the value to the consumer. Are the terms used in the ads correct or do the advertisers not expect a consumer to understand the medical jargon? Do they notice any misspellings or incorrect grammar?

- Have students visit an optician and report on the limitations of this specialist, the various types of correction lenses available, and the manner in which lenses are made. This gives the students a "real world" experience with the terminology they have been learning. Do the opticians use layman's terms? Did the students make the connection to the correct medical term?

- This last suggestion is not for the faint of heart. Cow eyes are readily available from local butchers. Using one to show the structure of the eyes is fascinating to many and "gross" to others. Poll your students before doing the demonstration to get an idea of their reactions. Medical assisting and other clinical students will probably have a more positive response than purely administrative students.

17

Teaching the Terminology of Otolaryngology/Ears, Nose, and Throat

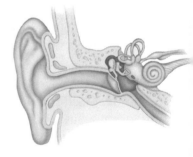

The specialty of ENT encompasses the ears, nose, and throat. The nose and throat are part of the respiratory system and the ears and the nose are part of the sensory system. For this reason, it may be easiest to examine each component individually. When using any of the following suggestions, incorporate all related terminology.

- Ask the students to try pronouncing the terms before you present them to the class.

- Using anatomy and physiology models, diagrams, or actual photos, point out the external and internal structures of each component.
- On the board, create three columns and list the prefixes, suffixes, roots, and combining forms for the ears, nose, and throat. Do the same with diagnostic tests, diseases and disorders, and surgical procedures.
- Since the oral cavity is also part of this system, examine the tonsils and adenoids and relate the terminology of the tonsillectomy and adenoidectomy.
- List any abbreviations that could have two meanings and show any combining forms that may be of both Greek and Latin origin.
- Invite an audiologist to speak to the class about hearing tests and the different types of hearing loss.
- Trace the pathway of sound through the structures of the ear while pointing out all terms.
- Discuss the dual role of the nose in both the sensory and respiratory systems. Explain the function of each structure as it pertains to both systems.
- When discussing the medications used to treat this system, point out that some come in more than one form. For example, a medication may be used both externally and internally.
- Ask for a student volunteer, and demonstrate how we are able to smell.
- Discuss the function of the nose, pharynx, and larynx and any diseases and disorders of each.

GROUP/INDIVIDUAL ACTIVITIES

- Bring a tympanic thermometer to class and demonstrate an aural temperature and allow the students to practice this method.
- Ask students to label separate anatomy and physiology diagrams of the ear, nose, and throat.
- Assign research on the different types of hearing loss and choose several students to present their information to the class while making a list of the terms included.
- Ask the students to watch a TV medical show and write down words pertaining to the ears, nose, and throat. Give a prize or bonus points for the most correct terms.
- Ask the students to surf the Internet and gather information and statistics on smokeless tobacco and oral cancer.
- Ask the students to gather information on hearing loss caused by exposure to noise. Make a list of common noises and the decibel level of each.
- Write statements on the board using ENT terminology and have the students give the common term for each medical term.
- Give the symptoms of a disease to the class and ask them to give the medical term for the disorder. This can also be done with treatment methods.
- Ask for a volunteer to do research and give a short presentation on the three different ways that sound is conducted, using the correct medical terminology.
- Create a crossword puzzle using ENT terms and word parts.
- On the board, write the two terms labyrinthectomy and labyrinthotomy. Have the students divide the words into parts and define each part.
- Divide the ear into outer, middle, and inner sections and ask the students to name and correctly spell the structures in each area.
- Ask the students to bring in an article on the ENT specialty.
- Ask if anyone in the class knows American Sign Language and if they would mind demonstrating some signs to the class. If not, give a handout of some of the common signs and have the students practice them.

18

Teaching the Terminology of Psychiatry

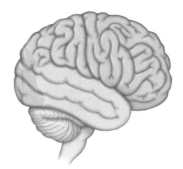

Psychiatry is the study and treatment of mental illness. The term is based on the word form "psyche," the Greek word for the mind and its processes.

Psychiatrists are medical doctors who specialize in researching, treating, and preventing mental illnesses. They may prescribe medications, psychotherapy or other methods of mental therapy. Psychologists are trained in the analysis and therapy of the mentally ill; they cannot prescribe drugs. Psychiatric technicians work in psychiatric care facilities, assisting the patient with various therapies and activities. In addition, there are other levels of counselors such as licensed social workers who work with substance abusers, sex offenders, and others who are mentally or emotionally challenged. The instructor should start out with defining each and describing the differences among the disciplines.

The basic word form, psych/o, is used in many terms regarding this science. Since it is not possible to relate these terms to a body system, the student needs to start with understanding the direction of current medicine regarding mental illness. Patients with mental illness had a stigma attached to their diagnosis; they were thought to be "weak" or simply resistant to "normal" behaviors. Today's psychology recognizes the effects that the imbalance of certain neurotransmitters that may be the cause of mental illnesses. As a result, patients are less likely to face the indignity that once was attached to mental illness.

Since the student will not be able to associate the terminology with specific anatomical structures, emphasis should be placed on the relationship of the brain and nervous systems to the psyche. Discussion should involve the concept of an imbalance in neurotransmitters directly linked to mental illness.

The terms within this particular section may be difficult to connect to a tangible concept and will be of a more indefinable nature. The instructor needs to be aware of the possible preconceptions that students will bring to the classroom. In addition, cultural differences and bias may cause the student to interpret some terminology in diverse ways. It is up to the instructor to be able to discern when this occurs and attempt to overcome any inaccuracies.

Correct spelling cannot be emphasized enough. Since many terms are similar but have very different meanings in the field of psychiatry—i.e., psychology vs. psychiatry—the accurate spelling may make a difference within the context of the material.

Emphasize that psychiatry is an evolving science, and improvements in treatment are often and many. Even so, the terminology will contain the same basic word elements. A comprehensive medical dictionary is very important to allow the student to check the specific definition of a psychiatric term, but may not be as current as one would like. The Internet is a valuable resource to keep up to date on therapies and drug modalities for the treatment of mental illness.

GROUP ACTIVITIES

Due to the very personal nature of the discussion of mental illness, the instructor must use tact and insight into the personality of the class. It is easy to overlook the societal taboos that are affiliated with the brain and its processes. Care must be taken when using humor when teaching this subject. In addition, do not expect students to openly discuss any personal or familial experiences with psychiatry. The students will probably not be willing to participate in class discussion as readily as they would with other subjects. The instructor should respect the privacy of students and not exert pressure on any student to share.

Quizzes such as depression indicators or mini-mental assessments may be used to familiarize the students with the language used in this specialty.

19
Teaching the Terminology of Oncology

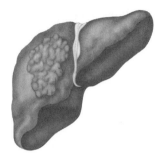

Oncology is the study of tumors, particularly malignant neoplasms (cancers) and the treatments available. It is constantly evolving branch of science, with new methods of therapy being discovered frequently. As a result, the terminology is changing with each new form of treatment.

When teaching this specialty, the instructor must be careful to differentiate between benign and malignant neoplasms. These differences are of particular importance in diagnosis coding.

Cancer can strike any body system. Most terms combine a suffix that describes the neoplasm with a combining form that relates to the body system affected. Thus, the student needs a strong knowledge of the body as a whole and the terms that concern each body system. However, since the change that indicates a malignancy begins at the cellular level, the instructor should review the cellular components and discuss the changes that occur in a cancerous cell.

Much statistical data is collected on the mortality and morbidity rates of various cancers. The use of such reports can be of great value when teaching this specialty. Current information can be found on the Internet. An assignment of a written report on a given type of cancer is an excellent way for the student to learn to recognize the suitable terms.

Since treatments for cancer are often new and complex, the terms involved may even be unfamiliar to the instructor. If this portion of the course is going to be comprehensive, be prepared. Read up on the most current treatments available.

Even though the therapies may change, the word roots contained within the names will be the same basic terms they have come to learn. Many surgeries and treatments are acronyms or eponyms; explaining the etymology of the name will help the student. Understanding the basis for a term enables the student to have a different viewpoint from which to grasp the concept.

Many treatments include chemotherapy and nuclear medicine components. Relating these to the specialty will give the student another view of the complexity of the science behind the medicine.

Correct spelling cannot be emphasized enough. If the student is going to use his/her newly gained knowledge in the form of diagnosis or procedure coding, the ability to spell accurately will facilitate the location of the proper code.

GROUP ACTIVITIES

Due to the complexity of the science of oncology, it is one of the most difficult sections to teach. The evolving nature of the treatments available makes it even harder. As with all group activities, insist that the students use the correct medical terminology and avoid the use of layman's terms. Verbal discussion, along with written reports, provides the instructor with a way to evaluate the pronunciation and true understanding of the terms.

- Have the students research a particular type of cancer. They should prepare a written report including appropriate terminology.
- Students could investigate the various types of therapies and the availability of them in a given geographical area. Of particular interest would be a hospital dedicated to the study and treatment of cancers. These cancer centers are becoming more common and therefore are more accessible.
- Since pathology is integral to the diagnosis of neoplasms, have the student research the manner in which histological specimens are processed.

20

Teaching the Terminology of Radiology and Nuclear Medicine

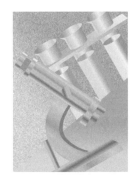

The instructor should differentiate between radiology and nuclear medicine. Radiology is the branch of medicine concerned with the study of anatomy and physiology, energy (x-rays, a magnetic field, sound waves), and radiation. It uses technology to create images of the internal structure of the body. Nuclear medicine is the medical specialty that uses radioactive substances to create images of internal structures of the body for the purpose of diagnosis.[1] When teaching this specialty, the instructor should start out with a discussion of the body as a whole and the difference between soft tissue, bones and how different modalities can create an image precise enough for the diagnosis of a disease process.

Imaging has come a long way from the simple bone x-ray developed by the Curies at the turn of the nineteenth century. Since then, science has discovered other "rays" and nuclear substances that can penetrate the body and give an image of soft tissue. The PET scan can go even further to produces images of the physiology and metabolism of an organ.

Since these techniques are based on science beyond simple anatomy and physiology, the terms used may not be derived from the basic word roots. Much of this science has been developed and named after researchers that were not necessarily from the field of medicine. Thus, many of the terms are acronyms of complicated expressions of nuclear science.

Having said that, the student should be able to break down and define a term by its roots, but with a twist. The anatomy (structure) of the body will be a standard term but the technological component may be unique to this science.

The easiest way to introduce and explain the process of radiology is to review the body planes, body regions and quadrants. Since most of the techniques used rely on the direction and angle of the penetrating ray, recognizing not only the anatomical part but its relationship to other surrounding structures is vital.

In addition to the various pieces of equipment involved, the techniques also utilize the infusion of many types of drugs or contrast materials. The students should be given a brief explanation of these substances and the response the body has to them.

[1]Definition from Susan Turley, *Medical Language*. Pearson/Prentice Hall, 2007.

Radiology reports can be long and complex. Using radiology reports to teach the terminology is very effective. The student not only learns the term, but discovers the connection between the anatomy and the technology.

GROUP ACTIVITIES

The complexity of this science creates its own set of difficulties for learning. The evolving nature of the techniques makes it imperative that the instructor be current in her/his knowledge of radiology and nuclear medicine.

- Have the students research the history of radiology. They should prepare a written report including appropriate terminology.
- Students may contact an imaging center and take a tour. Seeing the equipment helps to understand the terms used; the technician would be using the very terms the student is attempting to learn.
- Have the students make a poster listing various structures and which technique would be used to create an image most effectively.
- Students who have access to x-rays or other images could bring them into the class for viewing. Be sure, however, to obscure any manner of identification to prevent a breach of confidentiality.

21

Teaching the Terminology of Dentistry

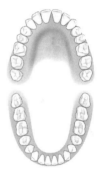

It is very rare to find a medical terminology textbook that includes a section on dentistry. The mouth and its components are most often covered in the gastroenterology/gastrointestinal section of most terminology texts.

Dentistry will include all components of the mouth and associated facial structures; following would be the different specialties associated with dentistry. Some students do not necessarily know the difference between general dentistry and endodontics. Some common specialties are pediodontics, endodontics, maxillofacial surgery, and orthodontics. It will help to break down the terms into word parts to teach the students the meaning behind the specialties. For example, endodontics: the suffix -ics means pertaining to; the prefix endo- means within, and the word root dont means tooth. So the meaning of endodontics is pertaining to within the tooth. You can then show the students how the meaning of the word connects to the specialty. Endodontics deals with the inside of the tooth (the root). You may ask your students what procedure(s) may be done by an endodontist.

A common problem when teaching the terminology of the mouth will be the surfaces of the teeth. There are many ways this can be approached, but with all of them it is vital to have some form of visual aid. The best will be a model of a tooth or mouth; diagrams will also be very valuable. As with all terminology, looking at the meaning will help the student to associate the term with its location, such as the buccal surface of the tooth. When the definition of buccal is established as pertaining to the cheek, it will help the student remember that the buccal surface of the tooth is the one next to the cheek. This process can be used with almost all of the surfaces. Once they have been instructed, repetition of the terms and their locations will help to solidify the material for the student.

Reading a dental report will assist the student with using the terms in context. It may be difficult to obtain these kinds of reports, but don't overlook their value.

GROUP ACTIVITIES

As with all group activities, insist that the students use the correct medical terminology and avoid the use of layman's terms. Verbal discussion, along with written reports, provides the instructor with a way to evaluate the pronunciation and true understanding of the terms.

Visuals are always one of the best ways to instruct. The mouth is one of the easiest parts of the body to visualize.

- Team students up to look at the structures of the mouth, and if students are comfortable, have them get up close with mirrors and look at the different shapes and name the tooth surfaces. Have students feel bones of the jaw and where they come together.

- Discussion of different dental maladies as a group can be fun for students and may help them to relate terms with the related problems. Most people have had some type of dental work done in their life, be it orthodonture or a root canal.

- If your students are going into the dental field, it may be helpful for them to spend some time in a dental office to hear the terms used in the actual setting. It will help to show the importance of using the correct terms.

- If the students are going to be billing for dental procedures, using the terms to find the appropriate billing codes can help them understand the material in context.

22

Teaching the Terminology of Dietetics

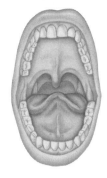

Dietetics is science of applying nutritional data to the regulation of the diet of healthy and sick individuals.[1] Dietetics and nutrition issues are usually covered under the body system of gastroenterology.

Reference materials can be found on the Internet, through various agencies that are dedicated to teaching good nutrition, and even through dentists. Instructors of basic medical terminology courses will probably not spend much time on this subject.

---

[1] *Taber's Cyclopedic Medical Dictionary*, 20th Edition. F.A. Davis, 2001.

23

Teaching the Terminology of Pharmacology

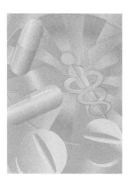

Pharmacology is the study of drugs, their origin, nature, properties and effects upon living organisms.[1] The terminology of this science is complicated and involves many chemical expressions that can be quite intimidating to students.

In most medical terminology courses, pharmacology is not a major section to be covered. In fact, some medical terminology textbooks do not devote a separate section to it. The instructor will need to do some research to be able to present the information in any detail. Due to the lack of special chapters, material will have to be presented from other reference material.

Pharmacological terms are primarily presented with each of the body systems. To have a specific segment of the course dedicated to the science may be redundant.

The primary research book for pharmacology should be the *Physician's Desk Reference.* Within its covers are the brand (trademarked) name, generic name and chemical name of all medications currently available.

Other forms of reference can be found on the Internet and pharmaceutical representatives.

In addition, methods of administration terms would be offered. The prefixes intra-, inter-, sub-, and trans- are common in relation to methods of administration of drugs. Terms that relate to the reaction of the body to a drug, such as idiosyncratic, adverse, and allergic should be emphasized.

In summary, the terminology of pharmacology may not be a major section of the course but should be referred to throughout the appropriate body systems.

---

[1]*Taber's Cyclopedic Medical Dictionary,* 20th Edition. F.A. Davis, 2001.

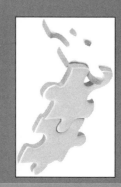

1

The Structure of Medical Language

Instructor Activity for the Beginning of Class

Dress in a surgical scrub suit or the top and pants used by medical assistants and dental assistants. Remind students that if they want to "walk the walk" of a career in health care, then they have to "talk the talk." In other words, they have to be serious about learning the medical language that they will need to use every day on the job. There is no other class in which they can do this, and now is the time to do it!

Classroom Activity for the Beginning of Class

While you are waiting for all students to arrive:

Pass around several copies of the "Deciphering Inscrutable Messages." Tell students to work in groups of two or three. This is a good icebreaker for students who don't know each other, and passes the time while waiting for all the students to arrive. Say: "Medical words are like puzzles that you will learn to decipher in this course. Sharpen your puzzle skills by seeing if you can figure out what this message says."

DECIPHERING
INSCRUTABLE MESSAGES

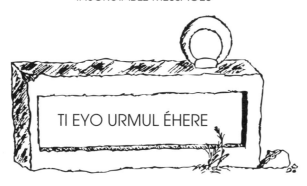

TI EYO URMUL ÉHERE

WHAT IS THE MESSAGE?

According to a letter in *Smithsonian* magazine, an expert in ancient languages was asked to examine this message found on a large stone that had an ancient metal ring embedded in it.

[The message says "Tie your mule here."]

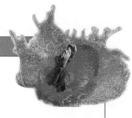

Instructor Activity for the Beginning of Class

The first day of a new class can be a time of anxiety for students, no matter what their age. Break the ice by telling students a little bit about yourself and your background in the healthcare field.

Then ask students to tell you a little bit about themselves. Ask them to take out a piece of paper and answer these questions as you dictate them one at a time.

1. What is your name? Your nickname?
2. Why are you taking this course?
3. What is one interesting fact about yourself? Hobbies? Job? Etc.?
4. Have you already purchased your textbook?
5. What is your greatest concern about this course?

Then have the students pass the papers in to you. As you look at each paper, call out the student's name and ask him/her to raise his/her hand so that you can put a face with the name and begin to memorize each student's name. Say: "I like to get to know my students and call them by name by the third week of class."

After reviewing all the papers, make a comment based on the collective answers to Question #2. For example, say: "Several of you are interested in careers in medical coding, others in nursing, and others as pharmacy technicians. We will be discussing various aspects of those healthcare fields throughout the course.

Also make a comment based on the collective answers to Question #5. Say something like, "I can see that some of you are concerned about not being able to remember everything or not being able to get a good grade. I will share memory aids with you and show you how to make the most of your study time. Some of you are concerned about being able to spell and pronounce medical words. We will have a lot of practice in those areas to help boost your confidence.

Finally, mention that not everyone has purchased the required course textbook yet and stress how important it is to get that right away so students can immediately do the Chapter 1 exercises.

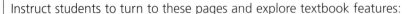

Classroom Activity for the Beginning of Class

Introduce students to the contents of the textbook and the chapter format. If this is not done on the first day of class and specifically emphasized, some students will never see or use all the features of the book.

Instruct students to turn to these pages and explore textbook features:

AT THE BEGINNING OF THE BOOK

p. iv	Textbook content at a glance, Chapters plus appendices
p. v	Comment by the author on the similarity of learning a foreign language and learning medical language
pp. vi–x	Features of the textbook, CD-ROM, and Companion Website
p. xxi	About the author and the illustrator
pp. xxiv–xxvi	Detailed Chapter Contents

AT THE END OF THE BOOK

p. A-1	Glossary of Medical Word Parts
p. A-17	Abbreviations Glossary
AK-1	Answer Key. Be sure students know that this is where they go to check their answers after completing the Chapter Review Exercises.
p. I-1	Index for looking up anything in the textbook.

CHAPTER FORMAT

Use Chapter 3 as an example.

pp. 86–87	Two-page chapter opener that introduces the body system and the medical specialty. Have students notice the photos and captions related to this chapter. Also point out the continuous timeline across the bottom of the two pages. Be sure to mention that the timeline is not specific to this chapter.
p. 88	Learning Objectives Remind students to review these from time to time as they study the chapter. Learning objectives are like landmarks on a road map; they help you stay on track and reach your destination.
pp. 89–98	Anatomy and physiology
pp. 99–102	Concise summary of anatomy and physiology for review and study purposes
pp. 103–104	Anatomy labeling exercises
pp. 105–106	Review of combining forms and practice building medical words
pp. 107–122	Diseases
pp. 123–126	Diagnostic procedures
pp. 127–132	Medical and surgical procedures
p. 133	Drug categories
p. 134	Abbreviations
p. 135	Career Focus. It's Greek to Me, which summarizes different combining forms that have the same meaning.
pp. 136–147	Chapter Review Exercises, including an actual medical report on p. 145. Mention that students are expected to complete these exercises and show the completed pages to the instructor at the beginning of class the following week.
pp. 148–150	Master pronunciation list for the chapter. Mention that students will be asked to pronounce 20 words as a test. All 20 words will be given to them ahead of time.
p. 151	Experience Multimedia. Checklist of CD-ROM learning activities for student to complete.

Classroom Activity for the Beginning of Class

Now let's lead by example. Say this to class: Let's begin our study of Chapter 1 the right way.

Turn with me to page 4 and let's read aloud together the learning objectives for this chapter.

Instructor Activity for the Beginning of Class

Say to students: "Medical words are like puzzles, and their word parts are like the pieces. If you put them together correctly, you can understand the meaning of the medical word. In this chapter, you'll explore medical language communication in all its forms. The pieces will all fall into place when you master this chapter.

Objective 1
Identify the five skills that make up medical language communication

- Text page(s) 5-6

Teaching Strategy

 Discuss the importance of proper communication of medical language.

Content Abstract

The five medical language skills are:

1. Reading
2. Listening
3. Thinking and analyzing
4. Speaking
5. Writing

Box 1-1: Classroom Activity
Have students repeat these five medical language skills out loud to reinforce their importance.

Box 1-2: Instructor Activity
MEDICAL LANGUAGE SKILLS Have students close their eyes while you read Scenario 1 on page 5. Then ask them to open their eyes and answer these questions: "What went wrong for the person in this scenario?" "How do you think this person feels about this outcome?" Have students close their eyes again while you read Scenario 2 on page 5. Then ask them these questions: "What was done differently that changed the outcome of this situation?" "How do you think this person feels about this outcome?" Stress this point: Medical language *is* a foreign language to you right now. Learning it will be like learning a foreign language. It will take time and patience, but there is no substitute for a thorough, working knowledge of medical language!

Objective 2
Describe three characteristics of each of these word parts: combining form, suffix, and prefix

- Text page(s) 7, 9, 15

Teaching Strategy

Explain to the students that each word part has a specific purpose. The combining form is the foundation of the word. It is usually based on a noun. The suffix is the word ending that further describes the combining form. The prefix is an optional word beginning that further describes the combining form.

Content Abstract

Characteristics of a combining form:

1. Every medical word contains a combining form.
2. A combining form is the foundation of a medical word and gives the word its medical meaning.
3. Sometimes a medical word contains two or more combining forms, one right after the other.
4. Prefixes and suffixes modify the meaning of the combining form.
5. A combining form is the first word part if there is no prefix. Otherwise, a combining form is positioned in the middle of a medical word between the prefix and the suffix.
6. A combining form contains two parts: a root and a combining vowel. The root is the part of the combining form that has medical meaning. The root is separated from the combining vowel by a forward slash. The combining vowel (usually an o, occasionally an i) is at the end of the combining form. (This item is not found in the textbook list. It relays information about Figure 1–3 on p. 7.)
7. A combining form always ends with a hyphen to show that it is a word part, not a complete word. The hyphen is deleted when the combining form joins with a suffix.

Box 1-3: Classroom Activity

WORD PARTS

Write different word parts (combining forms, prefixes, and suffixes) on the board and have students identify what each word part is. This will help students identify a combining form versus a prefix versus a suffix. Go around the room and have each student try to identify one of the word parts.

Box 1-4: Classroom Activity

WORD PARTS

Help students discover how much they already know about medical language word parts. Say these sentences and have students complete the blank. Write the medical word on the board as they give the answer.

If my tonsils are infected and red, I have _____.	[tonsillitis]
If my knee joints are stiff and hurt, I have _____.	[arthritis]
If I lose my voice, I have _____.	[laryngitis]
If my appendix is inflamed, I have _____.	[appendicitis]
Ask what is common to all these words.	[the suffix -itis]
Have students find the definition of -itis by looking in the Glossary of Medical Words Parts on page A-1.	[inflammation of]

Show how to begin with the meaning of the suffix and then go to the meaning of the first word part to define the meaning of a medical word.

Ask students to think of other -itis words.

[bronchitis, hepatitis, dermatitis, gastritis, colitis, encephalitis, tendonitis]

Then say these sentences and have students complete the blank. Write the medical word on the board as they give the answer.

If I have my appendix taken out, that is called an _____.	[appendectomy]
If a woman has her uterus taken out, that is a _____.	[hysterectomy]
If I have my tonsils taken out, that is a _____.	[tonsillectomy]
Ask what is common to all these words.	[the suffix -ectomy]
Have students find the definition of -ectomy in the Glossary of Medical Word Parts.	[surgical excision]

Again show how to begin with the meaning of the suffix and then go to the meaning of the first word part to define the meaning of a medical word.

Ask students to think of other -ectomy words.

[vasectomy, thyroidectomy, prostatectomy, salpingo-oophorectomy]

Box 1-5: Instructor Activity

COMBINING FORMS

Be sure to direct students' attention to the puzzle piece illustration of the parts of a combining form in Figure 1-3.

Characteristics of a suffix

- Every medical word contains a suffix.
- A suffix can be a single letter or a group of letters.
- A suffix cannot be the foundation of a medical word.
- A suffix is always positioned at the end of a medical word. Occasionally, a medical word contains two suffixes, one right after the other.
- A suffix attaches to the end of a combining form and modifies its meaning.
- A suffix always begins with a hyphen to show that it is a word part, not a complete word. The hyphen is deleted when the suffix joins the combining form.

Characteristics of a prefix

- Not every medical word contains a prefix. It is an optional word part.
- A prefix can be a single letter or a group of letters.
- A prefix cannot be the foundation of a medical word.
- When present, a prefix is always positioned at the beginning of a medical word. Occasionally, a medical word has two prefixes, one right after the other.
- A prefix attaches to the beginning of a combining form and modifies its meaning.
- A prefix always ends with a hyphen to show that it is a word part, not a complete word. The hyphen is deleted when the prefix joins the combining form.

Box 1-6: Instructor Activity

WORD PARTS

Mention that occasionally a student will encounter a word that seems to have no combining form. For example, "hypertrophy" seems to be composed of just the prefix "hyper-" and the suffix "-trophy." The textbook does list "-trophy" as a suffix. If you look closely, however, "-trophy" really contains the combining form "troph/o-" (development) plus the single-letter suffix "-y." The textbook does not list single-letter suffixes by themselves; they are united with the combining form to make a combination-type suffix.

Experience Multimedia

See the PowerPoint presentation on the accompanying Instructor's Media Library for a video on the topic of the elements of medical words.

Objective 3
Give the medical meaning of common combining forms, suffixes, and prefixes

- Text page(s) 8, 10–13, 16–19

Content Abstract

Combining Form	Medical Meaning
appendic/o-	appendix
arthr/o-	joint
cardi/o-	heart
cutane/o-	skin
esthes/o-	sensation, feeling
gastr/o-	stomach
hemat/o-	blood
hepat/o-	liver
laryng/o-	larynx (voice box)
mast/o-	breast; mastoid process
nas/o-	nose
nat/o-	birth
neur/o-	nerve
pneumon/o-	lung; air
psych/o-	mind
retin/o-	retina (of the eye)
tonsill/o-	tonsil
trache/o-	trachea (windpipe)
urin/o	urine; urinary system
ven/o	vein

Suffix	Medical Meaning
-ac	pertaining to
-al	pertaining to
-ar	pertaining to
-ary	pertaining to
-ation	a process; being or having
-ous	pertaining to
-tic	pertaining to
-ia	condition, state, thing
-ion	action; condition
-ism	process; disease from a specific cause
-itis	inflammation of
-megaly	enlargement

Suffix	Medical Meaning
-oma	tumor, mass
-osis	condition; abnormal condition; process
-pathy	disease, suffering
-ectomy	surgical excision
-graphy	process of recording
-scopy	process of using an instrument to examine
-iatry	medical treatment
-itian	a skilled professional or expert
-logy	the study of

Prefix	Medical Meaning
endo-	innermost, within
intra-	within
peri-	around
sub-	below; underneath; less than
an-	without, not
hyper-	above; more than normal
hypo-	below; deficient
poly-	many, much
brady-	slow
pre-	before, in front of
post-	after, behind
tachy-	fast
anti-	against
dys-	painful, difficult, abnormal

Box 1-7: Classroom Activity

PREFIXES

Have students think of English or common medical words that use some of the prefixes listed in the book.

Example: The prefix pre- is used in the English word predetermined.
Hyper- is used in the English word hyperactive.

[endogenous; interaction, interception, international, intersection; perimeter, periscope, subdivide, submarine, submissive, subterranean; anesthesia; hypodermic; polygraph, polyunsaturated; prelude, precursor, prenuptial; postgraduate, post-mark; antibiotic, antifreeze, antidepressant; dyslexia]

Objective 4
Demonstrate how to analyze and define word parts to build a medical word

- Text page(s) 7–19

Teaching Strategies

1. A combining vowel is attached to a root to comprise a combining form. The root cardi with the combining vowel o makes up the combining form cardi/o.
2. Review the rules for joining a combining form and a suffix to make a medical word and joining a prefix with a combining form and a suffix to make a medical word.

Content Abstract

Follow these three simple rules for joining a combining form and a suffix to make a medical word:

1. If the suffix begins with a vowel, delete the combining form's combining vowel before joining the two word parts.
2. If the suffix begins with a consonant, keep the combining form's combining vowel and join the two word parts.
3. If there are two combining forms, keep the combining vowel on the first combining form when joining it to the second combining form. Join the second combining form to the suffix as previously described.

Follow these two simple rules for joining a prefix to a combining form and suffix to make a medical word:

1. Follow all the rules for joining a combining form to a suffix, as previously stated.
2. Remove the hyphen from the prefix and join it to the beginning of the combining form.
   Note: Some medical words keep the hyphen if the last letter of the prefix is the same as the first letter of the combining form; other medical words do not.
   Example: intra- + abdominal = intra-abdominal
   Example: pre- + eclampsia = preeclampsia

Box 1-8: Classroom Activity

WORD PARTS

Buy or borrow a set of the mega-size Lego blocks that are suitable for toddlers. Tape various combining forms, suffixes, and prefixes from Chapter 1 on them. Give them out to students randomly and have them locate the students with other word part(s) that go with their Lego word part to form words mentioned in the chapter.

Then have students randomly put word parts together and see if they can come up with a definition to fit this imaginary medical word.

Example: tachy- + laryng/o- + -itis = inflammation of a fast voice box!

Objective 5
Demonstrate how to define and analyze medical words by dividing them into word parts

- Text page(s) 7–19

Content Abstract

Follow these three simple rules to define a medical word that contains a prefix, combining form, and a suffix:

1. Define each word part.
2. Put the definitions of the word parts in order, beginning with the suffix, followed by the prefix, and then the combining form.
3. Add small connecting words to make a correct and complete definition.

Medical Word	Word Type	Word Part	Word Part Meaning
laryngitis	suffix	-itis	inflammation of
	combining form	laryng/o-	larynx (voice box)

Medical Word Definition: inflammation of the larynx (voice box)

Medical Word	Word Type	Word Part	Word Part Meaning
cardiac	suffix	-ac	pertaining to
	combining form	cardi/o-	heart

Medical Word Definition: pertaining to the heart

Medical Word	Word Type	Word Part	Word Part Meaning
postnatal	suffix	-al	pertaining to
	prefix	post-	after, behind
	combining form	nat/o-	birth

Medical Word Definition: pertaining to after birth

WORD PARTS

1. Share this with students.

   Some medical words are very long. Why is that? Because the word is actually a short version of something much longer! Write "glomerulonephritis" on the board. Physicians will say the medical word glomerulonephritis so that they don't have to say "an inflammation of the microscopic filtration units of the kidney."

2. One of the longest medical words is otorhinolaryngologist at 21 letters! Write this word on the board. It might seem impossible to understand, but even the longest words follow the same rule for understanding the meaning of the word: Begin with the meaning of the suffix, then go to the meaning of the first word part, then the meanings of the other word parts.

   [Have students look up and call out the meaning of each word part after locating that word part in the Glossary of Medical Words Parts on page A-1 as you point to that word part.]

otorhinolaryngologist	-ist	[one who specializes in]
	ot/o-	[ear]
	rhin/o-	[nose]
	laryng/o-	[larynx (voice box)]
	log/o-	[the study of]

   So, beginning with the suffix, the meaning of this word is "one who specializes in the ear, nose, larynx study." In other words, an ENT specialist. If you can do that with the longest word, you can do it with every word.

WORD PARTS

Have students answer the question: Does medical terminology give you cephalgia?

Have them look in the Glossary of Medical Word Parts beginning on page A-1 to find the meaning of the medical word cephalalgia with the combining form cephal/o-, the combining form alg/o, and the suffix -ia.

Objective 6
Give six examples of common medical words derived from Latin, Greek, or other languages

- Text page(s) 20

Teaching Strategy

The majority of the word parts are derived from Greek and Latin. For this reason, learning medical terminology is like learning a new language.

Content Abstract

Etymology is the study of word origins and derivations. In medical language, many words have been taken from other languages.

Medical Word	Language of Origin	Definition
pelvis	Latin word *pelvis*	the hip bones
thorax	Greek word *thorax*	the chest and chest cavity
phobia	Greek word *phobos*	irrational fear
bladder	English word *blaedre*	hollow sac that holds urine
drug	Dutch word *droog*	medicine
physician	French word *physician*	doctor

Box 1-11: Instructor Activity

LATIN NAMES

Share this with students.

In the beginnings of modern science, much use was made of Latin and Greek to supply words for new discoveries. In biology, all students learn the Linnaean system that names each group of living things by its species and genus, etc. The names are nearly always in Latin. In astronomy, many stars are known by Latin names. In meteorology, some kinds of clouds are known by Latin names (cumulus). Law, too, is a subject whose vocabulary owes a great deal to Latin.

Source: "Study Advice Services," The University of Hull, www.studyadvice.hull.ac.uk

Just as we study our genealogy to learn about past generations, we can enrich our study of medical language by studying the etymology (or origin) of medical words. It is true that the meanings of some modern words bear little or no resemblance to the original meanings of their ancestors. This is in part because modern languages have evolved and borrowed from other languages . . . Still the study of etymology can pique our interest in the study of language, enrich our general knowledge, not only of language, but of ancient and modern cultures, and . . . help us remember and understand today's meanings and nuances of meaning.

Source: Drake, Ellen. "Using Storytelling to Teach and Learn Medical Terminology," *Perspectives on the Medical Transcription Profession,* Summer 2002, pp. 10.

Objective 7
Describe how to form the plural of common Latin and Greek singular nouns

- Text page(s) 21

Teaching Strategy

The best way to remember how to form plurals is to learn the rules, then remember one medical word that applies each rule. For example: For Latin feminine singular nouns, change -*a* to -*ae* (vertebra → vertebrae).

Content Abstract

Most English plurals are formed by adding -*s* or -*es* to a word. Follow the Latin and Greek rules that govern how plural nouns are formed.

Category	Singular Ending	How to Form the Plural	Example
Latin noun (feminine)	-*a*	change -*a* to -*ae*	vertebra → vertebrae
Latin noun (masculine)	-*us*	replace -*us* with -*i*	nucleus → nuclei
Latin noun (neuter)	-*um*	replace -*um* with -*a*	atrium → atria
Latin noun (other)	-*is*	replace -*is* with -*es*	testis → testes
	-*x*	replace -*ix* with -*ices*	helix → helices
		replace -*ex* with -*ices*	apex → apices
Greek noun	-*nx*	change -*nx* to -*nges*	phalanx → phalanges
	-*on*	replace -*on* with -*a*	ganglion → ganglia
	-*oma*	change -*oma* to -*omata*	carcinoma → carcinomata

Box 1-12: Classroom Activity

PLURAL WORDS

Divide the class into two groups. One student from Group A will come to the board and write a word in its singular form from the word list on page 21, then one student from Group B will write the word in its plural form on the board. Then the next student from Group B will write a singular word on the board and the next student from Group A will write its plural form, and so on.

Objective 8
Contrast the medical record with the health record, computerized patient record, and electronic patient record

- Text page(s) 22-24

Content Abstract

Medical Document	Definition
Medical record	Where healthcare professionals document all care provided to a patient, resident, or client in that healthcare setting.
Health record	Medical record that recently has become known as the health record; a reflection of the emphasis on preventive medicine.
Computerized patient record (CPR)	Record that provides immediate, simultaneous access by many healthcare providers to one patient's current and previous health records from the same healthcare facility.
Electronic patient record (EPR)	The most recent development in the overall plan to allow immediate, simultaneous, and seamless access to a patient's health records no matter where they were created or are currently located.

Types of Documents in the Health Record	Definition
Consent to treatment	Form that, when signed by the patient, gives physicians and other health-care providers the right to treat.
Informed consent	The physician describes the purpose of the proposed surgery, alternatives to the surgery, and explains the risks and possible complications of the surgery. When the patient signs, this shows consent to perform the surgery.
SOAP format	Uses the headings of subjective, objective, assessment, and plan. The subjective (S) category is for the patient's symptoms. The objective (O) category is for the results of the physical examination by the physician. The assessment (A) category is for the diagnosis. The plan (P) category is for the plan for follow-up care.

Experience Multimedia

See the PowerPoint presentation on the accompanying Instructor's Media Library for a video on the topic of taking patient histories.

Box 1-13: Instructor Activity

MEDICAL RECORDS

Share this information with students.

1. Call them electronic charts or electronic medical records: Whatever the name, the days of patients' medical conditions and diagnoses being written illegibly on paper and stored in manila folders are numbered. Medical records are going electronic. To help make that happen, the Institute of Electrical and Electronics Engineers (IEEE) has joined forces with the American Medical Association and eight other major nonprofit medical and engineering societies that represent over a million physicians, engineers, and computer professionals. The primary goal is nothing less than standardizing everything from medical terminology to networking protocols so that medical records can be stored electronically and sent instantly anywhere in the world—with absolute privacy, security, and understandability. Most doctors and hospitals rely on computers to bill for their services, but according to a U.S. study in early 2005, fewer than a third of hospitals and less than a fifth of private practice physicians use electronic medical records. One question to be addressed in the future is how medical records will be stored. Should all information be in a central database or could patients carry the records with them on an ID card (much like a driver's license) that could be scanned at every doctor's office?
    Source: The Institute (professional journal of IEEE), December 2005, Vol. 29, No. 4.

2. In 2004 in the State of the Union address, President George W. Bush called for the elimination of paper medical records within a decade. In January 2006, President Bush said he would ask for double the funding for this in the 2006 budget. Supporters say that electronic medical records could reduce medical costs as much as 20 percent. President Bush noted that electronic medical records can help change medicine, save money, and save lives.
    Source: The Washington Post, January 28, 2005.

3. Congress passed the Health Insurance Portability and Accountability Act (HIPAA) of 1996, which contained many provisions, to include:

    a. protection of health insurance coverage for workers when they change jobs
    b. national standards for electronic health care transactions
    c. national identifiers for providers, health plans, and employers
    d. security and privacy of health data
    e. widespread use of electronic data interchange in health care.

4. Medical Files Found in Landfill: Doctor's Old Records Meant for Destruction Turn Up in a Recycle Bin. Found recently amid the piles of old newspapers thrown into a paper recycling bin at. . .[the landfill] were slices of hundreds of lives— the discarded medical records of a cardiologist's former patients. An attorney for the physician said it was a mistake—a misunderstanding between the doctor and the person he hired to dispose of the records. But some former patients and their loved ones are upset about the potential invasion of privacy, and the state medical board is looking into the matter. The episode appears unusual, but raises the issue of what doctors do with old patient records and how they should or should not be discarded.
    Source: The Baltimore Sun Newspaper, November 29, 2000.

5. Susan Turley, the author, lives near a recycling plant and once when she was dropping off her paper to be recycled she saw a van pull up and dump cardboard boxes filled with medical records.

Box 1-14: Student Activity

MEDICAL RECORDS

Have students search the Internet for an article on the computerized patient record (CPR) or the electronic patient record (EPR). Discuss the latest developments in the movement toward the electronic medical record.

Box 1-15: Instructor Activity

MEDICAL RECORDS

1. Schedule a field trip to visit a hospital's health information management (medical record department) or a physician's office that is equipped with the technology of a computerized or electronic health record.

2. Have students look at the Abbreviations list at the end of Chapter 1. Point out the Word Alert box that explains how abbreviations can be misinterpreted and misunderstood. Point out that "CPR" has two meanings: "computerized patient record" and "cardiopulmonary resuscitation."

3. A Word Alert box appears with the abbreviation list at the end of each chapter in the textbook.

4. Share this information with students:

   Each hospital is required to have a comprehensive list of abbreviations that is acceptable to use in documents generated in that hospital. Each hospital decides what abbreviations are acceptable, and the abbreviations included on the list can vary from one hospital to the next.

   In 2004, the Joint Commission on Accreditation of Healthcare Organizations (JCAHO) created a "Do Not Use" list of abbreviations as part of their requirements for meeting the National Patient Safety Goal (NPSG). In 2005, JCAHO affirmed that same list. When JCAHO visits a hospital during the accreditation process, the JCAHO "Do Not Use" Abbreviation List is applied to all handwritten orders, handwritten medication-related documentation, and preprinted forms used by the hospital. Failure to substantially eliminate the use of these "Do Not Use" abbreviations accounts for 27%—the most frequent cause—of noncompliance found during a JCAHO accreditation survey.

   However, doctors and other healthcare professionals continue to use some of the abbreviations on the JCAHO "Do Not Use" Abbreviation List in their documentation in hospitals and other healthcare settings, and so students will see these "do not use" abbreviations used. In recognition of the danger associated with these abbreviations, the Word Alert box highlights these abbreviations, although the JCAHO rationale is not spelled out there. In addition, other confusing abbreviations not addressed by JCAHO are explained in each Word Alert box. As of May 2005, this is the official JCAHO "Do Not Use" Abbreviation List. This is actually a very short list, as seen on the following page.

   (continued)

The Structure of Medical Language | **17**

Box 1-15: Instructor Activity (*cont.*)

Official "Do Not Use" List[1]

Do Not Use	Potential Problem	Use Instead
U (unit)	Mistaken for "0" (zero), the number "4" (four) or "cc"	Write "unit"
IU (International Unit)	Mistaken for IV (intravenous) or the number 10 (ten)	Write "International Unit"
Q.D., QD, q.d., qd (daily)	Mistaken for each other	Write "daily"
Q.O.D., QOD, q.o.d, qod (every other day)	Period after the Q mistaken for "I" and the "O" mistaken for "I"	Write "every other day"
Trailing zero (X.0 mg)* Lack of leading zero (.X mg)	Decimal point is missed	Write X mg Write 0.X mg
MS	Can mean morphine sulfate or magnesium sulfate	Write "morphine sulfate" Write "magnesium sulfate"
MSO_4 and $MgSO_4$	Confused for one another	

[1]Applies to all orders and all medication-related documentation that is handwritten (including free-text computer entry) or on pre-printed forms.
***Exception:** A "trailing zero" may be used only where required to demonstrate the level of precision of the value being reported, such as for laboratory results, imaging studios that report size of lesions, or catheter/tube sizes. It may not be used in medication orders or other medication-related documentation.

In the future, JCAHO has said it might seek formal endorsement of the "Do Not Use" Abbreviation List from a variety of membership organizations for health-care professionals. In addition, JCAHO may possibly require these additional abbreviations be added to the "Do Not Use" list, as seen below.

Additional Abbreviations, Acronyms and Symbols
(For *possible* future inclusion in the Official "Do Not Use" List)

Do Not Use	Potential Problem	Use Instead
> (greater than)	Misinterpreted as the number	Write "greater than"
< (less than)	"7" (seven) or the letter "L"	Write "less than"
	Confused for one another	
Abbreviations for drug names	Misinterpreted due to similar abbreviations for multiple drugs	Write drug names in full
Apothecary units	Unfamiliar to many practitioners Confused with metric units	Use metric units
@	Mistaken for the number "2" (two)	Write "at"
cc	Mistaken for U (units) when poorly written	Write "ml" or "milliliters"
µg	Mistaken for mg (milligrams) resulting in one thousand-fold overdose	Write "mcg" or "micrograms"

In addition, the Institute for Safe Medication Practices (ISMP) has a list of "Do Not Use" drug name abbreviations and some symbols not included in the JCAHO "Do Not Use" Abbreviation List. The ISMP list is only a recommendation, however, and is not required for accreditation.

Objective 9
Correctly spell and pronounce medical words presented in this chapter

- Text page(s) 30

Teaching Strategies

1. Impress upon the students that medical words that are mispronounced are also probably going to be misspelled.
2. Encourage students to work on both pronunciation and spelling when studying.
3. Some medical words have more than one correct way to pronounce them. For example:

duodenum (DOO-oh-DEE-num) or (doo-AWD-ah-num)
cerebral (SER-eh-bral) or (seh-REE-bral)

Content Abstract

The "see and say" pronunciation guides are straightforward and easy to use. The syllables are separated by hyphens. Just say each syllable by following the phonetic spelling. Accented syllables are in all capital letters; secondary accented syllables are in smaller capital letters.

Medical Term	Pronunciation
appendectomy	(AP-pen-DEK-toh-mee)
cardiology	(KAR-dee-AWL-oh-jee)
gastritis	(gas-TRY-tis)
hepatomegaly	(HEP-ah-toh-MEG-ah-lee)
mastectomy	(mas-TEK-toh-mee)
neurology	(nyoo-RAWL-oh-jee)

Box 1-16: Classroom Activity

PRONUNCIATION

Use the comprehensive "see and say" pronunciation guides at the end of the chapter. Say the word and then have students repeat the correct pronunciation back to you.

Write a few of the pronunciation guides on the board and see if students can determine—without looking in the book—what the actual medical word is that goes with that pronunciation.

INTERESTING FACTS

Share this information with students.

1. The first horse-drawn ambulance service was established by Dr. Edward Dalton at Bellevue Hospital in New York City. The first motorized ambulance service was begun in Ohio.
2. In 1968, AT&T announced a new national emergency telephone number: 911.
3. In 1969, the first Shock Trauma Unit was established at the University of Maryland Hospital.

Objective 10
Test your knowledge of medical word structure by completing review exercises in the textbook and the CD-ROM learning activities

- Text page(s) 26-29, 31

At the end of class, give students this checklist to help them organize their course-related activities.

1. Purchase the textbook, if you have not already done so.
2. Read and study chapter 1.
3. Complete the Chapter Review Exercises by writing in the text. Be prepared to show your instructor these pages during the next class.
4. Check your answers in the Answer Key at the end of the book.
5. Make flashcards of all the word parts and their meanings and memorize them.
6. Call in the 20 pronunciation words to your instructor's answering machine.
7. Study for a chapter quiz, including spelling and abbreviations.

Experience Multimedia

See the PowerPoint presentation on the accompanying Instructor's Media Library for a video on the topic of a career as a paramedic.

Homework Activities

1. Make flashcards for all of the prefixes, suffixes, and combining forms given in the chapter. Using index cards allows you to carry them around to use to study. Flashcards can also be printed off the CD-ROM. Be sure to put the meaning of the word part on the reverse side of the card.

2. Look at the meanings and see if you can remember what the word part is that goes with that meaning.

3. Review the material provided in this chapter by completing the Chapter Review exercises. Refer to the Answer Key provided at the end of the book to check your answers.

4. Refer to the Experience Multimedia CD-ROM Learning Activities Checklist for a list of activities to complete on the interactive CD-ROM.

5. During class, the instructor will pick 20 words from the Pronunciation Checklist that you need to be able to pronounce correctly. Call your intructor's office phone number and leave a message on the answering machine, giving the correct pronunciations of those words.

6. Get extra credit by identifying five medical words in the chapter where the combining vowel (o) is dropped and three medical words where the combining vowel is retained when it is combined with a suffix.

7. Get extra credit by using a medical dictionary to write the definition of each of these words. Then write what it is that each of the words in this group has in common.

   Erythrocyte, cirrhosis, jaundice, chlorophyll, cyanosis, melanoma

   Adapted from Drake, Ellen. "Using Storytelling to Teach and Learn Medical Terminology," *Perspectives on the Medical Transcription Profession,* pp. 10–13.

8. Get extra credit by looking up 10 medical words in your medical dictionary and determining whether the origin of the word is Greek, Latin, or another language. Write the word, its origin, and its definition.

9. Get extra credit by completing the Word Search reproduced as handouts from the Instructor's Manual.

Word Search

Complete this word search puzzle that contains Chapter 1 words. Look for the following words as given in the list below. The number in parentheses indicates how many times the word is found in the puzzle.

communication   medical (2)
CPR   origin
EPR   patient
etymology (2)   prefix
Greek   record (2)
HIPAA   SOAP
language   suffix
Latin (3)   treatment
listen (2)   word (2)

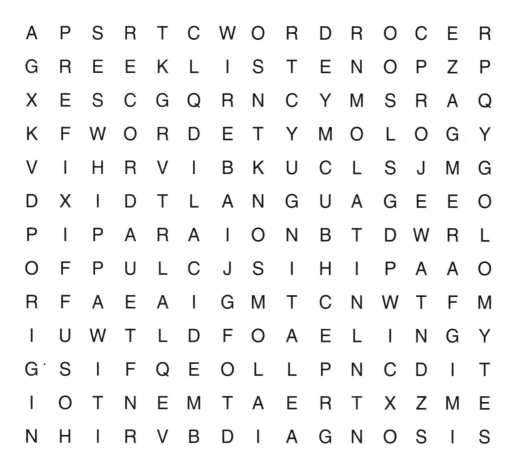

```
A  P  S  R  T  C  W  O  R  D  R  O  C  E  R
G  R  E  E  K  L  I  S  T  E  N  O  P  Z  P
X  E  S  C  G  Q  R  N  C  Y  M  S  R  A  Q
K  F  W  O  R  D  E  T  Y  M  O  L  O  G  Y
V  I  H  R  V  I  B  K  U  C  L  S  J  M  G
D  X  I  D  T  L  A  N  G  U  A  G  E  E  O
P  I  P  A  R  A  I  O  N  B  T  D  W  R  L
O  F  P  U  L  C  J  S  I  H  I  P  A  A  O
R  F  A  E  A  I  G  M  T  C  N  W  T  F  M
I  U  W  T  L  D  F  O  A  E  L  I  N  G  Y
G  S  I  F  Q  E  O  L  L  P  N  C  D  I  T
I  O  T  N  E  M  T  A  E  R  T  X  Z  M  E
N  H  I  R  V  B  D  I  A  G  N  O  S  I  S
```

The Structure of Medical Language | **23**

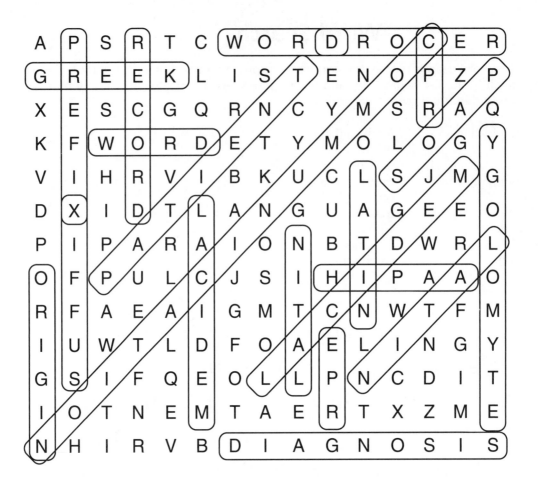

CHAPTER 2

The Body in Health and Disease

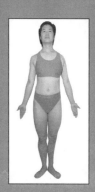

Instructor Activity for the Beginning of Class

[Equipment: Knife, cutting board, paper towel, two oranges, plastic bag (for disposing of the orange and its juices).]

Hold up a whole orange. Say, "If I wanted to study the structure of this orange, I would first examine the outside. But that wouldn't begin to reveal all the complexities of its structure, so then I would cut it in half to see what's inside." [Cut one orange in half from the stem end to the flower blossom end. Ask the students:] "With the orange cut like this, what might you conclude about the structure of an orange, if you had never seen one before?" [Wait for student answer: That it was composed of only two sections, one on each half of the orange.] "If you thought the orange only had two sections, that would not be accurate." [Now cut the other orange in half through the middle. Show the differences side by side of the two cut surfaces.] "Now you have a much more complete picture of the structure of the orange." [You might want to add: "That smells good! This course has a little bit of everything—even aromatherapy!"]

"An orange is a relatively simple structure and yet you can see how cutting it along two different planes reveals details of its structure that you couldn't see before. The human body is infinitely more complex. In order to study it, physicians had to devise ways to cut it along different planes to reveal its structure. Seeing the structure both macroscopically and microscopically sheds light on its physiology (function). That's what we are going to study today: how the human body can be divided for study in health and disease.

Classroom Activity for the Beginning of Class

REINFORCEMENT OF WEEK 1

Dictate a short quiz (no more than 5 to 10 questions) based on your course syllabus and the special features of the textbook that you discussed in Week 1. This should be an open-book, non-graded test in which the students can look in the textbook and at the course syllabus for answers. Many instructors say they have found this type of quiz to be very helpful in getting students on track from the very beginning of the course. Giving a quiz on this material shows the emphasis that you as a teacher place on the information in the syllabus and on being thoroughly acquainted with the course textbook.

Ask questions like these:

1. What is the e-mail address of the instructor?
2. What is the name of your textbook?
3. How many chapters are in your textbook?
4. On what page does the index begin?
5. If you wanted to look up the complete list of all the word parts presented in the textbook, what page would you go to?
6. Have you tried any of the activities on the CD-ROM yet?

Instructor Activity for the Beginning of Class

Share this information with students.

The first human dissection was performed about 2,500 years ago in Greece.

In this chapter you'll explore body positions, cavities, systems, and medical specialties. Then you'll be in a *position* to master the language of the body as a whole.

Objective 1
Describe seven approaches used to organize information about the human body

- Text page(s) 35–51

Teaching Strategy

Explain the importance of understanding the various approaches as they relate to the body as a whole. These approaches and their associated words are commonly used by healthcare professionals.

Content Abstract

There are many different approaches to studying the body. These include the

1. Body planes and body directions approach
2. Body cavities approach
3. Quadrants and regions approach
4. Anatomy and physiology approach
5. Microscopic-to-macroscopic approach
6. Body systems approach
7. Medical specialties approach

Box 2-1: Classroom Activity

ANATOMICAL POSITION

Ask all students to stand up, and then say: "Attention! Assume the position—the *anatomical position!* Stand up straight! Arms at your sides and palms forward. Look straight ahead. Now you are in anatomical position, the standard position that anatomists and physicians refer to when studing the human body. You can sit back down now."

Experience Multimedia

See the PowerPoint presentation on the accompanying Instructor's Media Library for an animation on the topic of body systems.

Objective 2
Identify body directions, body cavities, body systems, and medical specialties by correctly labeling them on anatomical illustrations

- Text page(s) 35–51

Teaching Strategy

Using a diagram or a skeleton model, show the location of the body cavities.

Content Abstract

Three planes of the body

Name of Plane	Synonym (also called)	Direction of Plane	Divides the Body into
Coronal	frontal	vertical	front and back sections (anterior and posterior sections) (ventral and dorsal sections)
Midsagittal	midline	vertical	right and left sides
Transverse	horizontal	horizontal	top and bottom sections (superior and inferior sections) (upper and lower halves)

Ten body directions

Prone	With the anterior section of the body down
Supine	With the posterior section of the body down
Medial	From the side of the body toward the midline
Lateral	From the midline toward the side of the body
Cephalad	Toward the head (superiorly)
Caudad	Toward the tailbone or the feet (inferiorly)
Superficial	On the surface of the body (external)
Deep	Below the surface and inside the body (internal)
Distal	From the body toward the end of a limb
Proximal	From the end of a limb toward where it is attached to the body

Note that *distal* and *proximal* are reserved for describing movement from one end of a limb to the other, *not* for describing movement on the torso of the body.

Five body cavities

Cranial	Cavity protected by the skull and containing the brain and cranial nerves
Spinal	Cavity protected by the vertebrae and containing the spinal cord and spinal nerves
Thoracic	Cavity protected by the breastbone (anteriorly), the ribs (laterally), and the spinal column (posteriorly), and containing the lungs, heart, trachea, and esophagus
Abdominal	Cavity within the abdomen and containing internal organs, collectively known as the viscera
Pelvic	A continuation of the abdominal cavity and containing viscera

Four abdominopelvic quadrants

RUQ	Right upper quadrant
LUQ	Left upper quadrant
LLQ	Left lower quadrant
RLQ	Right lower quadrant

Nine abdominopelvic regions

Right hypochondriac region
Epigastric region
Left hypochondriac region
Right lumbar region
Umbilical region
Left lumbar region
Right inguinal or iliac region
Hypogastric region
Left inguinal region

Anatomy—the study of the structures of the human body
Physiology—the study of the function and workings of those structures
Macroscopic—organs that can be seen with the naked eye
Microscopic—cells and cellular structures that can only be seen through a microscope

Fourteen body systems

Gastrointestinal system
Respiratory system
Cardiovascular system
Blood and lymphatic system
Integumentary system
Skeletal system
Muscular system
Nervous system
Urinary system
Male reproductive system
Female reproductive system
Endocrine system
Eyes
Ears, nose, and throat (ENT) system

Box 2-2: Instructor Activity

JCAHO

Share this information with students.

The Joint Commission for Accreditation of Hospitals (JCAHO) now requires doctors to sign their initials or write "yes" on the operative site after obtaining surgical consent from a patient before surgery. This requirement is in response to an alarming increase in operations on the wrong body part that confuse the right and left sides of the body and even on the wrong patient. Remember: When you face a patient, your right side corresponds to their left side.

Also, before the surgical procedure begins, the surgical team is required to take time to verify the identity of the patient and confirm the procedure to be performed.

Source: The Pittsburgh Post-Gazette, July 2004.

Box 2-3: Instructor Activity

RADIOGRAPHS

If possible, obtain one or more radiographs (x-rays), CT scans, or MRI scans to use as visual aids to demonstrate the application of one or all of these three planes of the body. These can be displayed for students to compare and contrast the differences of the images.

Examples	Demonstrates
PA chest x-ray	coronal (frontal) plane
Lateral chest x-ray	sagittal (lateral) plane
CT or MRI scan of abdomen	transverse (cross-sectional) plane

Share this information with students.

The radiology procedures of CT scans and MRI scans are able to "dissect" the body into slices of just 1/30 of an inch thick. CT stands for *computerized axial tomography*. *Tomography* means *the process of recording a cut, slice, or layer.*

Box 2-4: Classroom Activity

BODY PLANES

After discussing the three body planes, draw this table on the board. Fill in just one block to give students a clue.

Name of Plane	Also Called	Direction of Plane	Divides the Body into
1.			
2.	midline		
3.			

Then have one student at a time come to the board and fill in one of the blocks. Mention that the empty blocks can be filled in in any order and that this is an open book exercise.

[Answer Key]

Name of Plane	Also Called	Direction of Plane	Divides the Body into
1. Coronal	frontal	vertical	front and back sections (anterior and posterior sections) (ventral and dorsal sections)
2. Midsagittal	midline	vertical	right and left sides
3. Transverse	horizontal	horizontal	top and bottom sections (superior and inferior sections) (upper and lower halves)

Box 2-5: Classroom Activity

BODY DIRECTIONS

Have the students group together in pairs for this activity. Give each pair a card with one of the following statements written on it. On your signal, each pair works silently for just one minute to search pages 37–41 in Chapter 2 for the answer to their statement. Alternately, make this a "rapid response" exercise and only allow 30 seconds. Having a timer ticking away the seconds and buzzing loudly is a nice touch. When time is up, call on one pair at a time to present their statement and answer. Then one student in the pair reads the card aloud (this is also a pronunciation practice exercise) and the other student provides the correct answer. If the pair has not found the correct answer, the rest of the class can help.

1. Going in a cephalad direction from the lips brings you to the next facial feature of the _____. [nose]
2. Going inferiorly from the knee, the next joint you come to is the _____. [ankle]
3. The abdominal wall is located _____ to the intestines. [anterior or superficial]
4. If an x-ray passes through the back of the body to the front of the body, it is going in a _____ direction. [posteroanterior]
5. Sawing your body into top and bottom halves would correspond to dividing it with a _____ plane. [transverse]
6. Going from the elbow to the shoulder is moving in a _____ direction. [proximal]
7. Moving your arm out sideways from the side of your body is moving it in a _____ direction. [lateral]
8. Putting your leg in the air behind you like ice skater Michelle Kwan is moving it in a _____ and _____ direction. [posterior, superior]
9. Going from the elbow to the fingers is moving in a _____ direction. [distal]
10. Moving from inside your body toward your back is moving in a/an _____ direction. [dorsal or posterior or external]
11. Moving your arm forward and pointing to something in front of you means you moved your arm in a/an _____ direction. [anterior or ventral]
12. The intestines are located _____ to the abdominal wall. [posterior]
13. The lips are located _____ to the teeth. [anterior]
14. Swinging your arm backwards is moving it in a _____ direction. [posterior]
15. Raising your hand to answer a question is moving your hand and arm in a _____ direction. [superior]

Box 2-6: Instructor Activity

WORD ORIGINS

Share this information with students.

The meanings of words evolve over time. [Examples: caudad, hypochondriac.]

The word *caudad* originally meant *toward the tail*. In humans, who have no tail, it means *toward the tailbone.* The Greeks considered the two hypochondriac regions to be the seat of melancholy (sad feelings) because they contained the liver and spleen, which they thought released humors that caused different moods. Those regions kept that name even though we now know they do not cause moods. Later, the word *hypochondriac* evolved to mean a person who is depressed, worried, and talks excessively about imaginary illnesses.

Here are some examples of how well known English phrases came into being. In Old England, local folks started running out of places to bury people, so they would dig up coffins and take the bones to a "bone house" and then reuse the graves. When reopening these coffins, 1 out of 25 coffins were found to have scratch marks on the inside, and they realized they had been burying people alive. So they thought they would tie a string on the wrist of the body, lead it through the coffin and up through the ground and tie it to a bell! Someone would have to sit out in the graveyard all night ("the graveyard shift") to listen for the bell. Thus, someone who was buried but still alive could be "saved by the bell." If they were not alive, they were considered a "dead ringer."

Source: Urban Legends, www.snopes.com/language/phrases/1500.html

Box 2-7: Classroom Activity

QUADRANTS AND REGIONS

Have students draw two large outlines of a human body on a piece of paper. Have them draw and label the four abdominopelvic quadrants on one body and the nine abdominopelvic regions on the other body.

Memory aid: The *quad* in *quadrant* means *four.* There are four spaces to label for the abdominopelvic quadrants. Create the four spaces by drawing a large "plus sign (+)" over the abdomen from the rib cage to the groin. There are nine abdominopelvic regions. Create the nine regions by drawing a large tic-tac-toe board over the abdomen.

Box 2-8: Instructor Activity

DISSECTION OF THE HUMAN BODY

Share this information with students.

Dissection of the human body was performed regularly in the mid-1500s. Andreas Vesalius of Belgium dissected his first skeleton while in medical school by robbing the gallows after a public hanging. In 1543, he wrote and illustrated the first complete anatomy textbook.

In 1891, autopsies were performed routinely to discover the cause of death. Physicians gathered around the autopsy table were dressed in suits and bowties with just a covering apron. They wore no gloves and no masks to protect themselves from disease. Photographs often showed them smoking cigars. Why do you think they might be smoking? [To disguise the smell of the autopsy.]

Autopsies are still performed today, usually on patients who die unexpectedly or when the cause of death cannot be determined.

Box 2-9: Instructor Activity

DEATH SUMMARY

Share this information with students.

Once upon a time, there was an older physician who was thoughtful and thorough and who loved his vocation. Each patient to him was more than a set of organs or a disease. His patient was an elderly woman with the sad problems accompanying women of a certain age. I could tell the doctor respected his patient, Mrs. Dixon, and that he was determined to dictate for her the most complete and dignified death summary that he could. He carefully outlined the history of her last illness and he lingered more than usual on her social history. This was a woman of substance, a woman of means. She was a widow with several children, and I had the impression that she had led a full and contented life and was sensible to the end. Early on in the course of her hospitalization, she determined that she should have a "Do Not Resuscitate" status. She had one wish in life, one unfulfilled dream—to attend Harvard University. So she decided to will her body to science. And so the doctor finished her death summary by dictating, "And Mrs. Dixon went to Harvard."

Source: Judith Marshall, "Mrs. Dixon Goes to Harvard," *Perspectives on the Medical Transcription Profession,* Spring/Summer 1991.

Box 2-10: Instructor Activity

INTERESTING FACTS

Share this information with students.

1. In 1859, Louis Pasteur suggested that microscopic organisms caused disease.
2. In 1609, Galileo invented the microscope that included a magnifying lens and a focusing mechanism.

Medical Specialties and Body Systems

Medical Specialty	Body System	Structures	Function
gastroenterology	gastrointestinal	mouth, teeth, tongue, salivary glands, pharynx, esophagus, stomach, small intestine, large intestine, liver, gallbladder, pancreas	digestion, absorption, and elimination
pulmonology	respiratory	nose, pharynx, larynx, trachea, bronchi, lungs, alveoli	inhalation of oxygen and exhalation of carbon dioxide
cardiology	cardiovascular	heart, arteries, veins, capillaries	circulation of blood
hematology	blood	blood cells, plasma	transportation of oxygen to body, carbon dioxide to lungs, and waste products to kidneys
immunology	lymphatic	lymphatic vessels, lymph nodes, lymph, spleen, thymus, white blood cells	recognition and destruction of disease-causing organisms and abnormal cells
dermatology	integumentary	skin, hair, nails, sweat glands, oil glands	perception of pain, touch; protection of internal organs; regulation of body temperature
orthopedics	skeletal	bones, cartilage, ligaments, joints	maintenance of body support
orthopedics	muscular	muscles, tendons	production of body motion
neurology	nervous	brain, cranial nerves, spinal cord, spinal nerves, neurons	perception of pain, touch, temperature, body positions, taste, visual, smell, and auditory stimuli; coordination of movement; maintenance of memory and emotion
urology	urinary	kidneys, ureters, bladder, urethra, nephrons. In the male: urethra, penis	excretion of urine and waste products from body
male reproductive medicine	male reproductive	scrotum, testes, epididymides, vas deferens, seminal vesicles, prostate gland, urethra, penis	production of sperm and sex hormones, delivery of sperm to the female
gynecology and obstetrics	female genital and reproductive	breasts, ovaries, fallopian tubes, uterus, vagina, external genitalia	production of eggs and sex hormones; regulation of menstruation; pregnancy; and milk production after childbirth
endocrinology	endocrine	testes, ovaries, pancreas, adrenal glands, thymus, thyroid gland, parathyroid glands, pineal gland, pituitary gland	production and release of hormones; direction of activities of other organs
ophthalmology	eyes	eyes	perception of visual stimuli
otolaryngology	ears, nose, and throat	ears, nose, sinuses, throat, pharynx, larynx	perception of smell and auditory stimuli; production of speech

Other medical specialties

Psychiatry	study and treatment of the mind
Oncology	study and treatment of cancer
Radiology and nuclear medicine	use of x-rays, sound waves, and other forms of radiation and energy to diagnose and treat disease
Dentistry	study and treatment of the teeth and gums
Dietetics	study and use of nutrition, nutrients, and diet
Pharmacology	study and use of drugs as medicines
Neonatology	study and treatment of newborn infants
Pediatrics	study and treatment of infants and children
Geriatrics	study and treatment of the elderly

Box 2-11: Classroom Activities

MEDICAL SPECIALTIES

1. Name a body system and then have students identify a disease that affects that body system.
2. Have students think of the names of as many medical specialists as they can: urologist, pediatrician, etc. Write these in a list on the board.
3. Have students discuss what type of specialist a patient would see for various medical conditions, such as:

   a. pregnancy (gynecologist or obstetrician?)
   b. normal newborn (pediatrician or neonatologist?)
   c. colon cancer (oncologist or gastroenterologist?)

Objective 3
Define ten categories of diseases

- Text page(s) 62-63

Box 2-12: Instructor Activity

INTERNET SEARCH

Share this information with students.

If you type in the word *health* on the Google search engine, you will get references to more than 4,380,000,000 Web sites.

Content Abstract

Disease Type	Etiology
Congenital	Caused by an abnormality as the fetus develops or one that occurs during the birth process
Degenerative	Caused by the progressive destruction of cells due to disease or the aging process
Environmental	Caused by exposure to external substances
Hereditary	Caused by an inherited or spontaneous mutation in the genetic material of a cell
Iatrogenic	Caused by medicine or treatment given to a patient
Idiopathic	Having no identifiable cause
Infectious	Caused by a pathogen (disease-causing microorganism)
Nutritional	Caused by a lack of nutritious food, insufficient amounts of food, or an inability to utilize nutrients in the food
Neoplastic	Caused by the growth of benign or malignant tumors
Nosocomial	Caused by exposure to infection while the patient is in the hospital

Box 2-13: Instructor Activity

INTERESTING FACTS

Share this information with students.

> Physicians of the Utmost Fame
> Were called at once; but when they came
> They answered, as they took their Fees
> "There is no cure for this Disease."
>
> Hiliare Belloc (1870–1953)

According to a report issued by the Institute of Medicine, between 44,000 and 98,000 people die each year because of complications from hospital-caused infections, medical errors, or improper care.

Box 2-14: Classroom Activity

DISEASE CATEGORIES

Have students look at each one of the 10 disease categories and discuss/suggest ways to prevent each type of disease.

Objective 4
Describe four techniques used to perform a physical examination

- Text page(s) 64

Teaching Strategy

Explain the importance of the physical examination. The History and Physical Examination must be present on the medical record of all hospital patients prior to inpatient surgery.

Content Abstract

The physician uses the following techniques (as needed) during the physical examination:

1. Inspection   Using the eyes to examine the external surfaces of the body
2. Palpation   Using the fingers to push or press on a body part to feel masses and enlarged organs or detect tenderness
3. Auscultation Using a stethoscope to listen to sounds of the heart, lungs, or intestines
4. Percussion   Using the finger of one hand to tap on the finger of the other hand while the hand is spread over the thoracic or abdominal cavity

---

Box 2-15: Instructor Activity

INTERESTING FACTS

Share this information with students.

1. In 1714, the German physician Gabriel Fahrenheit invented the mercury thermometer. Today, digital thermometers are most commonly used in the physician's office and at home. Taking the temperature is part of every physical examination.
2. In 1816, Dr. Rene Laennec of France invented the first stethoscope. A stethoscope is used to do auscultation during the physical examination.

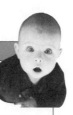

Did You Know?

About 70 percent of the useful diagnostic information utilized by a physician comes from the history and physical.

Experience Multimedia

See the PowerPoint presentation on the accompanying Instructor's Media Library for a video on the topic of physical examination techniques.

Objective 5
Describe three types of healthcare professionals

- Text page(s) 66-67

Content Abstract

Healthcare Professional	Definition
Physician or doctor	The leader of the healthcare team. He/she orders tests, diagnoses and treats diseases. Credentials include Doctor of Medicine (M.D.), Doctor of Osteopathy (D.O.), Doctor of Chiropractic (D.C.), Doctor of Optometry (O.D.), Doctor of Podiatric Medicine (D.P.M.), and Doctor of Dental Surgery (D.D.S.)
Surgeon	Physicians who completed additional training in surgery
Physician extenders	Perform some of the duties of a physician. Examples include Physicians' Assistant (PA), Nurse Practitioner (NP), Certified Nurse Midwive (CNM), and Certified Registered Nurse Anesthetist (CRNA)
Nurses	Examine patients, make nursing diagnoses, and administer treatments or drugs ordered by the physician. Examples are Registered Nurse (RN) and Licensed Practical Nurse (LPN)
Allied health professionals	Support the work of the physicians and nurses. Examples are technologists, technicians, therapists, and others

Box 2-16: Instructor Activity
BARBER'S POLE
Share this information with students.
The barber's pole dates back from the time when barbers were surgeons. It represents a red bandage wrapped around an injured arm.

HIPPOCRATES

Share this information with students.

In Greek medicine, the central historic figure is Hippocrates. He is known as the "Father of Medicine." He was born in 377 B.C. He provided an example of the ideal physician who focused on the physician's "duties" rather than his "rights." Centuries later, his greatest legacy lives on: the Hippocratic Oath which most physicians recite upon graduation from medical school. The traditional Hippocratic Oath contains references to swearing by the gods and goddesses and always honoring and caring for the physician who taught you the art of medicine, but it also contains the basic principles of integrity in treating the sick.

A modern version of the Hippocratic Oath was written in 1964 by Louis Lasagna, Academic Dean for the School of Medicine at Tufts University. In part, it reads:

> I swear to fulfill, to the best of my ability and judgment, this covenant. I will respect the hard-won scientific gains of those physicians in whose steps I walk and gladly share such knowledge as is mine with those who are to follow. I will remember that there is an art to medicine as well as science, and that warmth, sympathy, and understanding may outweigh the surgeon's knife or the chemist's drug. I will not be ashamed to say, "I know not," nor will I fail to call in my colleagues when the skills of another are needed for the patient's recovery. I will respect the privacy of my patients, for their problems are not disclosed to me that the world may know. Most especially must I tread with care in matters of life and death . . .

HEALTH PROFESSIONS

Invite a panel of guests to talk about their professions. The panel could include a physician's assistant, nurse practitioner, therapist, phlebotomist, etc. These practitioners could talk about what they do on the job. It would be interesting for the students to compare how their jobs are similar and different.

Objective 6
Describe seven settings where healthcare is provided

- Text page(s) 67–68

Teaching Strategy

Have students discuss what types of patients are seen in various healthcare settings.

Content Abstract

Healthcare Setting	Definition
Hospital	Provides healthcare services on an inpatient or outpatient basis
Physician's office	Most frequently used healthcare setting where patients are seen, diagnosed, treated, and counseled
Clinic	Provides healthcare services similar to that of a physician's office but for just one type of patient or one type of disease
Ambulatory surgery center	A facility where minor surgery is performed and the patient does not stay overnight (the patient is known as an outpatient)
Long-term care facility	Primarily a residential facility for elderly or disabled persons who are unable to care for themselves
Other healthcare settings	Examples include dialysis centers, physical therapy centers
Home health agency	Provides a range of healthcare services to persons in their homes
Hospice	A facility for patients who are dying (a physician has certified that the patient has less than six months to live)

Box 2-19: Instructor Activity
GUEST SPEAKER   Invite a guest speaker from a specific healthcare setting, such as a home health agency, hospice, a clinic, or a skilled nursing facility.

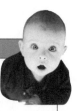

Did You Know?
Over 40 percent of all Americans will spend some time in a nursing home due to prolonged illness or a disability. The national average cost for nursing homes is approximately $105.00 per day. One year in a nursing home can cost $36,000 to $60,000.

Objective 7
Build medical words from combining forms, prefixes and suffixes

- Text page(s) 72–74

Teaching Strategy

Create a PowerPoint presentation with the combining forms, prefixes, and suffixes. The first slide would contain the combining form, prefix, or suffix. Then, the next slide would contain the meaning. This PowerPoint presentation could be utilized in class as a review prior to an exam.

Objective 8
Define common abbreviations for body systems, medical specialties, and healthcare professionals

- Text page(s) 74

Content Abstract

A&P	anatomy and physiology	Hx	history
AP	anteroposterior	LPN	licensed practical nurse
ASC	ambulatory surgery center	M.D.	Doctor of Medicine
CNM	certified nurse midwife	NP	nurse practitioner
CRNA	certified registered nurse anesthetist	OB	obstetrics
CV	cardiovascular	O.D.	Doctor of Optometry
D.C.	Doctor of Chiropractic	PA	physician's assistant
D.D.S.	Doctor of Dental Surgery	PA	posteroanterior
D.O.	Doctor of Osteopathy	PCP	primary care physician
D.P.M.	Doctor of Podiatric Medicine	PE	physical examination
Dr.	doctor	Pharm.D.	Doctor of Pharmacy
Dx	diagnosis	PT	physical therapy
ED	emergency department	RN	registered nurse
ENT	ears, nose, and throat	SNF	skilled nursing facility (pronounced "sniff")
GI	gastrointestinal		
GYN	gynecology	Sx	symptoms
H&P	history and physical examination	Tx	treatment

MEDICAL RECORDS

Obtain a copy of a complete medical record. Highlight all of the abbreviations used in the record and show students. Particularly note the abbreviation after the person's name who wrote (or dictated) and signed the report.

Did You Know?

The new designation for "Recovery Room" is "Postanesthesia Care Unit." This is abbreviated as PACU and pronounced as "PAK-yoo." The pediatric intensive care unit is abbreviated as PICU and pronounced as "PIK-yoo." The neonatal intensive care unit (as well as the neurologic intensive care unit) is abbreviated as NICU and pronounced as "NIK-yoo."

Objective 9
Correctly spell and pronounce medical words presented in this chapter

- Text page(s) 83–84

Teaching Strategies

1. Impress upon the students that medical words that are mispronounced are also probably going to be misspelled.
2. Encourage students to work on both pronunciation and spelling when studying.

Box 2-21: Classroom Activity

GROUP ACTIVITIES

1. Bring in a standard Scrabble game board set. The rules of the game are modified in that only medical words are allowed. Players may use a medical dictionary or the textbook to verify the correct spelling (but only half of the points are awarded). Option: Players can be required to define the words as they play them.

2. Using the comprehensive "see and say" pronunciation guide in the Pronunciation Checklist, say the word and then have the students as a group repeat the pronunciation back to you.

   Alternatively, say the pronunciation of one word and then have the students as a group say the pronunciation of the next word.

   Randomly pick and write a few of the "see and say" pronunciations on the board and see if students can determine—without looking in the book—what the actual medical word is that goes with that pronunciation—and then correctly spell it.

3. Show the Career Focus video clip about a health information manager. See the PowerPoint presentation on the accompanying Instructor's Media Library.

Objective 10
Test your knowledge of the body in health and disease by completing review exercises in the textbook and CD-ROM learning activities

- Text page(s) 76-82 (first complete all the in-chapter exercises on pages 57-61, 72 and 74)

Experience Multimedia
See PowerPoint presentation on the accompanying Instructor's Media Library for the videos on the topic of a career in health information management.

Homework Activities

1. Complete all of the exercises in the chapter, finishing with the Chapter Review exercises at the end of the chapter. Write in your textbook so that your instructor can verify that you did this work. See the Answer Key at the end of the book to check your answers.

2. Make flashcards for all of the prefixes, suffixes, and combining forms in the chapter. An index card makes a good homemade flashcard. One side of the flashcard should contain the word part and the other side should contain the meaning of the word part. Flashcards can also be printed from the CD-ROM. Flashcards can be carried everywhere and reviewed while waiting for a doctor's appointment, waiting for the bus, etc. Recruit family members, especially children, to help you study your flashcards.

   As an additional self-quiz, first look at the meaning of the word part and then remember what the word part is.

3. During class, your instructor assigned 20 words from the Pronunciation Checklist on pages 83-84. Practice the pronunciation of those words and then call your instructor's office or home phone number some time during the week and leave a message as you give your name and then pronounce each of the words.

4. Request a copy of your own medical record (from a hospital or doctor's office) and examine it to see how many abbreviations are used and what they mean.

5. Look in the newspaper and find an article that pertains to one of the types of healthcare facilities discussed in this chapter.

6. Complete the Word Search for Chapter 2.

7. Go to the Web site www.infoplease.com/pa/A0005110.html. See the list of the 10 leading causes of death in the United States. Copy this list and write after it the first names of anyone you know who has this disease. Then compare the 10 causes for men (in the middle of the chart) and the 10 causes for women (on the right side of the chart).

8. On the Internet, research one of the professions mentioned in the section Healthcare Professionals. For that profession, obtain the following information:
   1. Educational requirements/degree required
   2. Job opportunities available
   3. Salary ranges

9. Explore the Web site of the American Medical Association at www.ama.org. Learn more about physicians.

   Explore the Web site of the American Health Information Management Association at www.ahima.org. Learn more about health information management and coding professions.

   Explore the Web site of the American Association of Medical Transcription at www.aamt.org. Learn more about the medical transcription profession.

10. Visit an autopsy Web site at www.pathguy.com/autopsy.htm. This site is written by a pathologist and explains the steps involved in performing an autopsy. He explains that often the sign "This is the place where death rejoices to teach those who live" is hung where autopsies are performed because pathologists explore the anatomy of the body to seek to understand the cause of death and bring information and comfort to the family of the deceased.

11. Refer to the Experience Multimedia CD-ROM Learning Activities Checklist at the end of the chapter for a list of activities to complete on the interactive CD-ROM.

Word Search

Complete this word search puzzle that contains Chapter 2 words. Look for the following words as given in the list below. The number in parentheses indicates how many times the word appears in the puzzle.

acute
anatomy
anterior (2)
auscultation
body
caudad
cavity (2)
dorsal

etiology
health
hospice
hospitals
plane
prognosis
prone
sign

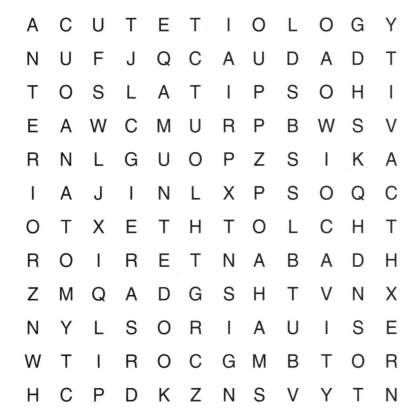

A C U T E T I O L O G Y
N U F J Q C A U D A D T
T O S L A T I P S O H I
E A W C M U R P B W S V
R N L G U O P Z S I K A
I A J I N L X P S O Q C
O T X E T H T O L C H T
R O I R E T N A B A D H
Z M Q A D G S H T V N X
N Y L S O R I A U I S E
W T I R O C G M B T O R
H C P D K Z N S V Y T N

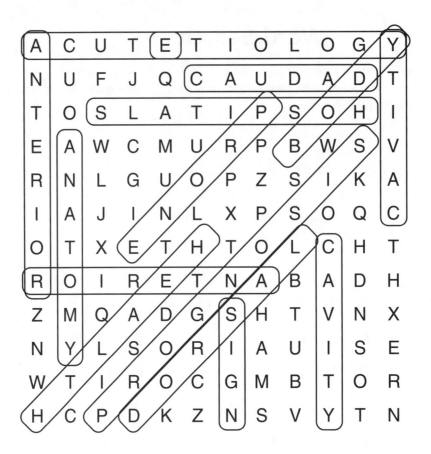

A	C	U	T	E	T	I	O	L	O	G	Y
N	U	F	J	Q	C	A	U	D	A	D	T
T	O	S	L	A	T	I	P	S	O	H	I
E	A	W	C	M	U	R	P	B	W	S	V
R	N	L	G	U	O	P	Z	S	I	K	A
I	A	J	I	N	L	X	P	S	O	Q	C
O	T	X	E	T	H	T	O	L	C	H	T
R	O	I	R	E	T	N	A	B	A	D	H
Z	M	Q	A	D	G	S	H	T	V	N	X
N	Y	L	S	O	R	I	A	U	I	S	E
W	T	I	R	O	C	G	M	B	T	O	R
H	C	P	D	K	Z	N	S	V	Y	T	N

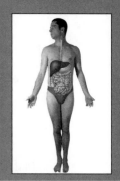

CHAPTER 3

Gastroenterology
Gastrointestinal System

Objective 1
Identify the anatomical structures of the gastrointestinal system by correctly labeling them on anatomical illustrations

- Text page(s) 89–96

Teaching Strategy

Explain the importance of learning the parts of the gastrointestinal system. Students should know the exact path that food takes, starting with the mouth and ending with the anus.

Content Abstract

Gastroenterology is the study of the stomach and the intestines. It is the healthcare specialty that studies the anatomy and physiology of the gastrointestinal system and uses diagnostic tests, medical and surgical procedures, and drugs to treat gastrointestinal diseases.

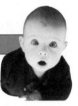

Did You Know?
Human intestines are 25 feet long, but horse intestines are 89 feet long.

 The anatomy of the gastrointestinal system includes:

1. mouth and throat
2. esophagus
3. stomach
4. small intestine
5. large intestine
6. abdomen and abdominopelvic cavity
7. liver
8. gallbladder
9. pancreas

Box 3-1: Instructor Activity

INTERESTING FACTS

1. Share this information with students.

   More than 500 strains of bacteria live in the human mouth.

   If the surfaces of all of the villi in the small intestine were flattened out, they would cover 5,400 square yards or about the area of a football field.

   Source: *The Human Body,* TimeLife Books.

   The Latin combining form *rect/o-* means *rectum,* but so does the Greek combining form *proct/o-*. The Greek form was used in the past (but seldom now) in such words as *proctitis* and *proctologist.*

   Up to 80 percent of the human liver can be removed without causing death. The remaining 20 percent will regenerate.

   Memory aids or "mnifty mnemonic devices" help you remember the order of the anatomical structures of the gastrointestinal system. These memory aids were created by students.

   To remember the parts of the colon (Ascending, transverse, descending, sigmoid) use this memory aid: All things down south.

   To remember the parts of the small intestine (duodenum; jejunum, ileum) Use any of these memory aids:

   > dogs eat junk and don't get ill
   > Dow Jones Industrial
   > Don't jump in

   To remember the parts of the large intestine (cecum, colon, rectum, anus) use any of these memory aids:

   > Cats eat canaries and run away
   > Call Cal Ripkin awesome
   > Credence Clearwater Revival Again

2. Share this with the class after you mention the "cardia" of the stomach.

   If you are over age 40, try to remember the first time someone talked to you about computers. You probably heard the words "mouse," "bites," and "windows." These words were familiar to you, but the meanings that you knew were incorrect in the context of computers. This is how it is with medical language. From your own living experience, you probably already have an idea as to the meanings of the words "gynecology" or "gastritis," but you may not know the correct or full meaning of these words.

Experience Multimedia

See the PowerPoint presentation on the accompanying Instructor's Media Library for animations showing the digestive system.

Objective 2
Describe the process of digestion

- Text page(s) 96–98

Teaching Strategies

1. Explain the importance of learning the parts of the digestive system and their functions in the process of digestion.
2. Explain the role of the pancreas, liver, and gallbladder during digestion.

Content Abstract

Digestion, which begins in the oral cavity, consists of two parts: mechanical and chemical. Mechanical digestion consists of

1. mastication—tearing, crushing, and grinding of food in the mouth
2. deglutition—swallowing
3. peristalsis in the esophagus, stomach, and intestines—mixing and moving of food

Chemical digestion consists of enzymes and acid that break down food into molecules of nutrients that can be absorbed and used by the body.

Absorption takes place in the ileum as food nutrients and water move through the intestinal wall into the blood. Absorption of water continues in the large intestine.

Elimination occurs when undigested food fibers and a small amount of remaining water are eliminated in the form of a solid waste known as feces or stool. Elimination is also known as bowel movement or defecation.

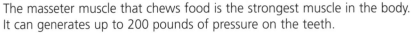

Did You Know?

The masseter muscle that chews food is the strongest muscle in the body. It can generates up to 200 pounds of pressure on the teeth.

Source: Fun Science Facts, www.hightechscience.org/funfacts.htm

The body produces about a quart of saliva each day and about 10,000 gallons over a lifetime.

Source: Fun Science Facts, www.hightechscience.org/funfacts.htm

Box 3-2: Instructor Activity

BEDSIDE COMMODE

If you are a particularly fearless instructor and your college has a medical assisting or nursing department, you might want to borrow a bedside commode—and deliver this part of your lecture while sitting on it (with the lid closed, of course!).

Box 3-3: Classroom Activity

DEMONSTRATIONS

1. Bring to class some Hunt Club or Ritz crackers, one for each student. Have students brush off the salt on the top of the cracker, place it in the mouth, and let it dissolve slowly. At some point, there will be a slight sweet taste. This occurs when the amylase in the saliva has broken down the starch (complex carbohydrate) in the cracker into simple sugar. As students swallow, have them place their hand on their anterior throat. Ask what is the structure that moves when they swallow. [larynx or voice box, also known as the Adam's apple] Tell students that the larynx must move upwards in order to close against the stationary epiglottis. The epiglottis acts as a lid to seal the opening of the larynx. Otherwise, the cracker they swallowed would have gone into the larynx and lungs instead of into the esophagus and stomach!

   When you think of the esophagus, think of a long snake that has swallowed food and you can actually see the bolus (bulge) of food slowly moving down the snake because of peristalsis.

   Source: Carol Rinzler, *Nutrition for Dummies.* Foster City, CA: IDA Books, 1997.

2. Bring something to class to demonstrate the total length of the small and large intestines: thin rope, string, beads, etc. Have the students stand around the room and each hold a segment of the total length.

3. To learn the process of digestion, give each student an individual sticky note that has an anatomical structure written on it. Have students arrange themselves in anatomical order to show the pathway that food takes from entering the body to being excreted.

Did You Know?

The popularized "taste map of the tongue" is incorrect. All regions of the tongue can detect different tastes such as bitter, sweet, salty, and sour. A newer taste known as unami is a savory taste such as in meat and soy sauce.

Objective 3
Build gastrointestinal words from combining forms, prefixes, and suffixes

- Text page(s) 105–106

Box 3-4: Classroom Activity

MEDICAL TERMINOLOGY BEE

Create a PowerPoint presentation with combining forms, prefixes, and suffixes with their meanings. Use this presentation in class. All students participate in a medical terminology bee. All students stand and take turns defining the combining form, prefix, or suffix displayed. If the student gets the answer right, the student remains standing and continues to play. If the student gets the answer wrong, the student will be seated and is out of the game. The last person standing is the winner. A prize could be given to the winner.

Objective 4
Describe common gastrointestinal diseases

- Text page(s) 107–122

Teaching Strategy

Invite a gastroenterologist or an internist to speak about the most common gastrointestinal diseases that young people (13-30 years old) are treated for.

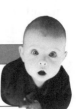

Did You Know?

Lactose intolerance is genetic and happens most often in people of African, Asian, and Mediterranean descent.

Content Abstract

Disease	Meaning
Anorexia	Decreased appetite
Dysphagia	Difficult or painful eating or swallowing
Cheilitis	Inflammation of the lips
Sialolithiasis	Stone in the salivary gland or duct
Stomatitis	Inflammation of the oral mucosa
Dyspepsia	Difficult or painful digestion
Varices	Varicose veins of the lower esophagus
Gastritis	Inflammation of the stomach
Gastroenteritis	Inflammation of the stomach and intestines
GERD	Chronic inflammation and irritation of the esophagus due to reflux of stomach acid back into the esophagus
Heartburn	Inflammation of the esophagus (see Box 3-6)
Hematemesis	Vomiting of blood
Hiatal hernia	Hernia of the esophagus or stomach through the diaphragm
Nausea and vomiting	Queasy feeling that progresses to throwing up
Peptic ulcer disease	Irritation, pain, and erosion of the stomach lining
Stomach cancer	Malignant tumor of the stomach
Ileus	Absense of peristalsis in the intestines
Intussusception	Telescoping of one segment of the intestine into another segment
Volvulus	Twisting of a loop of intestine around itself or another segment
Appendicitis	Inflammation and infection of the appendix
Colic	Crampy abdominal pain after eating
Colon cancer	Malignant tumor of the colon
Diverticulum	Pouch in the wall of the colon
Dysentery	Bacterial infection of the large intestine
Gluten enteropathy	Food allergy to the gluten in wheat
Inflammatory bowel syndrome	Diarrhea, bloody stools from unknown cause
Irritable bowel syndrome	Cramping, diarrhea, bloating
Polyps	Small, fleshy, benign, or precancerous growths in the colon
Hemorrhoids	Varicose veins of the rectum
Rectocele	Rectum pushes into the vaginal canal and blocks it
Constipation	Fewer than normal bowel movements
Diarrhea	Abnormally frequent and loose, watery stools
Fecalith	Hardened feces that becomes a stonelike mass

(continued)

Disease	Meaning
Flatulence	Excessive amounts of gas in the stomach or intestines
Hematochezia	Blood in the stool
Incontinence	Inability to voluntarily control bowel movements
Melena	Old blood in the stool from bleeding in the stomach
Steatorrhea	Fatty stools
Adhesions	Fibrous bands within the abdominal cavity
Hernia	Weakness in abdominal wall lets loops of bowel bulge out
Peritonitis	Infection in the peritoneum
Ascites	Excess fluid from liver disease accumulates in abdominal cavity
Cirrhosis	Inflammation and degeneration of the liver
Hepatitis	Infectious disease of the liver (see Box 3-7)
Hepatomegaly	Liver enlargement
Jaundice	Yellow skin color due to damaged liver
Liver cancer	Malignant tumor of the liver
Cholangitis	Inflammation of the bile ducts
Cholecystitis	Inflammation of the gallbladder
Cholelithiasis	Gallstones in the gallbladder
Pancreatic cancer	Malignant tumor in the pancreas
Pancreatitis	Inflammation of the pancreas

Box 3-5: Instructor Activity

REGURGITATION

From a novelty store, get a pile of rubber vomit. This can be brought out when the medical word "regurgitate" is discussed, but it can also be used to make the additional point that students should not just regurgitate facts back to the instructor. They should really seek to understand what they are learning!

Box 3-6: Instructor Activity

HEARTBURN

Share this information with students.

Chocolate, peppermint, coffee, carbonated beverages, alcoholic beverages, fatty foods and fried foods, citrus fruits and juices, pepper, vinegar, ketchup, and mustard are the foods most likely to cause heartburn.

Source: American Gastroenterological Association.

Box 3-7: Instructor and Classroom Activity

HEPATITIS

1. Share this information with students.

    Hepatitis C is the leading cause of liver failure and the major reason for liver transplants. About 25,000 Americans die each year while waiting for a liver transplant. This is partly due to the lack of available donor livers and to the fact that there is no way to mechanically sustain life as can be done with hemodialysis for a patient with kidney failure. One possible solution is surgery to split the liver of a living donor and give half to the patient in liver failure. This has been done successfully, and both the donated liver and the original liver continue to function while growing back to a normal size within the abdominal cavity.

    Source: ScienCentralNews at www.sciencentral.com, June 29, 2004.

2. When Susan Turley, the author, traveled to Vietnam to adopt her two daughters in 2001, she was warned about hepatitis. She and the other adoptive parents were told to drink bottled water or sodas from the can, never tap water or any drinks in a glass that contained ice cubes. When you brushed your teeth or rinsed out your toothbrush, you had to use bottled water. If you forgot and ran your toothbrush under tap water, you had to throw your toothbrush away!

3. Divide the class into five groups. Each group is assigned one type of hepatitis (Hepatitis A, B, C, D, or E). Have each group present the following information: symptoms of the disease, method of transmission, degree of damage, prognosis, and treatment. Write the information in a table drawn on the board. Along a vertical column on the left, list the five types of hepatitis. In a horizontal row across the top, the five headers given.

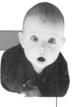

Did You Know?

The leading cause of acute liver failure in the United States is acetaminophen overdose. Acetaminophen has been sold as an over-the-counter drug since 1970. Its most popular brand name is Tylenol.

Box 3-8: Instructor Activity

SOUND-ALIKE WORDS

Dysphagia (difficult or painful eating) can be confused with dysphasia (difficult speech). Use this memory aid to help you remember the difference: dysphagia has to do with eating and it has the letters GI (gastrointestinal) in it.

Box 3-9: Instructor Activity

INTERESTING FACT

Some medical words have a musical quality that sounds something like the thing they represent (like the word "boom"). Pronounce these gastrointestinal disease words and write them on the board. Then give the meanings.

borborygmus	[BOHR-boh-RIG-mus]
singultus	[sing-GUL-tus]
intussuception	[IN-tus-suh-SEP-shun]

Adapted from Ellen Drake, "Using Storytelling to Teach and Learn Medical Terminology," *Perspectives on the Medical Transcription Profession,* Summer 2002, pp. 10–12.

Objective 5
Describe common gastrointestinal diagnostic laboratory and radiology tests

- Text page(s) 123–126

Did You Know?

The Heimlich maneuver was named after Dr. Harry J. Heimlich. He discovered that a simple series of movements can prevent choking to death in most cases. The movements involve placing arms around the patient's abdomen just below the diaphragm, grasping fists, and thrusting upward and inward to dislodge the item. Testimony from around the world affirms that this maneuver is put to good use every day.

Content Abstract

Test	Definition
Liver function test	Panel of individual blood tests; gives a comprehensive picture of liver function
Gastric analysis	Used to determine the amount of hydrochloric acid in the stomach
Barium enema	Dye is introduced in the rectum to take x-rays of colon and rectum
CT scan	X-rays (computed tomography) that create transverse images (thin successive slices of the abdomen)
Gallbladder ultrasound	Uses ultra high-frequency sound waves to create an image of the gallbladder
MRI	Magnetic resonance imaging that use a strong magnetic field to emit signals to form a series of images of the abdomen

Experience Multimedia

See the PowerPoint presentation on the accompanying Instructor's Media Library for animations and videos on the following topics covered in this chapter:

- MRIs
- Ultrasound

Objective 6
Describe common gastrointestinal medical and surgical procedures and drug categories

- Text page(s) 127–133

Teaching Strategy

Invite a gastroenterologist to speak about the newest technology in the GI field, specifically the capsule endoscopy.

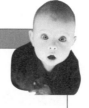

Did You Know?

Uvulectomy is a traditional surgery performed on infants and children throughout Africa and in some middle Eastern countries. It is done as a traditional treatment to prevent throat infections and normally is done early in infancy or the first or second year of life.

Content Abstract

Procedure	Definition
Appendectomy	Surgical procedure to remove the appendix
Biopsy	Surgical procedure to remove a small piece of tissue for examination to look for abnormal cells
Colostomy	Surgical procedure to remove the diseased part of the colon and create a new opening in the abdominal wall where feces can leave the body
Sigmoidoscopy	Visualization and examination of the rectum and sigmoid colon
Gastrectomy	Surgical procedure to remove part of the stomach
Herniorrhaphy	Surgical procedure that uses sutures to close a defect in a muscle wall where there is a hernia
Liver transplantation	Surgical procedure to remove a severely damaged liver from a patient with renal disease and insert a new liver from a donor

Drug Category	Description	Example
Antacid drugs	Treat heartburn and peptic ulcer disease	Maalox, Mylanta
Antibiotic drugs	Treat bacterial gastrointestinal infections	Ampicillin
Antiemetic drugs	Treat nausea, vomiting, and motion sickness	Antivert, Phenergan
Proton pump inhibitors	Treat peptic ulcers or GERD	Nexium, Prilosec

Box 3-10: Instructor Activity

MEDICAL HUMOR

Share with the students.

1. The amount of information in this chapter is substantial. I may not have succeeded in answering all your questions. Indeed, some of the answers only served to raise a whole new set of questions, some of which we didn't even know were questions! To sum it all up, in some ways you may feel confused, but you are now confused on a higher level and about more important things! (Adapted from a popular e-mail)
2. Ask students if they would like to have a sneak peek at one of the questions that will be on the test for this chapter. When they say "Yes," then say: There is only one question on the test. Here it is: "On your desk, you will find a scalpel and sutures. Remove your own appendix, and then close the incision. Your suturing technique will be checked for neatness."

Did You Know?

HEMORRHOIDS

The drug Preparation H for hemorrhoids contains shark's liver oil.

Experience Multimedia

See the PowerPoint presentation on the accompanying Instructor's Media Library for a video on the topic of sigmoidoscopy.

Objective 7
Define common gastrointestinal abbreviations

- Text page(s) 134

Teaching Strategy

Stress the importance of learning abbreviations and their full meanings.

Content Abstract

ABD	abdomen	**LLQ**	left lower quadrant
ALT	alanine aminotransferase	**LUQ**	left upper quadrant
AST	aspartate aminotransferase	**N&V**	nausea and vomiting
BE	barium enema	**NG**	nasogastric
BM	bowel movement	**NPO**	nothing by mouth (nil per os)
BRBPR	bright red blood per rectum	**(n.p.o.)**	
BS	bowel sounds	**OCG**	oral cholecystography
CBD	common bile duct	**O&P**	ova and parasites
EGD	esophagogastroduodenoscopy	**PEG**	percutaneous endoscopic gastrostomy
ERCP	endoscopic retrograde cholangiopancreatography	**PEJ**	percutaneous endoscopic jejunostomy
GERD	gastroesophageal reflux disease	**P.O.**	by mouth (per os)
GI	gastrointestinal	**(p.o.)**	
HAV	hepatitis A virus	**PTC**	percutaneous transhepatic cholangiography
HBV	hepatitis B virus	**PUD**	peptic ulcer disease
HCV	hepatitis C virus	**RLQ**	right lower quadrant
IBD	inflammatory bowel disease	**RUQ**	right upper quadrant
IBS	irritable bowel syndrome	**SGOT**	serum glutamic-oxaloacetic transaminase
IVC	intravenous cholangiography	**SGPT**	serum glutamic-pyruvic transaminase
LES	lower esophageal sphincter	**UGI**	upper gastrointestinal (series)
LFTs	liver function tests		

Box 3-11: Classroom Activity

ABBREVIATION GAME

Give students three minutes to study the abbreviation list. Then divide the class into two, three, or four teams and have them stand in separate lines. The instructor writes a common gastrointestinal abbreviation on the board. The first person on Team 1 must indicate what the abbreviation stands for. If correct, that person moves to the back of the team line. The first person on Team 2 will then define the next abbreviation written on the board by the instructor. If correct, that person moves to the end of the team line, and so on. If at any point a team member misses an abbreviation, that person is out of the game. The next team is given an opportunity to define the abbreviation. The winners are the team with the most players left at the end of the game.

Students not answering the question can continue to study the abbreviations list in the textbook until it is their turn.

Objective 8
Correctly spell and pronounce gastrointestinal words

- Text page(s) 148–150

<table>
<tr><td colspan="2">Chapter Spelling Test</td></tr>
<tr><td colspan="2">The chapter spelling test is included with the weekly chapter test. Dictate and spell (or Xerox a handout that contains) this list of 20 spelling words. For the chapter test, select just 10 of these words to test.</td></tr>
<tr><td>

1. anorexia
2. ascites
3. biliary
4. cholangiography
5. choledocholithiasis
6. cirrhosis
7. dysphagia
8. emesis
9. esophagus
10. hematochezia

</td><td>

11. hemorrhoidectomy
12. ileum
13. ileus
14. intussusception
15. jaundice
16. melena
17. pharynx
18. sialolithiasis
19. steatorrhea
20. umbilicus

</td></tr>
</table>

Teaching Strategies

1. Impress upon the students that medical words that are mispronounced are also probably going to be misspelled.
2. Encourage students to work on both pronunciation and spelling when studying.

Box 3-12: Classroom Activity

GAMES

1. From week to week, pick a different one of these spelling games to use during class. (The descriptions and instructions for the games are in the section "The Art and Craft of Teaching.")

   Beanbag Spelling Toss
   Scrabble
   Spelling Bee
   Gridlock
   Hangman

2. From week to week, pick a different one of these pronunciation games to use during class. (The descriptions and instructions for the games are in the section "The Art and Craft of Teaching.")

   Parroting
   Hieroglyphics
   Beach Ball Blast

Have students mark these 20 words listed in the Pronunciation Checklist for the chapter. During the week, they will call your office or home answering machine and pronounce each word.

1. anastomosis	11. gastroenterologist
2. ascites	12. hematochezia
3. bilirubin	13. hemorrhoidectomy
4. cholecystectomy	14. ileostomy
5. cholelithiasis	15. jaundice
6. colonoscope	16. jejunostomy
7. colonscopy	17. mesenteric
8. diverticulosis	18. pancreatitis
9. emesis	19. pharynx
10. exploratory laparotomy	20. steatorrhea

Objective 9
Apply your skills by analyzing a gastroenterology report

- Text page(s) 145-147

Box 3-13: Classroom Activity

In the medical report on page 145, circle all the medical words. Then list them and write their definitions. Rewrite the medical words in English as if you were explaining them to the patient.

Objective 10
Test your knowledge of gastroenterology by completing review exercises in the textbook and the CD-ROM learning activities

- Text page(s) 136-147 (first complete all the in-chapter exercises on pp. 103, 104, 105, and 106)

Teaching Strategies

1. Assign Chapter Review exercises in the textbook for homework. Refer to the Answer Key at the end of the book to check your answers.
2. Have the students complete the learning activities provided on the interactive CD-ROM.

Experience Multimedia
See the PowerPoint presentation on the accompanying Instructor's Media Library for a video on the topic of a career in medical assisting.

Homework Activities

1. Complete all of the exercises in the chapter, finishing with the chapter review exercises at the end of the chapter. Write in your textbook so that your instructor can verify that you did this work. See the Answer Key at the end of the book to check your answers.

2. Make flashcards for all of the prefixes, suffixes, and combining forms in the chapter. An index card makes a good homemade flashcard. One side of the flashcard should contain the word part and the other side should contain the meaning of the word part. Flashcards can also be printed from the CD-ROM. Flashcards can be carried everywhere and reviewed while waiting for a doctor's appointment, waiting for the bus, etc. Recruit family members, especially children, to help you study your flashcards.

   As an additional self-quiz, first look at the meaning of the word part and then remember what the word part is.

3. During class, your instructor assigned 20 words from the Pronunciation Checklist on pp. 148-150. Practice the pronunciation of those words and then call your instructor's office or home phone number some time during the week and leave a message, giving your name and then pronouncing each of the words.

4. Complete the Word Search for Chapter 3. (Your instructor will provide this as a handout.)

5. Refer to the Experience Multimedia CD-ROM Learning Activities Checklist for a list of activities to complete on the interactive CD-ROM.

6. Look up the definitions of these interesting-sounding words.

   borborygmi
   singultus
   intussuception

7. Use an English and a medical dictionary to answer a question about the etymology of this word.

   Why did appendicitis used to be called "typhilitis" in the 1800s?

8. Use water-soluble markers to draw the parts of the gastrointestinal system from the esophagus to the large intestine on a willing family member (spouse or child). Outline the edges of each organ or structure and then insert the first letter within it: Example: Draw a tubular shaped, vertical structure for the esophagus and write an "E" for "esophagus" in the center. That way, the sight of the "E" on the skin of the neck can be easily recalled and the word "esophagus" will come to mind. Take a photograph and show it to your instructor.

9. Look in your medicine cabinet at home and name all of the prescription and over-the-counter drugs that are used to treat symptoms of the GI tract. Be sure to spell the drug name correctly.

10. Write 10 sentences using 10 or more different abbreviations from the chapter.

11. Create a "mnifty mnemonic device" memory aid in the form of a rhyme, a word, or an abbreviation that helps you remember something about this body system.

12. Develop a crossword puzzle based on this chapter. Have some answers in the puzzle go from top to bottom (DOWN words) and others go from right to left (ACROSS WORDS). The words should intersect with each other at several points. Make one list of clues for DOWN words and another list of clues for ACROSS words.

13. Watch CSI, ER, or another medical show. Write down examples of three medical words (preferably from this chapter) and the sentences in which they were used in the show. Spell the words correctly and write their definitions.

14. Go to the American Gastroenterological Association Web site (www.gastro.org). Click on the public section, then click the digestive health resource center, and then choose a gastrointestinal disease site. Write a brief one-page summary of the information about that disease.

15. Keep a running list in your notebook of sound-alike words or combining forms that have the same meanings. Title this list of challenging words and word parts as "Perplexing Pairs." Begin by writing down the words or word parts found in the Word Alert boxes in this chapter. Then add the word parts found in the It's Greek to Me box at the end of this chapter.) Add any other words or word parts that you found particularly confusing. You will add to this list as you complete each chapter. Examples:

orth/o-	vs.	arthr/o-
myel/o-	vs.	my/o-
perine/o-	vs.	peritone/o-
cephal/o-	vs.	encephal/o-

Word Search

Complete this word search puzzle that contains Chapter 3 words. Look for the following words as given in the list below. The number in parentheses indicates how many times the word appears in the puzzle.

anal
bile (2)
cecum
digestion
duct
gastric
hemorrhoid
hernia
ileum

intestines
liver
oral
saliva
stomach
stool
uvula
vomit

```
D  B  F  M  U  C  E  C  I  H
D  I  G  E  S  T  I  O  N  Z
U  L  O  T  G  R  L  P  T  I
C  E  O  H  T  J  A  H  E  S
T  O  K  S  R  N  E  O  S  T
L  W  A  A  A  R  R  Q  T  O
I  G  V  L  N  A  O  K  I  M
V  C  B  I  L  E  U  M  N  A
E  L  A  V  O  M  I  T  E  C
R  X  J  A  L  U  V  U  S  H
```

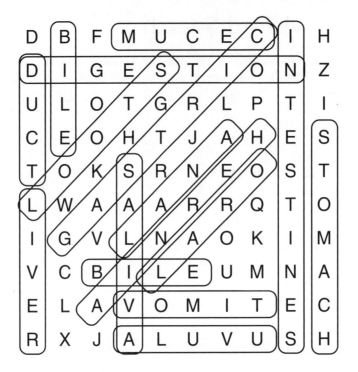

Pulmonology
Respiratory System

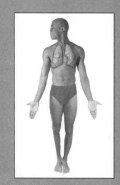

Blow up a large balloon but don't tie the end. Then let it go and let it fly all over the classroom to get everyone's attention. Then pose this question: How does air get into the lungs? Allow time for students to think and offer their suggestions. Some students quickly say that you breathe in. Then ask: "But what makes you breathe in?" Hint: Every motion begins with a muscle." Hint: What large muscle is involved in breathing? Some classes take quite a bit of time before they get the right answer. [The diaphragm contracts in response to nerve impulses sent from the respiratory center in the brain through the phrenic nerve.] A follow-up question might be: How do the lungs force the air out when you blow up a balloon? [The correct answer is that the muscles between the ribs contract, pulling the ribs together, decreasing the size of the rib cage. The muscular diaphragm also tenses. The size of the thoracic cavity quickly becomes smaller, forcing air out of the lungs and out of the body.] Give everyone in the class a balloon as a souvenir!

The average person breathes 300 million breaths in a lifetime. In the uterus, a fetus does not breathe. It takes its first breath at birth.

In this chapter you'll explore the respiratory system. You'll *breathe a sigh of relief* after you master the language of pulmonology!

Objective 1
Identify the anatomical structures of the respiratory system by correctly labeling them on anatomical illustrations

- Text page(s) 155–160

Teaching Strategy

Explain the importance of learning the parts of the respiratory system. Students should know the exact path that air takes as it moves into the lungs and from the lungs to the blood.

Content Abstract

Pulmonology is the study of the lungs. It is the healthcare specialty that studies the anatomy and physiology of the respiratory system and uses diagnostic tests, medical and surgical procedures, and drugs to treat respiratory diseases.

 The anatomy of the respiratory system includes:

1. nose and nasal cavity
2. pharynx
3. larynx
4. trachea
5. bronchi
6. lungs
7. thoracic cavity

Box 4-1: Instructor Activity
ALVEOLI Share this information with students. If all alveoli were laid out flat and stitched together like a patchwork quilt, they would be the size of a tennis court.

Box 4-2: Classroom Activity
THE ANATOMY OF THE RESPIRATORY SYSTEM To learn the anatomy of the respiratory system, give each student an individual sticky note that has an anatomical structure written on it. Have students arrange themselves in anatomical order to show the flow of air into the respiratory system.

Experience Multimedia
See the PowerPoint presentation on the accompanying Instructor's Media Library for an animation showing the respiratory system.

Objective 2
Describe the process of respiration

- Text page(s) 160–162

Teaching Strategy

Explain the importance of learning the process of respiration.

Content Abstract

The respiratory system serves the following basic functions:

1. It serves as a passageway for air to enter and leave the body.
2. It mechanically causes air to flow into the lungs.
3. It warms and moistens incoming air.
4. It traps and expels foreign particles, bacteria, and other pathogens in the incoming air.
5. It exchanges oxygen for carbon dioxide, which occurs in the lungs at the cellular level.

Respiration consists of breathing in and breathing out. Breathing in is called inhalation or inspiration. Breathing out is called exhalation or expiration. External respiration includes the physical process of inhalation and exhalation and what happens to the inhaled air. Internal respiration includes what happens to oxygen and carbon dioxide at the cellular level.

Box 4-3: Instructor Activity

BREATHING

Share this information with students.

The average person breathes over 23,000 times each day. Every minute, a person breathes in 13 pints of air. The average person will breathe approximately 75 million gallons of air in his or her lifetime.

Experience Multimedia

See the PowerPoint presentation on the accompanying Instructor's Media Library for videos on the following topics covered in this chapter:

- Vital signs
- Assessing respiratory rate

Objective 3
Build respiratory words from combining forms, prefixes, and suffixes

- Text page(s) 167–168

Objective 4
Describe common respiratory diseases

- Text page(s) 169–180

Content Abstract

Disease	Meaning
Asthma	Sudden onset of hyperreactivity of the bronchi and bronchioles with bronchospasm (see Box 4-5)
Bronchitis	Acute or chronic inflammation or infection of the bronchi
Bronchiectasis	Chronic enlargement and loss of elasticity of bronchioles
Abnormal breath sounds	Include pleural friction rub, rales, rhonchi, stridor, wheezes
Adult respiratory distress syndrome (ARDS)	Acute damage to the alveoli; they collapse with each breath
Atelectasis	Incomplete expansion or collapse of part or all of a lung due to tumor, mucus, or a foreign body that blocks the bronchus
Chronic obstructive pulmonary disease (COPD)	Chronic bronchitis plus emphysema (see Box 4-6)
Emphysema	Chronic, irreversibly damaged alveoli that create large air spaces in the lungs that trap air (see Box 4-7)
Cystic fibrosis (CF)	Genetic abnormality that produces excessive, constant coughing, thick mucus, and frequent bacterial infections
Influenza	Acute viral infection of the upper and lower respiratory tracts (see Box 4-8)
Empyema	Collection of pus in the thoracic cavity
Legionnaire's disease	Bacterial infection with severe pneumonia and liver and kidney failure
Lung cancer	Malignant tumor of the lungs (see Boxes 4-9 to 4-11)
Pneumonia	Inflammation or infection of some or all of the lobes of the lungs and the bronchi. Caused by bacteria, viruses, or other microorganisms.

Disease	Meaning
Pulmonary edema	Fluid in the lungs
Pulmonary embolism	Blockage of one of the pulmonary arteries to the lungs by an embolus (blood clot)
Severe acute respiratory syndrome (SARS)	Acute, severe viral infection of the lungs. It can be fatal.
Tuberculosis	Lung infection caused by the bacterium *Mycobacterium tuberculosis* and spread by airborne droplets, expelled by coughing (see Box 4-12)
Pleurisy	Inflammation of the pleura as a result of pneumonia or other infection, trauma, or tumor
Hemothorax	Blood in the thoracic cavity, usually from trauma
Pectus excavatum	Congenital deformity causing a hollow depression in the anterior chest wall
Pleural effusion	Fluid and inflammation in the pleural space
Pleurisy	Inflammation of the pleura. Also known as pleuritis.
Pneumothorax	Air in the pleural space that collapses the lung
Apnea	Absence of spontaneous respirations
Bradypnea	Abnormally slow rate of breathing
Dyspnea	Difficult, labored, or painful breathing
Orthopnea	Requiring a semi-upright position to breathe comfortably
Tachypnea	Abnormally fast rate of breathing
Anoxia	Lack of oxygen in the arterial blood and tissues
Sudden infant death syndrome (SIDS)	Unexpected death in an infant under 1 year old (see Boxes 4-13 and 4-14)
Cyanosis	Bluish discoloration of the skin due to low levels of oxygen
Hypercapnia	Abnormally high levels of carbon dioxide in the arterial blood
Hypoxemia	Abnormally low levels of oxygen in the arterial blood

Box 4-5: Instructor Activity

ASTHMA

Share this information with students.

Asthma Myths and Facts

1. *Children will outgrow asthma.* False. Asthma is a chronic condition. Some children experience fewer symptoms later in life; others experience more.
2. *Asthma is curable.* False. Asthma is a lifelong condition. There is no cure. However, with proper treatment, asthmatics can live a normal length and quality of life.
3. *Moving to the Southwest will help asthma.* False. Although symptoms may subside at first, new allergies to local plants soon develop.

Source: ScienCentralNews at www:sciencentral.com, January 16, 2005.

According to the National Center for Health Statistics, the incidence of asthma is rising, and asthma is the leading cause of school absenteeism.

Write this sequence on the board to show the relationship between these words:

    apnea ← bradypnea ← eupnea → tachpnea

Box 4-6: Instructor Activity

COPD

Share this information with students.

The author's (Susan Turley) father-in-law worked in coal mines his entire life. He had severe COPD with a barrel chest. If he ate a big meal, the pressure of his stomach contents would further compromise his lung capacity, and after dinner he would constantly cough and be so short of breath that he was unable to talk.

Box 4-7: Instructor Activity

EMPHYSEMA

Share this information with students.

1. Eight out of ten people with emphysema smoke.
2. If you put a lighted match several inches away from a person with severe emphysema, he or she will not be able to blow out the match because inhaled air is trapped in blebs in the lungs and cannot be completely exhaled. Light a single large kitchen match and hold it while you mention this fact.
3. Note the sound-alike words emphysema and empyema and their definitions.

Box 4-8: Instructor Activity

INFLUENZA

Share this information with students.

In 1918, influenza killed 15 million people around the world. A disease that affects many people is known as an epidemic. If an epidemic occurs over a wide geographic area it is called a pandemic. Today, scientists are concerned about the spread of bird flu, a form of influenza that originated in Asia. Although bird flu primary affects chickens and ducks, and millions of these have been destroyed, occasional cases in humans continue to occur. The possibility of the virus mutating into a form that is more easily contracted by humans could begin another pandemic that kills millions of people.

SMOKING

Share this information with students.

1. In the late 1800s, cigarettes were known as "coffin nails" and their health hazards were well known. In 1917, the sale of cigarettes was illegal in eight states; however, the onset of World War I caused an increase in sales as soldiers were allowed to smoke to calm and distract themselves.
2. In 1950, the first studies were published that linked smoking to cancer. In 1965, Congress required a warning label on cigarette packages to say that smoking was hazardous to your health.
3. The FDA removed nicotine lollipops and nicotine lip balm from the market in April 2002 because of the risk of their use by young people rather than just by adults who wanted to quit smoking.
4. In July 2002, the FDA denied a request from a California company to market NicoWater, a bottled water containing nicotine. Its advertising slogan was "a refreshing break to the smoking habit."

Source: Campaign for Tobacco-Free Kids.

5. In 1964, 44 percent of the people in the United States smoked.
6. According to the American Cancer Society, there are about 170,000 new cases of lung cancer each year. Smoking is the leading risk factor for lung cancer, causing about 8 out of every 10 cases.

Source: ScienCentralNews, www.sciencentral.com, August 18, 2004.

7. The cost of smoking to a 24-year-old woman who begins smoking and smokes throughout her life is $106,000 but the same for a 24-year-old male smoker is $220,000. These costs include the cost of the cigarettes, cost of medical and dental care, cost of medical insurance, loss of income due to smoking-related illnesses, and medical costs of family members due to second-hand smoke. That makes the cost of a single pack of cigarettes to actually be about $40.

Source: Frank Sloan, *The Price of Smoking.* MIT Press, 2004.

Box 4-10: Classroom Activity

SMOKING

1. Take a poll of the class (by secret ballot) asking how many of the students smoke, calculate the class percentage, and tell the class. Have students brainstorm as to why, with decreased advertising and more negative health information about smoking, smoking has increased.
2. Smoking history is given in a standard form as pack-years. This equals the number of packs smoked per day multiplied by the number of years smoking. Calculate the pack-years for a person who smoked 2 1/2 packs of cigarettes a day for 30 years.

Box 4-11: Instructor Activity

RADON GAS

Share this information with students.

Ten million homes in America contain dangerous levels of radon gas, an odorless, invisible gas. The Environmental Protection Agency (EPA) estimates that 21,000 Americans die of radon-induced lung cancer each year. This figure was revised upward by 150 percent from the EPA's estimate in 1994. Test kits for radon only cost $25, but many homebuyers forget to have the test done before they purchase a house. High levels of radon can be corrected by sealing cracks in the home's foundation where radon gas leaks in or by installing an exhaust system to pump out radon gas.

Source: The Baltimore Sun, August 22, 2004.

Box 4-12: Instructor Activity

TUBERCULOSIS

Share this information with students.

The old word for tuberculosis was "consumption" because of the way the disease chronically consumed body weight.

Box 4-13: Instructor Activity

PREMATURE BABIES

Share this information with students.

Each year, 60,000 babies in the United States are born so prematurely that they need assistance with breathing because their lungs do not have enough surfactant. Premature babies as young as 24 weeks' gestational age can survive, but must be treated with oxygen, mechanical ventilation, and surfactant. Even if they survive, they risk developing complications such as blindness, deafness, and cerebral palsy.

Source: The Baltimore Sun, July 7, 2005.

Box 4-14: Instructor Activity

SIDS

Share this information with students.

1. Sudden infant death syndrome affects about 2,200 infants between ages two and four months each year. The risk rises if the babies live with smokers.

   Source: The Baltimore Sun, August 2004.

2. The rate of SIDS (sudden infant death syndrome) has decreased by 40 percent due to the growing trend of placing infants on their backs while they sleep.

Box 4-15: Classroom Activity

RESPIRATORY DISEASES

Invite a guest speaker from the American Lung Society to speak to your class.

Box 4-16: Classroom Activity

MEDICAL WORDS CREATED FROM A PERSON'S NAME

Share this information with students.

1. Some medical words do not come from Greek or Latin combining forms, prefixes, or suffixes. Instead, they are derived from a person's name (often from the name of the physician who discovered the diagnosis or created a technique for a procedure). An example from this chapter includes Legionnaire's disease.
2. Ask students to think of other examples from any body system. (Down syndrome, Menière's disease, Alzheimer's disease, and Parkinson's disease).

Experience Multimedia

See the PowerPoint presentation on the accompanying Instructor's Media Library for animations and videos on the following topics covered in this chapter:

*   Pulmonary diseases
*   Asthma
*   Cystic fibrosis
*   Tuberculosis
*   Normal and abnormal breath sounds

Objective 5
Describe common respiratory diagnostic laboratory and radiology tests

*   Text page(s) 180-182

Content Abstract

Test	Definition
Pulmonary function test	Measures the capacity of the lungs and the volume of air that the lungs can move during inhalation and exhalation
Pulse oximetry	Measures the degree of oxygen saturation in the patient's blood and the heart rate from a device clipped on the fingertip
Sputum culture and sensitivity	Determines which bacterium is causing an infection and its sensitivity to particular antibiotics
Chest radiography	Radiography procedure that uses an x-ray beam to create an image of lung fields and thoracic cavity
CT scan and MRI scan	Radiology procedure that scans a narrow slice of tissue and creates an image

---

Box 4-17: Instructor Activity

TB TESTING

Have an employee of the local health department come to class to talk about the importance of a TB (tuberculosis) skin test.

Box 4-18: Instructor Activity

PULSE OXIMETRY

Invite a nurse to come to the class to demonstrate the use of a pulse oximetry.

Box 4-19: Instructor Activity

CHEST X-RAY

Share this information with students.

A chest x-ray is the most commonly performed diagnostic x-ray examination. Approximately half of all x-rays obtained in medical institutions are chest x-rays.

Box 4-20: Instructor Activity

CARBON DIOXIDE

Carbon dioxide is carried in three different forms in the blood:

1. On the hemoglobin molecule, which then becomes known as carbaminohemo-globin
2. In the form of bicarbonate ions in the blood
3. As carbon dioxide in the blood

Box 4-21: Instructor Activity

SPIROMETER

Purchase a plastic, disposable spirometer from a local medical supply store or over the Internet. Demonstrate in class how it is used.

Objective 6
Describe common respiratory medical and surgical procedures and drug categories

- Text page(s) 182–187

Content Abstract

Procedure	Definition
Auscultation	Medical procedure that uses a stethoscope to listen to the breath sounds in the various lobes of both lungs
Cardiopulmonary resuscitation (CPR)	Medical procedure to ventilate the lungs and artificially circulate the blood if the patient has stopped breathing and the heart has stopped (see Box 4-22)
Endotracheal intubation	Medical procedure that inserts an endotracheal tube between the vocal cords in the larynx and into the trachea in order to establish an airway for the patient to breathe through or to manually or mechanically ventilate the patient
Heimlich maneuver	Medical procedure to assist a choking victim with a complete obstruction somewhere between the pharynx and the lungs (see Boxes 4-23 and 4-24)
Bronchoscopy	Surgical procedure that uses a flexible, lighted bronchoscope that is inserted through the mouth and used to examine the trachea and bronchi
Lung resection	Surgical procedure that involves removal of part or all of a lung
Tracheostomy	Surgical procedure that makes an incision into the trachea and creation of a permanent opening
Incentive spirometry	Medical procedure to encourage patients to breathe deeply

Drug Category	Description	Example
Antibiotic drugs	Treat bacterial respiratory infections	Ampicillin
Bronchodilator drugs	Dilate constricted airways by relaxing the smooth muscles that surround the bronchioles and bronchi	Proventil, Serevent, Theophylline
Cortiocosteroid drugs	Block the immune system from causing inflammation	Azmacort, Flovent
Expectorant drugs	Reduce the thickness of sputum so that it can be coughed up	Guaifenesin

Box 4-22: Instructor Activity

VITAL SIGNS AND CPR

Share this information with students.

1. Think about the last time you went to the doctor's office. The medical assistant took your vital signs, which include your temperature, heart rate, respiratory rate, and blood pressure. You remember the thermometer in your mouth for your temperature, the medical assistant feeling the pulse in your wrist to take your heart rate, and the blood pressure cuff on your arm, but when did the medical assistant take your respiratory rate? [Answer: The medical assistant takes your respiratory rate after finishing your pulse rate but while still holding your wrist. That is to keep you from being self-conscious and altering the depth or rate of your respirations!]
2. In 1957, the ABC (airway, breathing, circulation) technique was developed that later gave rise to CPR (cardiopulmonary resuscitation).

Objective 7
Define common respiratory abbreviations

- Text page(s) 189

Teaching Strategies

1. Stress the importance of learning abbreviations and their full meanings.
2. Encourage students to make flashcards for abbreviations and their meanings as well as their usual flashcards for word parts and their meanings.

Content Abstract

ABG	arterial blood gases
AFB	acid-fast bacillus
A&P	auscultation and percussion
AP	anteroposterior (view on chest x-ray)
ARDS	adult respiratory distress syndrome; acute respiratory distress syndrome
bagged	manually ventilated with an Ambu bag (slang)
BS	breath sounds
C&S	culture and sensitivity
CF	cystic fibrosis
CO	carbon monoxide
CO$_2$	carbon dioxide
COPD	chronic obstructive pulmonary disease
CPAP	continuous positive airway pressure
CPR	cardiopulmonary resuscitation
CXR	chest x-ray
DOE	dyspnea on exertion
ETT	endotracheal tube
FEV$_1$	forced expiratory volume (in one second)
FiO$_2$	fraction (percentage) of inspired oxygen
FVC	forced vital capacity
HMD	hyaline membrane disease
LLL	left lower lobe (of the lung)
LUL	left upper lobe (of the lung)

MDI	metered-dose inhaler
O$_2$	oxygen
PA	posteroanterior (view on chest x-ray)
PCO$_2$	partial pressure of carbon dioxide (also pCO$_2$)
PCP	*Pneumocystis carinii* pneumonia
PFTs	pulmonary function tests
PND	paroxysmal noctural dyspnea
PO$_2$	partial pressure of oxygen (also pO$_2$)
PPD	protein purified derivative (TB test); packs per day (of cigarettes)
RA	room air (no supplemental oxygen)
RDS	respiratory distress syndrome
RLL	right lower lobe (of the lung)
RML	right middle lobe (of the lung)
RRT	registered respiratory therapist
RUL	right upper lobe (of the lung)
SARS	severe acute respiratory syndrome
SIDS	sudden infant death syndrome
SOB	shortness of breath
TB	tuberculosis
TPR	temperature, pulse, and respiration
trach	tracheostomy (slang)
URI	upper respiratory infection
V/Q	ventilation-perfusion (scan)

Box 4-27: Instructor Activity

SELMAN WAKSMAN

Share this information with students.

In 1944, the first drug was developed that was effective against tuberculosis. The microbiologist Selman Waksman (who discovered the antibiotic neomycin and the chemotherapy drug actinomycin D, and who coined the word *antibiotic*) was a professor at Rutgers University, where he studied soil bacteria. He was looking for a drug that would be effective against tuberculosis because the newly discovered wonder drug penicillin was not. He and his students examined 10,000 different soil samples looking for a substance that could kill tuberculosis bacteria. They examined a clump of dirt taken from the throat of a sick chicken. On it was growing the mold that would be found to kill tuberculosis. They called it streptomycin. Just before their discovery, however, a financial officer at Rutgers suggested Waksman be fired to cut down on expenses, stating that Wakman's work was obscure and his research would never repay the money invested in it. After the discovery of streptomycin, Waksman was offered $10 million. He gave it to Rutgers, which used it to build a new microbiology laboratory.

Source: Susan Turley, *Understanding Pharmacology for Health Professionals* (Prentice Hall).

Box 4-28: Classroom Activity

ABBREVIATIONS

Let the class have two minutes quickly to look over the list of chapter abbreviations and Word Alert box. Then they are to close their books. Divide the class into two, three, or four teams and have them stand in separate lines. Write a common pulmonary abbreviation on the board. The first student on Team 1 must give the meaning of the abbreviation. If the abbreviation also appears in the Word Alert box, the student must give all meanings of the abbreviation. If correct, that student moves to the back of the team line. Write another common pulmonary abbreviation on the board for the first student on Team 2. If correct, that student moves to the end of the team line. If at any point a student misses an abbreviation, that student is out of the game and must sit down. The student in the front of the line for the next team is given an opportunity to define the abbreviation. Continue writing abbreviations on the board until every student on every team has had at least one chance to play. The team with the most students left standing at the end of the game is the winner.

Objective 8
Correctly spell and pronounce respiratory words

- Text page(s) 201–202

Teaching Strategies

1. Impress upon the students that medical words that are mispronounced are also probably going to be misspelled.
2. Encourage students to work on both pronunciation and spelling when studying.

Chapter Spelling Test

The chapter spelling test is included with the weekly chapter test. Dictate and spell (or xerox a handout that contains) this list of 20 spelling words. Give the list to students the week before the test. For the chapter test, select just 10 of these words to test.

1. apnea
2. atelectasis
3. auscultation
4. bronchiectasis
5. bronchiole
6. cyanosis
7. diaphragm
8. dyspnea
9. emphysema
10. hemoptysis
11. laryngeal
12. larynx
13. mucosa
14. parenchyma
15. pleura
16. pneumonia
17. resuscitation
18. stethoscope
19. tachypneic
20. tracheostomy

Box 4-29: Classroom Activity

GAMES

1. From week to week, pick a different one of these spelling games to use during class. (The descriptions and instructions for the games are in the section "The Art and Craft of Teaching.")

   Beanbag Spelling Toss

   Scrabble

   Spelling Bee

   Gridlock

   Hangman

2. From week to week, pick a different one of these pronunciation games to use during class. (The descriptions and instructions for the games are in the section "The Art and Craft of Teaching.")

   Parroting

   Hieroglyphics

   Beach Ball Blast

Objective 9
Apply your skills by analyzing a pulmonology report

- Text page(s) 198–200

Content Abstract

Read the hospital Admission History and Physical Examination and Pathology Report and answer questions provided.

Box 4-30: Classroom Activity

MEDICAL REPORTS

Have students find and circle these words in the medical report: fatigue, appendectomy, bronchoscopy, biopsy, cyanosis, anteroposterior wheezes, rales, rhonchi, clubbing, pulse oximeter, sputum, C&S, apex, atelectasis, pneumonia, anthracosis. Have the students look in their book and write out a description or definition for each circled medical word. Then begin reading the report by having a student read the first header or sentence from the medical report on page 198. If one of the circled words occurs in that sentence, the student must also give their description or definition of that medical word. The next student reads the next header or sentence until the report is finished. This is to familiarize students with reading medical reports and analyzing words while also gaining practice in pronouncing words.

Objective 10
Test your knowledge of pulmonology by completing review exercises in the textbook and the CD-ROM learning activities

- Text page(s) 191-200 (first complete all the in-chapter exercises on pp. 166-168).

Teaching Strategies

1. Assign Chapter Review Exercises in the textbook for homework. Remind students to refer to the Answer Key at the end of the book to check their answers.
2. Refer to the CD-ROM Learning Activities in this section for multimedia learning experiences.

Experience Multimedia

See the PowerPoint presentation on the accompanying Instructor's Media Library for videos on the topic of careers in respiratory therapy.

Homework Activities

1. Complete all of the exercises in the chapter, finishing the Chapter Review Exercises at the end of the chapter. Write in your textbook so that your instructor can verify that you did this work. See the Answer Key at the end of the book to check your answers.

2. Make flashcards for all of the prefixes, suffixes, and combining forms in the chapter. An index card makes a good homemade flashcard. One side of the flashcard should contain the word part and the other side should contain the meaning of the word part. Flashcards can also be printed from the CD-ROM. Flashcards can be carried everywhere and reviewed while waiting for a doctor's appointment, waiting for the bus, etc. Recruit family members, especially children, to help you study your flashcards.

   As an additional self-quiz, first look at the meaning of the word part and then remember what the word part is.

3. During class, your instructor assigned 20 words from the Pronunciation Checklist on pp. 201–202. Practice the pronunciation of those words and then call your instructor's office or home phone number some time during the week and leave a message as you give your name and then pronounce each of the words.

4. Complete the Wordsearch for Chapter 4. (Reproduce this as a handout from the Instructor's Manual.)

5. Refer to the Experience Multimedia CD-ROM Learning Activities Checklist for a list of activities to complete on the interactive CD-ROM.

6. Create a "mnifty mnemonic device" memory aid in the form of a rhyme, a word, or an abbreviation that helps you remember something about this body system.

7. Develop a crossword puzzle based on this chapter. Have some answers in the puzzle go from top to bottom (DOWN words) and others go from right to left (ACROSS words). The words should intersect with each other at several points. Make one list of clues for DOWN words and another list of clues for ACROSS words.

8. Visit the Web site of the American Lung Association at www.lungusa.org. Explore their Web site and document at least three interesting facts, statistics, or personal stories about lungs and lung disease.

9. Visit the Web site of the Cystic Fibrosis Foundation at www.cff.org. Explore their Web site and document at least three interesting facts, statistics, or personal stories about cystic fibrosis.

10. Visit the Web site of the Philip Morris Company, found at www.philipmorris international.com. Why would a tobacco company want to stop youth from smoking? Explore their Web site.

11. Write a book report on the history of cigarettes and disease. One source you might want to consult would be Cassandra Tate, *Cigarette Wars: The Triumph of the Little White Slaver,* 2000.

12. Watch CSI, ER, or a medical documentary show. Write down examples of three medical words that you heard and the sentences in which they were used. Spell the words correctly. Write out the medical definition for each word.

13. Create an advertising campaign or brochure to decrease smoking.

14. Interview a smoker. Develop a list of questions to ask, such as: How long have you been smoking? Why do you smoke? Do you have any respiratory ailments? Could you quit smoking? Record the questions and the smoker's answers.

15. Visit a Web site that contains a dictionary of medical eponyms with a biography of the person. See www.whonamedit.com.

16. Listen to respiration sounds by going to the following Web site: www.rale.ca/Recordings.htm.

17. Write 10 sentences correctly using 10 or more different abbreviations from the chapter.

18. Visit a local pharmacy or drug store. Write down the names of all the over-the-counter drugs available to treat the common cold. Also make a list indicating the specific symptoms that the drug treats.

19. Use a PDR (*Physician's Desk Reference*) to look up some of the drugs used to treat respiratory diseases.

20. Explore the field of clinical respiratory therapy by visiting the Web site for the American Association for Respiratory Care at www.aarc.org or the Web site for the National Board of Respiratory Care at www.nbrc.org.

21. Keep a running list in your notebook of sound-alike words or combining forms that have the same meanings. Title this list of challenging words and word parts as "Perplexing Pairs." Begin by writing down the words or word parts found in the Word Alert boxes in this chapter. Then add the word parts found in the It's Greek to Me box at the end of this chapter. Add any other words or word parts that you found particularly confusing. You will add to this list as you complete each chapter. Examples:

orth/o-   vs.   arthr/o-
myel/o-   vs.   my/o-
perine/o-   vs.   peritone/o-
cephal/o-   vs.   encephal/o-

Word Search

Complete this word search puzzle that contains Chapter 4 words. Look for the following words as given in the list below.

apnea
asthma
breathe
bronchus
cilia
hilar
intubation
lumen
lungs
mucus

nasal
nose
oxygen
pharynx
pulmonary
ribs
SARS
thorax
URI

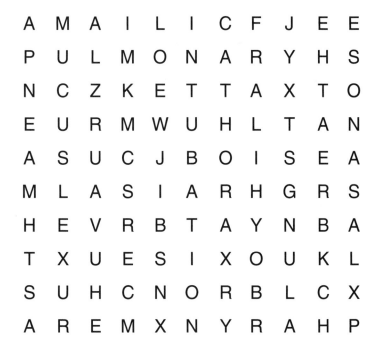

```
A  M  A  I  L  I  C  F  J  E  E
P  U  L  M  O  N  A  R  Y  H  S
N  C  Z  K  E  T  T  A  X  T  O
E  U  R  M  W  U  H  L  T  A  N
A  S  U  C  J  B  O  I  S  E  A
M  L  A  S  I  A  R  H  G  R  S
H  E  V  R  B  T  A  Y  N  B  A
T  X  U  E  S  I  X  O  U  K  L
S  U  H  C  N  O  R  B  L  C  X
A  R  E  M  X  N  Y  R  A  H  P
```

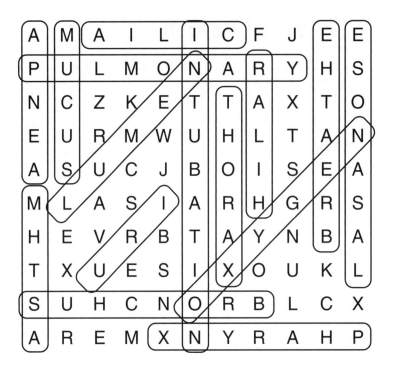

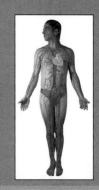

CHAPTER **5**

Cardiology
Cardiovascular System

Instructor Activity for the Beginning of Class

If you have been trained in how to correctly take a blood pressure, borrow a blood pressure cuff and stethoscope and demonstrate how to take a blood pressure. Bring alcohol swabs to wipe off the earpieces of the stethoscope and offer to let students hear the blood pressure sounds for themselves. Be sure to take the blood pressure only twice in the arm of each volunteer student. Taking the blood pressure repeatedly in the same arm gives an incorrect reading.

Mention that the blood pressure reading is written as the systolic reading over the diastolic reading. Explain that systole is the action of the heart contracting, and diastole is the time when the heart relaxes.

Classroom Activity for the Beginning of Class

Pass around the blood pressure cuff and have students examine the numbered gauge. Ask them to determine what unit of measurement is used to calibrate the gauge and measure blood pressure. After everyone has had a chance to examine the gauge, ask for the answer.

[Answer: mm Hg—millimeters of mercury. Hg is the chemical element name for mercury. Students may recall seeing a mercury blood pressure apparatus, but most offices and hospitals now use a circular (aneroid) gauge (*aneroid* means *without fluid*). The aneroid gauge contains a set of bellows, pins, and springs connected to each other and to the pointer on the face of the gauge.]

Instructor Activity for the Beginning of Class

Share this information with students.

Your heart will beat about 2.5 billion times in your life. Keep your *finger on the pulse* of medical language. You'll be *pumped up* once you master the language of cardiology.

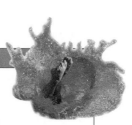

91

Objective 1

Identify the anatomical structures of the cardiovascular system by correctly labeling them on anatomical illustrations

- Text page(s) 206–214

Teaching Strategy

Explain the importance of learning the parts of the cardiovascular system.

Content Abstract

Cardiology is the study of the heart. It is the healthcare specialty that studies the anatomy and physiology of the cardiovascular system and uses diagnostic tests, medical and surgical procedures, and drugs to treat cardiovascular diseases.

The anatomy of the cardiovascular system includes the

1. Heart (heart chambers, heart valves, heart muscle)
2. Thoracic cavity and mediastinum
3. Blood vessels (arteries, capillaries, and veins)

Box 5-1: Classroom Activity
HEART
Bring a three-dimensional model of the heart to class and have the students identify the different parts.

Box 5-2: Instructor Activity
INTERESTING FACTS
Share this information with students.
1. The human heart beats 30 million times per year.
2. The heart of a whale weighs one ton. The heart of an elephant only beats 35 beats per minute. The heart of a mouse beats 700 beats per minute. The heart of a hummingbird beats 1,260 beats per minute (but slows down to 50 beats per minute at night).
3. The aorta is the largest artery in the body. It is more than one inch in diameter.
4. Remember that veins have one-way valves in them because both vein and valve begin with the letter v. Arteries do not contain valves.

Objective 2
Describe the process of circulation

- Text page(s) 215–218

Teaching Strategy

Explain the importance of learning the process of circulation.

Content Abstract

The blood circulates through two different pathways:

1. Systemic circulation — includes the arteries, capillaries, and veins everywhere in the body, except in the lungs.
2. Pulmonary circulation — includes the arteries, capillaries, and veins going to, within, and coming from the lungs.

The heartbeat occurs in two phases:

1. Systole — contraction of both atria followed by the simultaneous contraction of both ventricles.
2. Diastole — the resting period between contractions when the heart fills with blood.

Box 5-3: Instructor Activity

INTERESTING FACTS

Share this information with students.

1. In 1616, William Harvey, an English physician, described the circulation of the blood throughout the body.
2. There are approximately 60,000 miles of blood vessels in the human body. During the average lifetime, the heart beats 2.5 billion times. Each day, the heart pumps about 2,000 gallons of blood.

   Source: Discovery Health, www.discoveryhealth.com, September 2000.

3. When the body is resting, the heart pumps 5 to 6 quarts of blood each minute. Mild exercise increases this to 7 to 8 quarts of blood per minute. Strenuous exercise can increase this to almost 30 quarts of blood per minute.

   Source: The Human Body, TimeLife Books.

Box 5-4: Classroom Activity

PATH OF BLOOD CIRCULATION

To learn the anatomy of the heart and circulatory system, give each student an individual sticky note that has an anatomical structure written on it. Have students arrange themselves in a circle (to show the continuous path) and in anatomical order to show the path of blood circulation.

Box 5-5: Instructor Activity

PATH OF BLOOD CIRCULATION

Draw this simplified and clarified diagram on the board to help students remember the path of blood circulation around the body.

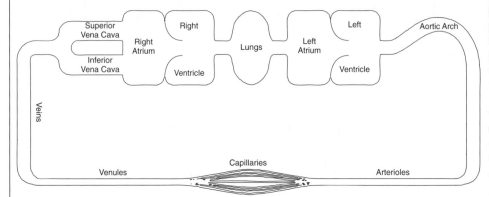

Tell students to think of the heart as a mechanical pump, an electrical pump, and a set of pipes.

Source: Stacey Long, Medical Terminology instructor.

Box 5-6: Classroom Activity

MYOCARDIUM

Remind students that the myocardium, like any other tissue in the body, needs oxygen in order to survive. Ask students where they think the myocardium gets its oxygen from. Ask if they think that the myocardium gets oxygen from the blood that passes through its chambers. [Answer: The myocardium cannot extract any oxygen from the blood that passes through its chambers. Its blood supply comes from the coronary arteries. These are the first to branch off the aorta as it leaves the heart. Blood flow through the coronary arteries is critical to the survival of the heart muscle cells. But these are very small arteries, whose lumen is about the size of the open end of a Bic "clicker" pen. Ask students to image how little plaque it would take to occlude such a small lumen. [If you have a Bic "clicker" pen, be sure to show it with the pen point retracted inside the pen to show the tiny hole.]

Experience Multimedia

See the PowerPoint presentation on the accompanying Instructor's Media Library for animations and videos on the following topics covered in this chapter:

- The cardiac cycle
- Capillary pressure
- Measuring blood pressure

Objective 3
Build cardiovascular words from combining forms, prefixes, and suffixes

- Text page(s) 226-228

Objective 4
Describe common cardiovascular diseases

- Text page(s) 229-241

Content Abstract

Disease	Meaning
Angina pectoris	Mild to severe chest pain caused by ischemia of the myocardium (see Box 5-7)
Cardiomegaly	Enlargement of the heart
Cardiomyopathy	Any condition of the heart that causes enlargement and heart failure
Congestive heart failure	Inability of the heart to pump sufficient amounts of blood (see Box 5-8)
Myocardial infarction	Death of myocardial cells due to severe ischemia (see Box 5-9)
Endocarditis	Bacterial infection of the endocardium and valves
Murmur	Abnormal heart sound created by turbulence as blood leaks past a defective heart valve
Pericarditis	Infection of the pericardial sac with fluid accumulation (see Box 5-10)
Rheumatic heart disease	Autoimmune response in which antibodies against a streptococcal infection begin to attack the body's own tissues
Mitral valve prolapse	Structural abnormality in which the leaflets of the mitral valve do not close tightly
Arrhythmia	Any type of irregularity in the rate or rhythm of the heart
Bradycardia	Slow heart rate
Cardiac arrest	Complete absence of a heartbeat
Flutter	Arrhythmia with a very fast (250 beats/minute) but regular rhythm
Fibrillation	Arrhythmia with a very fast, but uncoordinated rhythm
Heart block	Arrhythmia in which the AV impulses are blocked
Palpitation	An uncomfortable sensation felt in the chest during a premature contraction of the heart
Premature contraction	One or more extra contractions in one cardiac cycle
Sick sinus syndrome	Bradycardia alternating with tachycardia
Tachycardia	Fast (up to 200 beats/minute), but regular rhythm

(continued)

Disease	Meaning
Aneurysm	Area of dilatation and weakness in the wall of an artery (see Box 5-11)
Arteriosclerosis	Deposits of plaque that gradually clog an artery (see Box 5-12)
Bruit	Rushing sound of blood passing through a narrowed artery
Coronary artery disease	Arteriosclerosis of the coronary arteries
Hypertension	Elevated blood pressure (see Box 5-13)
Hypotension	Blood pressure that is below normal
Peripheral artery disease	Arteriosclerosis of the arteries of the legs
Peripheral vascular disease	Any disease of the arteries of the extremities
Phlebitis	Inflammation of a vein, usually with infection
Raynaud's disease	Severe vasoconstriction of arterioles in fingers and toes (see Box 5-14)
Varicose veins	Incompetent valves in the veins let blood collect and cause the veins to bulge. (see Box 5-15)
Hyperlipidemia	Elevated levels of blood lipids (see Box 5-16)

Box 5-7: Instructor Activity

ANGINA

Share this information with students.

In 1895, nitroglycerin was first used to treat angina. It was discovered to be effective when workers in a dynamite factory experienced relief of their chest pain. Nitroglycerin is an ingredient in dynamite.

Box 5-8: Classroom Activity

CONGESTIVE HEART FAILURE

Bring about 50 Legos (red color is best) with you to class. Also bring sticky notes. Use six sticky notes and put one anatomy word on each note: right ventricle, pulmonary artery, lung, left atrium, left ventricle, aorta. Have six students volunteer to stand at the front of the class. Give each of them a sticky note, keeping them in the order mentioned above. Stand next to the student who has the "right ventricle" label. Say "beat" to represent one heartbeat, and at that time you hand four red Lego blocks to the "right ventricle" student. The next time you say "beat," hand another four red Lego blocks to the "right ventricle student, who in turn hands his/her original four red Lego blocks to the "pulmonary artery" student. Keep slowly saying "beat," with each student handing their four red Lego blocks to the next student. Provide a box at the end where the "aorta" student can deposit Legos. Tell students that this demonstrates how the blood flows through a normal heart. Now begin the exercise again, but tell the "left ventricle" student that he/she is failing and can only accept three Legos at a time and can only pass on three Legos at a time to the aorta. Tell the "left atrium" student that he/she can only hold a maximum of four Legos at a time and cannot accept any more. Tell the "right ventricle" student and "pulmonary artery" student that they must continue to pass on the four red Lego blocks they are given. Tell the "lung" student that he/she must accept all Legos given to him/her. If all goes as planned, there will be a backup of excess Legos quickly developing with the "lung" student. This graphically illustrates how the blood backs up into the lungs in left-sided heart failure.

Box 5-9: Instructor Activity

HEART ATTACK

Share this information with students.

1. Sudden cardiac death from coronary heart disease occurs over 680 times per day in the United States.
2. There is a 40 percent higher risk of having a heart attack in the morning, especially in patients with hypertension because of early morning increases in blood pressure. There is a 53 percent higher risk of having a heart attack in the winter. Heart attacks occur more often in winter than in any other season.

   Source: Stephen Glasser, MD, Professor of Epidemiology, University of Minnesota.

3. Aspirin is recommended to prevent heart attacks, but a recent study found that aspirin works differently in men and women. In men, it is effective in preventing a heart attack, but in women it is more effective in preventing a stroke than a heart attack.

   Source: New England Journal of Medicine, as reported on the *ABC Nightly News,* January 17, 2006.

Box 5-10: Instructor Activity

PERICARDITIS

Susan Turley, the author, has a friend who, while he was doing woodworking and pressing hard to cut the wood with an X-acto knife, had the knife slip. The force drove the tip of the knife between his ribs and into the thoracic cavity. In the emergency department, he experienced shortness of breath, and an ultrasound of his heart (echocardiography) showed a pocket of blood in the pericardial sac. He was treated with antibiotic drugs to prevent pericarditis from developing.

Box 5-11: Instructor Activity

ANEURYSM

Share this information with students.

Israel's prime minister Ariel Sharon had an aneurysm in the septal wall within his heart. The aneurysm collected blood that clotted and the blood clot then moved to his brain and caused him to suffer a mild stroke on December 18, 2005. He also had a small hole in the septum of his heart that was to be repaired on January 5, 2005. On the evening before the scheduled surgical procedure, he suffered a massive stroke and became comatose.

Box 5-12: Instructor Activity

ARTERIOSCLEROSIS AND CORONARY ARTERY DISEASE

Share this information with students.

1. Examination of specimens of arteriosclerotic plaques taken from arteries show that 72 percent of them contain bacteria that are found in the mouth in periodontal disease (inflammation and infection of the gums and teeth). Cytomegalovirus was found in 38 percent of the specimens. This supports the theory that periodontal disease as well as other infections in the body may cause arteriosclerosis and other chronic illnesses. Source: *Scientific American,* May 2001.

2. Here are some examples of what a pathologist dictated when dissecting the bodies of various patients during their autopsies.

   Patient 1: The coronary arteries are distributed over the heart in the usual fashion and there is no significant atherosclerosis observed.

   Patient 2: Examination of the coronary arteries confirmed the presence of a complete occlusion of the right coronary artery by a thrombus in the area, with marked narrowing proximally by atherosclerotic plaque. The left coronary artery shows mild atherosclerotic plaque.

   Source: The SUM Program Pathology Module, Health Professions Institute.

Box 5-13: Instructor Activity

HYPERTENSION

Share this information with students.

1. African Americans of both sexes and Caucasian males have a higher rate of hypertension.
2. The Institute of Medicine urged Americans to cut their salt intake in half and have a more balanced intake of sodium and potassium to prevent high blood pressure. On average, women consume twice as much sodium as men. Three-quarters of the daily salt intake of Americans comes from sodium hidden in processed and restaurant foods. Food labels state the acceptable daily amount of sodium as 2,400 mg (a heaping teaspoon) per day, but the IOM recommendation is only 1,500 mg a day.
3. February 3 is national Wear Red Day. This campaign is to call attention to the fact that heart disease is the number one killer of women and claims the lives of ½ million women each year (www.goredforwomen.org).
4. Susan Turley, the author, recalls eating dinner with a friend who was on medication for high blood pressure. The friend proceeded to salt, and salt, and salt her green beans and never seemed concerned about how much salt she was using. It seemed like so much salt that it would have made the beans inedible. Our diet—particularly the hidden sodium in fast foods—accustoms us to tolerate high levels of salt and sodium, so much so that regularly seasoned food tastes bland in comparison.
5. Frozen dinners, spaghetti sauce, and soup seem to be a staple for the average student. These foods, though convenient and cheap, contain high levels of sodium. A physician for Penn State University Student Health Services noted that most people are eating 5,000 to 7,000 mg of sodium per day and, if they are eating fast foods, the number is probably higher! An average can of Campbell's Chunky Soup contains between 800 and 1,000 milligrams of sodium. Eat the whole can and you have consumed over the recommended daily value for sodium in just one sitting. A Big Mac contains 1,050 mg of sodium, and most people eat that with salty French fries.

   Source: The Digital Collegian, www.colleegian.psu.edu

Box 5-14: Instructor Activity

RAYNAUD'S DISEASE

Share this information with students.

Patients with Raynaud's disease are advised to wear gloves and socks as much as possible. If they need to reach into the freezer for food, they should put on oven mitts. They should also quit smoking because smoking further constricts the arteries.

Box 5-15: Instructor Activity

VARICOSE VEINS

Share this information with students.

Varicose veins of the rectum are known as hemorrhoids. Varicose veins of the esophagus and stomach are known as esophageal and gastric varices.

Box 5-16: Instructor Activity

HYPERLIPIDEMIA

Share this information with students.

Susan Turley, the author, used to work as a plasmapheresis nurse for a company that manufactures clotting factors. Unlike blood donation, which can only be done every 56 days, plasma donation can be done every few days because the body quickly replenishes the water and other contents in plasma. In the preliminary screening prior to the procedure, prospective donors are asked if they had fatty foods (eggs, sausage, etc.) for breakfast. If they answer "yes," they are not permitted to donate. The fat in the plasma interferes with the process of extracting clotting factors from the plasma. So how much fat is really in the blood after a fatty meal? The author saw for herself when a donor who had had a fatty breakfast denied that fact and proceeded to donate blood. After the unit of blood was centrifuged and the cells separated from the plasma, the plasma of this donor looked white and opaque (filled with fat) rather than clear and yellow in color! It takes the body several hours to clear this fat from the blood. Frequent fatty meals throughout the day cause the blood to constantly be in this condition, and this leads to the development of arteriosclerosis as the fat is deposited on the artery walls.

Experience Multimedia

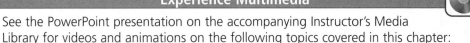

See the PowerPoint presentation on the accompanying Instructor's Media Library for videos and animations on the following topics covered in this chapter:

- Angina
- Congenital heart defects
- Coronary artery disease
- Heart attacks
- Dysrhythmia
- Aneurysm
- Ventricular fibrillation and AED
- Abnormal heart sounds
- Normal heart sounds

Objective 5
Describe common cardiovascular diagnostic laboratory and radiology tests

- Text page(s) 241-247

Content Abstract

Test	Definition
Cardiac enzymes	Blood test to measure the levels of enzymes that are released into the blood when myocardial cells die
Lipid profile	Blood test that provides a comprehensive picture of the levels of cholesterol, triglycerides, HDL, LDL, and VLDL (see Boxes 5-17, 5-18, and 5-19)
Cardiac catheterization	Diagnostic procedure performed to evaluate the right or left side of the heart
Electrocardiography	Diagnostic procedure that records the electrical activity of the heart during contractions and rest (see Box 5-20)
Holter monitor	Diagnostic procedure during which the patient's heart rate and rhythm are continuously monitored as an outpatient for 24 hours
Telemetry	Continuous monitoring of the patient's heart rhythm in the intensive care unit
Cardiac exercise stress test	Evaluation of the ECG response of the heart to exercise (see Box 5-21)
Angiography	Radiographic procedure in which radiopaque dye outlines an artery or vein
Aortography	Radiologic procedure in which radiopaque due outlines the aorta
Myocardial perfusion scan	Nuclear medicine procedure that uses a radioactive tracer during an exercise stress test
MUGA scan	Nuclear medicine procedure that uses a radioactive tracer bound to red blood cells to calculate the ejection fraction of the heart
Echocardiography	Ultrasound procedure that uses sound waves to show heart motion

Box 5-17: Instructor Activity
CARDIOVASCULAR TEST RESULTS Obtain various common cardiovascular test results (EKG, lipid profile, etc.) to circulate in class.

Box 5-18: Instructor Activity

CHOLESTEROL

Share this information with students.

1. In 2002, the federal government set a standard for the acceptable level of LDL cholesterol in the blood. In July 2004, the American Heart Association and the American College of Cardiologists recommended that patients who are in the moderate- to high-risk category for heart disease should be treated with cholesterol-lowering drugs to keep their LDL level less than 100. This recommendation dramatically increased the number of patients who should be considered for treatment with cholesterol-lowering drugs.

   Source: The Pittsburgh Post-Gazette, July 13, 2004.

2. A high intake of trans fat raises the level of LDL (the "bad" cholesterol). Trans fats are found in partially hydrogenated vegetable oils like margarine and shortening. They are also found in many processed foods like cookies, baked goods, fried foods, crackers, etc.

   Source: *USA Today,* September 16, 2005.

3. In addition to measuring the cholesterol, triglyceride, HDL, and LDL levels in the blood, homocysteine is now being measured. High levels of homocysteine have been shown to be a better predictor of heart disease than cholesterol. Eating foods rich in B vitamins helps to keep homocysteine levels low.

   Source: Labtestsonline.org, January 25, 2005.

Box 5-19: Classroom Activity

CHOLESTEROL

Ask students if they have heard all of the bad publicity about cholesterol. Ask them: Is there anything good about cholesterol? Does your body need cholesterol at all? Tell them they might be surprised to learn that the body does need cholesterol. The body even makes some of its own cholesterol to use as the basis for manufacturing hormones, even sex hormones! However, some people's bodies make too much cholesterol and other people eat too much cholesterol in their diets. Ask students: What in your diet gives you cholesterol? [Answer: Foods from animals. There is no cholesterol in plant foods.] Ask students if they have seen the TV ads for the cholesterol-lowering drug Vytorin. The ads picture an older relative on one side of the screen and a plate of food on the other side that somehow resembles the person. The ad makes clear that part of your cholesterol comes from your diet and part from your relatives (hereditary).

Box 5-20: Instructor Activity

ELECTROCARDIOGRAPHY

Share this information with students.

In 1889, British physiologist Augustus Waller performed the first electrocardiography (ECG).

EXERCISE STRESS TEST

Share this information with students. This is an excerpt from an actual exercise stress test report.

The patient recently had an episode of chest pain. He has had a coronary artery by-pass. A stress test was done. At that time he tolerated 13 minutes and 3 seconds of a modified Bruce protocol. He achieved a pulse rate that gradually increased up to 130. He reported no discomfort at that time. However, his EKG showed ST-segment elevation in leads II, III, and aVF. The test was considered to be possibly positive on the basis of this change.

Source: The SUM Program Cardiology Module, Health Professions Institute.

Experience Multimedia

See the PowerPoint presentation on the accompanying Instructor's Media Library for a video on the topic of the electrocardiogram.

Objective 6
Describe common cardiovascular medical and surgical procedures and drug categories

- Text page(s) 248-256

Content Abstract

Procedure	Definition
Auscultation	Using a stethoscope to listen to the heart sounds (see Box 5-22)
Cardioversion	Medical procedure to treat a life-threatening arrhythmia and restore the heart to a normal sinus rhythm (see Box 5-23)
Radiofrequency catheter ablation	Medical procedure that uses electrical impulses to destroy areas of the heart that are producing arrhythmias
Sclerotherapy	Sclerosing drug injected into a varicose vein to occlude it
Vital signs	Measurement of temperature, pulse, respirations, and blood pressure (see Box 5-24)
Aneurysmectomy	Surgical procedure to remove an aneurysm and repair the defect in the artery wall
Cardiopulmonary bypass	Technique used during open-heart surgery in which the patient's blood is rerouted through a cannula in the femoral vein to a heart-lung machine
Carotid endarterectomy	Surgical procedure to remove plaque from the carotid arteries

Procedure	Definition
Coronary artery bypass graft (CABG)	Surgical procedure to bypass an occluded coronary artery and restore blood flow to the myocardium (see Boxes 5-25 and 5-26)
Percutaneous transluminal coronary angioplasty (PTCA)	Surgical procedure to reconstruct an artery that is narrowed because of arteriosclerosis (see Box 5-27)
Heart transplantation	Surgical procedure to insert a donor heart into a patient (see Box 5-28)
Pacemaker insertion	Surgical procedure to insert a pacemaker to control the heart rate (see Box 5-29)
Pericardiocentesis	Surgical procedure to remove fluid buildup from the pericardium
Valvoplasty	Surgical procedure to correct a damaged heart valve
Valve replacement	Surgical procedure to insert a new, prosthetic heart valve

Drug Category	Description	Example
Antibiotic drugs	Treat bacterial infections of the heart and blood vessels	Ampicillin
Beta-blocker drugs	Treat angina pectoris and hypertension (see Box 5-30)	Inderal, Lopressor
Digitalis drugs	Treat congestive heart failure (see Box 5-31)	Digoxin
Drugs for hyperlipidemia	Treat hypercholesterolemia and hypertriglyceridemia	Lipitor, Vytorin, Zocor
Thrombolytic drugs	Treat a blood clot that is blocking blood flow through an artery	Activase

---

Box 5-22: Classroom Activity

AUSCULTATION AND THE PMI

Physicians often refer to the PMI when doing a physical examination. The point of maximal impulse (PMI) is the area where the heartbeat is the loudest and the heart sounds can best be heard. The physician places a stethoscope over this area. Its position is determined by finding the apex of the heart which is located at the intersection of the midclavicular line (a vertical line from the middle of the left collarbone) and the patient's fifth intercostal space (space between the fifth and sixth ribs).

Box 5-23: Instructor Activity

CARDIOVERSION, AED, AND CPR

Share this information with students.

1. The Food and Drug Administration (FDA) approved over-the-counter sales of automated external defibrillators (AED) in September 2004. Previously, these had only been available with a doctor's prescription. The device is about the size of a lunch box and weighs just three pounds. Pulling the handle on the top activates voice instructions that guide the user through each step. The patient needs to be hooked up to the machine, which then automatically analyzes his/her heart rhythm to determine if defibrillation is needed. AEDs have been available for some time in public places (airports, malls, sports stadiums). The *New England Journal of Medicine* reported that the number of people who survive cardiac arrest in public places could double if volunteers were trained to use AEDs and do CPR. Critics note that the home AEDs are expensive ($2,000) and that searching for a home AED might take the place of calling 911 or doing CPR.

   Source: The Baltimore Sun, "Defibrillator Home Use OK'd," October 18, 2004.

2. When defibrillation is provided within 5 to 7 minutes, the survival rate from cardiac arrest is as high as 49 percent.

3. It is found by researchers at the University of Arizona that performing continuous chest compression-only CPR while waiting for the paramedics to arrive is considerably better than doing nothing at all. It may even be as helpful as standard CPR. For more information on the advantages of continuous chest compression CPR (CCC-CPR), go to: http://www.heart.arizona.edu/publiced/lifesaver.htm.

Box 5-24: Classroom Activity

VITAL SIGNS

The radial pulse is the most common and convenient way to determine the heart rate. The radial pulse can be felt on the thumb side of the wrist area. It is where the radial artery goes over the radius bone of the lower arm. If the pulse has a regular rate, it can be counted for just 15 seconds and that number multiplied by 4 to obtain the number of heartbeats per minute. If the pulse is irregular, it must be counted for the full 60 seconds to obtain an accurate heart rate.

You will need a watch with a second hand. Have students find their own radial pulse by positioning their right hand with the palm up and then using the second, third, and fourth fingers of their left hand to feel along the wrist on the thumb side of their right hand. After they find the pulse, ask them if it has a regular rhythm. If so, tell them when to start counting and then time them for 15 seconds, then tell them to stop. Have them write down the number they obtained and multiply that by 4 to get their pulse rates.

In 1900, an Italian physician invented the sphygmomanometer for measuring blood pressure.

Box 5-25: Classroom Activity

CORONARY ARTERY BYPASS GRAFT

Susan Turley, the author, worked as a medical transcriptionist for a number of years. Once, she was transcribing a report in which the patient had had coronary artery bypass surgery in which a graft should have been sewn to one part of an artery, then around the blockage in that artery, and then back into the artery after the blockage. Instead, the graft was sewn to the artery and then into a vein, creating a fistula. The patient still was not receiving oxygenated blood and began to have chest pains as he recovered from the surgery. He had to be taken back to the operating room and the graft was redone. The diagnosis on this patient's medical record was "iatrogenic arteriovenous fistula." Look up the meaning of the word parts of "iatrogenic" in Appendix A of the textbook.

iatr/o- means _____

gen/o- means _____

-ic means _____

Box 5-26: Instructor Activity

CORONARY ARTERY BYPASS GRAFT

Share this information with students.

1. At age 58, former President Bill Clinton underwent quadruple coronary artery bypass graft surgery in September 2004. About 300,000 patients have this operation each year, and the survival rate is 99 percent. Clinton had had mild chest pains and shortness of breath. An angiogram showed blockages in four coronary arteries. His cholesterol level had been high in the past, and his doctors had put him on a cholesterol-lowering drug. His level of LDL was 177 (normal is less than 130). Clinton said that recently he had stopped taking his cholesterol medicine because he had gotten his cholesterol level lower.

   Source: www.cnn.com

2. Coronary artery bypass graft is abbreviated as CABG and often the slang word "cabbage" is used to pronounce the abbreviation!

Box 5-27: Instructor Activity

ANGIOPLASTY

Share this information with students.

This procedure is often called a balloon angioplasty because of the balloon that is inflated to press down the plaque.

After angioplasty and the insertion of a stent to correct a blocked coronary artery, 15 to 30 percent of the stents become blocked by tissue growing into them. A drug-coated stent known as Cypher prevents this tissue growth and decreases the rate of restenosis to just 5 percent.

Source: Family Circle magazine, September 7, 2004.

Box 5-28: Instructor Activity

HEART TRANSPLANTATION

Share this information with students.

1. In 1953, Dr. John Gibbon invented the first heart-lung machine to use during open heart surgery.
2. In 1967, Dr. Christiaan Barnard performed the first heart transplant operation.
3. In 1982, Barney Clark became the first person in the world to receive an implanted artificial heart, known as the Jarvik-7 for its creator, Dr. Robert Jarvik.
4. The Food and Drug Administration (FDA) approved the use of a temporary artificial heart in patients awaiting heart transplantation who are at risk of dying within 30 days. About 500 patients each year fall into this category.

Source: The Baltimore Sun, October 19, 2004.

Box 5-29: Instructor Activity

PACEMAKERS

Share this information with students.

1. In 1952, the first cardiac pacemaker was developed.
2. Cellular phones can interfere with pacemaker functioning. Digital phones are more likely to cause problems than analog phones. Keeping the cellular phone at least six inches away from the pacemaker may decrease the chances of problems. Issues regarding cellular phones should be discussed with the patient's heart doctor.

Box 5-30: Instructor Activity

HYPERTENSION DRUGS

The treatment of hypertension follows what is known as a stepped-care approach. First, life-style changes are suggested: Patients are asked to restrict the use of salt in cooking and at the table, or the physician may prescribe a low-salt diet to place a limit on total dietary sodium intake. If this does not work, a diuretic drug may be added to increase the excretion of sodium and water. If this does not work, an antihypertensive drug such as a beta blocker, calcium channel blocker, or ACE inhibitor may be added.

Box 5-31: Instructor Activity

DIGITALIS AND LIPITOR

Share this information with students.

1. In 1741, Dr. William Wuthering, an English physician, introduced the use of the foxglove plant as a drug for the heart. It contains the modern drug digitalis.
2. In a list of the drugs prescribed most frequently in 2004, Lipitor was number two, with 70,000,000 prescriptions written.

Source: RxList at www.rxlist.com

Experience Multimedia

See the PowerPoint presentation on the accompanying Instructor's Media Library for videos on the following topics covered in this chapter.
- Defibrillation
- Vital signs

Objective 7
Define common cardiovascular abbreviations

- Text page(s) 257

Teaching Strategy

Stress the importance of learning abbreviations and their full meanings.

Content Abstract

AAA	abdominal aortic aneurysm
ACE	angiotensin-converting enzyme (inhibitor)
ACS	acute coronary syndrome
AED	automatic external defibrillator
A fib	atrial fibrillation
AI	aortic insufficiency
AICD	automatic implantable cardioverter-defibrillator
AMI	acute myocardial infarction
AS	aortic stenosis
ASCVD	arteriosclerotic cardiovascular disease
ASD	atrial septal defect
ASHD	arteriosclerotic heart disease
AV	atrioventricular
BP	blood pressure
BPM, bpm	beats per minute
CABG	coronary artery bypass graft
CAD	coronary artery disease
cath	(cardiac) catheterization
CCU	coronary care unit
CHF	congestive heart failure
CK-MB	creatine kinase-M band
CPK-MB	creatine phosphokinase-M band
CPR	cardiopulmonary resuscitation
CRP	C-reactive protein
CV	cardiovascular
DSA	digital subtraction angiography
ECG	electrocardiography
echo	echocardiogram

EKG	electrocardiography
HDL	high-density lipoprotein
HTN	hypertension
JVD	jugular venous distention
LA	left atrium
LBBB	left bundle branch block
LDH	lactic dehydrogenase
LDL	low-density lipoprotein
LV	left ventricle
LVAD	left ventricular assist device
LVH	left ventricular hypertrophy
MI	myocardial infarction
mm Hg	millimeters of mercury
MR	mitral regurgitation
MUGA	multiple-gated acquisition (scan)
MVP	mitral valve prolapse
NSR	normal sinus rhythm
P	pulse
PAC	premature atrial contraction
PAD	peripheral artery disease
PDA	patent ductus arteriosus
PMI	point of maximum impulse
PTCA	percutaneous transluminal coronary angioplasty
PVC	premature ventricular contraction
PVD	peripheral vascular disease
RA	right atrium
RBBB	right bundle branch block
RFA	radiofrequency catheter ablation

RNV	radionuclide ventriculography		**SVT**	supraventricular tachycardia
RV	right ventricle		**TEE**	transesophageal echocardiogram
S$_1$	first heart sound		**TPR**	temperature, pulse, and respiration
S$_2$	second heart sound		**V fib**	ventricular fibrillation
S$_3$	third heart sound		**VLDL**	very low-density lipoprotein
S$_4$	fourth heart sound		**VSD**	ventricular septal defect
SA	sinoatrial		**V tach**	ventricular tachycardia
SBE	subacute bacterial endocarditis			
SPECT	single photon emission computerized tomography			

Objective 8
Correctly spell and pronounce cardiovascular words

- Text page(s) 270-272

Teaching Strategies

1. Impress upon the students that medical words that are mispronounced are also probably going to be misspelled.
2. Encourage students to work on both pronunciation and spelling when studying.

Box 5-32: Classroom Activity

GAMES

1. From week to week, pick a different one of these spelling games to use during class. (The descriptions and instructions for the games are in the section "The Art and Craft of Teaching.")

   Beanbag Spelling Toss
   Scrabble
   Spelling Bee
   Gridlock
   Hangman

2. From week to week, pick a different one of these pronunciation games to use during class. (The descriptions and instructions for the games are in the section "The Art and Craft of Teaching.")

   Parroting
   Hieroglyphics
   Beach Ball Blast

Chapter Spelling Test

The chapter spelling test is included with the weekly chapter test. Dictate and spell (or xerox a handout that contains) this list of 20 spelling words. For the chapter test, select just 10 of these words to test.

1. aneurysm
2. arrhythmia
3. arteriosclerosis
4. bradycardia
5. cardiopulmonary
6. defibrillator
7. diastolic
8. epinephrine
9. hypertriglyceridemia
10. lipoprotein
11. mediastinum
12. paroxysmal tachycardia
13. pericardiocentesis
14. peroneal artery
15. phlebitis
16. sphygmomanometer
17. systolic
18. telemetry
19. thrombophlebitis
20. trigeminy

Chapter Pronunciation Test

Have students mark these 20 words listed in the Pronunciation Checklist for the chapter. During the week, they will call your office or home answering machine and pronounce each word.

1. aneurysm
2. angina pectoris
3. angioplasty
4. arrhythmia
5. arteriosclerosis
6. atheromatous
7. cardiomyopathy
8. diastole
9. diastolic
10. hypertrophy
11. orthostatic
12. pericarditis
13. plaque
14. prosthetic valve
15. rheumatic heart disease
16. sphygmomanometer
17. systole
18. telemetry
19. thrombophlebitis
20. varicose veins

Objective 9
Apply your skills by analyzing a cardiology report

- Text page(s) 267-269

Content Abstract

Read the hospital Admission History and Physical Examination and answer the questions provided.

Objective 10
Test your knowledge of cardiology by completing review exercises in the textbook and the CD-ROM learning activities

- Text page(s) 259-269 (first complete all of the in-chapter exercises on pp. 224-228)

Teaching Strategies

1. Assign the Chapter Review Exercises in the textbook for homework. Remind students to refer to the Answer Key at the end of the textbook to check their answers.
2. Refer to the CD-ROM Learning Activities in this section for multimedia learning experiences.

Experience Multimedia

See the PowerPoint presentation on the accompanying Instructor's Media Library for videos on the topic of a career as a cardiac stress technologist.

Homework Activities

1. Do you know what your blood pressure usually is? Visit your local pharmacy or drug store and use the blood pressure testing machine to check your blood pressure. Record your blood pressure measurement, the date, and time.

2. Review the section on myocardial infarction in this chapter. Then interview someone who has had a heart attack. Prepare a list of questions to be used during the interview based on what you know from the chapter.

3. Use an English dictionary and a medical dictionary to show what the common meaning is between the origins of these word pairs.

   ventricle and ventriloquist
   digitalis and digit

   Adapted from Ellen Drake. "Using Storytelling to Teach and Learn Medical Terminology," *Perspectives on the Medical Transcription Profession,* pp. 10-13.

4. Look in your medicine cabinet. Find 10 prescription or over-the-counter drugs. List their drug names. Also look on the label and find any medical words. Write down these medical words and then look up and write their medical definitions.

5. Chemicals from the leech fight germs, widen veins, and restore blood circulation. Doctors are using leech saliva, a substance that keeps blood flowing freely and prevents clotting. Explore the Scholastic Web site at http://teacher.scholastic.com/researchtools/articlearchives/humanbody/grossmedicine.htm and read about how the old-fashioned remedies of leeches and maggots are making a comeback in removing blood trapped under the skin or removing tissue that has died due to a lack of blood flow.

6. Go to the Internet and type in "ways to decrease high blood pressure." Many Web sites will come up; visit several. Write down at least five different ways the sites suggest to decrease high blood pressure.

7. Use the Internet to research the link between pacemakers and microwaves. Write a summary of what you learn.

8. Keep a running list in your notebook of sound-alike words or combining forms that have the same meanings. Title this list of challenging words and word parts as "Perplexing Pairs." Begin by writing down the words or word parts found in the Word Alert boxes in this chapter. Then add the word parts found in the It's Greek to Me box at the end of this chapter. Add any other words or word parts that you found particularly confusing. You will add to this list as you complete each chapter. Examples:

orth/o-	vs.	arthr/o-
myel/o-	vs.	my/o-
perine/o-	vs.	peritone/o-
cephal/o-	vs.	encephal/o-

Word Search

Complete this word search puzzle that contains Chapter 5 words. Look for the following words as given in the list below.

angina
aorta
apex
arrhythmia
artery
atrium
bruit
heart (2)
ions

LBBB
LVH
murmur
node
pulse
telemetry
troponin
valve

```
R  U  M  R  U  M  L  C  X  A
X  J  E  S  L  U  P  V  I  Y
E  L  B  B  B  I  O  M  H  R
P  N  A  B  U  R  H  F  E  T
A  O  R  T  A  T  U  E  A  E
N  D  T  J  Y  A  H  I  R  M
I  E  E  H  H  E  A  R  T  E
G  T  R  O  P  O  N  I  N  L
N  R  Y  L  F  V  A  L  V  E
A  K  G  S  N  O  I  Q  F  T
```

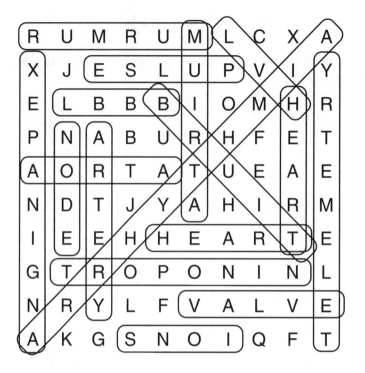

6

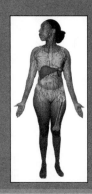

Hematology and Immunology
Blood and the Lymphatic System

Instructor Activity for the Beginning of Class

Contact the local chapter of the American Red Cross in your area. Request some blood donation marketing materials to display during class. If available, request a plastic banner that you can hang across the front of a table. It says, "American Red Cross, Donate Blood Today. Together, we can save a life." Also request a printed flyer that shows a person from your area who needed and received a blood transfusion.

If you are a regular blood donor, show the students your American Red Cross blood donor card. If you have organized local blood drives and have been given a red polo shirt and cap with the American Red Cross logo, wear those to teach class rather than your usual scrubs.

Instructor Activity for the Beginning of Class

Say this to students:

Raise your hand if you would like to get an a or A B in this course. How about an AB or an O? A, B, AB, and O are blood types we will study in this chapter. I can't guarantee you will get an A or a B—that's up to you, but I can guarantee that your knowledge will be flowing once you master the language of hematology and immunology!

Objective 1
Identify the anatomical structures of the blood and lymphatic system by correctly labeling them on anatomical illustrations

- Text page(s) 276-285, 287-289

Teaching Strategy

Explain the importance of learning the parts of the blood and lymphatic system.

Content Abstract

Hematology is the study of the blood. It is the healthcare specialty that studies the anatomy and physiology of the blood and uses diagnostic tests, medical and surgical procedures, and drugs to treat blood diseases.

Immunology is the study of the immune system. It is the healthcare specialty that studies the anatomy and physiology of the lymphatic system, the way the body distinguishes self from foreign, and uses diagnostic tests, medical and surgical procedures, and drugs to treat lymphatic and immune response diseases.

The blood can be divided into two component parts: plasma and blood cells. The fluid portion of blood is called plasma. Blood cells are suspended in the plasma (see Box 6-1).

There are three types of blood cells (see Box 6-2):

1. Erythrocytes (red blood cells)
2. Leukocytes (white blood cells) (see Box 6-3)
3. Thrombocytes (platelets)

Erythrocytes contain hemoglobin, which carries oxygen to the cells and carries carbon dioxide from the cells to the lungs, where it is exhaled. Carbon dioxide is carried in three different forms in the blood:

1. On the hemoglobin molecule, which then becomes known as carbamino-hemoglobin
2. In the form of bicarbonate ions in the blood
3. As carbon dioxide in the blood.

There are five different kinds of leukocytes (white blood cells). Many, many years ago, it was found that the different types of leukocytes could be differentiated from each other by applying chemical stains to a drop of blood spread on a glass slide. The stains brought out different structural features that made each leukocyte easier to identify. The red, acidic stain eosin is used as well as the blue, alkaline stain methylene blue. (See Table 6-1 on page 283). Notice how granules in the cytoplasm of the eosinophil take up the red eosin stain. The cell derives its name from this chemical reaction: The combining form *eosin/o-* means *eosin* (*acidic, red dye*) plus the suffix *-phil* means *attraction to or fondness for* (see Box 6-4). The granules in the cytoplasm of the basophil take up the methylene blue stain. The cell derives its name from this chemical reaction: The combining form *bas/o-* means *basic* (*alkaline*) plus the suffix *-phil* means *attraction to or fondness for.* A neutrophil also has granules in its cytoplasm, but these do not strongly take up either the red or the blue dye. The neutrophil is neutral in its reaction to these two colored stains.

The ABO blood group contains A, B, AB, and O antigens (see Boxes 6-5 and 6-6).

Box 6-1: Instructor Activity

PLASMA

Share this information with students.

Plasma is normally clear and yellow in color or straw-colored (see Figure 6-2 on page 277). If you look at a tube of blood that has been centrifuged (spun around so that gravity pulls the cells to the bottom), the plasma remains at the top and you can see right straight through it. Pique your students' interest by telling them that later in the class you will tell about an almost daily condition in which the plasma becomes as thick and opaque as milk!

Box 6-2: Instructor Activity

BLOOD CELLS

Share this information with students.

1. About 15 million blood cells are produced and destroyed in the body every second.

   Source: Fun Science Facts, www.hightechscience.org/funfacts.htm

2. Lobsters have blue blood.

   Source: Fun Science Facts, www.hightechscience.org/funfacts.htm

3. Do you know the city of Philadelphia? What does the word *Philadelphia* mean? What is the city's slogan? [The city of brotherly love.] The "phil" part of Philadelphia refers to love, just like the suffix -phil in eosinophil, basophil, and neutrophil refers to what stains those cells love.

Each type of leukocyte has a special shortened name. Students need to memorize these shortened names because they appear on laboratory test results.

Write these on the board:

Eosinophils	eos
Basophils	basos
Lymphocytes	lymphs
Monocytes	monos
Neutrophils	Many different shortened names, each of which describes something about the unique nucleus of this leukocyte. The highly visible nucleus is divided into more than three segments, hence the shortened names *segmented neutrophils, segs,* and *segmenters.* The segments of the nucleus are of different and varying shapes and sizes, hence the name *polymorphonuclear leukocytes* and the shortened name *polys* and the abbreviation *PMNs.*

Important: Do not confuse the shortened name *lymphs* with the medical word *lymph,* the fluid in the lymphatic system. Do not confuse the shortened name *monos* with the slang word *mono* that stands for the disease *mononucleosis.* Do not confuse the blood protein albumin with the egg white albumen.

Box 6-3: Classroom Activity

LEUKOCYTES

Write this partially completed table on the board. Divide students into four groups. Assign a specific leukocyte to each group. Have each group look on pages 280-282, plus page 289, read the description of their assigned leukocyte, and find the information needed to fill in the table. Have one student from each group come to the board to fill in the information for that leukocyte.

Leukocyte	Specific Function
Neutrophil	Destroys. . .
Eosinophil	Destroys. . .
	Destroys. . .
Basophil	Releases. . .
Lymphocyte	Destroys. . .
	Produces. . .
Monocyte	Destroys. . .
	Eats. . .

Leukocyte	Specific Function
Neutrophil	Destroys bacteria
Eosinophil	Destroys foreign cells like pollen and animal dander
	Destroys parasite worms/eggs
Basophil	Releases histamine and heparin
Lymphocyte	Destroys viruses and bacteria
	Produces antibodies (immunoglobulins)
Monocyte	Destroys pathogens and cancerous cells.
	Eats cellular debris and dead leukocytes

Note: You can increase the value of this activity by adding a middle vertical column with the header "Shortened Name" and have students fill in this information as well.

Box 6-4: Classroom Activity

PARASITIC INFECTIONS

Case History: The patient is a child with recurrent fevers, lethargy, and increased levels of eosinophils on the complete blood count. His symptoms would disappear and then return. Eosinophils are usually associated with an allergic reaction, but allergies are not associated with fevers. What other pathology is associated with increased levels of eosinophils?

[Have students read the paragraph on page 281 under Figure 6-5 to search for an answer.]

[Answer: Parasitic infections. The physician did some checking (after all, M.D. stands for "medical detective") and found that the child was crawling under the front porch of an old house and eating dog poop that contained parasites. The parasites' life cycle corresponded to the coming and going of the fevers.]

BLOOD TYPES

Ask students if they know their blood types. Go around the classroom and have each student say his/her blood type or "I don't know."

Write this table on the board.

Blood Type	Population (%)	Students
O	46	
A	40	
B	10	
AB	4	

Keep a tally of the number of each blood type. Have students calculate the percentage of each blood type by taking the number of students with that blood type and dividing it by the total number of students who knew their blood type. Fill in the student percentages in the table. Then compare the student totals to the general population.

Box 6-6: Instructor Activity

BLOOD TYPES

Share this information with students.

1. Even though blood type O negative is the universal donor and many units of this blood type are needed every day, only about 7 percent of people with blood type O are O negative. Most people with blood type O are O positive.
2. In 1940, the Rh blood group was identified by Dr. Karl Landsteiner of Austria.

Objective 2
Describe how the blood forms a clot

- Text page(s) 286-287

Teaching Strategy

Explain the importance of learning the physiology of blood clotting.

Content Abstract

After an injury, the body stops the flow of blood so that the person does not bleed to death. Immediately, the injured blood vessel constricts to decrease the amount of blood flow. Thrombocytes stick to the damaged area of the blood vessel wall and form clumps to block the blood flow. This is called platelet aggregation. Next, clotting factors in the plasma are activated and begin to produce strands of fibrin that trap erythrocytes and form a thrombus or blood clot. This is called coagulation.

The lymphatic system consists of the

1. lymphatic vessels
2. lymph nodes
3. lymph fluid
4. spleen
5. thymus.

Box 6-7: Instructor Activity

BLOOD CLOTTING

Share this information with students.

1. Thrombocytes (platelets) contain three clotting factors that help the blood to clot: Factor IV, Factor VIII, and Factor XIII. Factor II (prothrombin) is measured in laboratory tests. Factor VIII is missing in hemophiliac patients. The factors were named in the order of their discovery, but this does not correspond to the order in which they are activated to form a blood clot. There are 13 factors in all, but there is no Factor VI. Factor VI was later discovered to just be activated Factor V.

2. Standard gauze bandages do not control bleeding. They just become saturated with blood. Former Army surgeon LTC John Holcomb, now commander of the U.S. Armed Services Institute of Surgical Research, developed a bandage that contains small amounts of ground shrimp shells and vinegar. The combination clots the blood instantly and stops further bleeding. Chitosan, an ingredient in the shrimp shells, interacts with blood cells because its molecules are positively charged and the outer cell membrane of blood cells is negatively charged. The positive and negative charges attract each other, and the blood cells and chitosan form a clot. These bandages are currently in use by the U.S. Army in combat areas.

Source: ScienCentralNews.com, September 3, 2004.

Box 6-8: Classroom Activity

BLOOD CLOTTING

Ask students to brainstorm and answer these questions.

1. When is a blood clot a good thing?
2. When is a blood clot a bad thing? [Hint: Ask students if they have ever heard of a pulmonary embolism.]

[Answers: A blood clot is good when it controls superficial or internal bleeding that occurs after an injury. A blood clot is bad when it breaks away from the original site of injury and travels through the blood. It always becomes trapped when it tries to travel through a blood vessel that is slightly smaller than its size. If the clot is large and it blocks blood flow through a large blood vessel to the lung, it is known as a pulmonary embolus or pulmonary embolism. This can cause severe respiratory distress or even death.]

Box 6-9: Instructor Activity

LYMPHATIC SYSTEM

Share this information with students.

Unlike the circulatory system in which vessels form a continuous circuit, the lymphatic system has a beginning and an end. It begins in the tissues where microscopic lymphatic capillaries absorb tissue fluids. The lymphatic system ends in large lymphatic ducts that empty into large veins in the neck. We don't hear much about the lymphatic system until something goes wrong: infected tonsils and adenoids, lymph nodes containing cancer cells, a spleen ruptured during an automobile accident, and so forth.

Experience Multimedia

See the PowerPoint presentation on the accompanying Instructor's Media Library for an animation showing the lymphatic system.

Objective 3
Describe how the body's immune response functions

- Text page(s) 289-291

Content Abstract

The immune response involves a coordinated effort between the blood and the lymphatic system to destroy invading microorganisms and cancerous cells that arise internally. When microorganisms (such as bacteria, viruses, protozoa, fungi, yeast) or cancer cells are detected, the immune response attempts to destroy these pathogens.

When a pathogen is detected in the blood or lymphatic system, the body attacks it utilizing one of the following:

1. cytokines
2. neutrophils
3. eosinophils
4. basophils
5. monocytes
6. lymphocytes
7. antibodies
8. complement proteins

IMMUNE SYSTEM

Share this information with students.

1. Microorganisms that produce disease are known as pathogens. Pathogens include bacteria, viruses, retroviruses, fungi, and yeast. Allergens are plant particles (molds, pollen, or foods) or nonliving particles (dust, animal dander, smoke, chemicals) that cause allergic reactions.
2. Allergies are the sixth leading cause of chronic disease in the United States.
3. Research has shown that feelings of guilt may damage your immune system by lowering your immunoglobulin levels.

Objective 4
Build blood and lymphatic words from combining forms, prefixes, and suffixes

- Text page(s) 298–299

Objective 5
Describe common blood and lymphatic diseases

- Text page(s) 300–310

Content Abstract

Disease	Meaning
Blood dyscrasia	Any condition of the blood
Pancytopenia	Decreased numbers of all types of blood cells
Septicemia	Severe bacterial infection of the tissues that has also invaded the blood
Anisocytosis	Too large or too small erythrocytes
Poikilocytosis	Abnormal shapes of erythrocytes
Anemia	Decreased number of erythrocytes
Aplastic anemia	Anemia caused by destruction of bone marrow by disease, cancer, radiation, or chemotherapy
Iron deficiency anemia	Anemia from too little iron in the diet or loss of blood
Folic acid anemia	Anemia from too little folic acid in the diet (see Box 6-11)

Disease	Meaning
Pernicious anemia	Anemia from too little vitamin B_{12} in the diet or a lack of intrinsic factor secreted by the stomach (see Box 6-12)
Sickle cell anemia	Anemia in which the red blood cells can become sickled in shape because of a genetic defect (see Boxes 6-13 and 6-14)
Polycythemia vera	Condition in which the body makes too many red blood cells (see Box 6-15)
Thalassemia	Genetic abnormality in which the red blood cells are too small and lack iron (see Box 6-16)
Transfusion reaction	Reaction to transfusion of incompatible blood (see Box 6-17)
Acquired immunodeficiency syndrome (AIDS)	Severe infection caused by the human immunodeficiency virus (HIV) (see Boxes 6-18 and 6-19)
Leukemia	Cancer of the leukocytes (see Box 6-20)
Mononucleosis	Caused by the Epstein-Barr virus; also known as kissing disease
Multiple myeloma	Cancer of the plasma cells that produce antibodies (see Box 6-21)
Coagulopathy	Any disease affecting blood clotting
Deep vein thrombosis	A blood clot in one of the deep veins of the lower leg, often after surgery or in patients on bedrest
Disseminated intravascular coagulopathy (DIC)	Simultaneous clotting and bleeding disorder
Hemophilia	Inherited genetic abnormality of a gene on the X chromosome that causes an absence or deficiency of a specific clotting factor (see Box 6-22)
Thrombocytopenia	Decreased numbers of thrombocytes (platelets)
Graft-versus-host disease	Donor tissue or organ (a graft) reacts against the genetic difference of the patient's tissues
Lymphadenopathy	Enlarged lymph nodes (see Box 6-23)
Lymphedema	Swelling of the tissues after a lymph node chain has been removed (see Box 6-24)
Lymphoma	Cancerous tumor of the lymph nodes or lymphoid tissue
Splenomegaly	Enlargement of the spleen (see Box 6-25)
Thymoma	Benign tumor of the thymus
Autoimmune disease	Diseases of various parts of the body that all are caused when the body makes antibodies against its own tissues

Box 6-11: Instructor Activity

FOLIC ACID

Share this information with students.

A deficiency of folic acid can cause folic acid anemia, but it is also important in other ways. Folic acid is an extremely important vitamin during pregnancy. Pregnant mothers who do not have enough folic acid in their diets can give birth to babies with a defect of the spine known as meningomyelocele [see Figure 10-22 on page 547]. The baby is born with the spinal cord protruding out of the back. In severe cases, the baby will never have the use of its legs and will have bowel and bladder incontinence because of damage to the spinal nerves and spinal cord. Because of the extreme healthcare costs and care associated with this disease, the government mandated that cereals and breads be enriched with folic acid. Also, at the time of the first prenatal visit, a pregnant woman is given prenatal vitamins supplements that contain folic acid by her obstetrician. These measures have greatly reduced the incidence of this condition.

Box 6-12: Instructor Activity

PERNICIOUS ANEMIA AND INTRINSIC FACTOR

Share this information with students.

Just as your scalp produces fewer hairs as you get older, your stomach tends to produce less intrinsic factor. Without intrinsic factor, you cannot absorb vitamin B_{12} even if you have enough in your diet. For many years, the only treatment was to get weekly intramuscular injections of vitamin B_{12} for life. Now, vitamin B_{12} also comes as a nasal spray.

Box 6-13: Instructor Activity

SICKLE CELL ANEMIA

Share this information with students.

1. The sickle cells of sickle cell anemia were first seen under the microscope in 1904.

2. A sickle is an old-fashioned hand tool with a curved blade. It was used to harvest wheat before machines did the harvesting.

Box 6-14: Classroom Activity

SICKLE CELL DISORDER

Ask if anyone in the class knows someone with sickle cell disorder and would be willing to share some of the symptoms and signs.

Box 6-15: Instructor Activity

POLYCYTHEMIA VERA

Share this information with students.

Susan Turley, the author, has a friend who was an excellent athlete in his 40s—a bi-cyclist—when he began complaining of constant dizziness and fatigue. When he finally went to the doctor, his red blood cell count was very high and he was diagnosed with polycythemia vera. Now every month, he has to have his red blood cell count done. Based on the results, the physician usually has to withdraw a small or large amount of blood from his vein to decrease his total number of red blood cells. This blood, even if it is the equivalent of a unit of blood, is never given to someone else as a blood donation because of its abnormality.

Box 6-16: Instructor Activity

THALASSEMIA MINOR

Share this information with students.

Susan Turley, the author, adopted two daughters from Vietnam in 2001. One child has the mild form of the disease thalassemia minor. This medical condition was not reported on her medical records from Vietnam, but it was discovered when she had her first full pediatric visit and lab tests done in the United States. Then she was referred for a full workup with a hematologist at the University of Maryland Medical Center. Fortunately, she has a mild case and she is able to run and play normally and only occasionally complains of fatigue.

Box 6-17: Instructor Activity

TRANSFUSION REACTION

Share this information with students.

Susan Turley, the author, has a friend Linda whose mother was in the hospital. She had received too much anticoagulant drug and needed to receive clotting factors from a plasma transfusion. As Linda watched, the nurse hung a unit of plasma and was just about to open the roller clamp on the I.V. tubing to begin the transfusion when Linda realized that the label on the unit of plasma showed that it was from a donor who had type A blood. Linda knew that her mother had type B blood. [We know that the plasma of type A blood contains anti-B antibodies that would have caused a transfusion reaction if given to a patient with type B blood.] Linda quickly told the nurse. The nurse did not start the transfusion but insisted that the hospital lab would never make that kind of an error. Linda refused to allow the transfusion until her mother's blood type was rechecked. Finally, a lab technician was sent to draw a sample of her mother's blood to confirm her blood type. Fifteen minutes later, the lab called and said that there had been an error and not to proceed with the transfusion.

Box 6-18: Instructor Activity

HIV

Share this information with students.

1. The human immunodeficiency virus (HIV) is a special kind of virus known as a retrovirus. HIV infection officially becomes AIDS only when a patient's CD4 lymphocyte count falls below 200 and the patient has an opportunistic infection. The four main opportunistic infections are *Pneumocystis carinii* pneumonia, oral or esophageal candidiasis (a yeast infection), cytomegalovirus retinitis, and Kaposi's sarcoma (refer students to Figure 18-8 on page 960). In his book *And the Band Played On,* author Randy Shilts states that a French-Canadian flight attendant named Gaetan Dugas was the source of the AIDS epidemic because he had sexual intercourse with over 2,000 people in the United States, 40 of whom developed AIDS and passed it on to others.

2. In 1982, the phrase *acquired immunodeficiency syndrome* (AIDS) was first used.

3. In 1974, the drug AZT was synthesized and tested as a treatment for cancer, but it was not effective. Other uses for it were not investigated, and it was simply "shelved." In 1984, although there were only 3,000 reported cases of AIDS in the United States, researchers at the National Cancer Institute, including the codiscoverer of the AIDS virus, Dr. Robert Gallo, approached Burroughs Wellcome pharmaceutical company to develop a drug to treat AIDS. Other pharmaceutical companies were approached but declined to work with the deadly virus when there was an apparently limited need for a drug. Burroughs Wellcome agreed, and tested many different drugs, one of which was AZT. In 1984, AZT became the first drug used to treat human immunodeficiency virus. Its trade name, Retrovir, refers to the fact that HIV belongs to a class of viruses known as *retroviruses.* Now AZT has lost some of its effectiveness against HIV and must be given in conjunction with two other antiviral drugs.

   Source: Susan Turley, *Understanding Pharmacology for Health Professionals* (Prentice Hall).

4. A cure for AIDS seems less likely now that researchers have discovered that the human immunodeficiency virus (HIV) infects memory T cells where it lies dormant. These cells are the "memory" of the immune system. Memory T cells must survive to continue to protect the body into the future, and HIV survives too within the memory T cells. In 1996, when new drugs seemed to work so well, physicians cautiously speculated about eradicating HIV. But the following year it was discovered that even patients who had been treated with these drugs still had fully potent HIV within their memory T cells. The memory T cells serve as Trojan horses, concealing hoards of the virus.

   Source: "AIDS Research Focus Shifts from Cure to Control," *The Baltimore Sun,* April 29, 2001.

Box 6-19: Classroom Activity

AIDS

Invite someone who has AIDS to be a guest speaker or invite someone from a local agency that provides assistance to patients with AIDS to talk.

Box 6-20: Instructor Activity

LEUKEMIA

Share this information with students.

1. Survival rates for leukemia have increased from 14 percent in 1960 to more than 44 percent in the year 2000.
2. At the time of diagnosis of acute leukemia, 1 trillion cancer cells are generally present and widely distributed throughout the body of the patient. If an antileukemic drug were able to kill 99.9 percent of the cancer cells, the patient would show symptomatic improvement even though he or she would still harbor 1 billion cancer cells.

Source: Michael Gerald, *Pharmacology: An Introduction to Drugs.* Prentice Hall, out of print.

Box 6-21: Instructor Activity

MULTIPLE MYELOMA

Share this information with students.

Susan Turley's, the author, mother died from multiple myeloma. The average life expectancy after diagnosis is just 1 to 2 years. Her mother lived a few weeks short of 2 years after having undergone chemotherapy. Amazingly, her mother's best friend also developed multiple myeloma the previous year and died in about two years. Although multiple myeloma is a rare cancer that affects just 1 in every 4,300 Americans each year, epidemiologists did not think these two cases were related or were statistically significant. In other words, the fact that two women who were best friends and former neighbors had both developed multiple myeloma, a rare cancer, within a year of each other was labeled as just a coincidence.

Box 6-22: Instructor Activity

HEMOPHILIA

Share this information with students.

1. Hemophilia is the oldest known hereditary bleeding disorder.
2. Would you believe that the political climate we live in today was the indirect result of someone with hemophilia? Czar Nicholas II of Russia and his wife Alexandra had four female children before they finally had Alexei, the heir to the throne. Unfortunately, Alexei had hemophilia (his mother was the carrier of the hemophilia gene) and was frequently near death. Obsessed with their son's illness, Czar Nicholas and Alexandra paid little attention to the affairs of state, the widespread economic depression, and the rising call for political reform. Because of this, the entire family was executed during the Bolshevik Revolution, thus ending the czarist form of government forever in Russia and paving the way for Lenin and communism.

LYMPHADENOPATHY

Share this information with students.

1. Openings in the lymphatic capillaries are large enough to admit microorganisms and cancer cells from the tissues. These travel through the lymphatic vessel until they reach a lymph node. Lymphocytes and tissue macrophages that live in the lymph node work hard to destroy microorganisms and cancerous cells. However, a severe infection or cancer can overload one or more lymph nodes, causing them to enlarge.
2. Ask students: Think of the last time you went to the doctor's with a sore throat. After the doctor looked at your throat, what did he/she do to your neck? [Answer: Felt the lymph nodes in both sides of the neck.]
3. Ask students: When a woman performs a self-examination of the breasts, the breast tissue is palpated for lumps. What other area is also felt? [Answer: Under the arm where the axillary lymph nodes are located.]
4. Breast cancer cells that have spread or metastasized will become trapped in the axillary lymph nodes. In fact, the lymph nodes can be so full of cancer that they must be surgically removed along with the breast.

LYMPHEDEMA

Share this information with students.

Susan Turley's great aunt had breast cancer many years ago. At that time, the only surgical procedure offered was complete removal of the breast and all axillary lymph nodes. Although this great aunt has had no recurrence of breast cancer in 50 years, her arm still occasionally swells with lymphedema. Healthcare professionals also know never to take a blood pressure reading in that arm or start an intravenous line in that arm because of the compromised lymph flow.

SPLENOMEGALY

Share this information with students.

Notice that *spleen* is spelled with two *e*s but that in *splenomegaly* (and *splenectomy*) the second e has been deleted.

See the PowerPoint presentation on the accompanying Instructor's Media Library for animations and videos on the following topics covered in this chapter:

- HIV and AIDS
- Leukemia
- Sickle cell anemia

Objective 6
Describe common blood and lymphatic diagnostic laboratory and radiology tests

- Text page(s) 310-314

Teaching Strategy

Obtain copies of common blood and lymphatic diagnostic laboratory and radiology tests (blood typing and cross-matching, test for AIDS) to discuss and circulate in the classroom.

Content Abstract

Test	Definition
Blood type	Blood test that determines the blood type and the Rh factor of the patient's blood
Complete blood count (CBC) with differential	Group of blood tests that are performed automatically by machine to determine the number, type, and characteristics of various cells in the blood
ELISA	Serum screening test for antibodies against HIV
Western blot	Serum test for antibodies against HIV

Box 6-26: Instructor Activity

LABORATORY EQUIPMENT

Share this information with students.

In 1943, Becton Dickinson Company invented the vacuum tube with a rubber stopper (Vacutainer) for drawing blood.

Many years ago before the use of automated equipment in the hospital laboratory, technologists used to count the numbers and types of white blood cells by hand. Using a microscope and a drop of blood smeared onto a glass slide and stained to reveal the different white blood cells, the technologist would count 100 white cells and use a tally sheet to keep track of how many of each different type of white blood cell was seen. This was known as the WBC differential count.

Box 6-27: Classroom Activity

TALLY SHEET

A completed tally sheet might look something like this. [Draw this tally sheet on the board.]

Bands/Stabs	Neuthrophils	Eosinophils	Basophils	Lymphocytes	Monocytes
	40–60%	1–4%	0.5–1%	20–40%	2–4%
卌 卌	卌 卌 卌 卌 卌 卌 卌 卌 卌 卌 卌 卌 卌 卌	卜 丨	丨	卌 卌 卌 卌 卌 卌	丨丨丨丨

Explain this sheet. Have students notice the five categories of mature white blood cells listed across the top. Remind students that bands (also known as stabs) are not mature white blood cells; they are immature neutrophils.

Ask students:

- Which of the five types of mature leukocytes are normal in number?
  [Remind students that they are counting to a total of 100 white cells. The percentages at the top of each column are the normal range of values and are based on 100. So if the eosinophils are normally 1-4 percent, that would mean the technician would normally see anywhere from 1 to 4 eosinophils and make that many tally marks in that column.]
- How many eosinophils did the technologist see? [3]
- Would that be in the normal expected range of 1 to 4? [yes]
- How many basophils did the technologist see and was this normal? [1, yes]
- How many lymphocytes did the technologist see and was this normal? [30, yes]
- How many monocytes did the technologist see and was this normal? [4, yes]
- How many neutrophils did the technologist see and was this normal? [70, no]
- What type of microorganisms do neutrophils destroy? [bacteria]
- Why do you think the numbers of neutrophils are increased in this patient? [a bacterial infection]

Now, let's look at the left-hand column labeled Bands/Stabs.

When there is a severe bacterial infection and there are not enough mature neutrophils to fight it, the body does what some armies have done when there were not enough mature men to fight—they bring in children to fight. The body brings in immature neutrophils (bands/stabs). These appear in the blood and the technologist counts them. Normally, there should be no tally marks in this left-hand column. When there are tally marks (or today, when the electronic printout shows some bands/stabs), the doctor refers to this as a "shift to the left" because that column was traditionally on the left side of the tally sheet. So if your hear the phrase "shift to the left," it always indicates some type of severe bacterial infection.

Experience Multimedia

See the PowerPoint presentation on the accompanying Instructor's Media Library for a video on the topic of blood test basics.

Objective 7
Describe common blood and lymphatic medical and surgical procedures and drug categories

- Text page(s) 315-320

Content Abstract

Procedure	Definition
Bone marrow aspiration	Procedure to remove a specimen of red bone marrow from the posterior iliac crest of the hip bone
Phlebotomy	Medical procedure for drawing a sample of venous blood into a vacuum tube
Vaccination	Medical procedure that injects a vaccine into the body (see Boxes 6-30 through 6-32)
Blood donation	Medical procedure by which a unit of whole blood is collected from a volunteer donor (see Boxes 6-33 and 6-34)
Blood transfusion	Blood or component parts of blood given to a patient
Bone marrow transplantation	Medical procedure used to treat patients with leukemia and lymphoma
Plasmapheresis	Plasma is separated from donated whole blood and used to make plasma, albumin, and clotting factors (see Box 6-35)

(continued)

Procedure	Definition
Stem cell transplantation	Stem cells are used to treat leukemia or lymphoma (see Box 6-36)
Lymph node biopsy	Removal of part or all of a lymph node for diagnosis
Lymph node dissection	Removal of many lymph nodes affected by cancer
Splenectomy	Removal of the spleen after trauma ruptures it
Thymectomy	Removal of the thymus because of a tumor or to treat myasthenia gravis

Drug Category	Description	Example
Anticoagulant drugs	Prevent blood clot from forming by inhibiting the clotting factors or by inhibiting the production of vitamin K	Coumadin (oral), heparin (IM)
Corticosteroid drugs	Anti-inflammatory drugs given to suppress the immune responses and decrease inflammation	Decadron, Prednisone, Solu-Medrol

Box 6-29: Instructor Activity

BLOOD TEST RESULTS

Obtain copies of lab blood tests to show students how to read and interpret the results.

Box 6-30: Instructor Activity

POLIO

Share this information with students.

1. In 1921 at the age of 39, Franklin Delano Roosevelt contracted polio. He had been at his family's estate, helped to fight a forest fire, later took a swim and sat around in his wet bathing suit until he became chilled. The next day he felt like he had the flu, but he had contracted polio and was paralyzed from the waist down. He went on to become the 32nd president from 1933 to 1945, but concealed his illness because of societal views of the handicapped at that time.

2. Susan Turley, the author, remembers when polio was a dreaded disease. An epidemic in the United States during the early 1950s caused wide-spread fear and mothers kept their children home from school. Children on crutches and even in iron lungs (because the nerves that they used to breathe had been paralyzed) were evidence of the effects of polio. Dr. Jonas Salk developed the first polio vaccine in 1955. It was a solution of dead virus. Millions of American children were vaccinated in the upper arm and have a round scar remaining there. Then in 1961, Dr. Albert Sabin developed a weakened polio virus that could be given orally. It was administered on a sugar cube. Today, children receive an oral polio vaccine. Other childhood immunizations include injections of the vaccine for diphtheria, pertussis (whooping cough), and tetanus [DPT] plus measles, mumps, and rubella (German measles) [MMR].

Box 6-31: Instructor Activity

TETANUS

If you step on a rusty nail and haven't had a tetanus booster in years, you will be given a shot of tetanus immunoglobulins, antibodies against tetanus because you don't have time to develop your own antibodies.

Box 6-32: Instructor Activity

RABIES

If you are bitten by an unknown dog that is never caught, you will be given a shot of rabies immunoglobulins, antibodies against rabies because you don't have time to develop your own antibodies. Veterinarians, animal handlers, forest rangers, and hikers who go into caves (where there might be rabid bats) all have an increased risk of contracting rabies and so they are vaccinated ahead of time so that their body does develop its own antibodies against rabies.

Box 6-33: Instructor Activity

BLOOD DONATION

Share this information with students.

1. At 13 months of age, Paige was diagnosed with a brain tumor. What her parents had thought was a stomach virus ultimately resulted in multiple surgeries and six weeks of radiation therapy. A safe and adequate blood supply was necessary to provide Paige with the care she needed. Thanks to willing blood donors, she survived. Her father commented: "We know first-hand how blood donors can impact lives. The last thing any parent should have to worry about is if blood will be available when their child's life depends on it."

   Source: American Red Cross.

2. A single unit of blood can save the lives of up to 3 people. Surgical patients, trauma patients, cancer patients, organ transplant patients, and even premature newborns are among the 5 million Americans who receive some type of blood transfusion each year.

   Source: American Association of Blood Banks.

3. Each year 8 million people donate blood, and every two seconds someone needs a blood transfusion of some type.

   Source: ScienCentralNews at www.sciencentral.com, January 31, 2005.

4. January is National Blood Donor Month.

   Source: The American Red Cross.

5. Men who donate blood have a 30 percent reduced risk of heart disease compared to those who do not donate blood. The difference is thought to be due to a decrease in iron levels in donors.

6. Susan Turley, the author, has a blood type of O-positive. When she worked as a nurse in a neonatal intensive care unit in the late 1970s, she was sometimes asked to give blood to one of the premature babies. After her blood and the baby's were typed and crossmatched for compatibility, the unit's physician would insert a small needle in one of the veins of her hand and withdraw just a small volume of blood into a syringe. Then the blood, which was still warm, was injected into an intravenous line inserted into the baby.

7. Human blood substitutes derived from cow's blood are being developed for use in human surgeries.

Did You Know?

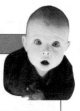

The first blood transfusion was performed in 1818 by Dr. James Blundell, a British obstetrician. A husband gave blood to save his wife, who was hemorrhaging after giving birth.

Box 6-35: Instructor Activity

CLOTTING FACTORS

Share this information with students.

1. Susan Turley, the author, used to work as a plasmapheresis nurse for a company that manufactures clotting factors. Unlike blood donation, which can only be done every 56 days, plasma donation can be done every few days because the body quickly replenishes the water and other contents in plasma. In the preliminary screening prior to the procedure, prospective donors are asked if they had fatty foods (eggs, sausage, etc.) for breakfast. If they answer "yes," they are not permitted to donate. The fat in the plasma interferes with the process of extracting clotting factors from the plasma. So how much fat is really in the blood after a fatty meal? The author saw for herself when a donor who had had a fatty breakfast would deny that fact and proceed to donate blood. After the unit of blood was centrifuged and the cells separated from the plasma, the plasma of this donor would look white and opaque (filled with fat) rather than clear and yellow in color! It takes the body several hours to clear this fat from the blood. Frequent fatty meals throughout the day cause the blood to constantly be in this condition, and this leads to the development of arteriosclerosis, as the fat is deposited on the artery walls.

2. In 1964, while watching a bag of frozen plasma thaw, Dr. Judith Pool, a Stanford University researcher, noticed stringy flakes settling to the bottom. These subsequently turned out to be Factor VIII and other clotting factors. Dr. Pool developed a method for separating the clotting factors from frozen plasma. Clotting factors are used to treat hemophiliac patients.

Box 6-36: Instructor Activity

STEM CELLS

Share this information with students.

South Korean scientists announced that they had cloned human stem cells. Human stem cell research is controversial because it involves the use of an actual human embryo. An alternative method known as parthenogenesis (parthen/o- means virgin) activates a cell that has not been fertilized by a sperm. In organisms like reptiles, fish, and insects, this is a common form of reproduction in which the female's egg begins to develop without union with a sperm.

Source: ScienCentralNews, www.sciencentral.com, February 12, 2004.

Experience Multimedia

See the PowerPoint presentation on the accompanying Instructor's Media Library for videos on the topic of phlebotomy.

Objective 8
Define common blood and lymphatic abbreviations

- Text page(s) 320

Teaching Strategy

Stress the importance of learning abbreviations and their full meanings.

Content Abstract

A	a blood type in the ABO blood group		**diff**	differential count of WBCs (slang)
AB	a blood type in the ABO blood group		**EBV**	Epstein-Barr virus
AIDS	acquired immunodeficiency syndrome		**ELISA**	enzyme-linked immunosorbent assay
ALL	acute lymphocytic leukemia		**eos**	eosinophils
AML	acute myelogenous leukemia		**G-CSF**	granulocyte colony-stimulating factor
B	a blood type in the ABO blood group		**GM-CSF**	granulocyte-macrophage colony-stimulating factor
basos	basophils		**GVHD**	graft-versus-host disease
BMT	bone marrow transplantation		**HCT**	hematocrit
CBC	complete blood count		**Hgb**	hemoglobin
CLL	chronic lymphocytic leukemia		**H&H**	hemoglobin and hematocrit
CML	chronic myelogenous leukemia		**HIV**	human immunodeficiency virus
cmm	cubic millimeter		**HLA**	human leukocyte antigen
DIC	disseminated intravascular coagulation		**IgA**	immunoglobulin A

(continued)

IgD	immunoglobulin D	**PMN**	polymorphonucleated leukocytes
IgE	immunoglobulin E	**polys**	polymorphonucleated leukocytes
IgG	immunoglobulin G	**PRBCs**	packed red blood cells
IgM	immunoglobulin M	**pro time**	prothrombin time (slang)
lymphs	lymphocytes	**PT**	prothrombin time
MCH	mean cell hemoglobin	**PTT**	partial thromboplastin time
MCHC	mean cell hemoglobin concentration	**RBC**	red blood cell
MCV	mean cell volume	**segs**	segmented neutrophils
mm³	cubic millimeter	**TNF**	tumor necrosis factor
mono	mononucleosis (slang)	**TPA**	tissue plasminogen activator (drug)
monos	monocytes	**WBC**	white blood cell
O	a blood type in the ABO blood group		

Box 6-38: Classroom Activity

ABBREVIATIONS

Divide the class into two, three, or four teams and have them stand in separate groups. Write a common blood and lymphatic abbreviation on the board. All of Team 1 can confer with each other (but cannot look in the textbook) to come up with the meaning of the abbreviation. Then the first student on Team 1 must come to the board and write the meaning of the abbreviation. If correct, that student goes back and rejoins the team. If incorrect, that student must sit down. Write another abbreviation on the board for Team 2 to answer, and so forth. The winners are the team with the most players left at the end of the game.

Objective 9
Correctly spell and pronounce blood and lymphatic words

- Text page(s) 333-334

Teaching Strategies

1. Impress upon the students that medical words that are mispronounced are also probably going to be misspelled.
2. Encourage students to work on both pronunciation and spelling when studying.

The chapter spelling test is included with the weekly chapter test. Dictate and spell (or xerox a handout that contains) this list of 20 spelling words. For the chapter test, select just 10 of these words to test.

1. anemia
2. coagulopathy
3. dyscrasia
4. electrophoresis
5. embolism
6. eosinophil
7. erythropoietin
8. hemolysis
9. hemophiliac
10. immunoglobulin
11. leukemia
12. lymphadenopathy
13. lymphocyte
14. macrophage
15. phlebotomy
16. purpura
17. splenectomy
18. thrombocytopenia
19. vaccination
20. venipuncture

Box 6-39: Classroom Activity

GAMES

1. From week to week, pick a different one of these spelling games to use during class. (The descriptions and instructions for the games are in the section "The Art and Craft of Teaching.")

   Beanbag Spelling Toss
   Scrabble
   Spelling Bee
   Gridlock
   Hangman

2. From week to week, pick a different one of these pronunciation games to use during class. (The descriptions and instructions for the games are in the section "The Art and Craft of Teaching.")

   Parroting
   Hieroglyphics
   Beach Ball Blast

Chapter Pronunciation Test

Have students mark these 20 words listed in the Pronunciation Checklist for the chapter. During the week, they will call your office or home answering machine and pronounce each word.

1. agglutination
2. autoimmune
3. coagulopathy
4. ecchymoses
5. fibrinogen
6. hemostasis
7. idiopathic
8. immunocompromised
9. lymphangiography
10. lymphoid
11. mononucleosis
12. morphology
13. myeloblast
14. pancytopenia
15. pernicious anemia
16. phlebotomy
17. plasmapheresis
18. polymorphonucleated leukocyte
19. reticulocyte
20. splenomegaly

Objective 10
Apply your skills by analyzing a hematology and immunology report

- Text page(s) 331–332

Content Abstract

Read the hospital Emergency Department Report and answer the questions provided.

Objective 11
Test your knowledge of hematology and immunology by completing review exercises in the textbook and the CD-ROM learning activities

- Text page(s) 322-332 (first complete all the in-chapter exercises on pp. 297-299)

Teaching Strategies

1. Assign the Chapter Review Exercises in the textbook for homework. Remind students to refer to the Answer Key at the end of the texbook to check their answers.
2. Refer to the CD-ROM Learning Activities in this section for multimedia learning experiences.

Experience Multimedia	
See the PowerPoint presentation on the accompanying Instructor's Media Library for a video on the topic of careers in phlebotomy.	

Homework Activities

1. Research a blood or lymphatic medical or surgical procedure (such as blood transfusion, bone marrow transplant, etc.) and submit a one-page typewritten report.

2. Call the national phone line for the American Red Cross Blood Donor Centers at 1-800-GIVE-LIFE. Indicate that you are a student in a medical terminology class. Ask them what qualifications a person must have to donate/who is able to donate. Who is not able to donate? Write a paper that has two lists: one that describes qualifications for donation and one that describes reasons for being unable to donate.

3. Make an appointment at a local blood donor center and donate a unit of blood. Write a one-page paper about the experience. If you have donated in the past, provide a photocopy of your blood donor card and describe a previous experience of donating blood.

4. Use an English and a medical dictionary to show what the common meaning is between the origins of these words: eosinophil, Philadelphia, and philanthropist

   Adapted from Ellen, Drake. "Using Storytelling to Teach and Learn Medical Terminology," *Perspectives on the Medical Transcription Profession,* Summer 2002, pp. 10-12.

5. Research and write a one-page paper about the personal story, symptoms, diagnosis, treatment, and aftermath of an immune system disorder as it affected one of these famous people.

   AIDS

Arthur Ashe	Tennis player
Rudy Galindo	Ice skater
Halston	Fashion designer
Rock Hudson	Actor
"Magic" Johnson	Basketball player
Liberace	Pianist entertainer
Greg Louganis	Olympic diver
Rudolf Nureyev	Ballet dancer

   Lymphoma

Dick Gregory	Civil rights activist and comedian
King Hussein	King of Jordan
Charles Lindbergh	Aviator
Mickey Mantle, Jr.	Baseball player
Roger Maris	Baseball player
Jackie Kennedy Onassis	Former first lady
Mr. T	Actor

6. Explore the National Immunization Program at the Centers for Disease Control's Web site at *http://www.cdc.gov/nip*. Research what immunizations are required and recommended. Then compare your own (or your child's) personal immunization record to determine if your immunizations are up to date.

7. Keep a running list in your notebook of sound-alike words or combining forms that have the same meanings. Title this list of challenging words and word parts as "Perplexing Pairs." Begin by writing down the words or word parts found in the Word Alert boxes in this chapter. Then add the word parts found in the It's Greek to Me box at the end of this chapter. Add any other words or word parts that you found particularly confusing. You will add to this list as you complete each chapter. Examples:

orth/o-	vs.	arthr/o-
myel/o-	vs.	my/o-
perine/o-	vs.	peritone/o-
cephal/o-	vs.	encephal/o-

8. Explore the Web site *www.afscme.org/health/faq.bbp.htm* and read about the Bloodborne Pathogens (BBP) Guidelines from the Occupational Safety and Health Administration (OSHA).

9. Visit this Web site and watch a video clip to see how to make a blood smear on a slide:

http://cal.vet.upenn.edu/dxendopar/techniques/bloodsmear.html

This activity requires Quick Time to play the video segment.

An introductory page comes up first. In the middle of that page, click on the underlined words

To view a Quick Time Video of the procedure, click here.

On the next page, click on the tiny arrow button at the bottom left below the picture with the hands. There is no sound to this video. The video clip will continue to repeat until you click on the double bar button at the bottom left to stop.

The blood smear technique is used to do a manual white blood cell count or to examine blood cell abnormalities. This technique requires time to master. A drop of blood is placed on one end of a glass slide. The drop is touched with the edge of a second glass slide that is held at an angle of 30 degrees. The blood is allowed to move across the entire edge of the angled slide. Then the technician quickly spreads the blood in one smooth motion so that if forms a layer across the slide. The resulting smear must be thinly and evenly spread with a "feathered" final edge where the blood cells are spread out and easy to examine. The slide is then allowed to air dry and fixative and stains are applied before the slide is viewed under the microscope.

10. Visit this Web site and do a computer-generated simulation of an electrophoresis laboratory test. Go to *www.rit.edu/~pac8612/electron/E_Sim.html* (note: after the /E_ there is an underline). Test an unknown protein against several known proteins to determine what it is.

Click on *Electrophoresis of Proteins,* which will take you to the next page.

Set the parameters on the left-hand side of the screen.

1. For the heading "Animation Speed," select "moderate."
2. For the "Unknown Protein," select "Unknown #4."
3. For "% Acrylamide" (the electrophoresis gel), select "7.5%."
4. For "Standards," click in every box in the vertical column to put a check mark. These will be the seven proteins whose electrophoresis pattern is already known. You will be comparing them to "Unknown #4."
5. For "Voltage," select "100V."
6. On the right side, look at the graphic that depicts the electrophoresis cell with gel in it. At the top left, notice the black negative electrode, and at the bottom right notice the red positive electrode. These create a current of electricity that pulls the known and unknown proteins through the gel.

Begin the electrophoresis.

1. Click on the box on the left labeled "Add Standard." Watch as a pipette appears and puts a solution of the seven known proteins (the "standards") in a well in the gel.
2. Click on the box labeled "Add Sample." Watch as a pipette appears and puts the solution of your "Unknown 4" protein in a different well in the gel.
3. Before you begin, find the vertical scale on the right side of the gel, and identify number 5 near the bottom.
4. Click on the box labeled "Start Run."
5. Watch as the seven different known proteins (different colored lines) begin to migrate through the gel at varying speeds toward the positive electrode. Also watch the black line representing the unknown protein as it moves through the gel.
6. Both the standards and the unknown begin with a purple line. When those purple lines reach the level of number 5 near the bottom of the gel, click on the box labeled "Stop Run."
7. Find the black line that represents the "Unknown #4" protein. See if it exactly matches the position of any of the colored lines of the "Standard" proteins. If so, then you have identified your unknown protein. Look in the key to find out what that colored line represents in the list of standard proteins. Your "Unknown" protein is actually that "Standard" protein.

Note: Do not let the two purple lines go off the edge of the gel. If this happens, or if you want to run the test again, just click on the box "Add Standard" and then on "Add Sample." Then click on "Start Run."

Word Search

Complete this word search puzzle that contains Chapter 6 words. Look for the following words as given in the list below. The number in parentheses indicates how many times the word is found in the puzzle.

anemia
baso
blood
cell
cells
clot
coagulation
erythrocyte
fibrin
heme

hemoglobin
immune
leukemia
lymphoma
mono
node (2)
plasma
seg (2)
serum
transfusion

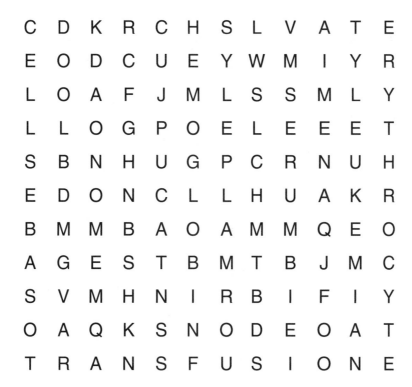

C D K R C H S L V A T E
E O D C U E Y W M I Y R
L O A F J M L S S M L Y
L L O G P O E L E E E T
S B N H U G P C R N U H
E D O N C L L H U A K R
B M M B A O A M M Q E O
A G E S T B M T B J M C
S V M H N I R B I F I Y
O A Q K S N O D E O A T
T R A N S F U S I O N E

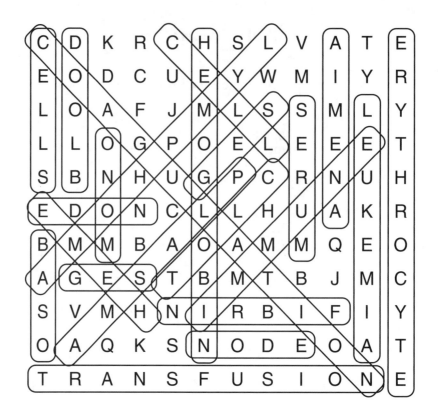

Dermatology
Integumentary System

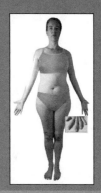

Share this information with students.

1. In 1959, author John Howard Griffin wrote *Black Like Me.* He was a middle-aged white man who, through a combination of exposure to ultraviolet light, oral medication, and skin dyes, was able to change the pigment of his skin over several weeks, so that eventually he appeared to be black. He traveled from his home in Texas to New Orleans where he posed as a black man. He was shocked by the level of racism and prejudice he encountered. After his skin color returned to white and his book was published, he received so many death threats that he moved his family to Mexico.

2. All races of people have the same number of pigment-producing cells (melanocytes) in their skin. The differences in skin color occur because of different levels of the production of melanin, a dark brown to black pigment. Even people who are albino have a normal number of melanocytes, but their cells do not produce any melanin.

3. Sunless tanners, also called self-tanners or tanning extenders, are chemicals that interact with amino acids on the skin's surface to make your skin look tan.

Are you ready to explore the *deeper layers* of knowledge? In this chapter you'll learn about the integumentary system. You'll move beyond *scratching the surface* once you master the medical language of dermatology.

Objective 1
Identify the anatomical structures of the integumentary system by correctly labeling them on anatomical illustrations

- Text page(s) 338-343

Teaching Strategy

Explain the importance of learning the parts of the integumentary system.

Content Abstract

Dermatology is the study of the skin. It is a healthcare specialty that studies the anatomy and physiology of the integumentary system and uses diagnostic tests, medical and surgical procedures, and drugs to treat integumentary diseases.

The integumentary system consists of the:

1. skin (epidermis, dermis, and subcutaneous tissue)
2. sebaceous and sweat glands
3. hair
4. nails

Box 7-1: Instructor Activity

INTERESTING FACTS

Share this information with students.

1. The skin is the largest organ in the human body.

2. Every minute, you shed between 30,000 and 40,000 dead skin cells from your body. Over the course of your lifetime, you will have shed 40 pounds of skin.

   Source: Fun Science Facts www.hightechscience.org/funfacts.htm

3. In the embryo, hair follicles and sweat glands form at 2 months before birth. At 4 months before birth, the hair begins to grow. At 5 months before birth, the nails begin to grow. At 6 months before birth, vernix caseosa and lanugo develop on the skin. The vernix caseosa protects the skin from constant exposure to amniotic fluid.

4. If your skin could be laid flat, it would cover about the area of a billiard table.

5. The average person has 5,000 hairs growing all over the body at the rate of about 1/2 inch per month. If those hairs were placed in a row end to end, they would have grown 37 miles by the end of a year. The only parts of your body where there are no hair follicles are the palms, soles, lips, tip of the penis (in men), and the clitoris and labia minora (in women).

   Source: *Reader's Digest,* "The Sense That Shapes Our Future," January 1992.

6. Fingernails grow at a rate of about 1 1/2 inches per year. Toenails grow at a rate of about 1/2 to 1 inch per year.

   Source: *The Human Body,* TimeLife Books.

7. Smoking causes wrinkles. Research has shown that cigarette smoke interferes with the body's ability to renew skin and causes premature aging.

8. It is the oil from the sebaceous glands that leave a fingerprint. Acetic acid can temporarily smooth out the fingerprints, but because they originate in the bottom, growing layer of the epidermis, they quickly return. The only way to permanently remove the fingerprints is to remove the skin on the tip of each finger and replace it with skin grafts. This painful and disfiguring operation was done on a few gangsters in the 1930s to avoid getting prosecuted for crimes. A positive fingerprint identification results in a conviction for a crime 93 percent of the time.

   Source: Simson Garfinkel, *Database Nation: The Death of Privacy in the 21st Century,* 2001.

9. A hippopotamus secretes thick, oily, pink-colored sweat.

10. Trichotillomania is the repetitive pulling out of hair from the head. *Trich/o-* means *hair, till/o-* means *to pull out,* and *-mania* means *a condition of frenzy.* Trichotillomania is not a dermatology disease; it is a psychiatric disease that falls in the category of impulse control disorders. This same category also includes kleptomania, pathological gambling, and fire-setting (pyromania).

11. Susan Turley, the author, recently drove an expensive rental car and was impressed by the gee-whiz Fingerprint Recognition Pad. Once the car's computer recognized her fingerprint, it world adjust the seat, mirror, etc., to suit her. Someone said, "But it would be fooled if you had an identical twin, wouldn't it?" He, like so many other people, wrongly thought that identical twins have identical fingerprints.

12. Are the fingerprints identical in identical twins? Interestingly, they are not! This can be explained by the fact their DNA is identical, but once they are separate, their DNA undergoes various micro-mutations as the embryo develops. Some things are programmed into DNA and express themselves identically in identical twins, while other things are more a product of the environment. The environment of the uterus can be slightly different for each twin. Fingerprints are created between the week 13 and 19 of gestation. If the fingertips of the fetus are compressed, they are more likely to develop an arch on the fingerprint. If the fingertips are swollen, they are more likely to develop a whorl pattern of ridges on the fingerprint.

    Source: ABC News, Great Moments in Science, at www.abc.net.au/science/k2/moments/s1234875.htm.

    Source: Howard Hughes Medical Institute, Ask a Scientist, at www.hhmi.org/cgi-bin/askascientist.html

13. Henry Faulds, a Scottish doctor, was the first person to solve a crime by using fingerprints. He described his technique in a letter to the scientific journal *Nature* in 1880.

    Source: ABC News, Great Moments in Science, at www.Abc.net.au/science/k2/moments/s1234875.htm.

Box 7-2: Classroom Activity

SUBCUTANEOUS LAYER

The subcutaneous tissue is a layer of fat beneath the skin. Find the thickness of the subcutaneous tissue in various parts of your body. First, use your fingers to pinch the skin on the back of your hand. Now use your fingers to pinch the skin on your abdomen. The subcutaneous tissue layer is thin in some areas and thick in other areas. If a person keeps eating more calories than the body needs, the excess calories are stored as fat in the lipocytes. Lipocytes do not divide; they just grow bigger and bigger.

The subcutaneous layer is what is removed when a patient undergoes liposuction and body sculpting.

Obesity in childhood is rising at an alarming rate. Over the past 30 years, the rate of obesity for children (ages 2 to 5) and adolescents (ages 12 to 19) has doubled, while the rate of obesity for children (ages 6 to 11) has more than tripled. As many as a third of 9-year-old girls have already tried dieting.

Source: Institute of Medicine (IOM), *Fact Sheet: Childhood Obesity in the United States,* September 2004.

Obese patients in the hospital who have abdominal surgery face the very real possibility of having their suture line dehisce. That means the sutures pull out because they had to be inserted through the fat layer which was very thick and not solid like skin, and the edges of the skin incision pull apart.

Objective 2
Describe the process of an allergic reaction

- Text page(s) 344

Teaching Strategy

Explain the physiology of an allergic reaction.

Content Abstract

 An allergy or allergic reaction is a hypersensitivity response to certain types of antigens known as allergens. A local reaction occurs when an allergen touches the skin or mucous membranes of a hypersensitive individual. A systemic reaction occurs when allergens are inhaled or ingested by or injected into a hypersensitive person, causing symptoms in one or more body systems.

Experience Multimedia
See the PowerPoint presentation on the accompanying Instructor's Media Library for animations and videos on the following topics covered in this chapter: • Inflammation • Shock

Objective 3
Build integumentary words from combining forms, prefixes, and suffixes

- Text page(s) 348-349

Box 7-3: Classroom Activity
MEDICAL TERMINOLOGY BEE Create a PowerPoint presentation with combining forms, prefixes, and suffixes with their meanings. Use this presentation in class. All students participate in a "medical terminology bee." All students stand and take turns defining the combining form, prefix, or suffix displayed. If the student gets the answer right, the student remains standing and continues to play. If the student gets the answer wrong, the student will be seated and is out of the game. The last person standing is the winner. A prize could be given to the winner.

Objective 4
Describe common integumentary diseases

- Text page(s) 350-369

Content Abstract

Disease	Meaning
Dermatitis	Any inflammation of the skin
Edema	Accumulation of excessive amounts of fluid in the skin
Hemorrhage	Bleeding in the skin
Lesion	Any area of damage or disease in the skin
Neoplasm	Any benign or malignant new growth that occurs on or in the skin (see Box 7-4)
Pruritus	Itching
Xeroderma	Excessive dryness of the skin
Albinism	Genetic condition where melanocytes do not produce melanin
Cyanosis	Bluish-gray discoloration of the skin and nails due to decreased oxygen levels in the blood (see Box 7-5)
Erythema	Reddish discoloration of the skin
Jaundice	Yellowish discoloration of the skin and whites of the eyes
Necrosis	Black discoloration of the skin due to tissue death
Pallor	Paleness of the skin due to a decreased flow of blood
Vitiligo	White, depigmented patches interspersed with normally pigmented skin (see Box 7-7)
Abrasion	Injury that removes the epidermis; a brush burn
Blister	Injury that separates the epidermis from the dermis and the area fills with tissue fluid
Burn	Damage to the skin caused by heat, electricity, chemicals, or radiation
Callus	Injury that causes the epidermis to gradually thicken
Cicatrix	Fibrous tissue composed of collagen that replaces injured skin tissue as the injury heals (see Box 7-9)
Decubitus ulcer	Injury in which the skin dies and breaks down to form a shallow or deep wound (see Box 7-10)
Laceration	Deep, penetrating wound across the skin
Abscess	Localized, pus-containing infection caused by bacteria
Cellulitis	Spreading infection of the skin and then connective tissue
Herpes	Viral infection of the skin
Tinea	Fungal infection of the skin in the warm, moist, environment of body creases and areas enclosed by clothing or shoes

(continued)

Disease	Meaning
Verruca	Rough lesions caused by the human papillomavirus; warts
Pediculosis	Infestation with lice (see Box 7-11)
Scabies	Infestation with mites
Contact dermatitis	Local reaction to contact with an allergen or irritant
Urticaria	Edema of the skin with wheals caused by an allergic reaction
Actinic keratoses	Rough, dry, raised areas from chronic sun exposure
Dysplastic nevus	Mole with irregular edges; it can develop into skin cancer
Hemangioma	Growth of superficial and dilated blood vessels
Lipoma	Tumor of adipose tissue
Nevus	Skin lesion present at birth that includes moles or port-wine stains
Papilloma	Soft, flesh-colored skin growth; skin tag
Senile lentigo	Flat, dark areas on the hands or face due to age and sun exposure
Syndactyly	Congenital abnormality in which the skin and soft tissues are joined between several fingers or toes
Xanthoma	Yellow plaque on the hands, elbows, knees, or feet
Cancer of the skin	Malignant condition of the epidermis (malignant melanoma, squamous cell carcinoma, or basal cell carcinoma) (see Box 7-12)
Kaposi's sarcoma	Cancer commonly seen only in AIDS patients (see Box 7-13)
Psoriasis	Autoimmune disease with continuous scaly silver plaques
Systemic lupus erythematosis	Autoimmune disease with degeneration of connective tissue
Scleroderma	Autoimmune disease with hardening of skin and internal organs
Acne vulgaris	Common acne of adolescence (see Box 7-14)
Acne rosacea	Acne of middle age with pustules and blotchy erythema; men can develop enlarged, lumpy noses (rhinophyma)
Alopecia	Acute or chronic loss of scalp hair (see Box 7-15)
Folliculitis	Infection of the hair follicles
Hirsutism	Excessive dark hair on the forearms and upper lip of a woman
Pilonidal sinus	Fistula that is a dimple on the skin of the sacrum and then continues through a hair follicle and into the subcutaneous tissue
Schizotrichia	Split ends on the hairs (not a disease)
Onychomyocosis	Fungal infection of the nails
Paronychia	Inflammation of the skin along the cuticle
Clubbing	Curved deformity of the nail due to chronic lack of oxygen

Box 7-4: Instructor Activity

METRIC SYSTEM

Share this information with students

While the United States uses inches to measure things, medical practice throughout the world uses the metric system. The size of a lesion, neoplasm, or tumor is expressed in centimeters or millimeters.

Box 7-5: Instructor Activity

SKIN COLOR

Share this information with students

The condition of the skin often reflects disease in a major organ of the body. Cyanosis of the skin is due to disease of the lungs. Refer to Figure 4-9 on page 171. Jaundice is due to underlying liver disease. The skin and the whites of the eyes become yellow. Refer to Figure 15-13 on page 823.

Box 7-6: Classroom Activity

DERMATOLOGY

Susan Turley, the author, once worked for a dermatologist who liked to impress her patients! When they would show her a rash on their skin and ask what it was, the dermatologist would say, "You have a macular papular erythematous rash." The patients thought this was a diagnosis when, in fact, it was more of a description of the rash. Can you describe the rash?

    Macular means _____
    Papular means _____
    Erythematous means _____

[This literally means "You have a sometimes flat, sometimes raised, reddish rash." It sounded impressively like a diagnosis, but it was really only a description.]

Box 7-7: Instructor Activity

VITILIGO

Share this information with students.

During a television interview with Oprah Winfrey, singer Michael Jackson stated that the paleness of his skin now compared to his skin when he was younger is due to the skin condition vitiligo.

Source: Wikipedia, the free Encyclopedia on the Internet.

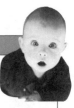

PEDICOLOSIS

Share this information with students

Head lice are common among schoolchildren because kids tend to share combs and hats. Scabies in humans is caused by the same parasite that causes mange in dogs.

SKIN CANCER

Share this information with students.

1. More than one million Americans develop skin cancer each year. It is now the most common type of cancer.

   Source: ScienCentralNews at www.sciencentral.com, January 16, 2005.

2. As a young woman, Shonda Schilling loved the sun. She'd spend hours at the beach. In college as a journalism major, she found that a tanning booth could help her maintain her beautiful bronze look all year round. She met baseball player Curt Schilling and had three children. Then when she was 33 and her children were all under the age of six, she was diagnosed with skin cancer. She has had seven surgeries to remove malignant melanomas from her back, legs, chest, and arms. Fortunately, in each case the cancer had not spread elsewhere in her body. She says, "Malignant melanoma is the leading cancer killer of women ages 20 to 29. People are blown away by that when we tell them." Fair-skinned people are 20 times more likely to develop skin cancer than African-Americans. According to a Florida dermatologist, the incidence of skin cancer has triped between 1980 and 2003, due in part to the availability of tanning booths since the 1980s. Their rays are equally as destructive as those of the sun. One out of every five children will develop skin cancer.

   Source: Linell Smith, "More Than Skin Deep," *The Baltimore Sun,* September 23, 2005.

3. Everyone has heard the warnings about not spending long amounts of time in the sun without the use of sunscreen. However, getting too little sun actually increases your risk of colon, prostate, breast, and digestive tract cancer by up to 30 times because the cancer-preventing effect of vitamin D is not present. It is now recommended that you spend 15 minutes in the sun (without sunscreen) three or four times a week to generate vitamin D in your skin.

   Source: Parade Magazine (Sunday newspaper supplement), 2005.

KAPOSI'S SARCOMA

Share this information with students.

Kaposi's sarcoma (refer students to Figure 18-8 on page 960) is an opportunistic cancer that is seen nearly exclusively in AIDS patients.

Box 7-14: Instructor Activity

ACNE

Share this information with students.

1. Although today we think of something vulgar as being disgusting or obscene, the word *vulgar* had a different meaning in the Middle Ages. *Vulgar* meant *common.* There were the noblemen and everyone else was considered to be common or vulgar.
2. Acne rosacea was well known in the Middle Ages as shown in the painting, *Portrait of an Old Man and a Young Boy* by Italian Renaissance painter Domenico Ghirlandaio (1449-1494). The old man has the enlarged and lumpy nose characteristic of rhinophyma, a complication of acne rosacea.

Box 7-15: Instructor Activity

ALOPECIA

Share this information with students.

For thousands of years, men have smeared smelly stuff on their scalps in a vain attempt to treat baldness. Cleopatra reportedly put a concoction of bear grease, burned mice, deer marrow, and horse teeth on Caesar. Other remedies have included pigeon droppings, horseradish, and buffalo dung. Minoxidil (Rogaine) was the first medicine shown actually to stimulate hair growth.

Source: Susan Turley, *Understanding Pharmacology for Health Professionals.* Prentice Hall.

Experience Multimedia

See the PowerPoint presentation on the accompanying Instructor's Media Library for animations and videos on the following topics covered in this chapter:

- Acne
- Integumentary repair
- Eczema
- Pressure ulcers
- Decubitus ulcers
- Herpes
- Skin cancer

Objective 5
Describe common integumentary diagnostic laboratory tests

- Text page(s) 369-370

Content Abstract

Test	Definition
Allergy skin testing	Various antigens are given by intradermal injections in the forearm
Culture and sensitivity	A specimen of the exudate from an ulcer, wound, burn, or laceration or the pus from an infection is cultured in a Petri dish to diagnose a bacterial infection
Skin scraping	Done with the edge of a scalpel to obtain material from certain skin lesions, examine it under a microscope, and make a diagnosis

Objective 6
Describe common integumentary medical and surgical procedures and drug categories

- Text page(s) 370-375

Content Abstract

Procedure	Definition
Botox injections	Medical procedure to release deep wrinkles (see Box 7-16)
Collagen injections	Medical procedure to decrease the depth of wrinkles or scars
Cryosurgery	Medical procedure with liquid nitrogen to freeze a benign or malignant lesion
Curettage	Medical procedure that involves using a curette to scrape off the superficial part of a skin lesion
Debridement	Medical or surgical procedure in which necrotic tissue is debrided from a burn, wound, or ulcer
Electrosurgery	Medical procedure that uses electrical current to remove a small lesion or benign or malignant tumor
Incision and drainage	Medical procedure that makes an incision to let out fluid or pus
Laser surgery	Medical procedure that uses a laser to remove lesions
Skin resurfacing	Medical procedure that uses chemicals, a wire brush, crystals, or a laser to smooth the skin surface
Suturing	Medical procedure to bring together the cut edges of a laceration

(continued)

Procedure	Definition
Biopsy	Surgical procedure to remove some or all of a lesion by using a scalpel, needle, punch, or razor blade
Dermatoplasty	Any type of plastic surgery procedure on the skin
Liposuction	Surgical procedure to remove adipose fat through a cannula (see Box 7-20)
Mohs' surgery	Surgical procedure to remove skin cancer
Rhytidectomy	Surgical procedure to tighten the skin and remove wrinkles
Skin grafting	Surgical procedure to use human, animal, or artificial skin to cover a burn

Drug Category	Description	Example
Antibiotic drugs	Treat bacterial infections of the skin (see Box 7-22)	Bacitracin, Neomycin
Antifungal drugs	Treat ringworm	Desenex, Lamisil AT, Lotrimin, Tinactin
Antipruritic drugs	Decrease itching	Benadryl, Caladryl
Antiviral drugs	Treat herpes simplex	Famvir, Valtrex, Zovirax

Box 7-16: Instructor Activity

BOTOX

Share this information with students.

Gordon Nelson is the first brave soul to go under the needle, surrounded by a group of curious women sipping Diet Coke or red wine and eating strawberries. He's a pleasant, fit-looking man in his late 30s whose whole face is relatively un-lined by the standards of most of the people gathered here at the salon and day spa. But those pesky furrows across his forehead bother him, so he's having them injected with Botox, the hottest weapon in the fight against Father Time. [In 2002] the Food and Drug Administration approved Botox Cosmetic for one specific use, to soften the vertical frown lines between the eyebrows. With that approval, people have become more comfortable with the idea of using botulinum toxin type A—the same deadly poison that might be found in a soup can with a bulging lid—as an anti-aging drug. For therapeutic and cosmetic use, of course, the toxin has been purified and diluted. Botox temporarily relaxes the muscles that cause wrinkle lines. This costs about $300 but needs to be repeated three or four times every year . . . Botox injections have become a part of our culture. Botox parties [like the one described above] include a brief lecture by a physician and a question and answer session and then injections for those who want them, either privately or in front of the group.

Source: Elizabeth Large, "Botox: A Shot of Youth," *The Baltimore Sun,* May 26, 2002.

Box 7-17: Instructor Activity

BAND-AID

Share this information with students.

In 1920, the Band-Aid was invented by an employee of Johnson & Johnson.

Box 7-18: Instructor Activity

MAGGOTS

The Food and Drug Administration (FDA) approved the sale of maggots as medical devices to remove dead tissue from ulcers and nonhealing surgical wounds and the sale of leeches to remove collections of blood under the skin.

Source: The Pittsburgh Post-Gazette Newspaper, July 13, 2004.

Box 7-19: Instructor Activity

MOLE REMOVAL

Share this information with students.

Susan Turley, the author, worked for a dermatologist at one time. Once a patient came in to have a mole removed from her back. The patient laid on the examination table with her face to the wall. After the mole was removed, the doctor held it with tweezers to transfer it to a small pathology specimen jar to be sent to the laboratory. Unfortunately, she missed the container and dropped the mole on the floor. It rolled right under the examining table, and the author had to get on her hands and knees to retrieve it. It was covered with some hairs and dust, but was washed off and then inserted in the specimen jar.

Box 7-20: Instructor Activity

LIPOSUCTION

Share this information with students.

In 2003, over 300,000 Americans had liposuction.

Source: ScienCentralNews, www.sciencentral.com

Box 7-21: Instructor Activity

ACCUTANE

Share this information with students.

The drug isotretinoin (Accutane) is used to treat severe cystic acne. However, it has also been linked to side effects of suicide attempts.

> On that snowy January day, Brandon Troppman seemed to be loving life. He put on a new shirt and combed his hair just so before heading to the mall to hang out with his high school sweetheart . . . At 6:30 that evening, he talked on the phone with his best friend, laughing and making his friend laugh. An hour later, he hanged himself from a rod in his bedroom closet.

> Congressman Bart Stupak from Michigan publicly blamed the drug for his 17-year-old son's suicide. During his own investigation, he found an internal FDA memo that stated: "Given all of the pieces of evidence available, it is difficult to avoid the conclusion that Accutane use is associated with severe psychiatric disease in some patients."

Source: Susan Turley, *Understanding Pharmacology for Health Professionals.* Prentice Hall.

Box 7-22: Instructor Activity

INTEGUMENTARY DRUGS

Share this information with students.

1. In 1979, Ciba-Geigy introduced the first transdermal (through the skin) patch drug delivery system. The drug was scopolamine for motion sickness.

   Source: Susan Turley, *Understanding Pharmacology for Health Professionals.* Prentice Hall.

2. In 1928, the Scottish bacteriologist Alexander Fleming concluded experiments looking for drugs that would inhibit the growth of staphylococcus, a common bacterium on the skin. He left for vacation and instructed an assistant to wash the culture plates that were soaking in the sink. When Fleming returned from his vacation, the plates had not been washed. One culture plate remained above the water, and on it had grown a blue-green mold which clearly had killed the staphylococcus. Fleming called this mold *Penicillium notatum.* However, Fleming was unable to extract a drug from it. (The mold itself contained only one part penicillin per two million parts mold.) He wrote a paper about his findings but they remained largely unknown in the scientific world. During World War II, however, there were two researchers in England working with the penicillin mold. They were afraid that their entire supply might be destroyed in the bombings of London. Therefore, they smeared some of the mold inside their coat jackets and brought it to the United States to be produced. A 43-year-old policeman was the first person to be injected with penicillin. He was dying from septicemia (blood poisoning) that had begun as an abscess when he scratched his face on a rosebush. Penicillin was in such short supply that his urine had to be saved each day, and the penicillin extracted from it for the next day's drug dose. He was given the world's entire supply of penicillin. He responded well, but on the fifth day of treatment the supply of penicillin ran out. He relapsed and died. Later researchers discovered a different strain of *Penicillium* on a moldy cantaloupe in Peoria, Illinois. It was approximately 20 times stronger than the original strain and could be grown in large vats. By 1945, penicillin had become a household word and the word *antibiotic* was coined as well.

3. In 1934, a German researcher was screening chemicals for possible medicinal use. A red dye used to color cloth was tested and seemed to cure streptococcal infections in mice. The researcher's own daughter was dying of streptococcal septicemia from pricking her finger. In desperation, he injected her with the dye and she recovered. The red dye was converted in the body into the anti-infective drug sulfanilamide and became the first of the sulfa drugs.

   Source: Susan Turley, *Understanding Pharmacology for Health Professionals.* Prentice Hall.

4. The drug coal tar is often used to treat psoriasis. Coal tar is a by-product of the processing of bituminous coal. It contains over 10,000 different chemicals and has been used since the 1800s to treat psoriasis.

   Source: Susan Turley, *Understanding Pharmacology for Health Professionals.* Prentice Hall.

5. Nonprescription drugs used to treat lice contain the active ingredient pyrethrin, which is derived from chrysanthemums. The drug acts on the nervous system of the parasite to paralyze it. Pyrethrin is also a common ingredient in flea powder for dogs and cats. The word *nitpicking,* meaning *to point out tiny details,* comes from the process of picking through the hair looking for lice eggs, which are called *nits.*

   Source: Susan Turley, *Understanding Pharmacology for Health Professionals.* Prentice Hall.

Objective 7
Define common integumentary abbreviations

- Text page(s) 377

Teaching Strategies

1. Stress the importance of learning abbreviations and their full meanings.
2. Encourage students to make flashcards for abbreviations and their meanings as well as their usual flashcards for word parts and their meanings.

Content Abstract

Bx	biopsy
Ca	cancer (slang)
C&S	culture and sensitivity
Derm	dermatology (slang)
HSV	herpes simplex virus

I&D	incision and drainage
PDT	photodynamic therapy
PUVA	psoralen drug and ultraviolet A light (therapy)
SLE	systemic lupus erythematosus
SQ, subcu, subQ	subcutaneous

Objective 8
Correctly spell and pronounce integumentary words

- Text page(s) 391-392

Teaching Strategies

1. Impress upon the students that medical words that are mispronounced are also probably going to be misspelled.
2. Encourage students to work on both pronunciation and spelling when studying.

Chapter Spelling Test

The chapter spelling test is included with the weekly chapter test. Dictate and spell (or xerox a handout that contains) this list of 20 spelling words. Give the list to students the week before the test. For the chapter test, select just 10 of these words to test.

1. adipose
2. anaphylaxis
3. cutaneous
4. sebaceous
5. vesicle
6. pruritus
7. xeroderma
8. cyanosis
9. erythema
10. callus
11. cicatrix
12. decubitus ulcer
13. abscess
14. tinea pedis
15. pediculosis
16. psoriasis
17. seborrhea
18. alopecia
19. onychomycosis
20. rhytidectomy

Box 7-23: Classroom Activity

GAMES

1. From week to week, pick a different one of these spelling games to use during class. (The descriptions and instructions for the games are in the section "The Art and Craft of Teaching.")

   Beanbag Spelling Toss

   Scrabble

   Spelling Bee

   Gridlock

   Hangman

2. From week to week, pick a different one of these pronunciation games to use during class. (The descriptions and instructions for the games are in the section "The Art and Craft of Teaching.")

   Parroting

   Hieroglyphics

   Beach Ball Blast

Chapter Pronunciation Test

Have students mark these 20 words listed in the Pronunciation Checklist for the chapter. During the week, they will call your office or home answering machine and pronounce each word.

1. alopecia
2. anaphylaxis
3. blepharoplasty
4. cicatrix
5. comedo
6. curettage
7. debridement
8. diaphoresis
9. ecchymosis
10. eczema
11. erythematous
12. Kaposi's sarcoma
13. onychomycosis
14. paronychia
15. psoralens
16. rhytidectomy
17. seborrheic
18. urticaria
19. xanthelasma
20. xeroderma

Objective 9
Apply your skills by analyzing a dermatology report

- Text page(s) 388-390

Content Abstract

Read the two office chart notes and answer the questions provided.

Box 7-24: Classroom Activity

MEDICAL REPORTS

Have students find and circle these words in the medical report: pruritus, erythema, erythematous, nodule, edematous, cellulitis, urticaria. Have the students look in their book and write out a description or definition for each circled medical word. Then begin reading the report by having a student read the first header or sentence from the medical reports on pages 388 and 389. If one of the circled words occurs in that sentence, the student must also give their description or definition of that medical word. The next student reads the next header or sentence until the report is finished. This is to familiarize students with reading medical reports and analyzing words while also gaining practice in pronouncing words.

Objective 10
Test your knowledge of dermatology by completing review exercises in the textbook and the CD-ROM learning activities

- Text page(s) 380-390

Teaching Strategies

1. Assign the Chapter Review Exercises in the textbook for homework. Remind students to refer to the Answer Key at the end of the textbook to check their answers.
2. Refer to the CD-ROM Learning Activities in this section for multimedia learning experiences.

Experience Multimedia

See the PowerPoint presentation on the accompanying Instructor's Media Library for videos on the topic of careers in physician assisting.

Homework Activities

1. Write 10 sentences that contain abbreviations from this chapter or any of the previous chapters. On a separate page, write an answer key that gives what each abbreviation stands for. In class, exchange papers with a student near you. Translate the abbreviations in the paper you have been given and write them down. After a few minutes, exchange answer keys. Check to see if you gave the correct meaning of the abbreviations.

2. Make a list of tanning salons in your local area. Call one salon and inquire as to the safeness of tanning with respect to skin cancer.

3. Watch a plastic surgery or cosmetic makeover show on television and write down all the medical words you hear. Then write definitions for those words.

4. Visit the Internet and gather information about the Rule of Nines System for describing burns. Draw a figure (front and back) showing the Rule of Nines System.

5. Keep a running list in your notebook of sound-alike words or combining forms that have the same meanings. Title this list of challenging words and word parts as "Perplexing Pairs." Begin by writing down the words or word parts found in the Word Alert boxes in this chapter. Then add the word parts found in the It's Greek to Me box at the end of this chapter. Add any other words or word parts that you found particularly confusing. You will add to this list as you complete each chapter. Examples:

orth/o-	vs.	arthr/o-
myel/o-	vs.	my/o-
perine/o-	vs.	peritone/o-
cephal/o-	vs.	encephal/o-

6. Look in your medicine cabinet. Find 10 prescription or over-the-counter drugs. List their drug names. Also look on the label and find any medical words. Write down these medical words and then look up and write their medical definitions.

7. Interview someone who has undergone allergy skin testing. Prepare a list of questions to be used during the interview based on this chapter and on your Internet research. Submit a one-page paper.

Word Search

Complete this word search puzzle that contains Chapter 7 words. Look for the following words as given in the list below.

adipose
burn
callus
collagen
cuticles
cyst
dermis
hair
herpes
integument
keloids

nail
necrosis
rash
sebum
skin
subcutaneous
tinea
tissues
ulcer
wheal
wound

```
S U O E N A T U C B U S
F K X R W D T N U H F U
O K I M N I I R N A I L
E A Q N S P N Z A T S L
H K P S V O E S N S W A
D C U I R S A E E D H C
B E W L E E M B C I E U
S H R P C U D U R O A T
G F R M G E G M O L L I
U E L E I T R Z S E D C
H B T L J S F D I K B L
D N U O W N E T S Y C E
I S K N E G A L L O C S
```

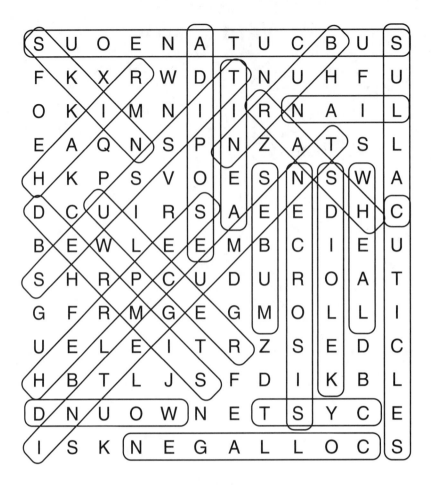

CHAPTER 8

Orthopedics

Skeletal System

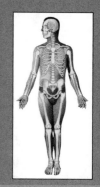

Instructor Activity for the Beginning of Class

Have students look at the anatomical illustration by Andreas Vesalius in Figure 8-8 on page 404. Note that Andreas Vesalius, who was an excellent illustrator of anatomy and whose illustrations were the first to be used in any medical book, also had a sense of humor as evidenced by this illustration of a skeleton contemplating a skull. He also included a lot of scenery in his drawings. However, this drawing of the skeleton has an artistic error. The lines of perspective are not drawn correctly. The edge of the table closest to the skeleton's chest and the edge of the base of the table by the skeleton's feet should be parallel in their orientation to correctly go to the vanishing point of the picture.

Share this information with students.

Do you want to discover just the *hard facts*? Then you'll want to study the bones of the skeletal system. You'll have *structure and support* once you master the language of the skeletal system.

Objective 1
Identify the anatomical structures of the skeletal system by correctly labeling them on anatomical illustrations

- Text page(s) 396-412

Teaching Strategy

Explain the importance of learning the parts of the skeletal system.

Content Abstract

Orthopedics is the study of the bones and joints. It is the healthcare specialty that studies the anatomy and physiology of the skeletal system and uses diagnostic tests, medical and surgical procedures, and drugs to treat skeletal diseases.

The skeleton can be divided into the axial skeleton and the appendicular skeleton. The skeletal system is composed of bones of the

1. head (cranium, facial bones, other bones of the head)
2. chest
3. neck and back
4. shoulders
5. arms
6. wrists, hands, and fingers
7. hips
8. legs
9. ankles, feet, and toes
10. joints, cartilage, and ligaments

Box 8-1: Instructor Activity

AXIAL SKELETON

Share this information with students.

1. The axial skeleton is like the axle of a car. The axle is the steady part while the wheel spins around it. The axial skeleton is the steady part while the appendicular skeleton moves around it. To remember appendicular, think of the sound-alike word appendix. The appendix is the long, hanging part that is attached to the intestine. Similarly, the four limbs are long, hanging parts attached to the axial skeleton.

2. Animal antlers are made of bone and are shed and regrown each year, while horns are made of keratin (like fingernails) and are kept for life.

Box 8-2: Classroom Activity

NAMING BONES

Create three identical pads of sticky notes with 15-20 bone names, one bone name on each sheet. Divide the class into three groups. Give one pad of sticky notes to each group. Have the group pick one person in their group who will be the anatomical model to stand with arms out and legs part. The sticky notes are divided among the group members. When the instructor says "Go," each group should stick the bone name sticky sheet to the correct location on the anatomical model. (Provide a roll of tape for each group to use if the sticky notes do not adhere well.) This is an open-book activity, so students can look up unfamiliar bones in the textbook. The first group to apply all their bone name sticky notes calls out "Stop" to end the activity. The instructor reviews the placement of their bone name sticky notes. If all are accurately placed, then that group is the winner. However, if one sheet is in the wrong spot, whichever group accurately placed the most sticky notes is the winner.

Box 8-3: Instructor Activity

BONES

Use a model skeleton, if available, to point to when talking about each bone.

Share this information with students.

1. The names of the bones of the cranium correspond to the names of the lobes of the brain which are studied in Chapter 10.

2. There are three tiny bones in the middle ear. Schoolchildren call them the hammer, anvil, and stirrup because their shapes resemble those common items. The medical names for these bones are the malleus, incus, and stapes. These bones are studied in Chapter 16.

3. The smallest bone in the body is the stapes in the middle ear. It is only 0.11 inch long.

   Source: Fun Science Facts, www.hightechscience.org/funfacts.htm

4. There is another bone in the body called the malleolus. Ask students what the difference is between the malleus and the malleolus.

5. Susan Turley, the author, once worked in the office of an ear, nose, and throat (ENT) specialist. He was a demanding employer, who usually worked right through lunch and expected his staff to do the same. He was also an avid scuba diver who went all over the world to scuba dive and take underwater pictures. He would regularly dictate letters to be transcribed and sent to the editor of *Scuba Diver* magazine about the ENT problems associated with deep sea diving. In one letter, he dictated a comment about the "malleolus" in the middle ear. As the author transcribed the letter, she looked up "malleolus" in the medical dictionary and found that it was a bony projection on the distal end of the lower leg! With much anxiety, she took her medical dictionary and presented this information to the physician, stating that he must surely have meant to say "malleus" instead of "malleolus." He examined the dictionary entries carefully and then said, "I have been saying this incorrectly for years and I didn't even know it."

6. *Clavicle* is Latin for *small key.* Early Roman physicians compared the shape of a clavicle to the S-shape of an old Roman key. The clavicle (collar bone) is the most fractured bone.

   Source: www.emedx.com

7. The xiphoid bone is the small pointed tip of the sternum. *Xiph/o-* means *sword* and *-oid* means *resembling.* Remember the name of this bone by thinking of Zorro, who used his sword to make a "Z." Imaging him using his sword to make an "X."

8. Cervical vertebrae are at the top of the neck. Ask the class if the word "cervical" sounds familiar and if they have heard it used with any other body structure. At least one student is certain to answer that it is used in relation to the female genital system. Draw this figure on the board.

   Point to the round part of the drawing and call it the uterus. State that the cervix is the neck or narrow part below the uterus. Cervix means neck. The *cervix* is the location where *cervical* cancer occurs.

   Point to the round part of the drawing again and this time call it the head. State that there is no cervix associated with the head and neck, but the cervical vertebrae are located in the neck area. The late actor Christopher Reeve broke his neck at the cervical level and the broken bone severed the spinal cord at that level.

   (continued)

Box 8-3: Instructor Activity *(continued)*

9. Remind students that Latin feminine nouns form the plural by changing -a (vertebra) to -ae (vertebrae).

10. Use these "mnifty mnemonic devices" or memory aids as you study the skeletal system. Remember the order of the cervical, thoracic, lumbar, and sacral vertebrae and coccyx and the how many **c**ervical (7), **t**horacic (12), **l**umbar (5), and **s**acral (5), and **c**occyx (4) bones there are by using this memory aid: "**C**ome **T**o **L**ovely **S**outh **C**arolina 712554."

11. The spines of the Skylab astronauts lengthened about 1 1/2 to 2 1/4 inches due to the expansion of the disks and the effect of zero gravity.

    Source: Fun Science Facts, www.hightechscience.org/funfacts.htm

12. Humerus: Refer to the Word Alert box and cartoon on page 407 and review the other words that can be confused with the name of this bone.

13. Radius and ulna: Tell students that they need to remember which of the two bones of the forearm is on the thumb side of the forearm. Ask students to show you where you a healthcare worker takes your pulse. Mention that this is by the base of the thumb. Ask if they know what the name of that pulse is. Usually one student will know that this is the radial pulse. Mention that it is called the radial pulse because it is taken in a blood vessel that goes along the radius bone. So the radius bone is on the thumb side of the forearm. The ulna is along the little finger side of the arm (and its other end contains the large square-shaped bone that forms the elbow).

Box 8-4: Classroom Activity

REVIEWING WORD PARTS

Have students look in the Glossary of Word Parts in the Appendix of the textbook. Look up the combining form radi/o- and say its three definitions. Ask them: When you see the word "radial" in an orthopedic report, which of those three definitions is the correct one? [Answer: Radius.]

Box 8-5: Instructor Activity

BONES

Share this information with students.

Carpal bones are the bones of the wrist joint. Point out that these can be confused with the sound-alike tarsal bones of the ankle joint. Use this mnifty mnemonic device to help you remember the difference between the carpal bones of the wrist and the tarsal bones of the ankle. The **car**pal bones are in the hand and **car**penters use their hands. Also you use the **carpal** bones when you **carpool** and turn the steering wheel as you drive kids to school. Whereas, the **t**arsal bones are next to the **t**oes.

Metacarpal bones. Remember that meta- means subsequent to. So these bones occur subsequent to the carpal bones as you travel down the arm toward the fingers.

Phalanges is a Greek word that means *a line of soldiers*. It refers to either the fingers or the toes. The "ph" sound in *phalanges* is the same as the "f" sound in *fingers*.

Surgeons in France made history in 1998 by performing the world's first hand transplant on a patient from New Zealand. The procedure involved connecting the bones as well as many small muscles, nerves, and blood vessels. Because the patient was not compliant with taking his immunosuppressant drugs and going to physical therapy, the hand transplant was rejected by his body. The patient asked to have the hand transplant removed, and British surgeons did this procedure in 2001.

Ilium: Refer to the Word Alert box on page 408 and review the other words that can be confused with the name of this bone.

Box 8-6: Classroom Activity

HIP BONES

Have students stand up and position their hands on their hips at the waist with their thumbs pointing posteriorly. In this position, their fingers are over the anterior-superior iliac spines, and their thumbs are over the posterior iliac crests. Have them sit down and slide their hands under their buttocks. The large, rounded bones they feel are the right and left ischium.

Box 8-7: Instructor Activity

INTERESTING FACTS ABOUT BONES

Share this information with students.

1. Coccyx. The word *coccyx* is Greek for *cuckoo bird*. The Greeks thought that the bone shape looked like the beak of the cuckoo. Not very many people today know what the beak of a cuckoo looks like!

2. Femur. The femur or thigh bone makes up about one-quarter of a person's height.

3. Patella. The patella in an infant is completely cartilage. It begins to become bone between three and five years of age and is not completely bone until the end of adolescence.

   An elephant is the only animal with four knees. (A knee bends anteriorly, while the hock of a horse or cow bends posteriorly.)

   Source: Backwoodsbound.com, Amazing Animal Facts.

4. Lateral malleolus and medial malleolus. These bones of the lower leg can be confused with the middle ear bone, the malleus.

5. Tarsal bones in the ankle joint. Remember the difference between carpal bones in the wrist and tarsal bones in the foot because *tarsal* begins with a "t" and *toes* begins with a "t."

Box 8-8: Classroom Activity

BLACKBOARD ACTIVITY

Write this incomplete table on the board. Have students fill in the blanks in the Characteristics and Example columns.

Joint Name	Characteristics	Example
Suture joint		
Symphysis joint		
Synovial joint		

Box 8-9: Instructor Activity

Share this information with students.

1. *Articul/o-* is Latin for *joint,* and *arthr/o-* is Greek for *joint.*
2. "Mnifty" mnemonic aid: You can remember that the **e**piphysis is at the **e**nd of the bone because they both begin with the letter **e.** You can remember that the diaphysis is the shaft of the bone because "diaph" rhymes with "shaft."
3. The medullary cavity is filled with yellow marrow. If a large bone like the femur is badly fractured, a piece of the yellow marrow may escape into the blood. This fat globule is known as an embolus. It travels through the blood, through the right side of the heart, but becomes lodged in one of the pulmonary arteries traveling to the lungs. Then it is known as a pulmonary embolus. Symptoms include dyspnea and chest pain.

Experience Multimedia

See the PowerPoint presentation on the accompanying Instructor's Media Library for animations on the following topics covered in this chapter:

- Classification of joints and joint movement
- Skeletal movement

Objective 2
Describe the process of growth

- Text page(s) 413-414

Teaching Strategy

Explain the importance of learning about the process of growth.

Content Abstract

Cartilaginous tissue is gradually replaced by bone in a process known as ossification. Also, new bone is formed along the epiphysial growth plates at the ends of long bones as the body grows taller.

Box 8-10: Instructor Activity

INTERESTING FACTS

Share this information with students.

1. Normally, a baby doubles its birth weight in the first four to six months and triples its birth weight by the time it is one year old.
   Source: Dr. Greene's HouseCalls: Pediatric Wisdom for the Information Age, www.drgreene.com
2. When the baby is growing, it utilizes calcium and phosphorus pulled from the mother's bones, which is why prenatal nutrition is such an important topic to discuss with pregnant women.
3. Martial arts masters are able to break concrete blocks because bones are able to withstand 40 times the force that breaks concrete.

Experience Multimedia

See the PowerPoint presentation on the accompanying Instructor's Media Library for an animation showing bone healing.

Objective 3
Build skeletal words from combining forms, prefixes and suffixes

- Text page(s) 422-423

Objective 4
Describe common skeletal diseases

- Text page(s) 424-435

Content Abstract

Disease	Meaning
Avascular necrosis	Death of cells in the epiphysis at the end of long bone
Bone tumor	Benign or malignant growth in a bone
Chondroma	Benign tumor of cartilage
Chondromalacia patellae	Abnormal softening of the patella (see Box 8-11)
Fracture	Broken bone due to an accident, injury, or disease process
Osteomalacia	Abnormal softening of bone
Osteomyelitis	Infection of the bone and bone marrow
Osteoporosis	Abnormal thinning of the bone structure (see Box 8-12)
Ankylosing spondylitis	Inflammation of the vertebrae with stiffening of the spine
Kyphosis	Abnormal, excessive, posterior curvature of the thoracic spine (see Box 8-14)
Lordosis	Abnormal, excessive, anterior curvature of the lumbar spine (see Box 8-13)
Scoliosis	Abnormal, excessive, lateral, S-shaped curvature of the spine (see Box 8-13)
Spondylolisthesis	Slipping out of alignment of one vertebra onto another (see Box 8-14)
Arthralgia	Pain in the joint
Arthropathy	Disease of a joint from any cause
Dislocation	Displacement of a bone end from its normal position in the joint
Gout	Metabolic disorder with excess uric acid in the blood with crystals in the joints and soft tissues
Hemarthrosis	Blood in the joint cavity
Lyme disease	Arthritis from the bite of an infected deer tick
Osteoarthritis	Chronic inflammatory disease of the joints (see Box 8-15)
Rheumatoid arthritis	Autoimmune disease with inflammation and deformity of the joints (see Box 8-15)
Sprain	Overstretching or tearing of a ligament
Torn meniscus	Tear of the cartilage pad of the knee
Pectus excavatum	Congenital deformity with the xiphoid process bent inward (see Box 8-16)
Genu varum	Lower legs are bent toward the midline; bowleg.
Genu valgum	Lower legs are bent outward from the midline; knocknee.
Hallux valgus	Great toe is angled laterally toward the other toes, often causing a bunion at the base of the great toe.
Talipes equinovarus	Clubfoot

Box 8-11: Instructor Activity

CHONDROMALACIA PATELLAE

Share this information with students.

In the phrase *chondromalacia patellae,* the word *patellae* is actually in the form of the genitive case, a Latin case that shows possession. So the phrase means *a condition of softening of the cartilage of the patella. Of the patella* is the phrase that shows possession. The genitive case is sometimes confused with the Latin feminine plural (which would also be *patellae*) but would not have a noun in front of it.

Box 8-12: Instructor Activity

OSTEOPOROSIS

Share this information with students.

1. Osteoporosis produces thinning bone structure that can cause a spontaneous fracture. When disease causes the fracture, it is known as a pathological fracture. *Path/o-* means disease. Often, an elderly person will fall and think that caused a fracture when, in reality, a spontaneous pathological fracture actually caused the person to fall.
2. An estimated 1.3 million fractures due to osteoporosis occur annually in the United States; 25 percent of postmenopausal women have spinal compression fractures from osteoporosis and 15 percent have hip fractures. Supermodel Lauren Hutton was featured in drug advertisements for hormone replacement therapy (a treatment for osteoporosis). She states that she disregarded her physician's advice to begin hormone replacement therapy when she experienced hot flashes at the onset of menopause. The following year, when she found her height had decreased by 1 inch (due to bone loss), she started hormone replacement therapy.

   Source: Susan Turley, *Understanding Pharmacology for Health Professionals.* Prentice Hall.

Box 8-13: Instructor Activity

LORDOSIS AND SCOLIOSIS

Share this information with students.

How can you remember the difference between lordosis, scoliosis, and kyphosis? **L**ordosis begins with an "L," as does "**l**umbar region" and "**l**ower back" where this curvature is located. **S**coliosis begins with an "S," as does "**s**ideways," which describes the way the curvature goes and "**s**choolchildren" who are routinely screened for scoliosis by the school nurse.

Box 8-14: Instructor Activity

KYPHOSIS AND SPONDYLOLISTHESIS

Share this information with students.

Susan Turley, the author, has an elderly relative who is 93 years old and suffers from kyphosis and spondylolisthesis. Her spinal x-ray shows severe deformity with several vertebrae out of alignment. The spinal nerves are pinched because of this malalignment, and she must apply a Duragesic patch every few days (it contains a narcotic) to get relief from the pain.

Box 8-15: Instructor Activity

OSTEOARTHRITIS AND RHEUMATOID ARTHRITIS

Share this information with students.

1. Two chemists from the University of Newcastle gave volunteers copper bracelets to wear for a month. At the end of the month, they gave them new bracelets that looked the same but were not made of copper. Three out of four volunteers felt better with the copper bracelets on, according to the study results published in the Swiss journal *Agents and Actions*. This could show a therapeutic effect of copper or it could be due to the placebo effect.
2. Rheumatoid arthritis affects about 2.1 million Americans and affects more women than men between the ages of 20 and 50.

Box 8-16: Instructor Activity

PECTUS EXCAVATUM

Share this information with students.

Because this condition involves a deep, curving deformity of the chest wall, it is sometimes mistakenly spelled as "excurvatum." Think of it rather as a cave that is excavated or dug out.

Experience Multimedia

See the PowerPoint presentation on the accompanying Instructor's Media Library for videos on the following topics covered in this chapter:

- Arthritis
- Osteoporosis

Objective 5
Describe common skeletal diagnostic laboratory and radiology tests

- Text page(s) 434-435

Teaching Strategy

Obtain a copy of a patient's bone density test for routine screening for osteoporosis.

Content Abstract

Test	Definition
Rheumatoid factor	Blood test that is positive in patients with rheumatoid arthritis
Arthrography	Radiologic procedure that uses a radiopaque contrast dye that is injected into a joint
Bone density tests	Radiologic procedure that measures the bone mineral density (BMD) to determine if demineralization from osteoporosis has occurred
X-ray	Radiologic procedure that uses x-rays to diagnose bony abnormalities of any part of the body

Objective 6
Describe common skeletal medical and surgical procedures and drug categories

- Text page(s) 436-441

Content Abstract

Procedure	Definition
Cast	Plaster or fiberglass is used to encase and immobilize a fracture
Closed reduction	Ends of a displaced fracture are manipulated back into alignment
Cortisone injection	Cortisone is injected into the joint for pain relief
Extracorporeal shock wave therapy (ESWT)	Sound waves are used to break up bone spurs
Goniometry	A goniometer is used to measure the angle of the joints and range of motion

(continued)

Procedure	Definition
Orthosis	Brace, splint, or collar to immobilize
Physical therapy	Active or passive range of motion to improve patient's condition
Prosthesis	Orthopedic device like an artificial leg
Traction	Weights pull apart the bone ends of a fracture to correct the alignment
Amputation	Surgical removal of all or part of an extremity (see Box 8-17)
Arthrocentesis	Surgical procedure to remove excess fluid from a joint
Arthrodesis	Surgical procedure to fuse the bones in a degenerated, unstable joint
Arthroscopy	Surgical procedure that uses a scope to look into a joint
Bone graft	Surgical procedure that uses whole bone or bone chips to repair fractures or bone cancer with extensive bone loss
Cartilage transplant	Surgical procedure alternative to total knee replacement
Bunionectomy	Surgical procedure to remove a bunion
External fixation	Surgical procedure to immobilize a complicated fracture or lengthen a congenitally short leg
Joint replacement surgery	Surgical procedure to replace a joint that has been destroyed by inflammation (see Box 8-18)
Open reduction and internal fixation (ORIF)	Surgical procedure that uses an open incision plus screws, nails, and plates to immobilize a complicated fracture of several pieces

Drug Category	Description	Example
Analgesic drugs	Over-the-counter drugs used to suppress inflammation and decrease pain	Ecotrin, Bayer, Tylenol
Corticosteroid drugs	Suppress inflammation	Hydocortisone, Prednisone
Nonsteroidal anti-inflammatory drugs	Suppress inflammation and decrease pain	Ibuprofen, Motrin

Box 8-17: Instructor Activity

AMPUTATION

Share this information with students.

1. In 1529, French physician Ambroise Paré devised amputation to save the lives of soldiers on the battlefield. He also created the first artificial leg.

2. During the first half of the 1800s, surgery was still performed without the benefit of general anesthesia. During the PBS television series *Treasure Houses of Great Britain,* the story was told of the Marquis de Angelcy, whose leg was destroyed by cannon shot during the battle of Waterloo (1815). His leg was then amputated. The surgeon wrote afterward that he was amazed that the patient's pulse did not vary during the operation. The Marquis' only recorded comment was, "I do not think the saw was very sharp."

Source: Susan Turley, *Understanding Pharmacology for Health Professionals.* Prentice Hall.

Box 8-18: Instructor Activity

HIP REPLACEMENT

Share this information with students.

1. Hip replacement surgery was traditionally done through a 12-inch to 18-inch incision in the hip, cutting large leg muscles to remove the head of the femur from the acetabulum. Now, using minimally invasive surgery, the procedure can be done using two 1 1/2-inch incisions and working around the muscles.
2. According to the National Center for Health Statistics, about 550,000 Americans undergo joint replacement surgery each year. This is expected to increase dramatically as the baby boomer generation reaches middle age. The problem with current joint replacements made with stainless steel or titanium is that they can wear down after just 10 years and the replacement surgery is far costlier than the original surgery. Now a researcher at the University of Alabama has found a way to grow a very thin layer of diamond (the hardest known substance) on the metal implant to make a joint replacement that could last for 40 years. In 2001, the researchers were producing diamonds but they would not stick to metal and they were rough. Then one day their lab's gas reactor sprang a leak, adding a little air to the carefully controlled combination of hydrogen and methane that they used to make the diamonds. Amazingly, they found that the diamond layer was smooth and only a few nanometers thick and that it adhered to the metal. It is hoped this type of joint replacement will be available in the future.

Source: ScienCentralNews at www.sciencentral.com, June 29, 2004.

Box 8-19: Instructor Activity

ORTHOPEDIC SURGEONS

Share this information with students.

1. Orthopedic surgeons perform surgery on bones, but usually not on the cranial bones, facial bones, or ear bones. Podiatrists, or Doctors of Podiatric Medicine (D.P.M.), are only licensed to perform surgery on the bones of the foot and ankle.
2. Susan Turley, the author, has transcribed many orthopedic surgical reports. She noticed that an orthopedic surgeon performing a bunionectomy on the foot will dictate about two paragraphs for the surgical procedure, while it is not uncommon for a podiatrist performing a bunionectomy to dictate a two-page report! Podiatrists are foot doctors who perform surgical procedures on the foot and ankle, but not on other body parts.
3. Orthopedic physicians use many of the same tools as carpenters: they use sterile hammers, chisels, gouges, rongeurs, shavers, nails, screws, plates, and so forth!

Box 8-20: Classroom Activity

ORTHOPEDIC DICTATION

Hand out the sheet with blanks on it to each student (see the following page). Then dictate from the Instructor's Answer Sheet. Students are to fill in the missing words, spelling these words correctly.

ORTHOPEDIC MEDICAL DICTATION

1. The patient was seen by me in _____ follow-up and my tentative _____ was _____ of the left ankle. Now it would appear that a more definitive _____ would be _____ at the _____ and _____ aspects of the left ankle. She is currently having throbbing pain through the central _____. She is tender along the _____ _____ _____ and along the _____ _____ behind the _____ and _____ _____ of the left ankle.

2. The patient has a painful _____ On physical examination, she has a moderately severe _____ _____ of the left great toe and _____ of the midfoot. X-rays show a large deviation at the _____ joint. Otherwise, there are no signs of degenerative _____.

3. On exam, he has some tenderness along the _____ joint line. X-rays show a cyst in the _____.

4. Plan: Diagnostic _____ to be done in the near future.

5. Findings at this time are consistent with right _____ of the right _____.

6. X-rays of the right hip show a total hip replacement _____ and no evident _____ destructive process.

7. X-ray of the right foot shows a _____ fracture of the _____ portion of the first _____. There is degenerative _____ present. There is an old _____ fracture noted.

ORTHOPEDIC MEDICAL DICTATION

Instructor Answer Sheet

1. The patient was seen by me in ORTHOPEDIC follow-up and my tentative DIAGNOSIS was SPRAIN of the left ankle. Now it would appear that a more definitive DIAGNOSIS would be TENDONITIS at the MEDIAL and LATERAL aspects of the left ankle. She is currently having throbbing pain through the central RAYS. She is tender along the POSTERIOR TIBIAL TENDON and along the PERONEAL TENDON behind the MEDIAL and LATERAL MALLEOLI of the left ankle.

2. The patient has a painful BUNION. On physical examination, she has a moderately severe HALLUX VALGUS of the left great toe and PRONATION of the midfoot. X-rays show a large deviation at the METATARSOPHALANGEAL joint. Otherwise, there are no signs of degenerative ARTHRITIS.

3. On exam, he has some tenderness along the ANTEROLATERAL joint line. X-rays show a cyst in the TALUS.

4. Plan: Diagnostic ARTHROSCOPY to be done in the near future.

5. Findings at this time are consistent with CHONDROMALACIA of the right PATELLA.

6. X-rays of the right hip show a total hip replacement PROSTHESIS and no evident OSSEOUS destructive process.

7. X-ray of the right foot shows a TRANSVERSE fracture of the PROXIMAL portion of the first PHALANX. There is degenerative OSTEOARTHRITIS present. There is an old CALCANEAL fracture noted.

Objective 7
Define common skeletal abbreviations

- Text page(s) 442

Content Abstract

AKA	above-the-knee amputation	**MCP**	metacarpophalangeal (joint)
AP	anteroposterior	**NSAID**	nonsteroidal anti-inflammatory drug
ASIS	anterior-superior iliac spine	**OA**	osteoarthritis
BKA	below-the-knee amputation	**ortho**	orthopedics (slang)
BMD	bone mineral density	**P**	phosphorus
C1-C7	cervical vertebrae	**PIP**	proximal interphalangeal (joint)
Ca	calcium	**PT**	physical therapy/therapist
CDH	congenital dislocation of the hip	**QCT**	quantitative computerized tomography
DEXA, DXA	dual-energy x-ray absorptiometry	**RA**	rheumatoid arthritis
		RLE	right lower extremity
DIP	distal interphalangeal (joint)	**ROM**	range of motion
DJD	degenerative joint disease	**RUE**	right upper extremity
ESWT	extracorporeal shock wave therapy	**S1**	first sacral vertebra
fib	fibula (slang)	**T1-T12**	thoracic vertebrae
Fx	fracture	**THR**	total hip replacement
L1-L5	lumbar vertebrae	**tib**	tibia (slang)
LLE	left lower extremity		
LUE	left upper extremity		

Teaching Strategies

1. Remind students to make flash cards for all the abbreviations and their meanings.
2. There is a combined skeletal and muscular abbreviation student activity in Chapter 9, Orthopedics (Muscular).

Objective 8
Correctly spell and pronounce skeletal words

- Text page(s) 453-454

Teaching Strategies

1. Impress upon the students that medical words that are mispronounced are also probably going to be misspelled.
2. Encourage students to work on both pronunciation and spelling when studying.

Chapter Spelling Test

The chapter spelling test is included with the weekly chapter test. Dictate and spell (or xerox a handout that contains) this list of 20 spelling words. Give the list to students the week before the test. For the chapter test, select just 10 of these words to test.

1. ankylosing spondylitis
2. arthralgia
3. cancellous bone
4. cartilaginous
5. coccyx
6. diaphysis
7. hemarthrosis
8. ilium (hip bone)
9. malalignment
10. malleolus
11. meniscus
12. osseous
13. osteomyelitis
14. pectus excavatum
15. peroneal
16. phalanx
17. scoliosis
18. symphysis pubis
19. xiphoid
20. zygoma

Box 8-21: Classroom Activity

GAMES

From week to week, pick a different one of these spelling games to use during class. (The descriptions and instructions for the games are in the section "The Art and Craft of Teaching.")

Beanbag Spelling Toss
Scrabble
Spelling Bee
Gridlock
Hangman

From week to week, pick a different one of these pronunciation games to use during class. (The descriptions and instructions for the games are in the section "The Art and Craft of Teaching.")

Parroting
Hieroglyphics
Beach Ball Blast

Objective 9
Apply your skills by analyzing an orthopedic (skeletal) report

- Text page(s) 451–452

Content Abstract

Read the Chart Note and answer the questions provided.

Objective 10
Test your knowledge of orthopedics (skeletal) by completing review exercises in the textbook and the CD-ROM learning activities

- Text page(s) 444–450

Teaching Strategies

1. Assign the Chapter Review Exercises in the textbook for homework. Remind students to refer to the Answer Key at the end of the textbook to check their answers.
2. Refer to the CD-ROM Learning Activities in this section for multimedia learning experiences.

X-RAY

If you have had an x-ray recently, you can obtain a copy of the actual film from the facility where it was taken. Just go to the facility and request the x-ray film. You will be asked to sign it out and take responsibility for bringing it back to the facility. Patients are often asked to go the radiology facility and obtain their x-ray and carry it themselves when they are referred to the office of a specialist. Obtain radiographs (x-rays) and use them as visual aids during class, pointing out the various bones on the x-ray.

Experience Multimedia

See the PowerPoint presentation on the accompanying Instructor's Media Library for videos on the topic of careers in physical therapy.

Homework Activities

1. Visit the Web site for the Arthritis Foundation at www.arthritis.org and explore the various sections on the site.

2. Using water-soluble markers, draw the bones on a willing family member (spouse or child). Rather than just drawing a long line for a bone, interrupt the line with the first letter of the bone. For example, draw a line down the upper arm and write an "H" for "humerus" on the line. That way, the sight of the "H" on the skin of the upper arm can be easily recalled and the word "humerus" will come to mind. Take a photograph to show your instructor.

3. Interview someone who has had a skeletal disease or injury or surgery (examples: fractured bone, arthritis, joint replacement surgery). Read the description of that disease, injury, or surgery in the textbook and then prepare a list of appropriate questions to ask the person during the interview. Write out your questions and the person's answers for homework.

4. Keep a running list in your notebook of sound-alike words or combining forms that have the same meanings. Title this list of challenging words and word parts as "Perplexing Pairs." Begin by writing down the words or word parts found in the Word Alert boxes in this chapter. Then add the word parts found in the It's Greek to Me box at the end of this chapter. Add any other words or word parts that you found particularly confusing. You will add to this list as you complete each chapter. Examples:

   orth/o-   vs.   arthr/o-
   myel/o-   vs.   my/o-
   perine/o-   vs.   peritone/o-
   cephal/o-   vs.   encephal/o-

Word Search

Complete this word search puzzle that contains Chapter 8 words. Look for the following words as given in the list below.

bone
bones
cast
digits
disk
femur
fracture
joint
maxilla
ossification
osteal

osteoporosis
osteosarcoma
pelvis
rib
sacrum
scapula
skull
spinal
tibia
ulna
vertebrae

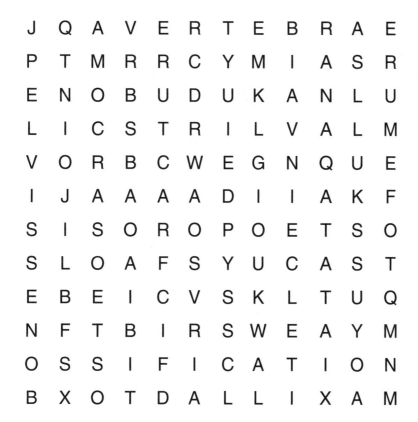

```
J  Q  A  V  E  R  T  E  B  R  A  E
P  T  M  R  R  C  Y  M  I  A  S  R
E  N  O  B  U  D  U  K  A  N  L  U
L  I  C  S  T  R  I  L  V  A  L  M
V  O  R  B  C  W  E  G  N  Q  U  E
I  J  A  A  A  D  I  I  A  K  F
S  I  S  O  R  O  P  O  E  T  S  O
S  L  O  A  F  S  Y  U  C  A  S  T
E  B  E  I  C  V  S  K  L  T  U  Q
N  F  T  B  I  R  S  W  E  A  Y  M
O  S  S  I  F  I  C  A  T  I  O  N
B  X  O  T  D  A  L  L  I  X  A  M
```

```
J Q A V E R T E B R A E
P T M R R C Y M I A S R
E N O B U D U K A N L U
L I C S T R I L V A L M
V O R B C W E G N Q U E
I J A A A A D I I A K F
S I S O R O P O E T S O
S L O A F S Y U C A S T
E B E I C V S K L T U Q
N F T B I R S W E A Y M
O S S I F I C A T I O N
B X O T D A L L I X A M
```

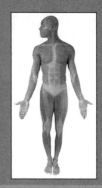

Orthopedics

Muscular System

Objective 1
Identify the anatomical structures of the muscular system by correctly labeling them on anatomical illustrations

- Text page(s) 466-471

Teaching Strategies

1. Explain the importance of learning the muscles of the body.
2. Using a diagram or model, identify each muscle in the body as it is discussed.

Content Abstract

 Orthopedics is the study of the muscles and bones. It is the healthcare specialty that studies the anatomy and physiology of the muscular and skeletal systems and uses diagnostic tests, medical and surgical procedures, and drugs to treat muscular and skeletal diseases.

There are three types of muscles in the body:

1. skeletal muscles
2. cardiac muscles
3. smooth muscles

The origin or beginning of a muscle is where it is attached to a stationary or nearly stationary bone of the skeleton. The insertion or ending point is where the muscle attaches to the bone that it moves when it contracts and relaxes.

Muscle names describe where the muscle is located, what shape it is, what size it is, or what action it performs.

The skeletal system is composed of muscles of the

1. head and neck
2. shoulders, chest, and back
3. arms and hands
4. abdomen
5. legs and buttocks

Box 9-1: Instructor Activity

INTERESTING FACTS

Share this information with students.

1. Eye muscles may contract more than 10,000 times each day.
2. The largest muscle is the gluteus maximus muscle of the buttocks.
3. The following misinformation actually appeared in a medical terminology textbook: "The gastrocnemius muscles move food into the stomach." That author confused the muscle name *gastrocnemius* with the combining form *gastr/o-* that means *stomach*.
4. *Quadriceps femoris* is the collective name for four muscles on the anterior and lateral aspects of the thigh. All of these muscles—the rectus femoris, vastus lateralis, vastus intermedius (beneath the vastus lateralis), and the vastus medialis—have tendons that insert at the patella. Contraction of the four muscles straightens the lower leg in extension.
5. *Hamstrings* is the collective name for three muscles on the posterior aspect of the thigh. The tendons of all of these muscles—the biceps femoris, semitendinosus, and semimembranosus—form two tendon groups, one on each side of the popliteal space at the back of the knee. Contraction of these muscles moves the upper leg posteriorly and bends the lower leg toward the buttocks in flexion.
6. A cat has 32 muscles in its ear.
   Source: Fun Science Facts, www.hightechscience.org/funfacts.htm
7. The masseter muscle that is used for chewing is the strongest muscle in the body. It can exert 200 pounds of pressure on the teeth.
8. There are tiny erector muscles at the base of each hair follicle. When the skin is cold, these muscles contract to form goose bumps.

---

9. The smallest muscle in the body is the stapedius muscle that controls the stapes bone in the middle ear; it is only 5/100 inch in length.

10. The longest muscle in the body is the sartorius muscle in the leg.

11. The muscle with the longest name—*musculus levator labii superioris alaeque nasi*—makes the top lip curl upward and makes the nostrils flare.

12. It is common practice to mix the English and Latin names of anatomical parts, e.g., using English for the noun and Latin for the adjectives. In the phrase "latissimus dorsi muscle," the first two words are in Latin and the third word (the noun) is in English.

    Source: The American Association for Medical Transcription Book of Style, page 25.

13. Skeletal muscle is the most abundant tissue in the human body and also one of the most adaptable. Vigorous training with weights can double or triple a muscle's size, whereas disuse (as during space travel) can shrink muscles by 20 percent in two weeks. . . . Everyone knows that when we age, our muscles weaken and our movements become slower. But why is that so? With aging comes a number of changes to the skeletal muscles. Most marked is the loss of mass, which begins as early as 25 years of age. By age 50, the skeletal muscle mass is often reduced by 10 percent, and by age 80 approximately 50 percent of the muscle mass is gone. This age-related reduction is caused mainly by a loss of muscle fibers. Weightlifting can stave off the loss of mass from the muscle as a whole by greatly thickening the individual muscles fibers, but it appears to have no major effect on the loss of fibers.

    Source: "Muscle, Genes, and Athletic Performance," *Scientific American*, September 2000, page 54.

Experience Multimedia

See the PowerPoint presentation on the accompanying Instructor's Media Library for animations showing various muscles in the body.

Objective 2
Describe how muscles contract and produce movement

- Text page(s) 463-465, 472–473

Teaching Strategies

1. Explain the importance of learning the various types of muscle movements.

2. Explain the importance of learning the physiology of a muscular contraction.

3. Demonstrate how muscles contract and coordinate movement using your body as an example.

MEMORY TOOLS

Share this information with students.

The position of the forearm when it is **sup**ination (pronounced soo-pih-NAY-shun) is the same position that you must use to carry a bowl of **soup.** Also, the palms are **up.**

To remember that **plant**ar flexion moves the foot so the toes are pointing down, think of plantar warts that occur on the sole of the foot.

You can remember that the latissimus dorsi muscle is in the back because *dorsi* is related to the word *dorsal,* which means *back.* Remember, the dorsal fin on the back of a shark is the one that sticks out of the water.

If a form asked you "What is your country of origin?" what would you answer? Your country of origin is where you were born, where you had your beginning, where you originated from, or your place of birth. You can never change your place of birth. Where you were born (originated) will always be the same (fixed). The origin of a muscle is on a stationary (fixed) bone that never changes or moves.

Have students stand up. Tell them to listen to each command for a specific muscle movement and then quickly do it. Say these commands quickly to get the students moving and thinking.

> Extend your right leg
> Rotate your head to the left
> Put your palms in supination
> Flex your right arm
> Flex your left leg
> Abduct your left arm
> Dorsiflex your right foot
> Rotate your head to the right
> Abduct and then adduct your left leg
> Plantar flex your right foot
> Flex your neck
> Pronate your left hand
> Extend your right arm
> Flex your right hip
> Do extension of your neck

Content Abstract

There are various types of muscle movement, such as flexion, extension, abduction, adduction, rotation, supination, pronation, eversion, and inversion. The type of muscle can be any of the following: flexor, extensor, abductor, adductor, rotator, supinator, pronator, evertor, or invertor.

The main function of the muscles is to produce movement for the body. A muscle will only contract because of an electrical impulse from a nerve. Each muscle fiber is connected to a single nerve cell at the neuromuscular junction. When the electrical impulse reaches the end of the nerve cell, the nerve cell releases the neurotransmitter acetylcholine. This is a chemical messenger that moves across the neuromuscular junction and acts as a key to unlock receptors on the muscle fiber. Calcium ions cause the thin filaments (actin) to slide between the thick filaments (myosin), shortening the muscle and producing a muscle contraction.

Box 9-3: Instructor Activity

INTERESTING FACTS

Share this information with students.

1. It takes the coordination of over 200 muscles to walk. It takes 17 muscles to smile, and 43 muscle to frown.
   Source: Bit of Fun, www.bitoffun.com
2. An ant can lift 50 times its own weight and pull 300 times its own weight.
   Source: doghouse.com
3. Fleas can jump 130 times higher than their own height. In human terms, this is like a 6-foot person jumping 780 feet into the air.
   Source: Fun Science Facts, www.hightechscience.org/funfacts.htm
4. The burning sensation in muscles as you exercise is not caused by fatigue. It is caused by lactic acid building up inside the muscle fibers.
   Source: The Baltimore Sun, August 30, 2004.

Experience Multimedia

See the PowerPoint presentation on the accompanying Instructor's Media Library for an animation showing muscle contraction.

Objective 3
Build muscular words from combining forms, prefixes, and suffixes

- Text page(s) 480-481

Box 9-4: Classroom Activity

MEDICAL TERMINOLOGY BEE

Create a PowerPoint presentation with combining forms, prefixes, and suffixes with their meanings. Use this presentation in class. All students participate in a "medical terminology bee." All students stand and take turns defining the combining form, prefix, or suffix displayed. If the student gets the answer right, the student remains standing and continues to play. If the student gets the answer wrong, the student will be seated and is out of the game. The last person standing is the winner. A prize could be given to the winner.

Objective 4
Describe common muscular diseases

- Text page(s) 482-488

Teaching Strategy

Invite someone from the Muscular Dystrophy Association (MDA) to speak about the different types of muscular dystrophy.

Patients with muscular dystrophy lack a gene that controls the production of the protein dystrophin. Without dystrophin muscles weaken and the heart and breathing muscles fail, usually by age 25. Now researchers are testing a new therapy for the disease. The missing gene is inseated into a virus. The virus acts like a cargo ship, carrying the gene through the blood, and unloading the gene when it comes in contact with a body cell. Through the blood, the virus is able to reach every muscle cell in the body and supply it with the missing gene.

Source: ScienCentralNews, "Muscular Dystrophy Gene Therapy," At www.sciencentral .com/articles/view.php3?Article_id=218392770

Contrast muscular dystrophy with myasthenia gravis.

Disease	Onset	Defect	Weakness
Muscular dystrophy	Childhood	Lack of dystrophin	Slowly progresses over years
Myasthenia gravis	Adulthood	Antibodies against acetylcholine receptors	Worsens during day, better with rest

Content Abstract

Disease	Meaning
Atrophy	Loss of muscle bulk in one or more muscles
Avulsion	Muscle tears away from the tendon or the tendon tears away from the bone
Compartment syndrome	Crushing injury or blunt trauma releases blood that builds up pressure in the enveloping fascia
Contracture	Inactivity or paralysis with continued nerve impulses progressively flexes the muscle until it becomes nearly immovable
Fibromyalgia	Pain along trigger points that are tender to the touch
Hyperextension-hyperflexion injury	Car accident injury in which person's head snaps backward and then forward
Muscle contusion	Bruise; blunt trauma causes bleeding in the muscle
Muscle spasm	Sudden, severe, involuntary, prolonged contraction of a muscle
Muscle strain	Overstretching of a muscle, often due to physical overexertion
Muscular dystrophy	Genetic inherited disease due to a mutation of the gene that makes the muscle protein dystrophin
Myalgia	Pain in one or more muscles due to injury or muscle disease
Myasthenia gravis	Abnormal and rapid fatigue of muscles, particularly in the face
Myopathy	Any disease of the muscles
Myositis	Inflammation of a muscle with localized swelling and tenderness
Repetitive strain injury	Trauma from repetitive movements over an extended period of time (see Box 9-5)
Rhabdomyoma	Benign tumor that arises from striated muscle tissue
Rhabdomyosarcoma	Cancerous tumor of the muscle
Rotator cuff tear	Tear of the rotator muscle of the shoulder
Torticollis	Painful contraction of the muscles of one side of the neck
Ataxia	Incoordination of the muscles during movement
Bradykinesia	Abnormally slow muscle movements or decrease in the number of spontaneous muscle movements
Dyskinesia	Difficulty controlling voluntary muscle movements with resulting tics, jerking, or writhing
Hyperkinesia	Increased muscle movements, restlessness
Tremor	Small, involuntary, back-and-forth movements of the hands, head, or extremities
Restless legs syndrome	Restlessness and twitching with tingling of the muscles of the legs, particularly at night
Bursitis	Inflammation of a bursal sac due to repetitive movement
Dupuytren's contracture	Fascia of the palm of the hand becomes shortened and causes a flexion deformity of the fingers

(continued)

Disease	Meaning
Ganglion	Cyst on a tendon, usually on the wrist, hand, or foot
Golfer's elbow	Overuse injury of the flexor and pronator muscles of the forearm and their tendons to the elbow
Shin splints	Overuse injury with inflammation of the tendons of the flexor muscles of the lower leg
Tendonitis	Inflammation of any tendon, usually from overuse
Tennis elbow	Overuse injury of the extensor and supinator muscles of the forearm and their tendons to the elbow
Tenosynovitis	Overuse injury and inflammation of any tendon and tendon sheath

Box 9-5: Instructor Activity

REPETITIVE STRAIN INJURY

Share this information with students.

1. Repetitive strain injury (RSI) affects the muscles, tendons, and nerves. It is caused by trauma from an occupation that requires a repetitive movement, such as typing and medical transcription. The Occupational Safety and Health Administration works to prevent workplace-related injuries of all types. However, there are no specific guidelines for ergonomics to prevent repetitive strain disorder. Guidelines were signed in 2000 by then-President Clinton, but several weeks later Congress repealed those ergonomic standards because of the cost to employers. Repetitive strain disorder is the single largest cause of occupational health problems.
2. Housemaid's knee is a form of bursitis and carries the medical name prepatellar bursitis. The common name is thought to have originated because of damage to the knees that occurred when maids knelt to scrub floors.

Experience Multimedia

See the PowerPoint presentation on the accompanying Instructor's Media Library for videos on the following topics covered in this chapter:

- Muscular dystrophy
- Muscle atrophy

Objective 5
Describe common muscular diagnostic laboratory tests

- Text page(s) 489

Teaching Strategy

Obtain copies of common muscular diagnostic laboratory and radiology tests (EMG, etc.) to discuss and circulate in the classroom.

Content Abstract

Test	Definition
Acetylcholine receptor antibodies	Blood test for myasthenia gravis
CPK-MM	Blood test that shows destruction of muscles, as in muscular dystrophy
Electromyography	Diagnostic procedure to diagnose muscle disease or nerve damage
Tensilon test	Diagnostic procedure in which the drug Tensilon is given to confirm a diagnosis of myasthenia gravis

Objective 6
Describe common muscular medical and surgical procedures and drug categories

- Text page(s) 490-494

Content Abstract

Procedure	Definition
Muscle strength test	Medical procedure used to test the strength of certain muscle groups
Trigger point injections	Anesthetic and corticosteroid drugs are injected into trigger points in patients with fibromyalgia
Fasciectomy	Surgical procedure to remove fascia causing Dupuytren's contracture
Ganglionectomy	Surgical procedure to remove a ganglion from a tendon
Muscle biopsy	Surgical procedure to remove a piece of muscle to diagnose a muscle disease
Tenorrhaphy	Surgical procedure of suturing together the torn ends of a tendon following an injury
Thymectomy	Surgical excision of the thymus gland

Drug Category	Description	Example
Analgesic drugs	Over-the-counter drugs used to suppress inflammation and decrease pain	Bayer aspirin, Ecotrin, Tylenol
Beta-blocker drugs	Block the action of epinephrine to suppress essential familial tremor	Inderal
Muscle relaxant drugs	Relieve muscle spasm and stiffness	Flexeril, Parafon Forte, Soma
Nonsteroidal anti-inflammatory drugs (NSAIDs)	Suppress inflammation and decrease pain	Ibuprofen, Motrin

Experience Multimedia

See the PowerPoint presentation on the accompanying Instructor's Media Library for a video on the topic of intramuscular injections.

Objective 7
Define common muscular abbreviations

- Text page(s) 495

Teaching Strategies

1. Stress the importance of learning abbreviations and their full meanings.
2. Encourage students to make flashcards for abbreviations and their meanings as well their usual flashcards for word parts and their meanings.

Content Abstract

ADA	Americans with Disabilities Act
ADLs	activities of daily living
COTA	certified occupational therapy assistant
CPK-MM	creatine phosphokinase (MM bands)
CTD	cumulative trauma disorder
DTRs	deep tendon reflexes
EMG	electromyography
IM	intramuscular
LLE	left lower extremity
LUE	left upper extremity
MD	muscular dystrophy
NSAID	nonsteroidal anti-inflammatory drug

OOB	out of bed
ortho	orthopedics (slang)
OSHA	Occupational Safety and Health Administration
OT	occupational therapy/therapist
PM&R	physical medicine and rehabilitation
PT	physical therapy/therapist
rehab	rehabilitation (slang)
RLE	right lower extremity
ROM	range of motion
RUE	right upper extremity
RSI	repetitive strain injury

Box 9-6: Classroom Activity

ABBREVIATION GAME

Let the class have two minutes to quickly look over the lists of abbreviations in Chapters 8 and 9 and the Word Alert boxes. Then they are to close their books. Divide the class into two, three, or four teams and have them stand in separate lines. Write a common skeletal or muscular abbreviation on the board. The first student on Team 1 must give the meaning of the abbreviation. If the abbreviation also appears in the Word Alert box, the student must give all meanings of the abbreviation. If correct, that student moves to the back of the team line. Write another common skeletal or muscular abbreviation on the board for the first student on Team 2. If correct, that student moves to the end of the team line. If at any point a student misses an abbreviation, that student is out of the game and must sit down. The student in the front of the line for the next team is given an opportunity to define the abbreviation. Continue writing abbreviations on the board until every student on every team has had at least one chance to play. The team with the most students left standing at the end of the game is the winner.

Objective 8
Correctly spell and pronounce muscular words

- Text page(s) 507-508

Teaching Strategies

1. Impress upon the students that medical words that are mispronounced are also probably going to be misspelled.
2. Encourage students to work on both pronunciation and spelling when studying.

Chapter Spelling Test

The chapter spelling test is included with the weekly chapter test. Dictate and spell (or xerox a handout that contains) this list of 20 spelling words. Give the list to students the week before the test. For the chapter test, select just 10 of these words to test.

1. abduction
2. analgesic
3. biceps brachii muscle
4. chiropractor
5. dermatomyositis
6. Dupuytren's contracture
7. fascia
8. fibromyalgia
9. ganglionectomy
10. gluteus maximus muscle
11. latissimus dorsi muscle
12. musculoskeletal
13. myasthenia gravis
14. ptosis
15. rhabdomyosarcoma
16. sternocleidomastoid muscle
17. tendinous
18. tenosynovitis
19. torticollis
20. tremor

GAMES

1. From week to week, pick a different one of these spelling games to use during class. (The descriptions and instructions for the games are in the section "The Art and Craft of Teaching.")

   Beanbag Spelling Toss

   Scrabble

   Spelling Bee

   Gridlock

   Hangman

2. From week to week, pick a different one of these pronunciation games to use during class. (The descriptions and instructions for the games are in the section "The Art and Craft of Teaching.")

   Parroting

   Hieroglyphics

   Beach Ball Blast

Chapter Pronunciation Test

Have students mark these 20 words listed in the Pronunciation Checklist for the chapter. During the week, they will call your office or home answering machine and pronounce each word.

1. acetylcholine
2. atrophy
3. atrophic
4. biceps brachii muscle
5. bradykinesia
6. chiropractor
7. creatine phophokinase
8. dermatomyositis
9. electromyography
10. fibromyalgia
11. ganglionectomy
12. gluteus maximus muscle
13. latissimus dorsi muscle
14. myasthenia gravis
15. neurotransmitter
16. rectus abdominis muscle
17. rhabdomyosarcoma
18. sternocleidomastoid muscle
19. tenosynovitis
20. trapezius muscle

Objective 9
Apply your skills by analyzing an orthopedic (muscular) report

- Text page(s) 504-506

Content Abstract

Read the hospital Operative Report and the Pathology Report and answer questions provided.

Box 9-8: Classroom Activity

MEDICAL REPORT

In the medical report, circle all the medical words. Then list them and write their definitions. Rewrite the medical words in English as if you were explaining them to the patient.

Objective 10
Test your knowledge of orthopedics by completing review exercises in the textbook and the CD-ROM learning activities

- Text page(s) 497-503 (first complete all the in-chapter exercises on pp. 478–481)

Teaching Strategies

1. Assign the Chapter Review Exercises in the textbook for homework. Remind students to refer to the Answer Key at the end of the book to check their answers.
2. Refer to the CD-ROM Learning Activities in this section for multimedia learning experiences.

Experience Multimedia

See the PowerPoint presentation on the accompanying Instructor's Media Library for videos on the topic of careers in massage therapy.

Homework Activities

1. Using water-soluble markers, draw the muscles on a willing family helper (spouse or child), a friend, or fellow student. Outline the edges of the muscle and insert the first letter of the muscle: Draw a triangular-shaped outline at the lateral aspect of the upper arm and write a "D" for "deltoid" in the center. That way, the sight of the "D" on the skin of the upper arm can be easily recalled and the word "deltoid" will come to mind. Take a photograph to show your instructor.

2. Watch a physical therapist at work. Describe and correctly name the various muscle movements seen.

3. Visit the Web site for the New York Committee for Occupational Safety and Health at www.wtcexams.org/pdfs/nycosh_repetitive_stress_injuries.pdf.

   List eight factors that tend to cause job-related RSI. List nine jobs that carry a high risk for repetitive strain injury (RSI).

4. Keep a running list in your notebook of sound-alike words or combining forms that have the same meanings. Title this list of challenging words and word parts as "Perplexing Pairs." Begin by writing down the words or word parts found in the Word Alert boxes in this chapter. Then add the word parts found in the It's Greek to Me box at the end of this chapter. Add any other words or word parts that you found particularly confusing. You will add to this list as you complete each chapter. Examples:

orth/o-	vs.	arthr/o-
myel/o-	vs.	my/o-
perine/o-	vs.	peritone/o-
cephal/o-	vs.	encephal/o-

5. Look in your medicine cabinet. Find 10 prescription or over-the-counter drugs. List their drug names. Also look on the label and find any medical words. Write down these medical words and then look up and write their medical definitions.

6. Write 10 sentences correctly using 10 or more abbreviations from the chapter.

Word Search

Complete this word search puzzle that contains Chapter 9 words. Look for the following words as given in the list below.

aponeurosis
ataxia
atrophy
belly
biceps
bursa
DTR
dyskinesia
EMG
evertors
exercise
fascia

fiber
flexors
gastrocnemius
muscular
myalgia
NSAID
origin
ptosis
strain
tendon
tremor
triceps

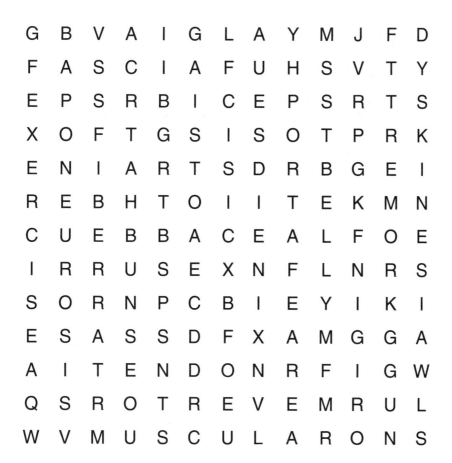

```
G B V A I G L A Y M J F D
F A S C I A F U H S V T Y
E P S R B I C E P S R T S
X O F T G S I S O T P R K
E N I A R T S D R B G E I
R E B H T O I I T E K M N
C U E B B A C E A L F O E
I R R U S E X N F L N R S
S O R N P C B I E Y I K I
E S A S S D F X A M G G A
A I T E N D O N R F I G W
Q S R O T R E V E M R U L
W V M U S C U L A R O N S
```

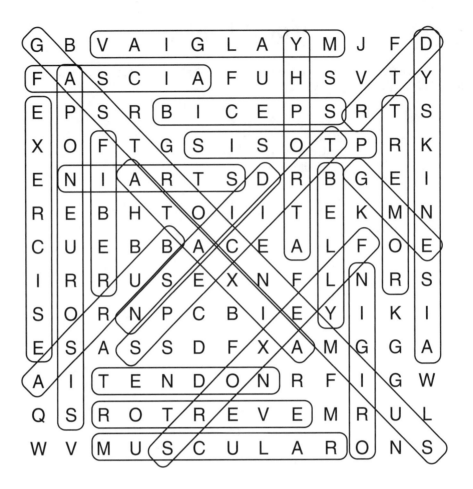

G	B	V	A	I	G	L	A	Y	M	J	F	D
F	A	S	C	I	A	F	U	H	S	V	T	Y
E	P	S	R	B	I	C	E	P	S	R	T	S
X	O	F	T	G	S	I	S	O	T	P	R	K
E	N	I	A	R	T	S	D	R	B	G	E	I
R	E	B	H	T	O	I	I	T	E	K	M	N
C	U	E	B	B	A	C	E	A	L	F	O	E
I	R	R	U	S	E	X	N	F	L	N	R	S
S	O	R	N	P	C	B	I	E	Y	I	K	I
E	S	A	S	S	D	F	X	A	M	G	G	A
A	I	T	E	N	D	O	N	R	F	I	G	W
Q	S	R	O	T	R	E	V	E	M	R	U	L
W	V	M	U	S	C	U	L	A	R	O	N	S

CHAPTER 10

Neurology

Nervous System

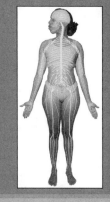

Instructor Activity for the Beginning of Class

Bring in a small musical instrument, like a recorder or a child's xylophone. Play the note "C" and ask students "What color is this sound?" Then hold up a book and ask "What does this taste like?"
People who can hear colors and taste or smell sights have synesthesia. This genetic condition affects one in every 2,000 persons. For one person with synesthesia, the musical note C is always red, and F sharp is blue. For another person, the number two is always green and five is always blue. For another person, the spoken word "table" tastes like apricots, the word "book" tastes like tomato soup, and the word "telephone" tastes like earwax! How does this occur? The person with synesthesia has a crosswiring of these sections of the brain.

Source: www.youramazingbrain.org.uk

Do you have the *impulse* to learn more? Don't be *nervous!* You'll get the *message* once you master the language of neurology!

Objective 1
Identify the anatomical structures of the nervous system by correctly labeling them on anatomical illustrations

- Text page(s) 512-523

Teaching Strategies

1. Explain the importance of learning the parts of the nervous system.
2. Use a model or diagram to show students the various parts of the nervous system as they are discussed.
3. To learn the anatomy of the nervous system, have students label its parts on an anatomical diagram.
4. When you discuss dermatomes on page 521, refer students to the illustration of body dermatomes on page 341.

Content Abstract

Neurology is the healthcare specialty that studies the anatomy and physiology of the nervous system and uses diagnostic tests, medical and surgical procedures, and drugs to treat nervous system diseases.

 The anatomy of the nervous system can be divided into the central nervous system and the peripheral nervous system. The central nervous system consists of the brain and the spinal cord. The peripheral nervous system consists of the cranial nerves and the spinal nerves.

 The brain consists of the cerebrum, ventricles, thalamus, hypothalamus, brainstem, and cerebellum.

There are 12 pairs of cranial nerves that originate in the brain and carry impulses between the brain and the face, head, neck, upper back and abdomen. There are 31 pairs of spinal nerves that originate at regular intervals along the spinal cord.

Box 10-1: Instructor Activity

INTERESTING FACTS

Share this information with students.

1. [Copy this Egyptian hieroglyphic onto the board.]

   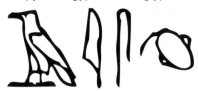 This is an Egyptian hieroglyphic that means *brain*. The Greek philosopher Aristotle thought the heart, not the brain, was the location of intelligence and thought. The ancient Egyptians did not think much of the brain. In fact, when creating a mummy, the Egyptians scooped out the brain through the nostrils and threw it away. However, the heart and other internal organs were removed carefully and preserved, and then put back into the body or into jars that were set next to the body. Nevertheless, the ancient Egyptians are responsible for the oldest written record using the word *brain*. It appears on a papyrus dated 1700 B.C. but is based on texts that go back to about 3000 B.C. This document is considered to be the first medical document in the history of mankind.

   Source: "Neuroscience for Kids," University of Washington Web site, http://staff.washington.edu/chudler/papy.html

2. As the brain grows in the developing fetus inside the mother, new neurons are created at the rate of 250,000 per minute.

   Source: The Human Body, TimeLife Books.

3. A newborn baby's brain increases to almost three times its size in the first year of life.

4. The adult brain has 100 billion neurons.

5. The average brain weights three pounds. Some can be larger, but the size of the brain has no relevance to performance.

6. How to remember the names of the cranial nerves: This mnifty mnemonic device was thought of by medical students many years ago: "On Old Olympus' Towering Tops, a Finn and German Viewed Some Hops." You can remember that the first "O" is for "olfactory" because you have one nose, and that the second "O" is for "optic" because you have two eyes.

7. Because it has no backbone, an octopus can squeeze through a hole no larger than a silver dollar.

   Source: Backwoodsbound.com, Amazing Animal Facts.

Box 10-2: Instructor Activity

MEMBRANES

Share this information with students.

How can you remember the names of the three lining membranes over the brain?

1. The first lining membrane, the dura mater, is very tough to protect the brain in case the cranial bone is broken. *Dura mater* is a Latin phrase that means *tough mother.*
2. The middle layer, the arachnoid, holds many branching blood vessels that give it a spider web-like appearance. Arachnida is the class of insects that includes spiders, scorpions, etc. The Greek combining form *arachn/o-* means *spider or spider web* and the suffix *-oid* means *resembling.*
3. The layer closest to the delicate tissues of the brain is the pia mater. *Pia mater* is a Latin phrase that means *tender mother.*

Box 10-3: Instructor Activity

CRANIAL NERVES

You can categorize the cranial nerves into three broad categories:

1. Senses (smell, vision, taste, hearing, and equilibrium)
2. Movement (iris, lens, eyeballs, eyelids, facial expression, chewing, speaking, salivary gland contraction, sneezing, coughing, vocal cords, movement of the neck and upper back; plus beating of the heart, breathing, and peristalsis of GI tract via the vagus nerve)
3. Sensation (scalp, face, mouth, ears, throat, neck, chest, internal organs of the abdomen)

Cranial nerve X, the vagus nerve is the only cranial nerve that leaves the area of the head and upper body. It goes to the heart, the diaphragm, and the internal organs of the abdominal cavity. *Vagus* is a Latin word that means *wandering.*

Experience Multimedia

See the PowerPoint presentation on the accompanying Instructor's Media Library for animations on the following topics covered in this chapter:

- Brain
- Autonomic nervous system

Objective 2
Describe the process of nerve transmission

- Text page(s) 524-525

Teaching Strategy

Explain the importance of learning the process of nerve transmission.

Content Abstract

 Each neuron consists of the dendrites, the cell body, and the axon. The dendrites receive a neurotransmitter from the previous neuron, convert it into an electrical impulse and send it to the cell body. The cell body contains the nucleus that directs cellular activities and provides energy for the cell. The cytoplasm around the nucleus contains structures that produce neurotransmitters. The cell body sends the electrical impulse to the axon. The axon is covered by a fatty, white insulating layer of myelin that keeps the electrical impulse intact as it travels. There is a space or synapse between the axon of one neuron and the dendrites of the next neuron. It is the neurotransmitter that crosses this space. The traveling of the electrical and chemical impulses from one neuron to the next, and so forth, takes a fraction of a second.

Box 10-4: Instructor Activity
NERVE IMPULSE Share this information with students. 1. A nerve impulse travels at about 300 miles per hour. 2. Scientists have found that it is impossible to tickle yourself. The cerebellum, a region in the posterior portion of the brain, warns the rest of your brain when you are attempting to tickle yourself.

Experience Multimedia	
See the PowerPoint presentation on the accompanying Instructor's Media Library for an animation showing a neurosynapse.	

Objective 3
Build nervous system words from combining forms, prefixes, and suffixes

- Text page(s) 533-535

Objective 4
Describe common nervous system diseases

- Text page(s) 536-552

Content Abstract

Disease	Meaning
Amnesia	Partial or total loss of memory of recent or past experiences
Anencephaly	Rare congenital condition in which some or all of the cranium and cerebrum are missing in a newborn
Aphasia	Loss of the ability to communicate verbally or in writing
Arteriovenous malformation	Arteries in the brain connect directly to veins rather than capillaries
Brain tumor	Benign or malignant tumor of the brain
Cephalalgia	Headache (see Box 10-15)
Cerebral palsy	Lack of oxygen to the brain during birth, producing spastic muscles and lack of coordination
Cerebrovascular accident	Disruption or blockage of blood flow to the brain, which causes tissue death and an area of necrosis known as an infarct (see Box 10-13)
Coma	Deep state of unconsciousness and unresponsiveness caused by trauma or disease in the brain
Concussion	Traumatic injury to the brain that results in the immediate loss of consciousness for a brief or prolonged period of time
Dementia	Gradual decline in mental abilities; one type is Alzheimer's disease (see Box 10-8)
Down syndrome	Congenital genetic defect in which there are three of chromosome 21 instead of the normal two, causing mental retandation (see Box 10-9)
Dyslexia	Difficulty reading and writing, with letters read or written backwards or out of order
Encephalitis	Inflammation of the brain due to a virus
Epilepsy	Recurring condition in which a group of neurons in the brain spontaneously sends out electrical impulses in an abnormal, uncontrolled way (see Box 10-10)
Hematoma	Localized collection of blood inside the cranium
Huntington's chorea	Inherited degenerative disorder of the brain
Hydrocephalus	Excessive amount of cerebrospinal fluid. Usually associated with meningomyelocele
Meningitis	Inflammation of the meninges due to bacteria or viruses (see Box 10-11)

(continued)

Disease	Meaning
Migraine headache	Sudden, throbbing headache with photophobia and nausea; caused by arteries constricting then dilating in the brain
Narcolepsy	Involuntary episodes of falling asleep during the day
Parkinson's disease	Chronic, degenerative disease due to an imbalance in the levels of the neurotransmitters dopamine and acetylcholine in the brain
Syncope	Temporary loss of consciousness
Neural tube defect	Congenital abnormality of the vertebrae with failure to close; the spinal cord and nerves can protrude out of the back (see Box 10-12)
Radiculopathy	Pain along the distribution of the sciatic nerve because of a herniated nucleus pulposus in the spine
Spinal cord injury	Trauma to the spinal cord with a partial or complete transection of the cord
Amyotrophic lateral sclerosis	Progressive disease of motor neurons with muscle wasting and paralysis
Anesthesia	Lack of sensation
Bell's palsy	Inflammation of cranial nerve VII with weakness and paralysis on one side of the face
Carpal tunnel syndrome	Chronic condition with tingling in the hand because of inflammation and swelling of the tendons that go through the carpal tunnel of the wrist bones to reach the hand
Guillain-Barré syndrome	Temporary, acute weakness; an autoimmune disorder in which the body makes antibodies against myelin
Hyperesthesia	Abnormal heightened awareness to touch and pain
Multiple sclerosis	Chronic, progressive weakness and fatigue; a degenerative autoimmune disease in which the body makes antibodies against myelin (see Box 10–16)
Neuralgia	Pain along the path of a nerve
Neuritis	Inflammation of a nerve
Neurofibromatosis	Hereditary disease with benign tumors on the peripheral nerves
Neuroma	Benign nerve tumor
Neuropathy	Any disease or injury of the nerves
Paresthesia	Abnormal sensations of tingling, burning of the skin

Box 10-6: Classroom Activity

DISEASES

Draw this table on the board and have students complete it.

Disease	Symptoms and Signs	Cause
Hemiparesis of the right side Hemiplegia of the left side Paraplegia Quadriplegia		

[Answer Key]

Disease	Symptoms and Signs	Cause
Hemiparesis of the right side	Muscle weakness on the right side of the body	Small stroke/cerebrovascular accident on the left side of the brain
Hemiplegia of the left side	Anesthesia and paralysis on the left side of the body	Stroke/cerebrovascular accident on the right side of the brain
Paraplegia	Anesthesia and paralysis below the waist	Spinal cord injury to the lower spinal cord
Quadriplegia	Anesthesia and paralysis below the neck	Spinal cord injury to the upper spinal cord

Box 10-7: Instructor Activity

ADHD

Attention-deficit hyperactivity disorder (ADHD) is described in Chapter 17, Psychiatry, on page 911.

Box 10-8: Instructor Activity

ALZHEIMER'S DISEASE

1. Alzheimer's disease (AD) is everyone's greatest fear as they grow older. . . . Alzheimer's currently affects 4.5 million Americans . . . that's considerably more than in 1980, and the numbers are growing. . . . We now know that Alzheimer's is a disease, regardless of the age at which it appears. Although it most often accompanies the aging process, growing older does not cause this disease.

   Those with senile dementia do not necessarily have AD. . . . An experimental vaccine has been developed that seems to be able to [prevent the formation of the characteristic plaques and tangles] in animals.. . . . Most recent speculation about the cause of Alzheimer's implicates insulin. . . . Insulin concentrations in the brain drop dramatically in early Alzheimer's and continue to fall as the disease progresses . . . This may contribute to cell death and the tangles characteristic of AD. Another hallmark of Alzheimer's—low levels of acetylcholine—also is directly linked to loss of insulin, all of which suggests that Alzheimer's may be a form of diabetes."

   Source: Parade Magazine, January 15, 2006; "Health on Parade."

(continued)

Box 10-8: Instructor Activity (*cont.*)

2. Alzheimer's disease affects more than 4 million Americans. Nearly half of all people over age 85 have Alzheimer's disease. The National Institutes of Health (NIH) is funding a clinical trial using gene therapy with nerve growth factor (NGF) to treat Alzheimer's disease. In the first phase, Alzheimer's patients had special genetically engineered cells that produce NGF injected into their brains. These patients showed far less intellectual decline compared to patients on Alzheimer's drugs. In the next clinical trial, a harmless virus, will be used to carry the NGF gene directly to the brain cells affected by Alzheimer's disease, and then the brain cells will begin to produce NGF.

   Source: ScienCentralNews, www.sciencentral.com, August 5, 2004.

3. Alzheimer's disease can only be diagnosed after death by performing an autopsy that shows the presence of neurofibrillary tangles. However, researchers have found that the same beta amyloid protein that composes neurofibrillary tangles in the brain can also be found in the eye. Patients with Alzheimer's disease show evidence of beta amyloid protein along the edges of the lens of the eye, forming an unusual type of cataract. This can be detected by a pulse of infrared laser in a noninvasive, brief test done in the doctor's office. Eye drops that bind to the beta amyloid protein and fluoresce are also being used. This test, if approved by the FDA, could detect the first signs of Alzheimer's disease years before the deterioration of mental ability occurs.

   Source: ScienCentralNews, www.sciencentral.com, November 1, 2005.

4. Researchers at the New York University School of Medicine found that a significant decrease in the size of the brain, particularly in the middle part of the temporal lobe and the hippocampus, occurs several years before signs of memory impairment. This change in size can be easily seen on an MRI scan.

   Source: ScienCentralNews, www.sciencentral.com, August 5, 2004.

5. Early Alzheimer's disease may be able to be detected sooner because researchers have found that patients first lose their ability to distinguish different smells. The area in the brain that processes smells is one of the first to be affected by Alzheimer's buildup of abnormal proteins. Once a year for five years, healthy persons and patients with mild memory loss were asked to scratch and sniff 10 different smells (lemon, strawberry, smoke, soap, menthol, clove, pineapple, natural gas, lilac, and leather). Patients with mild memory loss who scored low on this test were much more likely to develop Alzheimer's disease.

   Source: ScienCentralNews, www.sciencentral.com, January 16, 2005.

6. Researchers at Duke University have identified a gene that controls the onset of both Alzheimer's and Parkinson's disease. It controls when the symptoms of these diseases begin to appear. If this gene could be controlled, it might be possible to delay the onset of the disease for years.

   Source: ScienCentralNews, www.sciencentral.com, August 5, 2004.

Box 10-9: Instructor Activity

DOWN SYNDROME

In 1959, patients with Down syndrome and mental retardation were found to have an abnormal number of chromosomes.

Box 10-10: Instructor Activity

EPILEPSY

1. [Put a paper grocery bag over your head. Then ask students this question.] What disease did doctors once think this was useful for? To treat social phobia? To prevent influenza? Or to treat epilepsy? [Answer: To treat epilepsy.]

2. About 2.5 million Americans have epilepsy. Most cases begin in childhood. Children are of normal intelligence and healthy. Seizures are controlled in 60 percent to 70 percent of children and adults. Patients who have seizures that are not controlled by drugs continue to have seizures an average of 22 years before considering surgery. However, continued severe seizures have been shown to damage the brain. An operation that severs the nerves connecting the right and left hemispheres of the brain can cure epilepsy in two thirds of the patients.

   Source: Parade Magazine (Sunday supplement), September 18, 2005.

3. Efforts to control epilepsy were largely in vain for centuries. The cause was attributed to supernatural forces, poison, and so forth. Phenobarbital was the first drug found to be effective in treating epilepsy. It was introduced in 1912. In 1923, young Tracy Putnam was a resident in neurology. He became intrigued with the possibility that epilepsy might be caused by a chemical abnormality in the brain. He noted, for example, that patients who rebreathed their own exhaled carbon dioxide by putting a bag over their heads got some relief from seizures. He thought that an institution might be built next to a brewery to treat epilepsy because there would be increased carbon dioxide in the air. Putnam later abandoned this idea and instead began searching for drug cures. "I combed the catalog," Putnam later wrote, "for suitable compounds that were not obviously poisonous." He was looking for a drug with a structure similar to that of phenobarbital. "Parke-Davis wrote back to me that it had on hand samples of 19 different compounds similar to Phenobarbital and that I was welcome to them." Of the 19 compounds in the shipment, all were inactive and ineffective except one—phenytoin (Dilantin) was introduced in 1938 and is still the drug of choice for treating adult tonic-clonic seizures.

   Source: Susan Turley, *Understanding Pharmacology for Health Professionals* (Prentice Hall).

Box 10-11: Instruction Activity

MENINGITIS

Do not confuse these sound-alike phrases.

Nuchal rigidity is neck stiffness that can be a sign of meningitis.

Nuchal cord is a condition in which the umbilical cord is wrapped around the baby's neck. If it is wrapped tightly it can cut off the supply of blood and cause brain damage or even death.

Box 10-12: Instructor Activity

NEURAL TUBE DEFECT

[Hold up a box of cornflakes and a bottle of vitamins. Then ask students this question.] What was added to these to prevent a specific disease in newborns? [Answer: Folic acid to prevent neural tube defects.]

After folic acid supplementation in cereals and prenatal vitamins began in 1998, the occurrence of neural tube defects dropped by 34 percent and the occurrence of anencephaly dropped by 16 percent.

Box 10-13: Instructor Activity

CEREBROVASCULAR ACCIDENTS, STROKE, OR BRAIN ATTACK

1. The old word for a stroke was "apoplexy."
2. Doctors at the University of New York at Buffalo found that the presence of periodontal disease created twice the risk of stroke compared to someone with healthy teeth and gums.

   Source: Parade Magazine (Sunday newspaper supplement), February 21, 2001.

3. Review the similarities between a brain attack and a heart attack.
   a. A brain attack is often preceded by a transient ischemic attack (TIA), weakness and loss of sensation due to a temporary lack of oxygenated blood to the brain cells. A heart attack is often preceded by angina pectoris, chest pain due to a temporary lack of oxygenated blood to the heart cells.
   b. Both a brain attack and a heart attack are caused by a combination of arteriosclerosis and/or a blood clot.
   c. Both a brain attack and a heart attack result in the death of cells. Symptoms and signs vary depending on how many cells died.
4. Nearly 700,000 Americans have a stroke every year. Physical therapy is used to treat the resulting weakness and paralysis. The American Stroke Association says that a new type of physical therapy—forced-use therapy—is better at improving the amount and the quality of movement. Forced-use therapy immobilizes the normal arm and forces the stroke patient to use the arm affected by the stroke.

   Source: Baltimore Sun, "Treatment for Stroke Shows Promise," February 19, 2006.

Box 10-14: Instructor Activity

POLIOMYELITIS

In 1921, outbreaks of poliomyelitis plagued America. That summer, a young politician named Franklin Delano Roosevelt was vacationing with his family at their private estate. After an exhausting day fighting a local forest fire, taking a cold swim, and then lounging in a wet swimming suit at home, he went to bed feeling as though he had a cold. In a few days, he found out he had polio. The virus enters the nose or mouth and incubates for a few days in the intestines. Then the patient develops a headache, nausea and vomiting, and a fever. Then the virus enters the bloodstream. The body makes antibodies against it and most people recover and have a lifetime immunity against polio. Only about 1 percent are left with paralysis. Roosevelt was among that 1 percent. His legs were permanently paralyzed. He continued his political career and eventually became president. There was an understanding with the press never to photograph his braces. He was occasionally photographed standing (with support that was not obvious), but mostly while seated. He led the fight against polio by helping to found the March of Dimes and promoted polio research while not revealing his own illness. An outbreak of polio in the 1950s resulted in posters with pictures of affected children on crutches or in iron lungs to breathe. The first polio vaccine was not developed until 1955 by Dr. Jonas Salk.

Box 10-15: Classroom Activity

CEPHALALGIA

Ask students: Does medical terminology give you cephalalgia? Ask students to name the three word parts in this medical word and give their definitions.

Box 10-16: Instructor Activity

MULTIPLE SCLEROSIS

When Susan Turley, the author, moved into a new house, she left many unopened moving boxes in the basement. At one point, a heavy rainstorm caused a leak in the basement, and some of the boxes got slightly wet. When she unpacked those boxes several days later, she found that many of the books had mold on them and she threw those away and cleaned up the others. Two days later, she experienced severe flu-like symptoms. These symptoms continued for several weeks and did not subside. They included extreme fatigue and muscle weakness and muscle achiness. She was evaluated at Johns Hopkins and tentatively diagnosed as having multiple sclerosis, even though a lumbar puncture was negative for oligoclonal bands. For months she was unable to return to work as a medical transcriptionist because she was unable to keep her hands and arms up to stay in position on the keyboard. Very gradually over a year the symptoms subsided but her muscles always fatigued easily and she would have recurrences, particularly in the spring. Several years later, she was tested by an allergist and found to be extremely allergic to molds. She was begun on weekly allergy shots. Even the weakest dilution of mold extracts. reproduced her symptoms of muscle weakness and fatigue. Multiple sclerosis is a progressive disease that can only be diagnosed by seeing plagues in the brain on an MRI scan. She had an MRI scan of the brain several years later, and it showed no evidence of multiple sclerosis.

Experience Multimedia	

See the PowerPoint presentation on the accompanying Instructor's Media Library for animations and videos on the following topics in this chapter:

- Carpal tunnel syndrome
- Epilepsy
- Down syndrome
- Parkinson's disease
- Multiple sclerosis
- Seizures

Objective 5
Describe common nervous system diagnostic laboratory and radiology tests

- Text page(s) 553-555

Content Abstract

Test	Definition
Cerebrospinal fluid exam	Lab test that examines the CSF macroscopically for clarity and color, microscopically for cells, and chemically for proteins and other substances
Cerebral angiography	Radiologic procedure in which a radiopaque contrast dye is injected into the carotid arteries, and an x-ray is taken to visualize the arterial circulation in the brain
Computed axial tomography	Radiologic procedure that uses x-rays to create many individual, closely spaced images
Magnetic resonance imaging	Radiologic procedure that uses a magnetic field and radiowaves to align the protons in the body and cause them to emit signals
Electroencephalography	Diagnostic procedure to record the electrical activity of the brain
Nerve conduction study	Medical procedure to measure the speed that an electrical impulse travels along a nerve

---

Box 10-17: Instructor Activity

EEG

Share this information with students.

Do not confuse EEG (the abbreviation for electroencephalography) with ECG or EKG (abbreviations for electrocardiography). An EEG records the electrical activity of the brain, while an ECG or EKG records the electrical activity of the heart.

Experience Multimedia

See the PowerPoint presentation on the accompanying Instructor's Media Library for animations and videos on the following topics covered in this chapter:

- Brain scans
- C-spine immobilization

Objective 6
Describe common nervous system medical and surgical procedures and drug categories

- Text page(s) 556-561

Content Abstract

Procedure	Definition
Lumbar puncture	Medical procedure to obtain cerebrospinal fluid (CSF) for testing
Biopsy	Surgical procedure to remove a tumor or mass from the brain or other part of the nervous system
Craniotomy	Surgical incision into the skull to expose the brain tissue
Diskectomy	Surgical excision of part or all of the herniated nucleus pulposus from an intervertebral disk
Laminectomy	Surgical excision of the lamina (the flat area of the arch of the vertebra)
Stereotactic neurosurgery	Surgical procedure that uses a specialized technique that allows three-dimensional excision of a deep tumor within the cerebrum

Drug Category	Description	Example
Antiepileptic drugs	Prevent the seizures of epilepsy	Dilantin, Tegretol
COMT inhibitor drugs	Treat Parkinson's disease by inhibiting the enzyme that metabolizes the drug levodopa	Comtan, Tasmar
Corticosteroid drugs	Used to suppress inflammation in chronic pain conditions and multiple sclerosis	Hydrocortisone, Medrol, Prednisone

---

Box 10-18: Instructor Activity

ARTIFICIAL DISKS

Share this information with students.

The Food and Drug Administration (FDA) approved an artificial spinal disk made of plastic and metal. The artificial disk replaces a ruptured disk between two spinal vertebrae in patients with severe lower back pain. It is an alternative procedure to a spinal fusion.

Source: The Baltimore Sun, October 2004.

Objective 7
Define common nervous system abbreviations

- Text page(s) 562

Teaching Strategy

Stress the importance of learning abbreviations and their full meanings.

Content Abstract

AFP	alpha fetoprotein		**HNP**	herniated nucleus pulposus
ALS	amyotrophic lateral sclerosis		**ICP**	intracranial pressure
AVM	arteriovenous malformation		**LP**	lumbar puncture
BAEP	brainstem auditory evoked potential		**MRI**	magnetic resonance imaging
BAER	brainstem auditory evoked response		**MS**	multiple sclerosis
CNS	central nervous system		**NICU**	neurologic intensive care unit
COMT	catechol-*O*-methyltransferase		**PET**	positron emission scan
CP	cerebral palsy		**RIND**	reversible ischemic neurological deficit
CRPS	chronic regional pain syndrome		**SCI**	spinal cord injury
CSF	cerebrospinal fluid		**SSEP**	somatosensory evoked potential
CT	computed tomography		**SSER**	somatosensory evoked response
CTS	carpal tunnel syndrome		**TENS**	transcutaneous electrical nerve stimulation (unit)
CVA	cerebrovascular accident		**TIA**	transient ischemic attack
EEG	electroencephalography		**VEP**	visual evoked potential
END	electroneurodiagnostic (technician)		**VER**	visual evoked response
GCS	Glasgow Coma Scale (or Score)			

Objective 8
Correctly spell and pronounce nervous system words

- Text page(s) 576-578

Box 10-19: Classroom Activity

GAMES

1. From week to week, pick a different one of these spelling games to use during class. (The descriptions and instructions for the games are in the section "The Art and Craft of Teaching.")

   Beanbag Spelling Toss

   Scrabble

   Spelling Bee

   Gridlock

   Hangman

2. From week to week, pick a different one of these pronunciation games to use during class. (The descriptions and instructions for the games are in the section "The Art and Craft of Teaching.")

   Parroting

   Hieroglyphics

   Beach Ball Blast

Teaching Strategies

1. Impress upon the students that medical words that are mispronounced are also probably going to be misspelled.
2. Encourage students to work on both pronunciation and spelling when studying.

Objective 9
Apply your skills by analyzing a neurology report

- Text page(s) 573-575

Content Abstract

Read the neurologic office consultation and answer questions provided.

Objective 10
Test your knowledge of neurology by completing the review exercises in the textbook and the CD-ROM learning activities

- Text page(s) 564-575

Teaching Strategies

1. Assign the Chapter Review Exercises in the textbook for homework. Remind students to refer to the Answer Key at the end of the textbook to check their answers.
2. Have the students complete the learning activities provided by the interactive CD-ROM.

Experience Multimedia
See the PowerPoint presentation on the accompanying Instructor's Media Library for videos on the topic of careers in pharmacy and speech pathology.

Homework Activities

1. Complete all of the exercises in the chapter, finishing the Chapter Review Exercises at the end of the chapter. Write in your textbook so that your instructor can verify that you did this work. See the Answer Key at the end of the book to check your answers.

2. Make flashcards for all of the prefixes, suffixes, and combining forms in the chapter. An index card makes a good homemade flashcard. One side of the flashcard should contain the word part and the other side should contain the meaning of the word part. Flashcards can also be printed from the CD-ROM. Flashcards can be carried everywhere and reviewed while waiting for a doctor's appointment, waiting for the bus, etc. Recruit family members, especially children, to help you study your flashcards.

   As an additional self-quiz, first look at the meaning of the word part and then remember what the word part is.

3. During class, your instructor assigned 20 words from the Pronunciation Checklist on pages 576-578. Practice the pronunciation of those words and then call your instructor's office or home phone number some time during the week and leave a message as you give your name and then pronounce each of the words.

4. Complete the Word Search for Chapter 10.

5. Refer to the Experience Multimedia CD-ROM Learning Activities Checklist for a list of activities to complete on the interactive CD-ROM.

6. Create a "mnifty mnemonic device" memory aid in the form of a rhyme, a word, or an abbreviation that helps you remember something about this body system.

7. Develop a crossword puzzle based on this chapter. Have some answers in the puzzle go from top to bottom (DOWN words) and others go from right to left (ACROSS words). The words should intersect with each other at several points. Make one list of clues for DOWN words and another list of clues for ACROSS words.

8. Use an English dictionary and a medical dictionary to show what the common meaning is between the origins of this pair of words.

   Arachnoid membrane and arachnophobia

   Adapted from Ellen Drake, "Using Storytelling to Teach and Learn Medical Terminology," *Perspectives on the Medical Transcription Profession*, pp. 10-13.

9. Interview someone who has had a stroke or interview a healthcare professional who works with stroke patients. Prepare a list of questions to be used during the interview. Ask about symptoms and signs, level of functioning after a stroke, and types of rehabilitation equipment used.

10. Research and write a one-page report on the personal story, symptoms, diagnosis, treatment, and aftermath of neurologic disease as it affected one of these famous people.

Dick Clark, entertainer	Stroke
Michael J. Fox, actor	Parkinson's disease
Annette Funicello, actress	Multiple sclerosis
Lou Gehrig, baseball player	Lou Gehrig's disease (amyotrophic lateral sclerosis)
Danny Glover, actor	Epilepsy
Steven Hawking, scientist	Amyotrophic lateral sclerosis
Itzhak Perlman, violinist	Paraplegia
Ronald Reagan, President	Dementia
Christopher Reeve, actor	Quadriplegia

Wilma Rudolph, Olympic sprinter	Postpolio syndrome
Ariel Sharon, Prime Minister of Israel	Stroke
Mohammed Ali, boxer	Parkinson's disease

11. Visit the Web site for the Alzheimer's Association at www.alz.org and explore the various sections on the site.

12. This Web site has an interesting hieroglyphics picture/word puzzle where you read the hieroglyphics and try to see what neurology word it is saying. See http://faculty.washington.edu/chudler/hiro.html#hiro23

13. Visit the Web site for Your Amazing Brain. Go to www.youramazingbrain.org.uk/ supersenses/default.htm. Click on the headings Optical Illusions and Upside Down Face and see all of the different ways that your brain can be tricked!

14. Keep a running list in your notebook of sound-alike words or combining forms that have the same meanings. Title this list of challenging words and word parts as "Perplexing Pairs." Begin by writing down the words or word parts found in the Word Alert boxes in this chapter. Then add the word parts found in the It's Greek to Me box at the end of this chapter. Add any other words or word parts that you found particularly confusing. You will add to this list as you complete each chapter. Examples:

orth/o-	vs.	arthr/o-
myel/o-	vs.	my/o-
perine/o-	vs.	peritone/o-
cephal/o-	vs.	encephal/o-

Word Search

Complete this word search puzzle that contains Chapter 10 words. Look for the following words as given in the list below. The number in parentheses indicates how many times the word appears in the puzzle.

aphasia
auras
axon
brain (2)
cerebellum
CNS
coma
cortex
dementia
dural
EEG
epilepsy

glioma
gyrus
hemiparesis
lobe
myelin
nerve
nervous
pons
RIND
sulcus
TENS

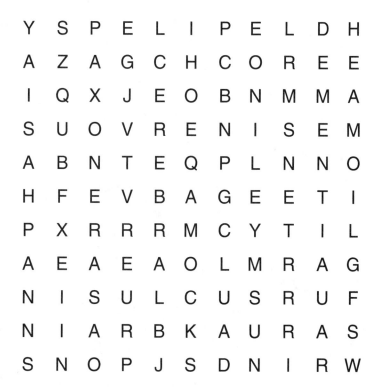

Y S P E L I P E L D H
A Z A G C H C O R E E
I Q X J E O B N M M A
S U O V R E N I S E M
A B N T E Q P L N N O
H F E V B A G E E T I
P X R R R M C Y T I L
A E A E A O L M R A G
N I S U L C U S R U F
N I A R B K A U R A S
S N O P J S D N I R W

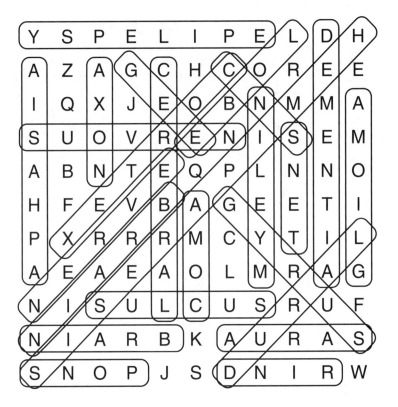

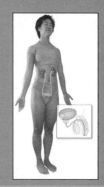

CHAPTER 11

Urology

Urinary System

Objective 1
Identify the anatomical structures of the urinary system by correctly labeling them on anatomical illustrations

- Text page(s) 582-587

Teaching Strategies

1. Explain the importance of learning the parts of the urinary system.
2. Using a visual aid, discuss the anatomy of the urinary system.
3. To learn the anatomy of the urinary system, have the students label the structures on an anatomical diagram.

Content Abstract

Urology is the study of the kidneys and urinary system. It is the healthcare specialty that studies the anatomy and physiology of the urinary system and uses diagnostic tests, medical and surgical procedures, and drugs to treat urinary diseases.

 The anatomy of the urinary system includes:

1. kidneys
2. ureters
3. bladder
4. urethra

Box 11-1: Classroom Activity

RETROPERITONEAL SPACE AND LUMBAR AREA

1. The retroperitoneal space is just a small area, not a body cavity like those discussed in Chapter 2. It is a small space behind the peritoneal cavity. The prefix *retro-* means *behind or backward.* You can remember the meaning of *retro-* by recalling how some people will comment, "Oh, that's so retro," meaning a throwback to years past (a "blast from the past").

   If the kidneys and the beginnings of the ureters are in the retroperitoneal space and the bladder is in the abdominopelvic cavity, when do the ureters make the transition from the retroperitoneal space? They don't! The ureters continue along the outside of the abdominopelvic cavity until they enter the posterior wall of the bladder. The posterior wall of the bladder is outside the abdominopelvic cavity, and so the ureters never actually enter the abdominopelvic cavity.

2. Susan Turley, the author, had a relative who was having severe pain. She had a history of degenerative joint disease of the sacrum and hip that gave her pain. She also often had pain because of a duodenal ulcer. Her present pain was sharp and constant. The author asked her to point to where her pain was located. She pointed to her right flank. Ask students to point to their right flank. [Answer: The right flank is in the right midback in an area on and just below the lower edge of the rib cage.] Ask students what organ is located there. [Answer: The right kidney.] Mention that most people are very surprised to learn that their kidneys are located so high in the body, with the tops actually under the lower edge of the posterior rib cage. Most people picture their kidneys much lower and closer to the bladder. The author's relative then went to the doctor. A urine test showed blood and pus in her urine from a kidney infection, which was causing her pain.

Box 11-2: Instructor Activity

KIDNEY

Share this information with students.

1. Each kidney contains more than one million individual nephrons. If these were laid end to end, they would be 80 miles in length.

2. Approximately 440 gallons of blood flow through the renal arteries to be filtered by the kidneys every day.

3. Word Alert: Do not confuse the bony pelvis of the hip with the renal pelvis in the kidney.

BLADDER

Have students look at Figure 11-6 on page 587. Have them find the bladder on this illustration. Now have them find the uterus. Ask them to complete this sentence with an anatomical direction: The bladder is _____ to the uterus. The uterus is _____ to the bladder. [Answer: inferior, superior]. Ask students what do they think happens to the bladder over nine months during pregnancy. [Answer: The pregnant uterus continues to expand and press down on the bladder. This causes the characteristic frequency and urgency of urination experienced by pregnant women.]

Experience Multimedia

See the PowerPoint presentation on the accompanying Instructor's Media Library for animations on the following topics covered in this chapter:

- Urinary system
- Kidneys

Objective 2
Describe the process of the production of urine

- Text page(s) 588-590

Teaching Strategy

Explain the importance of learning the function of the kidneys in the production of urine.

Content Abstract

The nephron is the functional unit of the kidney and the site of urine production. The blood that enters the nephron contains waste products from the body's metabolic processes. If these waste products were not excreted in the urine, they would quickly reach toxic levels in the blood. The pressure of the blood in the capillary system pushes water, waste products, electrolytes, glucose, and other substances through pores in the glomerulus and out into Bowman's capsule. This process is called filtration. The filtrate (or solution of water) in Bowman's capsule then flows into the proximal convoluted tubule of the nephron. Some of the water and nonwaste substances move out of the tubule and into the blood in a nearby capillary. This process is known as reabsorption.

The process of eliminating urine from the body is described in several ways: urination, micturition, voiding, or passing water.

Objective 3
Build urinary words from combining forms, prefixes, and suffixes

- Text page(s) 595-596

Teaching Strategy

Create a PowerPoint presentation with combining forms, prefixes, and suffixes with their meanings. Use this presentation in class. Have students participate in a "medical terminology bee." All students stand and take turns defining the combining form, prefix, or suffix displayed. If the student gets the answer right, the student remains standing and continues to play. If the student gets the answer wrong, the student will be seated and is out of the game. The last person standing is the winner. A prize could be given to the winner.

Objective 4
Describe common urinary diseases

- Text page(s) 597-605

Content Abstract

Disease	Meaning
Glomerulonephritis	Complication after a streptococcal or viral infection in which the body's antibodies combine with the microorganism and clog the pores of the glomeruli
Hydronephrosis	Enlarged kidney from pressure of backed-up urine
Nephrolithiasis	Kidney stone or calculus formation in the urinary system (see Box 11-4)
Nephropathy	General word for any disease process involving the kidney
Nephroptosis	Abnormally low position of a kidney
Nephrotic syndrome	Damaged glomeruli allow albumin to leak into the urine; this changes the osmotic pressure of the blood and produces edema.
Polycystic kidney disease	Congenital disease characterized by cysts in the kidney that eventually cause kidney failure
Pyelonephritis	Infection of the pelves of the kidneys
Renal cell cancer	Cancer of the nephrons
Renal failure	Kidney function progressively decreases and then urine production stops
Uremia	Excessive amounts of urea in the blood during kidney failure
Wilm's tumor	Cancerous tumor of the kidney that occurs in children and arises from residual embryonic tissue

Disease	Meaning
Bladder cancer	Malignant tumor of the bladder (see Box 11-6)
Cystitis	Inflammation or infection of the bladder (see Box 11-8)
Cystocele	Hernia in which the bladder bulges through a weakness in the muscular wall of the vagina or rectum
Neurogenic bladder	Urinary retention due to lack of nerve innervation to the bladder
Overactive bladder	Urinary urgency and frequency due to involuntary contractions of the bladder wall as the bladder fills with urine
Urinary retention	Inability to empty the bladder because of an obstruction, nerve damage, or as a side effect of certain types of drugs
Vesicovaginal fistula	Abnormal passageway connecting the bladder to the vagina
Epispadias	Congenital abnormality in which the urethral opening is incorrectly positioned above its normal location
Hypospadias	Congenital abnormality in which the male urethral opening is incorrectly positioned on the underside of the penis
Urethritis	Inflammation or infection of the urethra
Albuminuria	Albumin in the urine because of damage to the glomeruli
Anuria	Absence of urine production by the kidney
Bacteriuria	Bacteria in the urine
Dysuria	Difficult or painful urination
Enuresis	Involuntary urination during sleep (see Box 11-7)
Frequency	Urinating often because of an infection, kidney stone, or prostatic enlargement (see Box 11–10)
Glycosuria	Glucose in the urine because of diabetes mellitus
Hematuria	Blood in the urine because of an infection, kidney stone, cancer, or cystitis
Hesitancy	Inability to initiate a normal stream of urine
Hypokalemia	Decreased potassium in the blood because of the action of a diuretic drug
Incontinence	Inability to voluntarily keep urine in the bladder
Ketonuria	Ketone bodies in the urine because of diabetes mellitus or malnutrition
Nocturia	Increased urination at night
Oliguria	Decreased production of urine associated with kidney failure
Polyuria	Increased urine production with diabetes mellitus, diabetes insipidus (see Box 11-5)
Pyuria	White blood cells (pus) in the urine because of infection
Urgency	Strong urge to urinate because of infection, kidney stone, or prostatic enlargement
Urinary tract infection	Infection anywhere in the urinary tract (see Box 11-9)

Box 11-4: Instructor Activity

NEPHROLITHIASIS

Share this information with students.

1. Egyptian mummies have been found to have kidney stones.
2. Susan Turley, the author, has had three kidney stones. The first episode began like the pain of a backache. She laid on the bed with a heating pad. After one day, she made an appointment to see the doctor, who gave her an antibiotic drug for a presumed kidney infection. He told her to call back if she was not feeling better in two days. The pain continued and worsened. She had the setting on the heating pad so high that it nearly burned her skin. When she couldn't stand it any longer, she contacted the physician on call, who advised her to go to the emergency department. There, she was diagnosed with a kidney stone, which later passed in the urine. It was found to be a calcium oxylate stone.

   The second episode came while she was out of state doing a seminar for teachers. After her plane flight, she began to feel a distinct ache in her back. She took a hot shower, but nothing helped. She told her roommate and fellow seminar presenter that she needed to go to the emergency department. Once there, she became very nauseated and proceeded to throw up in the wastebasket of the emergency department secretary who was taking her insurance information. After two doses of intravenous morphine, the pain subsided and she was taken for an IVP. The IVP dye apparently washed the stone into the bladder (as it often is known to do) and it was excreted. She took a taxi back to the hotel, all the while talking nonsense because of the morphine. The next day she felt fine and gave her seminar presentation.

   The third episode included severe abdominal pain, nausea, and diarrhea. In the emergency room, the resident performed a pelvic examination to look for any gynecologic problems. A urine specimen showed blood but no white cells (no infection). A CT scan was negative, but the diagnosis was presumed kidney stone after her history of kidney stones was known.
3. Word Alert: *Calculus* is the Latin word for *kidney stone.* It actually means *a pebble.* Calculus is also an advanced form of algebra; a small stone was used in calculations in ancient times.

Box 11-5: Instructor Activity

POLYURIA

Polyuria is a symptom of both diabetes mellitus and diabetes insipidus.

Box 11-6: Instructor Activity

BLADDER CANCER

The bladder is the most common site of malignancy of the urinary system.

Box 11-7: Instructor Activity

ENURESIS

Word Alert: Do not confuse anuresis (the absence of urine production) with enuresis (bedwetting).

Bedwetting: Forty percent of children age 3 wet the bed, but only 2-3 percent of children ages 12-15 continue to wet the bed. Eighty-five percent of children who wet the bed have a relative who wets the bed. Bedwetting can be due to a combination of all these things:

1. Overproduction of urine at night
2. Small bladder capacity
3. Deep sleep
4. Underdevelopment of the nervous system that sends signals when the bladder is full
5. Heredity

Box 11-8: Instructor Activity

INTERSTITIAL CYSTITIS

Interstitial cystitis affects about a million people, the majority of whom are women. It causes such severe pain in the bladder and pelvic region and urgency that about one-half of the patients with it are unable to continue to work. Scientists at the University of Maryland have found a substance (antiproliferative factor) in the urine of most patients with interstitial cystitis; it inhibits the growth of epithelial cells in the bladder. Now that this factor has been identified, scientists want to develop a diagnostic test to detect it and then hopefully develop a treatment.

Source: *The Baltimore Sun,* August 2004.

Box 11-9: Instructor Activity

URINARY TRACT INFECTIONS

Urinary tract infections are more common in women than in men because the female urethra is much closer to the rectum. The rectum contains the bacterium *Escherichia coli* (E. coli), the most common cause of urinary tract infections.

Box 11-10: Instructor Activity

FREQUENCY

Share this information with students.

As a person ages, some nephrons deteriorate and die. As the number of nephrons decreases, kidney function decreases proportionally. Why then do many older people have urinary frequency? In women, it is often because the uterus has prolapsed and presses on the bladder. This decreases the capacity of the bladder. In men, enlargement of the prostate gland prevents the bladder from emptying fully. In both men and women, the bladder muscle itself contracts less forcefully. This keeps the bladder from emptying fully. It also takes less time for the bladder to fill to capacity again.

Objective 5
Describe common urinary diagnostic laboratory and radiology tests

- Text page(s) 606-611

Content Abstract

Test	Definition
Blood urea nitrogen	Blood test that measures the amount of urea
Culture and sensitivity	Urine test that puts urine onto culture medium in a Petri dish to identify the cause of a urinary tract infection
Drug screening	Urine test performed on a group of employees or athletes to detect any individual who is using illegal, addictive, or performance-enhancing drugs
Urinalysis	Urine test to describe the characteristics of the urine and detect substances in it (see Box 11-11)
Renal angiography	Radiologic procedure that uses x-rays and radiopaque contrast dye to detect blockage of the renal artery
Cystometry	Diagnostic procedure that evaluates the function of the nerves to the bladder

Box 11-11: Instructor Activity

URINALYSIS

Obtain a copy of a urinalysis and discuss the findings with the class.

Physicians in the Middle Ages routinely examined the urine, held up in a flask to the light, to diagnose diseases. In 1637, Thomas Brian wrote the book *The Pisse-Prophet* that ridiculed this medical practice. Physicians also tasted the urine and, in the case of diabetes mellitus in which the urine tastes sweet, this did help them make the diagnosis.

The Dropsical Woman is a famous painting done by Gerard Dou in 1663. It shows a physician holding up a flask of urine to the light and examining it. The patient had dropsy, the old medical word for congestive heart failure.

Objective 6
Describe common urinary medical and surgical procedures and drug categories

- Text page(s) 612-619

Content Abstract

Procedure	Definition
Catheterization	Procedure in which a catheter is inserted through the urethra and into the bladder to drain urine (see Box 11-12)
Dialysis	Procedure to remove waste products from the blood of patients with renal failure
Intake and output	Nursing procedure that documents the total amount of fluid intake and the total amount of fluid output (see Box 11-13)
Cystectomy	Surgical procedure to remove the bladder because of bladder cancer
Cystoscopy	Surgical procedure that uses a cystoscope inserted through the urethra in order to examine the bladder
Lithotripsy	Procedure that uses sound waves to break up a kidney stone (see Boxes 11-14 and 11-15)
Renal biopsy	Surgical procedure in which a small piece of kidney is excised for microscopic analysis

Drug Category	Description	Example
Antibiotic drugs	Used to treat urinary tract infections	Gantrisin, Macrobid
Chemotherapy drugs	Kill rapidly dividing cancer cells in the bladder or kidney	Adriamycin, Vincasar
Diuretic drugs	Used to block sodium from being absorbed from the tubule back into the blood	Aldactone, Esidrix, Hygroton, Lasix, Zaroxolyn
Urinary analgesic drugs	Exert a pain-relieving effect on the mucosa of the urinary tract	Pyridium, Urogesic

Box 11-12: Classroom Activity

CATHETERIZATION

1. Purchase a Foley catheter kit from a medical supply house (these are inexpensive) or borrow one from your school's nursing or medical assistant department.

2. Describe how a catheter without a balloon at its tip would slide out of the bladder and would not be useful for continuous drainage of urine.

3. Show how the syringe is used to insert air and inflate the balloon once the catheter is in the bladder. Show how the syringe is used to deflate the balloon when the catheter needs to be changed or discontinued.

Box 11-13: Instructor Activity

URINE OUTPUT

Eccentric aviator, inventor, and business man Howard Hughes became a recluse in his later years. He kept the drapes of his home closed, refused to see visitors, and had his servants save all of his urine, stored in container after container, all numbered and cataloged!

Box 11-14: Classroom Activity

KIDNEY STONE TREATMENT

Discuss the advantages and disadvantages of these treatment options for kidney stones. Draw this table on the board and have students complete the blank areas.

Kidney Stone Treatment	Advantages and Disadvantages
Strain the urine	
Extracorporeal shock wave lithotripsy	
Percutaneous ultrasonic lithotripsy	
Nephrolithotomy	
Stone basketing	

[Answer Key]

Kidney Stone Treatment	Advantages and Disadvantages
Strain the urine	Medical procedure. No need for surgery, but cannot remove the stone; only catches the stone after it is passed.
Extracorporeal shock wave lithotripsy	Medical procedure done in the radiology department. It uses sound waves to break up the stone. Requires specialized equipment, but no surgery and no incision.
Percutaneous ultrasonic lithotripsy	Surgical procedure that must be done in an operating room. A skin incision is made and an endoscope inserted through the skin and into the kidney. Ultrasonic probe inserted to break up the kidney stone with sounds waves. Incision increases the risk of infection.
Nephrolithotomy	Surgical procedure that must be done in an operating room. A skin incision is made and an endoscope inserted through the skin and into the kidney. Instruments are used to cut kidney tissue to remove the stone. Damage to kidney tissue. Incision increases the risk of infection.
Stone basketing	Surgical procedure that must be done in an operating room, but no incision is required. A cystoscope is inserted into the bladder. A stone basket is passed through the cystoscope to snare the stone and remove it.

Box 11-15: Instructor Activity

KIDNEY STONES

Share this information with students.

Barbers and surgeons in the Middle Ages who specialized in removing kidney stones were called stonecutters. Because little was known of the internal anatomy of the urinary system at that time, attempts to remove stones frequently resulted in complications or even death.

Box 11-16: Instructor Activity

KIDNEY TRANSPLANTATION

1. The first successful kidney transplantation occurred in 1954 between identical twins. It was not until the FDA approved the anti-rejection drug cyclosporine in 1984 that transplantation of kidneys (and other organs) from cadavers or unrelated living donors could be performed successfully.

   Source: Susan Turley, *Understanding Pharmacology for Health Professionals.* Prentice Hall.

2. The health of a kidney donor is not affected by losing one kidney. In fact, the remaining kidney enlarges to take over almost full function.

3. Organ transplant surgeons use a sophisticated computer program to find scarce organ donors of medically compatible kidneys for desperately ill patients. The mathematical algorithm that is the basis for the computer program was developed by Dr. Dorry Segev, a Johns Hopkins transplant surgeon, and his wife, Dr. Sommer Gentry, a professor of math at the U.S. Naval Academy. Their work was the basis for a January 2006 *Numb3rs* episode on television in which the FBI used the mathematics in reverse to track down the recipient of a kidney sold on the black market. The black market issue is an ongoing concern because often a patient in need of a kidney does not match any friends or relatives willing to donate a kidney. The mathematical algorithm is being used to increase the number of donor kidneys available through legitimate channels by creating a paired organ donation system in which a donor gives a kidney to a patient who is a stranger while another donor who is a stranger but a tissue match gives a kidney to the first donor's friend or relative.

   Source: The Baltimore Sun, January 27, 2006.

Box 11-17: Instructor Activity

DRUGS

Share this information with students.

1. Obtain a copy of a urine culture and sensitivity report and discuss the findings with the class.

2. Botox, the toxin that kills people with food poisoning and, in a greatly diluted form, is injected into the skin to smooth wrinkles, is now being tested for enlarged prostate glands. When injected, it reduced urinary frequency by 65 percent.

   Source: Parade Magazine (Sunday newspaper supplement), June 19, 2005.

   (continued)

Box 11-17: Instructor Activity (*cont.*)

Most drugs are metabolized by the liver and transformed into an inactive substance, which is then excreted by the kidneys. However, the drug Neurontin is one of the few drugs that is not metabolized by the liver. It is excreted in its original active form by the kidneys. Susan Turley, the author, had an elderly relative who was on Neurontin to treat mild seizures associated with dementia. She had been on it for about one year. During that time, her kidney function slowly decreased without anyone being aware of it. Then her level of seizures required that she begin to take a higher dose of Neurontin. Soon after that, she developed symptoms of nausea and a rash. She was admitted to the hospital. Blood tests showed only decreased kidney function. Her symptoms continued to increase. She had nausea, dizziness, headache, an increase in her normally present head and neck tremor, increased confusion, fever, constant coughing, fatigue, and blisters in the mouth. She also had an extremely itchy and red rash spreading over her skin that appeared to be a herpes infection. She was placed in an isolation room because of concerns that she had an infectious disease. Finally, the author researched all of her relative's medications in the definitive source *Drug Facts and Comparisons*. The author found that Neurontin is excreted unchanged by the kidneys. The normal half-life of the drug is 5 to 7 hours (the time it takes for half of the dose to be excreted by the kidneys), but in patients with decreased kidney function, the half-life can be as long as 52 hours. That meant that multiple doses of the active, unmetabolized drug continued to be in the patient's system with more added each day, and the increased drug levels were causing drug side effects. The documented side effects of this drug matched the patient's symptoms and signs. When this information was communicated to the physician, he immediately discontinued the patient's Neurontin. Within days, her symptoms disappeared, and she was well enough to be discharged from the hospital.

Experience Multimedia

See the PowerPoint presentation on the accompanying Instructor's Media Library for an animation and video on the following topics in this chapter:

- Catherization
- Continuous bladder irrigation

Objective 7
Define common urinary abbreviations

- Text page(s) 619

Teaching Strategies

1. Stress the importance of learning abbreviations and their full meanings.
2. Encourage students to make flashcards for abbreviations and their meanings as well as their usual flashcards for word parts and their meanings.

Content Abstract

ARF	acute renal failure		**I&O**	intake and output
BUN	blood urea nitrogen		**IVP**	intravenous pyelogram
CAPD	continuous ambulatory peritoneal dialysis		**K or K⁺**	potassium
cath	catheterize or catheterization (slang)		**KUB**	kidneys, ureters, bladder
cc	cubic centimeter (measure of volume)		**mL**	milliliter (measure of volume)
CCPD	continuous cycling peritoneal dialysis		**pH**	potential of hydrogen (acidity or alkalinity)
C&S	culture and sensitivity		**RBC**	red blood cell
CRF	chronic renal failure		**SG,**	specific gravity
cysto	cystoscopy (slang)		**sp gr**	
epis	epithelial cells (in the urine specimen) (slang)		**TNTC**	too numerous to count
ESWL	extracorporeal shock wave lithotripsy		**TURBT**	transurethral resection of bladder tumor
ESRD	end-stage renal disease		**UA**	urinalysis
GU	genitourinary		**UTI**	urinary tract infection
	gonococcal urethritis		**VMA**	vanillylmandelic acid
hpf	high-power field		**WBC**	white blood cell

Objective 8
Correctly spell and pronounce urinary words

* Text page(s) 631–632

Teaching Strategies

1. Impress upon the students that medical words that are mispronounced are also probably going to be misspelled.
2. Encourage students to work on both pronunciation and spelling when studying.

Chapter Spelling Test

The chapter spelling test is included with the weekly chapter test. Dictate and spell (or xerox a handout that contains) this list of 20 spelling words. Give the list to students the week before the test. For the chapter test, select just 10 of these words to test.

1. albuminuria
2. catheterization
3. creatinine
4. cystitis
5. cystoscopy
6. diuretic drug
7. glomerulonephritis
8. hemodialysis
9. hypospadias
10. incontinence
11. intravesical chemotherapy
12. lithotripsy
13. nephrolithiasis
14. nephroptosis
15. nocturia
16. pyelonephritis
17. retroperitoneal space
18. ureter
19. urethra
20. urinalysis

Box 11-18: Classroom Activity

GAMES

1. From week to week, pick a different one of these spelling games to use during class. (The descriptions and instructions for the games are in the section "The Art and Craft of Teaching.")

   Beanbag Spelling Toss

   Scrabble

   Spelling Bee

   Gridlock

   Hangman

2. From week to week, pick a different one of these pronunciation games to use during class. (The descriptions and instructions for the games are in the section "The Art and Craft of Teaching.")

   Parroting

   Hieroglyphics

   Beach Ball Blast

Chapter Pronunciation Test

Have students mark these 20 words listed in the Pronunciation Checklist for the chapter. During the week, they will call your office or home answering machine and pronounce each word.

1. caliectasis	11. incontinence
2. catheterization	12. lithotripsy
3. creatinine	13. nephrolithiasis
4. cystitis	14. nephrologist
5. cystocele	15. nocturia
6. dysuria	16. pyelonephritis
7. epispadias	17. retroperitoneal space
8. glomerulonephritis	18. ureter
9. hemodialysis	19. urethra
10. hydronephrosis	20. urinalysis

Objective 9
Apply your skills by analyzing a urology report

- Text page(s) 629-630

Content Abstract

Read the emergency department report and answer the questions provided.

Objective 10
Test your knowledge of urology by completing the review exercises in the textbook and the CD-ROM learning activities

- Text page(s) 621-630 (first complete all the in-chapter exercises on pp. 594-596).

Teaching Strategies

1. Assign the Chapter Review Exercises in the textbook for homework. Remind students to refer to the Answer Key at the end of the textbook to check their answers.
2. Have the students complete the learning activities provided by the interactive CD-ROM.

Experience Multimedia

See the PowerPoint presentation on the accompanying Instructor's Media Library for videos on the topic of a career as a dialysis nurse.

Homework Activities

1. Complete all of the exercises in the chapter, finishing the Chapter Review Exercises at the end of the chapter. Write in your textbook so that your instructor can verify that you did this work. See the Answer Key at the end of the book to check your answers.

2. Make flashcards for all of the prefixes, suffixes, and combining forms in the chapter. An index card makes a good homemade flashcard. One side of the flashcard should contain the word part and the other side should contain the meaning of the word part. Flashcards can also be printed from the CD-ROM. Flashcards can be carried everywhere and reviewed while waiting for a doctor's appointment, waiting for the bus, etc. Recruit family members, especially children, to help you study with your flashcards.

   As an additional self-quiz, first look at the meaning of the word part and then remember what the word part is.

3. During class, your instructor assigned 20 words from the Pronunciation Checklist on pp. 631-632. Practice the pronunciation of those words and then call your instructor's office or home phone number some time during the week and leave a message as you give your name and then pronounce each of the words.

4. Complete the Wordsearch for Chapter 11.

5. Refer to the Experience Multimedia CD-ROM Learning Activities Checklist for a list of activities to complete on the interactive CD-ROM.

6. Create a "mnifty mnemonic device" memory aid in the form of a rhyme, a word, or an abbreviation that helps you remember something about this body system.

7. Develop a crossword puzzle based on this chapter. Have some answers in the puzzle go from top to bottom (DOWN words) and others go from right to left (ACROSS Words). The words should intersect with each other at several points. Make one list of clues for DOWN words and another list of clues for ACROSS words.

8. Get extra credit by using English and medical dictionaries to show what the common meaning is between the origins of this pair of words: cryptorchism and orchid. What is the meaning of the word orchidology?

   Adapted from Ellen Drake, "Using Storytelling to Teach and Learn Medical Terminology," *Perspectives on the Medical Transcription Profession,* pp. 10-13.

9. More kidney transplantations are performed each year than transplantations of any other organ. Visit the Web site Decision: Donation at www.organdonor.gov/student/access/organs.asp

   Also, find out how to become an organ donor in your state. Many if not all states will ask you if you want to become an organ donor when you renew your driver's license; if you say yes, this is noted in a special box on your license.

10. Keep a running list in your notebook of sound-alike words or combining forms that have the same meanings. Title this list of challenging words and word parts as "Perplexing Pairs." Begin by writing down the words or word parts found in the Word Alert boxes in this chapter. Then add the word parts found in the It's Greek to Me box at the end of this chapter. Add any other words or word parts that you found particularly confusing. You will add to this list as you complete each chapter. Examples:

orth/o-   vs.   arthr/o-
myel/o-   vs.   my/o-
perine/o-   vs.   peritone/o-
cephal/o-   vs.   encephal/o-

11. Look in your medicine cabinet. Find 10 prescription or over-the-counter drugs. List their drug names. Also look on the label and find any medical words. Write down these medical words and then look up and write their medical definitions.

Word Search

Complete this word search puzzle that contains Chapter 11 words. Look for the following words as given in the list below. The number in parentheses indicates how many times the word appears in the puzzle.

anuria
bladder
BUN
cystitis
enuresis
ESRD
hilum
IVP
kidneys

pyuria
renal (2)
renin
rugae
urea
ureter
urinalysis
urine
UTI

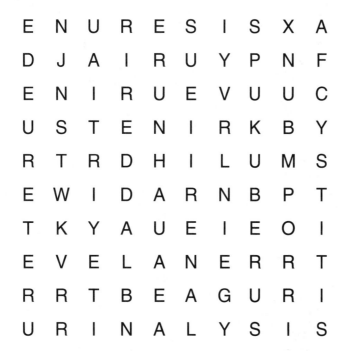

```
E  N  U  R  E  S  I  S  X  A
D  J  A  I  R  U  Y  P  N  F
E  N  I  R  U  E  V  U  U  C
U  S  T  E  N  I  R  K  B  Y
R  T  R  D  H  I  L  U  M  S
E  W  I  D  A  R  N  B  P  T
T  K  Y  A  U  E  I  E  O  I
E  V  E  L  A  N  E  R  R  T
R  R  T  B  E  A  G  U  R  I
U  R  I  N  A  L  Y  S  I  S
```

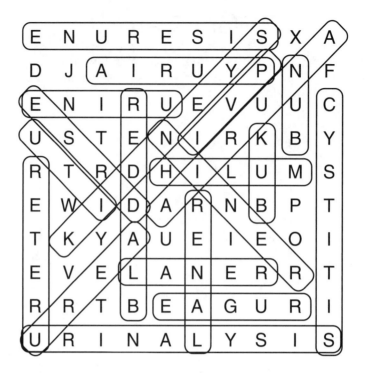

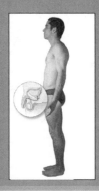

CHAPTER 12

Male Reproductive Medicine

Male Genitourinary System

Objective 1
Identify the anatomical structures of the male genitourinary system by correctly labeling them on an anatomical illustration

- Text page(s) 636-641

Teaching Strategies

1. Explain the importance of learning the parts of the male reproductive system.
2. Using a diagram or model, identify each part of the male reproductive system as it is discussed.
3. To learn the anatomy of the male reproductive system, have the students label them on an anatomical diagram.

Content Abstract

Male reproductive medicine is the medical specialty that studies the anatomy and physiology of the male genitourinary system and uses diagnostic tests, medical and surgical procedures, and drugs to treat male reproductive diseases.

 The anatomy of the male reproductive system consists of

1. scrotum
2. testis
3. epididymis
4. vas deferens
5. seminal vesicles
6. ejaculatory duct
7. prostate gland
8. bulbourethral glands
9. penis

Box 12-1: Instructor Activity

INTERESTING FACTS

Share this information with students.

1. Word Alert
   prostate   A genitourinary gland being studied in this chapter
   prostrate   Lying in a face-down position

2. The following announcement appeared in a local newspaper: "PROSTRATE CANCER EXHIBIT. North Arundel Hospital's exhibition area at Arundel Mills Mall will present an educational exhibit on prostrate cancer on September 11 from 8:30 to 10:00 a.m."

3. The Latin word *testis* means a *witness* or *one who testifies*. In Roman courts, no man was allowed to act as a witness unless he could prove his testes were intact. He was required to take an oath with his hand on his testes.

4. Early Greek scholars noted the resemblance of the testes to the bulb of an orchid plant. Due to this resemblance, they believed the orchid bulb had medicinal value and used it to treat diseases of the testes, including sterility. Hence, the combining form *orchid/o-* means *testis*.

5. *Testosterone* is a combination of the combining form *test/o-* (testis), the letters *ster* from *sterol* (a category of chemicals), and the suffix *-one* (a chemical structure).

6. Notice these combining forms:

   pen/o-   Latin, meaning *a tail*
   balan/o-   Greek, meaning *acorn*
   phall/o-   Greek, meaning *penis*

7. Both the Romans and the Greeks thought the tip of the penis resembled an acorn. The Greek combining form *balan/o-* means *acorn*, and the Latin word *glans* (glans penis) means *acorn*.

8. The Greek *phall/o-* in the phrase *phallic symbol* is used in psychiatry. The plural of the Latin word *semen* is *semina*. It means *seed*.

9. Chinook salmon are the largest salmon in the Pacific Ocean. When they are four years old, they return to the stream where they were born. There they mate and then die. Researchers are studying the salmon because their numbers are declining. Now they have found that 84 percent of the salmon that appear to be females actually have the chromosomes of a male. The population of true females might actually disappear. They are investigating whether female hormone–type pesticides in the water or the nightly release of cold water from hydroelectric plants could be the cause.

Source: Science News Online at www.sciencenews.org

Experience Multimedia

See the PowerPoint presentation on the accompanying Instructor's Media Library for an animation showing the male pelvis.

Objective 2
Describe the processes of spermatogenesis and ejaculation

- Text page(s) 642-643

Teaching Strategy

Explain the importance of learning the process of the production of sperm and the act of ejaculation.

Content Abstract

During childhood, the seminiferous tubules contain immature cells called spermatocytes. At puberty, the anterior pituitary gland begins to secrete hormones to stimulate the testes. The hormones stimulate the spermatocytes to begin to divide and cause the interstitial cells to begin to produce testosterone. The 46 chromosomes in the immature spermatocyte duplicate by mitosis, and the duplicated chromosomes group together and randomly exchange genetic material. Then the spermatocyte divides 2 more times into 4 individual spermatozoon, each with 23 chromosomes (or half the usual number). Each spermatozoon is composed of a head that contains the 23 chromosomes and a tail or flagellum that propels it; it is also called a gamete. The process of forming mature spermatozoa is known as spermatogenesis.

The process of ejaculation begins in response to thoughts or sensations that initiate sexual arousal. The smooth muscles in the penis relax, allowing increased blood flow to the penis, producing an erection. Contractions occur and spermatozoa in the vas deferens move into the ejaculatory duct. Fluid from the seminal vesicles is mixed with the spermatozoa, which then move into the urethra. The bulbourethral glands and the prostate gland also contribute fluid to the semen. A series of contractions of the muscles around the penis cause the semen to be expelled through the urethral meatus. This process is known as ejaculation.

Objective 3
Build male genitourinary words from combining forms, prefixes, and suffixes

- Text page(s) 647-648

Teaching Strategy

Create a PowerPoint presentation with combining forms, prefixes, and suffixes with their meanings. Use this presentation in class. All students participate in a "medical terminology bee." All students stand and take turns defining the combining form, prefix, or suffix displayed. If the student gets the answer right, the student remains standing and continues to play. If the student gets the answer wrong, the student will be seated and is out of the game. The last person standing is the winner. A prize could be given to the winner.

Objective 4
Describe common male genitourinary diseases

- Text page(s) 649-653

Content Abstract

Disease	Meaning
Cryptorchism	Failure of one or both of the testicles to descend through the inguinal canal into the scrotum
Epididymitis	Bacterial infection of the epididymis, usually caused by a sexually transmitted disease
Infertility	Failure to conceive after at least one year of regular intercourse (see Box 12-2)
Oligospermia	Less than the normal amount of spermatozoa produced by the testes
Orchitis	Infection of the testes by bacteria or the mumps virus; also can be inflammation due to trauma
Testicular cancer	Malignant tumor of the testis, arising from abnormal spermatozoa
Varicocele	Varicose vein in the spermatic cord to the testis

Disease	Meaning
Benign prostatic hypertrophy	Enlargement of the prostate gland
Cancer of the prostate	Malignant tumor of the prostate gland (see Box 12-3)
Prostatitis	Acute or chronic bacterial infection of the prostate gland
Balanitis	Inflammation and infection of the glans penis
Chordee	Congenital downward curvature of the penis due to a constricting band of tissue
Dyspareunia	Painful or difficult sexual intercourse
Erectile dysfunction	Inability to achieve or sustain an erection of the penis
Phimosis	Congenital condition in which the opening of the foreskin is too small to allow the foreskin to pull back over the glans penis
Premature ejaculation	Ejaculation of semen before the penis is fully erect
Priapism	Continued, painful erection due to spinal cord injury or from taking drugs to treat erectile dysfunction
Sexually transmitted diseases	Contagious diseases that are contracted during intercourse with an infected individual (see Box 12-4)
Gynecomastia	Enlargement of the breasts in a male

Box 12-2: Instructor Activity

INFERTILITY

Share this information with students.

1. About 6.5 million couples (10 percent of the reproductive-age population) have infertility.

   Source: The Baltimore Sun, September 2000.

2. Susan Turley, the author, had a diagnosis of infertility because she and her husband were unable to conceive for seven years. They both had an infertility workup at the Reproductive Medicine Clinic of a very large and famous medical center. Her husband first had a semen analysis, in which the sperm were normal in amount, shape, and activity. Then, because of complaints of dyspareunia, the doctors suspected that she might have endometriosis. They performed a laparoscopy to view the abdominal organs, but no endometriosis was found. Then they performed a hysterosalpingography to look for blockage in the fallopian tubes, but it, too, was normal. The doctors were unable to give any reason for the infertility. A year later, because of allergy symptoms, the author visited a physician (M.D.) who specialized in natural medicine. She also mentioned that she had not been able to get pregnant and had had a complete infertility workup with no reason found. This physician suggested an elimination diet to pinpoint the foods she was most allergic to, but did not directly address the infertility issue. The elimination diet showed that she was highly allergic to dairy products, oranges, chocolate, and other foods—most of which were her favorite foods. She stopped eating these foods. Her allergy symptoms improved significantly and, within three menstrual cycles, she was pregnant! The physician explained that the constant allergic irritation to her body may have prevented a fertilized egg from implanting in the uterus.

Objective 5
Describe common male genitourinary diagnostic laboratory and radiology tests

- Text page(s) 653-654

Content Abstract

Test	Definition
Hormone testing	Blood test to determine the levels of FSH and LH from the anterior pituitary gland and testosterone from the testes
Prostate-specific antigen	Blood test that detects a glycoprotein from cells of the prostate gland
DNA analysis	Semen is compared to other samples of known DNA in a criminal database
Semen analysis	Microscopic examination of the spermatozoa as part of infertility testing or to determine the effectiveness of a vasectomy

Objective 6

Describe common male genitourinary medical and surgical procedures and drug categories

- Text page(s) 655-657

Content Abstract

Procedure	Definition
Digital rectal examination	Procedure to palpate the prostate gland
Biopsy	Surgical procedure to remove tissue from the prostate to diagnose prostatic cancer
Circumcision	Surgical procedure to remove the prepuce (foreskin) of the glans penis (see Box 12-8)
Orchiectomy	Surgical procedure to remove a testis because of testicular cancer (see Box 12-9)
Vasectomy	Surgical procedure in the male to prevent pregnancy in the female

Drug Category	Description	Example
Androgen drugs	Treat lack of production of testosterone by the testes because of cryptorchism	Testroderm, Virilon
Antiviral drugs	Treat viral infection that causes genital herpes and condylomata acuminatae	Aldara, Condylox, Zovirax
Drugs that produce an erection	Inhibit a substance that limits the process of blood flow into the penis	Cialis, Levitra, Viagra

---

Box 12-7: Instructor Activity

HUMOR

Here are some amusing answers to questions that sixth grade children put on history tests. This made the rounds as a popular e-mail.

> The nineteenth century was a time of a great many thoughts and inventions. People stopped reproducing by hand and started reproducing by machine. Cyrus McCormick invented the McCormick raper, which did the work of a hundred men.

> Charles Darwin was a naturalist who wrote "The Organ of the Species."

> Sir Francis Drake circumcised the world with a 100-foot clipper.

Box 12-8: Instructor Activity

CIRCUMCISION

The National Center for Health Statistics estimates that 65 percent of newborn males undergo circumcision. There is a slightly higher incidence of urinary tract infections and cancer of the penis in boys who are not circumcised; however, the American Academy of Pediatrics (AAP) does not feel these potential benefits are great enough to recommend circumcision for all newborn males. Circumcision is usually performed in the hospital by the obstetrician who delivered the baby. For many years, newborn circumcision was performed without any anesthesia. The rationale was that it was a quick procedure and that, although the baby cried, he quickly forgot about the pain. This thinking has changed. AAP now recommends using a topical anesthetic drug of numbing cream or a local anesthetic drug injected in several locations around the penis to provide anesthesia prior to a circumcision.

Box 12-9: Instructor Activity

ORCHIECTOMY

Orchiectomy is the surgical excision of the testicles. It is also known as castration. When a male is castrated before puberty, he is known as a eunuch; male secondary sex characteristics fail to develop. Castration was a common practice when a king would conquer a neighboring country and bring male captives back to his kingdom.

TREATMENT FOR AN ENLARGED PROSTATE

Newer surgeries to decrease the size of an enlarged prostate gland:

1. Transurethral microwave thermotherapy (TUMT). A microwave device is inserted into the urethra and microwaves are directed toward the prostate. This heats up the prostatic tissue until it dies.
2. Transurethral needle ablation (TUNA). Tiny needles are inserted into the prostate gland. Low-level energy delivered through the needles heats the prostatic tissue to 200 degrees. This destroys prostatic cells.
3. Transurethral ultrasound-guided laser-induced prostatectomy (TULIP). Ultrasound is used to locate the prostate gland and guide a laser which destroys prostatic cells. The laser also coagulates bleeding blood vessels as it destroys prostatic tissue.

| Box 12-11: Instructor Activity |

VIAGRA

Share this information with students.

The drug Viagra was introduced in 1998 as a treatment for erectile dysfunction (ED). Former senator and presidential candidate Bob Dole appeared in television commercials candidly discussing ED and urging viewers to see their doctors.

Source: Susan Turley, *Understanding Pharmacology for Health Professionals.* Prentice Hall.

| Experience Multimedia |

See the PowerPoint presentation on the accompanying Instructor's Media Library for videos on the following topics covered in this chapter:

- Circumcision
- Vasectomy

Objective 7
Define common male genitourinary abbreviations

- Text page(s) 658

Teaching Strategies

1. Stress the importance of learning abbreviations and their full meanings.
2. Encourage students to make flashcards for abbreviations and their meanings as well as their usual flashcards for word parts and their meanings.

Content Abstract

AIDS	acquired immunodeficiency syndrome	**LH**	luteinizing hormone
BPH	benign prostatic hypertrophy	**PAP**	prostatic acid phosphatase
CDCP	Centers for Disease Control and Prevention	**PSA**	prostate-specific antigen
DRE	digital rectal examination	**RPR**	rapid plasma reagin (test for syphilis)
ED	erectile dysfunction	**STD**	sexually transmitted disease
FSH	follicle-stimulating hormone	**TRUS**	transrectal ultrasound
GC	gonococcus (*Neisseria gonorrhoeae*)	**TSE**	testicular self-examination
GU	genitourinary	**TURP**	transurethral resection of the prostate
HIV	human immunodeficiency virus	**VD**	venereal disease
HPV	human papillomavirus	**VDRL**	Venereal Disease Research Laboratory (test for syphilis)
HSV	herpes simplex virus		

Objective 8
Correctly spell and pronounce male genitourinary words

- Text page(s) 669–670

Teaching Strategies

1. Impress upon the students that medical words that are mispronounced are also probably going to be misspelled.
2. Encourage students to work on both pronunciation and spelling when studying.

Chapter Spelling Test

The chapter spelling test is included with the weekly chapter test. Dictate and spell (or xerox a handout that contains) this list of 20 spelling words. Give the list to students the week before the test. For the chapter test, select just 10 of these words to test.

1. adolescence
2. balanitis
3. chancre
4. chordee
5. circumcision
6. ductus deferens
7. dyspareunia
8. epididymitis
9. genitalia
10. glans penis
11. gonorrhea
12. gynecomastia
13. orchiectomy
14. perineum
15. phimosis
16. prostate gland
17. seminal vesicle
18. spermatozoon
19. testis
20. varicocele

Chapter Pronunciation Test

Have students mark these 20 words listed in the Pronunciation Checklist for the chapter. During the week, they will call your office or home answering machine and pronounce each word.

1. balanitis
2. chancre
3. chordee
4. circumcision
5. ductus deferens
6. dyspareunia
7. epididymis
8. genitalia
9. gonorrhea
10. gynecomastia
11. orchiectomy
12. perineum
13. phimosis
14. seminal vesicle
15. sonogram
16. spermatozoon
17. testis
18. varicocele
19. vasectomy
20. venereal disease

Objective 9
Apply your skills by analyzing a male reproductive medicine report

- Text page(s) 667-668

Content Abstract

Read the hospital Operative Report and answer the questions provided.

Objective 10
Test your knowledge of male reproductive medicine by completing review exercises in the textbook and the CD-ROM learning activities

- Text page(s) 660-666 (first complete all the in-chapter exercises on pp. 646-648)

Teaching Strategies

1. Assign the Chapter Review Exercises in the textbook for homework.
2. Remind students to refer to the Answer Key at the end of the textbook to check their answers.
3. Refer to the CD-ROM Learning Activities in this section for multimedia learning experiences.

Experience Multimedia
See the PowerPoint presentation on the accompanying Instructor's Media Library for videos on the topic of careers in medical technology.

Homework Activities

1. Complete all of the exercises in the chapter, finishing the Chapter Review Exercises at the end of the chapter. Write in your textbook so that your instructor can verify that you did this work. See the Answer Key at the end of the book to check your answers.

2. Make flashcards for all of the prefixes, suffixes, and combining forms in the chapter. An index card makes a good homemade flashcard. One side of the flashcard should contain the word part and the other side should contain the meaning of the word part. Flashcards can also be printed from the CD-ROM. Flashcards can be carried everywhere and reviewed while waiting for a doctor's appointment, waiting for the bus, etc. Recruit family members, especially children, to help you study with your flashcards.

   As an additional self-quiz, first look at the meaning of the word part and then remember what the word part is.

3. During class, your instructor assigned 20 words from the Pronunciation Checklist on pp. 669-670. Practice the pronunciation of those words and then call your instructor's office or home phone number some time during the week and leave a message as you give your name and then pronounce each of the words.

4. Complete the Word Search for Chapter 12.

5. Refer to the Experience Multimedia CD-ROM Learning Activities Checklist for a list of activities to complete on the interactive CD-ROM.

6. Research and write a one-page paper about the personal story, symptoms, diagnosis, treatment, and aftermath of prostate or testicular cancer as it affected one of these famous people.

Prostate Cancer

Harry Bellafonte	Singer
Ben Carson	Surgeon
Bob Dole	Former U.S. senator and presidential candidate
Robert Goulet	Singer
Rudy Giuliani	Former mayor of New York City
Bob Kerry	Former U.S. senator and presidential candidate
Nelson Mandela	Former President of South Africa
Arnold Palmer	Golfer
Linus Pauling	Nobel Prize winner
Colin Powell	Former secretary of state
Telly Savalas	Actor
Norman Schwarzkopf	Army general

Testicular Cancer

Lance Armstrong	Bicycle racer
Scott Hamilton	Ice skater

7. Keep a running list in your notebook of sound-alike words or combining forms that have the same meanings. Title this list of challenging words and word parts as "Perplexing Pairs." Begin by writing down the words or word parts found in the Word Alert boxes in this chapter. Then add the word parts found in the It's Greek to Me box at the end of this chapter. Add any other words or word parts that you found particularly confusing. You will add to this list as you complete each chapter. Examples:

orth/o-   vs.   arthr/o-
myel/o-   vs.   my/o-
perine/o-   vs.   peritone/o-
cephal/o-   vs.   encephal/o-

8. Use a PDR (*Physican's Desk Reference*) or other drug reference book available in the library or do a search on the Internet and complete a list of the drugs available to treat erectile dysfunction (ED). Indicate whether these are prescription drugs or herbal drugs, etc. Also gather newspaper ads or describe TV ads dealing with drugs to treat erectile dysfunction.

9. Investigate the Web site Paternity Experts at www.paternityexperts.com. This Web site offers personal DNA paternity testing for one father and one child for $138. This test can be performed in the privacy of your own home. How is the DNA sample taken?

10. Research the medical, cultural, and religious issues dealing with circumcision.

11. Visit Planned Parenthood's Web site at www.plannedparenthood.org. In the Search window at the bottom of the page, type in *vasectomy*. Read some of the articles, questions, and answers about vasectomy.

12. Develop a plan for disseminating information about STDs (sexually transmitted diseases). Some of the topics to be covered include the following: What is the age range of the target audience? What type of written information should be provided? Where and how should the information be disseminated?

Word Search

Complete this word search puzzle that contains Chapter 12 words. Look for the following words as given in the list below. The number in parentheses indicates how many times the word appears in the puzzle.

AIDS
biopsy
duct
genitalia
glans penis
gonads
orchitis
penis
prostate
scrotum

semen
sexual
sperm
spermatozoa
STD
syphilis
testes (2)
TURP
vasectomy
virus

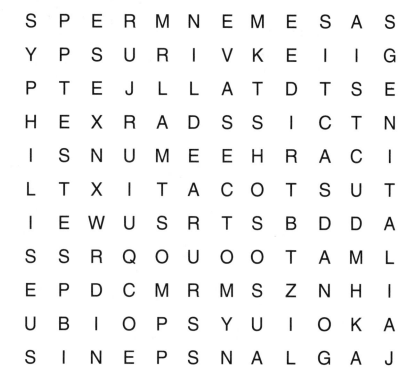

```
S  P  E  R  M  N  E  M  E  S  A  S
Y  P  S  U  R  I  V  K  E  I  I  G
P  T  E  J  L  L  A  T  D  T  S  E
H  E  X  R  A  D  S  S  I  C  T  N
I  S  N  U  M  E  E  H  R  A  C  I
L  T  X  I  T  A  C  O  T  S  U  T
I  E  W  U  S  R  T  S  B  D  D  A
S  S  R  Q  O  U  O  O  T  A  M  L
E  P  D  C  M  R  M  S  Z  N  H  I
U  B  I  O  P  S  Y  U  I  O  K  A
S  I  N  E  P  S  N  A  L  G  A  J
```

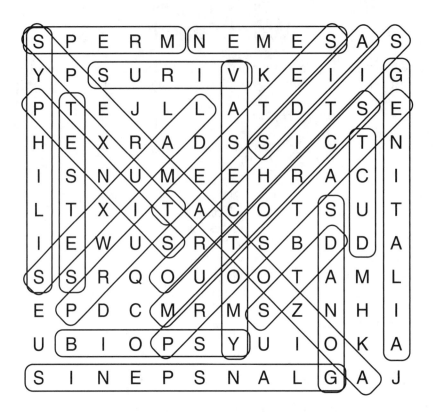

CHAPTER 13
Gynecology and Obstetrics
Female Reproductive System

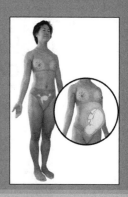

Instructor Activity for the Beginning of Class

Print out the image below and pass it around the class. Tell students that this is what a state-of-the-art sonogram looked like in 1982. Ask students to see if they can identify the head, flexed arm, and abdomen of the fetus. Locate someone who has recently been pregnant and has had a now state-of-the-art three-dimensional ultrasonography done. Borrow the picture of that test or refer students to Figure 13–27 on page 719 to see the difference.

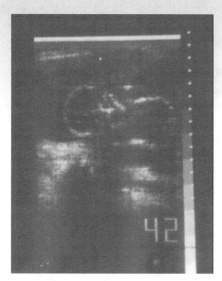

Are you ready for a chapter that really *delivers?* Let's begin the female reproductive chapter. You'll have a *fertile* mind once you master the language of gynecology and obstetrics.

Objective 1
Identify the anatomical structures of the female genital and reproductive system by correctly labeling them on anatomical illustrations

- Text page(s) 674–682

Teaching Strategies

1. Explain the importance of learning the parts of the female reproductive system.
2. To learn the anatomy of the female reproductive system, have the students label them on an anatomical diagram.

Content Abstract

Gynecology is the study of the female genital and reproductive system. It is the healthcare specialty that studies the anatomy and physiology of the female genital and reproductive system and uses diagnostic tests, medical and surgical procedures, and drugs to treat diseases.

Obstetrics is the study of the pregnant female reproductive system. It is the healthcare specialty that studies the anatomy and physiology of the female reproductive system during pregnancy and childbirth and uses diagnostic tests, medical and surgical procedures, and drugs to treat diseases.

The anatomy of the female reproductive system consists of:

1. ovaries
2. fallopian tubes
3. uterus
4. vagina
5. external genitalia
6. breasts

Box 13-1: Instructor Activity

INTERESTING FACTS

Share this information with students.

1. The ovum is about 1/180 of an inch in diameter.
   Source: Bit of Fun, www.bitoffun.com
2. An unfertilized ostrich egg is the largest known single cell.

Experience Multimedia

See the PowerPoint presentation on the accompanying Instructor's Media Library for animations showing the female pelvis.

Objective 2
Describe the processes of oogenesis, menstruation, and conception

- Text page(s) 683–687

Teaching Strategies

1. Explain the importance of learning the process of menstruation and conception.
2. Discuss the stages of pregnancy from conception to delivery.

Content Abstract

Each menstruation cycle takes 28 days and includes these four phases:

1. Menstrual phase
2. Proliferative phase
3. Secretory phase
4. Ischemic phase

Once semen is deposited in the female vagina by ejaculation from the penis during sexual intercourse, only some spermatozoa are able to reach the ovum in the fallopian tube. When one spermatozoon penetrates the ovum, this moment of penetration is called fertilization or conception, and pregnancy begins. The fertilized ovum travels to the intrauterine cavity. The development of the amniotic cavity, placenta, and umbilical cord occur. After four days of development, the fertilized ovum is known as an embryo. After eight weeks, it is known as a fetus. The moment of conception to the moment of birth is known as gestation. The gestational period is about nine months. Gestation can be divided into three trimesters; each trimester contains three months.

Box 13-2: Instructor Activity

INTERESTING FACTS

Share this information with students.

1. One Chinese character for menstruation means *little red sister has come;* another means *the red general has grasped the door.* The first disposable pad for menstrual bleeding was developed by Kotex in 1921. The Egyptians invented the first tampon, which was composed of softened and rolled papyrus. The tampon invented by the ancient Greeks consisted of lint wrapped around a small wood stick. The first modern tampon was created by a male physician and marketed by Tampax in 1931. His patent description called it a "catamenial device." *Tampon* is a French word that means *to stop up.* Ask your students about the words their families used for menstruation. Examples: Auntie Flo, the curse, red flag, fall off the roof.

(continued)

Box 13-2: Instructor Activity (*cont.*)

2. A woman's best chance of becoming pregnant is between ages 18 and 25. By age 40, she has only a 15 percent chance and after age 44 there is only a 1 percent chance of becoming pregnant each month.

   Source: Isadore Rosenfeld, "The Fertility Factor," *Parade Magazine* (Sunday paper supplement), October 12, 2003.

3. In the developing world, fertility rates often vary in inverse proportion to literacy rates. Afghanistan's female literacy rate is 8 percent with a fertility rate of 6.9 per 1,000 population. Thailand's female literacy rate is 88 percent with a fertility rate of 2.6 per 1,000 population.

4. From the size of the fertilized egg to the size of the newborn baby is an increase in growth of two billion times.

   Source: The Human Body, TimeLife Books.

5. Identical twins develop when a single fertilized ovum (a zygote) splits into two and creates two separate but identical zygotes. The question is this: Are the fingerprints identical in identical twins? Interestingly, they are not! This can be explained by the fact their DNA is identical, but once they separate, their DNA undergoes various micromutations as the embryo develops. Some things are programmed into DNA and express themselves identically in identical twins, while other things are more a product of the environment. The environment of the uterus can be slightly different for each twin. Fingerprints are created between weeks 13 and 19 of gestation. If the fingertips of the fetus are compressed, they are more likely to develop an arch on the fingerprint. If the fingertips are swollen, they are more likely to develop a whorl pattern on the fingerprint. We don't often realize it, but identical twins do have other nonidentical features. Their facial features are just slightly different, their arms may be longer, etc. (although these differences might not be obvious except with the most exact measurements).

6. Print out the Milestones in Embryo and Fetal Development chart on the following page to share with students, if desired.

Experience Multimedia

See the PowerPoint presentation on the accompanying Instructor's Media Library for animations on the following topics covered in this chapter:

- Conception
- Oogenesis

Objective 3
Describe the process of labor and delivery

- Text page(s) 687-689

Teaching Strategies

1. Explain the importance of learning the process of labor and delivery.
2. Show a video of an actual delivery.

Milestones in Embryo and Fetal Development

Month	Trimester	Designation	Description
1	1	Embryo	Heart begins to beat at three weeks.
			Lungs, trachea, liver, pancreas, and intestines form.
2	1	Embryo	Sweat glands and hair follicles form.
			Kidneys form and begin to produce urine.
			Umbilical cord forms.
3	1	Fetus	Spinal cord and brain begin to form.
			Gallbladder and genitalia form.
4	2	Fetus	Hair begins to grow; facial features form.
			The fetus swallows amniotic fluid.
			Eyes and ears begin to form.
			Mother feels first fetal movements (quickening).
5	2	Fetus	Nails begin to grow on fingers and toes.
			Tonsils form.
6	2	Fetus	Spleen, adrenal glands, and bone marrow form.
			Vernix caseosa and lanugo develop on skin
7	3	Fetus	Eyelids open; testes begin to descend.

Content Abstract

Between 38 and 42 weeks' gestation, labor begins. The uterus begins to contract regularly and the cervix softens; this process is known as cervical ripening. The process of labor and childbirth is known as parturition and is divided into three stages:

1. First stage of labor—dilation, effacement and rupture of membranes occur
2. Second stage of labor—crowning and delivery of newborn occurs
3. Third stage of labor—delivery of placenta occurs

Box 13-3: Instructor Activity

INTERESTING FACTS

Share this information with students.

1. A study published in the *New England Journal of Medicine* found that one to three cups of coffee per day increases the risk of miscarriage by 30 percent, while three to five cups per day increases the risk of miscarriage by 40 percent. Tea, cocoa, and sodas normally contain less caffeine than coffee but can also contribute to miscarriage, as can caffeine-containing medications.

   Source: The Baltimore Sun, December 30, 2000.

2. Elvis Presley had a twin brother who died at birth.

Experience Multimedia

See the PowerPoint presentation on the accompanying Instructor's Media Library for videos on the topic of labor and delivery.

Objective 4
Describe normal and abnormal findings in the neonate

- Text page(s) 690

Teaching Strategy

Explain the importance of learning the normal and abnormal findings in the neonate.

Content Abstract

A newborn born between 38 and 42 weeks' gestation is called a neonate. A newborn between 28 and 37 weeks' gestation is called a preterm or premature newborn. At one year of age, the neonate becomes an infant. The skin of the neonate is covered with vernix caseosa. The baby's head can exhibit molding, which is a temporary reshaping of the cranium that occurs to facilitate passage through the mother's bony pelvis. On the top of the head, there is a large area known as the anterior fontanel or soft spot. This spot is only covered by the dura mater, not by cranial bone. It closes at about two years of age. Acrocyanosis is a temporary condition in which the neonate's face, hands, and feet are bluish. The first stool is a greenish-black, thick, sticky substance known as meconium.

Box 13-4: Instructor Activity

NEONATE

Share this information with students.

1. The family of Fyodor Vassilyev from Russia had a record number of children. His wife gave birth to 16 sets of twins. They also had 7 sets of triplets and 4 sets of quads.
2. Heaviest single birth: Anna Bates gave birth to a 23-pound, 12-ounce boy in Seville, Ohio, in 1879.

   Source: Guinness Book of World Records.
3. Lowest birth weight for a surviving infant: Marian Taggart (née Chapman) was born 6 weeks prematurely in England in 1938. She weighed just 10 ounces and was fed with brandy, glucose (sugar), and water through a fountain pen filter.

   Source: Guinness Book of World Records.
4. One in every nine babies is born prematurely. This is partly due to the multiple births resulting from assisted reproduction techniques.

   Source: The Baltimore Sun, November 2000.
5. Breast-milk fed babies have less gastroenteritis, necrotizing enterocolitis, neonatal sepsis, and otitis media compared to formula-fed babies and may be at lower risk for immunologically based diseases such as type 1 diabetes mellitus and Crohn's disease.
6. About 64 percent of American women breastfeed during the first month after birth. That number is up from 50 percent in the late 1990s, but is less than the recommended goal of 75 percent. Even fewer mothers continue to breastfeed for six months.

   Source: The Baltimore Sun, November 2000.
7. In 1948, Dr. Virginia Apgar developed the Apgar score, an assessment tool for assigning a number score to newborns after birth.
8. Many years ago, it was believed that the placenta formed a natural barrier that protected the fetus from harmful substances taken by the mother. Now we know this is not true, and even occaisional use of alcohol or drugs can affect the fetus.
9. The placenta is a flat, pancake-like structure. It is slippery and rubbery. One side has a surface of gnarled blood vessels and the umbilical cord. The other surface, where it pulled away from the wall of the uterus, is like raw meat. Susan Turley, the author, has a small farm. She has helped deliver many baby goats over the years and was always amazed when the mother goat ate the placenta. This is a protective mechanism with animals to remove the scent of the placenta so as not to attract predators who might also harm the babies. It also provides nourishment for the mother, but it is amazing to see how the large, rubbery placenta (which stays in one piece) could be swallowed!

Box 13-5: Classroom Activity

CONGENITAL ABNORMALITIES OF THE NEONATE

Draw the following table on the board. Then ask students to fill in the blanks based on their knowledge of congenital abnormalities that they have studied in the previous chapters or from life experience.

Congenital Abnormalities of the Neonate

Body System	Abnormalities
1. Ears, nose, throat	
2. Eyes	
3. Cardiovascular system	
4. Gastrointestinal system	
5. Genitourinary system	
6. Nervous system	
7. Integumentary system	

[Answer Key]

Congenital Abnormalities of the Neonate

Body System	Abnormalities
1. Ears, nose, throat	Cleft lip, cleft palate, deafness
2. Eyes	Blindness, strabismus
3. Cardiovascular system	Patent ductus arteriosus, atrial or septal defect, tetralogy of Fallot
4. Gastrointestinal system	Esophageal atresia, umbilical or inguinal hernia, imperforate anus
5. Genitourinary system	Undescended testes, epispadias, hypospadias
6. Nervous system	Anencephaly, Down syndrome, myelomeningocele
7. Integumentary system	Skin tag, port wine stain, hemangioma, syndactyly, polydactyly

Experience Multimedia	

See the PowerPoint presentation on the accompanying Instructor's Media Library for a video on the topic of assessment of a newborn.

Objective 5
Build female genital and reproductive words from combining forms, prefixes, and suffixes

- Text page(s) 698–700

Teaching Strategy

Create a PowerPoint presentation with combining forms, prefixes, and suffixes with their meanings. Use this presentation in class. All students participate in a "medical terminology bee." All students stand and take turns defining the combining form, prefix, or suffix displayed. If the student gets the answer right, the student remains standing and continues to play. If the student gets the answer wrong, the student will be seated and is out of the game. The last person standing is the winner. A prize could be given to the winner.

Objective 6
Describe common female genital and reproductive diseases

- Text page(s) 701-713

Content Abstract

Disease	Meaning
Anovulation	Failure of the ovaries to release a mature ovum at the time of ovulation
Ovarian cancer	Malignant tumor of the ovary
Polycystic ovary syndrome	Multiple cysts of the ovaries that enlarge with each menstrual cycle and cause pain
Salpingitis	Inflammation and infection of the fallopian tube
Endometrial cancer	Malignant tumor of the endometrium of the uterus
Endometriosis	Endometrial tissue implanted in abnormal places on the outer surfaces of reproductive organs and on the abdominal wall
Hydatidiform mole	Union of ovum and spermatozoon that only produces hundreds of fluid-filled sacs
Leiomyoma	Benign tumor of the myometrium
Leiomyosarcoma	Malignant tumor of the myometrium
Myometritis	Infection of the myometrium
Pelvic inflammatory disease	Infection of the cervix and then the uterus, tubes, and ovaries, often from a sexually transmitted disease
Retroflexion of uterus	Abnormal bending backwards position of the uterus
Uterine prolapse	Descent of the uterus from its normal position
Amenorrhea	Absence of monthly menstrual periods
Dysfunctional uterine bleeding	Menstrual bleeding without a true menstrual period, associated with anovulation
Dysmenorrhea	Painful menstruation
Menopause	Normal cessation of menstrual periods occurring around age 40
Menorrhagia	Menstrual flow that is excessive or lasts longer than 7 days
Oligomenorrhea	Light menstrual flow or infrequent menstrual periods
Premenstrual syndrome	Breast tenderness, fluid retention, bloating, and mild mood changes prior to menstruation (see Box 13-6)

(continued)

Disease	Meaning
Premenstrual dysphoric disorder	Symptoms of premenstrual syndrome plus depression, eating and sleep disturbances, and pain
Cervical cancer	Malignant tumor of the cervix
Cervical dysplasia	Abnormal squamous cells in the epithelium of the cervix
Incompetent cervix	Cervix dilates during pregnancy, which sometimes results in a spontaneous abortion
Bacterial vaginosis	Vaginal bacterial infection due to *Gardnerella vaginalis*
Candidiasis	Vaginal yeast infection due to *Candida albicans*
Cystocele	Herniation of the bladder through a weakness in the vaginal wall
Dyspareunia	Painful sexual intercourse due to an intact hymen or infection
Rectocele	Herniation of the rectum through a weakness in the vaginal wall
Vaginitis	Irritation of the vagina from chemicals or infection of the vagina
Breast cancer	Malignant tumor of the breast (see Box 13-7)
Failure of lactation	Lack of enough milk production to breastfeed
Fibrocystic disease	Benign condition of fluid-filled cysts of the breast
Galactorrhea	Discharge of breast milk when the patient is not pregnant or breastfeeding, due to a tumor in the anterior pituitary gland
Abnormal presentation	Abnormal birth position in which the head is not the presenting part
Abruptio placentae	Separation of the placenta from the uterus prior to delivery of the fetus (see Box 13-8)
Arrest of labor	Cessation of or prolonging of labor
Cephalopelvic disproportion	Fetal head size exceeds the opening in the mother's pelvis (see Box 13-9)
Dystocia	Difficult or abnormal labor or delivery
Ectopic pregnancy	Fertilized ovum implants in the fallopian tube
Gestational diabetes mellitus	Temporary disorder of glucose metabolism that only occurs during pregnancy
Mastitis	Inflammation or infection of the breast
Morning sickness	Nausea and vomiting during the first trimester of pregnancy (see Box 13-10)
Oligohydramnios	Decreased volume of amniotic fluid
Placenta previa	Placenta partially or completely covers the cervix
Polyhydramnios	Increased volume of amniotic fluid
Postpartum hemorrhage	Excessive uterine bleeding after birth
Preeclampsia	Increased weight gain, hypertension, and protein in the urine that can lead to seizures (eclampsia)
Premature labor	Regular uterine contractions before 38-42 weeks' gestation (see Box 13-11)
Premature rupture of membranes	Rupture of the amniotic sac before labor begins

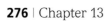

Disease	Meaning
Prolapsed cord	Umbilical cord caught between the fetal presenting part and the birth canal
Spontaneous abortion	Loss of pregnancy before full gestation
Uterine inertia	Weak, uncoordinated contractions
Apnea	Temporary or permanent cessation of breathing after birth (see Box 13-12)
Fetal distress	Bradycardia and passage of meconium due to decreased oxygen
Jaundice	Yellowish discoloration of the skin
Meconium aspiration	Breathing in of meconium passed in utero because of fetal distress (see Box 13-13)
Nuchal cord	Umbilical cord wrapped around the neck (see Box 13-14)
Respiratory distress syndrome	Difficulty inflating the lungs in a premature infant (see Box 13-15)

Box 13-6: Instructor Activity

PMS

The symptoms of premenstrual syndrome (PMS) can vary from mild to severe. The aching joints, dysmenorrhea, headache, bloating, and irritability can make 1-2 days each month nonproductive days for some women. Premenstrual dysphoric disorder (PMDD) is actually a psychiatric diagnosis because of the overlay of depression and anxiety on pre-existing premenstrual symptoms.

Box 13-7: Instructor Activity

BREAST CANCER

Share this information with students.

1. The average American woman has a one in seven chance of developing breast cancer during her lifetime. If she inherits the BRCA-1 or BRCA-2 gene, her risk increases to one in two chances.

   Source: CBS News "HealthWatch," July 28, 2004.

2. Women who work night shifts may increase their risk of breast cancer and colon cancer by 35 percent or more, depending on how long they work that shift. Researchers found that bright light in the dark hours of the night decreases melatonin secretion and increases estrogen levels. Normal levels of melatonin appear to inhibit the growth of tumors. These findings are of particular interest to medical terminology students, who will soon be healthcare professionals who are often asked to work the night shift.

   Source: Brigham and Women's Hospital press release, June 3, 2003.

Box 13-8: Instructor Activity

ABRUPTIO PLACENTAE

In the phrase *abruptio placentae,* the word *placentae* is actually in the form of the genitive case, a Latin case that shows possession. So the phrase means *a breaking off of the placenta. Of the placenta* is the phrase that shows possession. The genitive case is sometimes confused with the Latin feminine plural (which would also be *placentae,* but would not have a noun in front of it).

Box 13-9: Instructor Activity

CEPHALOPELVIC DISPROPORTION

Egyptian mummies have been found with the skull of the fetus firmly wedged in the mother's bony pelvis, a case of cephalopelvic disproportion. Until the development of cesarean section surgery, there was no treatment for cephalopelvic disproportion and it resulted in the death of both the mother and the baby.

Box 13-10: Instructor Activity

MORNING SICKNESS

Morning sickness is a relatively mild and temporary condition. Severe, continued morning sickness is known by the Latin phrase *hyperemesis gravidarum*. The prefix *hyper-* means *above* or *more than normal,* and the suffix *-emesis* means *vomiting.* The word *gravidarum* is a Latin genitive form that means *of pregnancy.*

Box 13-11: Instructor Activity

PREMATURE LABOR AND PREMATURE INFANTS

Susan Turley, the author, worked for many years in the neonatal intensive care unit (NICU). This abbreviation is pronounced as "NIK-yoo." She routinely took care of extremely small premature infants, weighing less than two pounds. Her favorite size of babies was between three to four pounds. They were extremely active, skinny, very alert, and often had few medical problems except that they needed to gain weight. In contrast, occasionally the infant of a diabetic mother would be brought into the NICU to be observed. This baby, who weighed over 10 pounds, would be placed in an incubator, where it seemed like a whale in a jar compared to the tiny two-pound babies. Why was it so big? Because the mother's gestational diabetes mellitus had not been controlled; her blood sugar had been high many times because of not watching her diet or taking antidiabetic medication. This high level of glucose in the blood was transmitted through the placenta to the baby whose pancreas was just fine and had no trouble making large amounts of insulin to metabolize the large amounts of glucose it was receiving. However, after delivery, the baby, who had been used to constant high levels of glucose, now had to survive on a first feeding of sterile water followed by a small amount of milk or breastmilk. This caused the baby's blood sugar level to suddenly fall. This baby, who had been active and crying, would suddenly become floppy and cyanotic and could even stop breathing!

Box 13-12: Instructor Activity

APNEA

Premature babies who are prone to episodes of apnea are sent home on an apnea monitor. It sounds an alarm whenever the baby's breathing pauses for a certain length of time.

Objective 7
Describe common female genital and reproductive diagnostic laboratory and radiology tests

- Text page(s) 714-719

Content Abstract

Test	Definition
Biopsy	Diagnostic and medical or surgical procedure to remove tissue for analysis for suspected cancer
Pap smear	Cytology test used as a screening test to detect abnormal and possibly cancerous cells in the cervix
Amniocentesis	Amniotic fluid test
Pregnancy test	Blood test to detect human chorionic gonadotropin (HCG) secreted by the fertilized ovum
Mammography	Radiologic procedure that uses x-rays to create an image of the breast

Box 13-16: Instructor Activity

PAP SMEAR

Share this information with students.

1. In 1943, the Pap test for cervical cancer was invented by George Papanicolaou.
2. The American Cancer Society recommends annual Pap smears (screening test for cervical cancer) by age 20.
3. There are 50 million Pap smears performed annually in the United States. Of these, only about 4,000 detect new cases of cervical cancer. Cervical cancer is almost always caused by the sexually transmitted disease of the human papillomavirus (HPV). There are more than 100 types of HPV that fall into two main categories: HPV types that are a high risk for causing cervical cancer and HPV types that are a low risk of causing cervical cancer (but do cause genital warts). Now the DNA with Pap test can show whether the abnormal cells on a Pap smear belong to the high-risk catetory of HPV.

Source: Parade Magazine (Sunday newspaper supplement), October 10, 2004.

Box 13-17: Instructor Activity

MAMMOGRAPHY

Share this information with students.

1. In 1969, the first mammography of the breast was performed.
2. Annual mammography is recommended for all women, with ultrasound follow-up of suspicious areas on mammography. However, magnetic resonance imaging (MRI) can spot nearly twice as many cancers as mammography, and so is recommended for women in the high-risk category.

Source: CBS News "HealthWatch," July 28, 2004.

3. On regular mammography, an estimated 15–20 percent of cancers are missed. In a controversial move in 2003, the American Cancer Society (ACS) recommended stopping breast self-examination because research did not show that it saved lives. The ACS does recommend annual mammography for women over age 40. The National Cancer Institute and the Institute of Medicine recommend mammography every one to two years.

Source: Family Circle Magazine, October 19, 2004.

Objective 8
Describe common female genital and reproductive medical and surgical procedures and drug categories

- Text page(s) 720-731

Content Abstract

Procedure	Definition
Cryosurgery	Medical procedure to destroy small areas of abnormal tissue on the cervix
Gynecologic examination	Medical procedure to examine the external and internal genitalia
Colporrhaphy	Surgical procedure to suture a weakness in the vaginal wall
Endometrial ablation	Surgical procedure that uses heat or cold to destroy the endometrium
Hysterectomy	Surgical procedure to remove the uterus
Laparoscopy	Surgical procedure to visualize the pelvic cavity, uterus, fallopian tubes, and ovaries for diagnosis, biopsy, or surgery to remove or repair
Tubal ligation	Surgical procedure to prevent pregnancy (see Box 13-19)
Mammaplasty	Surgical procedure to change the size, shape, or position of the breast (see Box 13-18)
Version	Medical procedure to correct a breech or other malpresentation prior to delivery
Cerclage	Surgical procedure to place sutures fashioned into a loop around the cervix

Drug Category	Description	Example
Antibiotic drugs	Treat bacterial infections of the breasts, internal organs, external female genitalia	Ampicillin
Drugs for dysmenorrhea	Treat the pain associated with dysmenorrhea	Motrin, Ponstel
Hormone replacement therapy	Treat the symptoms of menopause	Estraderm, Estratest, Premarin, Prempro (see Box 13–23)

Box 13-18: Instructor Activity

MAMMAPLASTY AND BREAST IMPLANTS

Share this information with students.

In 1961, the first breast silicone implant surgery was performed. The Food and Drug Administration (FDA) banned silicone breast implants in 1992 after concerns that their rupture could result in multiple sclerosis and other immune disorders. However, they are reconsidering lifting the ban, and the American Society of Plastic Surgeons supports the resumption of silicone breast implants.

Source: The Baltimore Sun, August 5, 2005.

Box 13-19: Instructor Activity

TUBAL LIGATION

Share this information with students.

1. Approximately 700,000 women have a tubal ligation for birth control annually in the United States.

   Source: Centers for Disease Control and Prevention.

2. Tubal ligation is a surgical procedure performed under general anesthesia and requires several days of recuperation. A new procedure, the hysteroscopic tubal occlusion, was recently approved by the Food and Drug Administration and can be performed under local anesthesia; the patient can immediately resume her normal activities. A hysteroscope is inserted through the cervix and uterus, and a catheter inserted into the fallopian tube releases a spring device. Tissue grows around the device and blocks the fallopian tube within three months to prevent a pregnancy.

   Source: Baylor College of Medicine in Houston, Texas, 2003.

Box 13-20: Instructor Activity

EPISIOTOMY

Episiotomies were first performed in the early 1900s. They quickly became a standard obstetrical procedure. Now the American College of Obstetricians and Gynecologists has recommended not doing an episiotomy. A study in the *Journal of the American Medical Association* reported there was no evidence that having an episiotomy gave women better sexual function or less bowel or bladder incontinence after birth.

Source: The Baltimore Sun, "Episiotomy Should be the Exception, not Rule," March 31, 2006.

Box 13-21: Instructor Activity

CESAREAN SECTION

Share this information with students.

1. Historically, cesarean sections were not done except in an emergency because of the lack of anesthesia. The discovery of ether and chloroform in the mid-1800s changed that. Queen Victoria had both of her children by cesarean section: Leopold in 1853 and Beatrice in 1857.

   Source: www.emedicine.com

2. In 2001, 25 percent of all babies born in the United States were born by cesarean section.

   Source: Time magazine, August 2002.

3. In the past, it was thought that once a woman had a cesarean section, she could not have a vaginal delivery for a subsequent pregnancy because of the risk that the surgical scar in the uterus could rupture during labor. That was disproved, and in the 1980s and early 1990s, the trend was to have a vaginal birth after cesarean section (VBAC). Now that trend is reversing. Vaginal births carry a lower risk of medical complications, but cesarean sections are increasing because patients can schedule the birth; obstetricians are agreeing to cesarean sections because there is always a risk of a lawsuit if something happens during a prolonged vaginal birth, and because the stress of labor can cause physical problems in the mother after birth. The Centers for Disease Control and Prevention has set a goal for 2010 to have 37 percent of women who have had a cesarean section to have a subsequent vaginal birth. Right now, only 22 percent have a subsequent vaginal birth.

   Source: The Baltimore Sun, December 30, 2000.

Box 13-22: Instructor Activity

IN VITRO FERTILIZATION

Share this information with students.

1. In 1978, Louise Brown of Great Britain became the first baby to be conceived by *in vitro* fertilization techniques. She was nicknamed "the test tube baby." Baby Louise weighed 5 pounds, 12 ounces.

2. The first birth of a child from a frozen embryo was in Australia in 1984. Baby Zoe weighed 5 pounds, 13 ounces.

   Source: Guinness Book of World Records, 2004.

Box 13-23: Instructor Activity

PREMARIN

Share this information with students.

The estrogen hormone replacement therapy drug Premarin, which is taken when menopause begins, is made from the urine of pregnant mares. The name is derived from that also: **pre**gnant **ma**res' u**rin**e.

Source: Susan Turley, *Understanding Pharmacology for Health Professionals.* Prentice Hall.

Box 13-24: Instructor Activity

CONTRACEPTIVES

Share this information with students.

1. In 1960, the first oral contraceptive pill was introduced.

2. The drug Ortho Evra, introduced in 2001, was the first transdermal patch contraceptive.

Box 13-25: Instructor Activity

OVULATION-STIMULATING DRUGS

Share this information with students.

Bobbi McCaughey, age 29, of Carlisle, Iowa, took Pergonal (an ovulation-stimulating drug used to treat infertility). She became pregnant and delivered the world's only surviving set of septuplets on November 20, 1997. The four boys and three girls were born at 30 weeks' gestation and each weighed from 2 pounds 5 ounces to 3 pounds 4 ounces.

Source: Susan Turley, *Understanding Pharmacology for Health Professionals.* Prentice Hall.

Experience Multimedia

See the PowerPoint presentation on the accompanying Instructor's Media Library for a video on the topic of C-sections.

Objective 9
Define common female genital and reproductive abbreviations

- Text page(s) 731–732

Teaching Strategies

1. Stress the importance of learning abbreviations and their full meanings.
2. Divide the class into two, three, or four teams and have them stand in separate lines. The instructor writes a common female reproductive abbreviation on the board. The first person on Team 1 must indicate what the abbreviation stands for. If correct, that person moves to the back of the team line. The first person on Team 2 will then define the next abbreviation written on the board by the instructor. If correct, that person moves to the end of the team line, and so on. If at any point, a team member misses an abbreviation, that person is out of the game. The next team is given an opportunity to define the abbreviation. The winners are the team with the most players left at the end of the game.

Content Abstract

AB, Ab	abortion		**EDB**	estimated date of birth
AFP	alpha fetoprotein		**EDC**	estimated date of confinement
AGA	appropriate for gestational age		**EGA**	estimated gestational age
ASC-H	atypical squamous cells, cannot exclude HSIL		**EMB**	endometrial biopsy
ASC-US	atypical squamous cells of undetermined significance		**FHR**	fetal heart rate
			FSH	follicle-stimulating hormone
BBT	basal body temperature		**G**	gravida
BPD	biparietal diameter (of fetal head)		**GIFT**	gamete intrafallopian transfer
BPP	biophysical profile		**G/TPAL**	see *G* and *TPAL*
BRCA	breast cancer (gene)		**GYN**	gynecology
BSE	breast self-examination		**HCG,**	human chorionic gonadotropin
BSO	bilateral salpingo-oophorectomy		**hCG**	
Bx	biopsy		**HPV**	human papillomavirus
Ca	cancer, carcinoma		**HRT**	hormone replacement therapy
CIN	cervical intraepithelial neoplasia (grading system on Pap smear)		**HSG**	hysterosalpingography
			HSIL	high-grade squamous intraepithelial lesion
CIS	carcinoma in situ		**ICSI**	intracytoplasmic sperm injection
CNM	certified nurse midwife		**IUGR**	intrauterine growth retardation
CPD	cephalopelvic disproportion		**IVF**	*in vitro* fertilization
CS	cesarean section ("C-section")		**L&D**	labor and delivery
CVS	chorionic villus sampling		**LEEP**	loop electrocautery excision procedure
D&C	dilation and curettage		**LGA**	large for gestational age
DUB	dysfunctional uterine bleeding			

LH	luteinizing hormone	**ROM**	rupture of membranes
LMP	last menstrual period	**SAB**	spontaneous abortion
L/S	lecithin/sphingomyelin (ratio)	**SCC**	squamous cell carcinoma
LSIL	low-grade squamous intraepithelial lesion	**SGA**	small for gestational age
NB	newborn	**STD**	sexually transmitted disease
NICU	neonatal intensive care unit	**TAB**	therapeutic abortion
NST	nonstress test	**TAH-BSO**	total abdominal hysterectomy and bilateral salpingo-oophorectomy
NSVD	normal spontaneous vaginal delivery	**TPAL**	term (newborns), premature (newborns), abortions, living (children)
OB	obstetrics		
OCP	oral contraceptive pill	**TRAM**	transverse rectus abdominis muscle (flap)
P	para	**TVH**	total vaginal hysterectomy
Pap	Papanicolaou (smear or test)	**VBAC**	vaginal birth after ceserean section ("V-back")
PID	pelvic inflammatory disease		
PMDD	premenstrual dysphoric disorder	**ZIFT**	zygote intrafallopian transfer
PMS	premenstrual syndrome		
PROM	premature rupture of membranes		

Objective 10
Correctly spell and pronounce female genital and reproductive words

- Text page(s) 746–748

Teaching Strategies

1. Impress upon the students that medical words that are mispronounced are also probably going to be misspelled.
2. Encourage students to work on both pronunciation and spelling when studying.

Chapter Spelling Test

The chapter spelling test is included with the weekly chapter test. Dictate and spell (or xerox a handout that contains) this list of 20 spelling words. Give the list to students the week before the test. For the chapter test, select just 10 of these words to test.

1. amniocentesis
2. areola
3. cerclage
4. cesarean section
5. culdoscopy
6. dysmenorrhea
7. dystocia
8. embryo
9. endometriosis
10. fallopian tube
11. genitalia
12. gravida
13. hysterectomy
14. intrauterine
15. laparoscopy
16. lochia
17. mammography
18. menstruation
19. preeclampsia
20. salpingo-oophorectomy

GAMES

1. From week to week, pick a different one of these spelling games to use during class. (The descriptions and instructions for the games are in the section "The Art and Craft of Teaching.")

   Beanbag Spelling Toss
   Scrabble
   Spelling Bee
   Gridlock
   Hangman

2. From week to week, pick a different one of these pronunciation games to use during class. (The descriptions and instructions for the games are in the section "The Art and Craft of Teaching.")

   Parroting
   Hieroglyphics
   Beach Ball Blast

Chapter Pronunciation Test

Have students mark these 20 words listed in the Pronunciation Checklist for the chapter. During the week, they will call your office or home answering machine and pronounce each word.

1. adnexal	11. genitalia
2. amenorrhea	12. hemosalpinx
3. amniocentesis	13. hysterectomy
4. carcinoma *in situ*	14. intrauterine
5. cerclage	15. laparoscopy
6. colostrum	16. lochia
7. culdoscopy	17. menarche
8. dystocia	18. multiparous
9. effacement	19. oxytocin
10. endometriosis	20. salpingo-oophorectomy

Objective 11
Apply your skills by analyzing a gynecology report

- Text page(s) 744–745

Content Abstract

Read the hospital History and Physical Examination and answer questions provided.

Objective 12
Test your knowledge of gynecology and obstetrics by completing review exercises in the textbook and the CD-ROM learning activities

- Text page(s) 734–743 (first complete all the in-chapter exercises on pp. 697–700)

Teaching Strategies

1. Assign the Chapter Review Exercises in the textbook for homework.
2. Remind students to refer to the Answer Key at the end of the textbook to check their answers.
3. Refer to the CD-ROM Learning Activities in this section for multimedia learning experiences.

Experience Multimedia

See the PowerPoint presentation on the accompanying Instructor's Media Library for videos on the topic of a career as a nurse midwife.

Homework Activities

1. Complete all of the exercises in the chapter, finishing the Chapter Review Exercises at the end of the chapter. Write in your textbook so that your instructor can verify that you did this work. See the Answer Key at the end of the book to check your answers.

2. Make flashcards for all of the prefixes, suffixes, and combining forms in the chapter. An index card makes a good homemade flashcard. One side of the flashcard should contain the word part and the other side should contain the meaning of the word part. Flashcards can also be printed from the CD-ROM. Flashcards can be carried everywhere and reviewed while waiting for a doctor's appointment, waiting for the bus, etc. Recruit family members, especially children, to help you study with your flashcards.

   As an additional self-quiz, first look at the meaning of the word part and then remember what the word part is.

3. During class, your instructor assigned 20 words from the Pronunciation Checklist on pp. 746–748. Practice the pronunciation of those words and then call your instructor's office or home phone number some time during the week and leave a message as you give your name and then pronounce each of the words.

4. Complete the Word Search for Chapter 13.

5. Refer to the Experience Multimedia CD-ROM Learning Activities Checklist for a list of activities to complete on the interactive CD-ROM.

6. Create a "mnifty mnemonic device" memory aid in the form of a rhyme, a word, or an abbreviation that helps you remember something about this body system.

7. Develop a crossword puzzle based on this chapter. Have some answers in the puzzle go from top to bottom (DOWN words) and others go from right to left (ACROSS words). The words should intersect with each other at several points. Make one list of clues for DOWN words and another list of clues for ACROSS words.

8. Write 10 sentences correctly using 10 or more different abbreviations from the chapter.

9. Interview a woman who has given birth. Ask her to walk you through the process step by step and describe the events to you from her personal perspective.

10. Prepare a chronological log of events that depicts what should occur in the pregnant woman during each week of pregnancy (40 weeks).

11. Research and write a one-page paper about the personal story, symptoms, diagnosis, treatment, and aftermath of breast cancer as it affected one of these famous people.

Shirley Temple Black	Child actress, diplomat
Julia Child	TV chef
Betty Ford	Former First Lady
Peggy Fleming	Olympic ice skater and TV commentator
Linda Ellerbee	TV journalist
Olivia Newton-John	Singer, actress
Sandra Day O'Connor	Supreme Court Justice
Nancy Reagan	Former First Lady
Cokie Roberts	TV journalist
Carly Simon	Singer
Suzanne Somers	Actress

12. The American Cancer Society has an on-line mammogram reminder. This interactive tool sends an e-mail message each year as a reminder to schedule your mammogram. To register yourself or someone you love, go to http://www.cancer.org/docroot/PED/content/PED_2_3x_Mammogram_Reminder.asp.

13. Keep a running list in your notebook of sound-alike words or combining forms that have the same meanings. Title this list of challenging words and word parts as "Perplexing Pairs." Begin by writing down the words or word parts found in the Word Alert boxes in this chapter. Then add the word parts found in the It's Greek to Me box at the end of this chapter. Add any other words or word parts that you found particularly confusing. You will add to this list as you complete each chapter. Examples:

orth/o-	vs.	arthr/o-
myel/o-	vs.	my/o-
perine/o-	vs.	peritone/o-
cephal/o-	vs.	encephal/o-

14. Research all of the methods of female birth control (contraception) and draw a table comparing and contrasting each.

15. Go to PBS NOVA online at http://www.pbs.org/wgbh/nova/miracle/, to view "Life's Greatest Miracle," the sequel to the award-winning film "The Miracle of Life," which showed the first color photographs of a fetus in the uterus.

16. Write a one-page summary of a newspaper article about female genital or reproductive health issues.

Word Search

Complete this word search puzzle that contains Chapter 13 words. Look for the following words as given in the list below. The number in parentheses indicates how many times the word appears in the puzzle.

amniocentesis
breast
cesarean
clitoris
contraception
corpus
CPD
EGA
fetal
fetus
gonad
gravida
labial

menses
neonate
NICU
ovum
para
pica
placenta
PMS (2)
pregnancies
pubic
uterus
vernix
zygote

```
A  L  C  R  L  A  G  E  J  X  P  D  N
X  M  O  D  L  A  T  K  I  U  R  A  E
E  P  N  A  R  B  B  N  C  L  E  N  O
V  O  T  I  R  Z  R  I  E  R  G  O  N
C  E  R  E  O  E  N  D  A  C  N  G  A
F  W  A  T  V  C  Z  S  C  L  A  Y  T
E  S  C  P  D  Y  E  O  L  D  N  L  E
T  U  E  U  G  C  R  N  I  A  C  I  P
U  Q  P  O  T  P  Y  V  T  D  I  N  M
S  M  T  U  U  E  A  A  O  E  E  C  S
S  E  I  S  B  R  R  E  R  V  S  Q  P
L  W  O  K  G  I  T  U  U  A  U  I  J
M  E  N  S  E  S  C  B  S  W  P  M  S
```

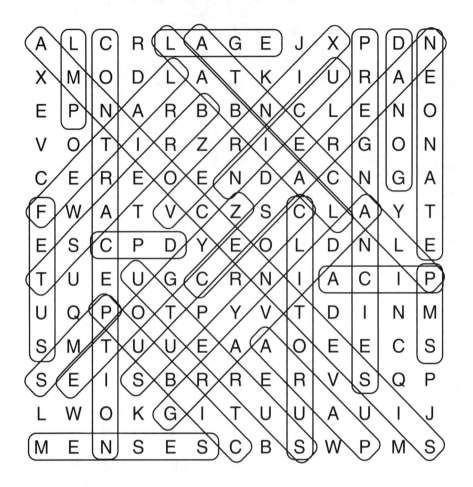

CHAPTER **14**

Endocrinology

Endocrine System

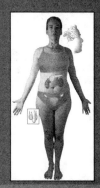

Instructor Activity for the Beginning of Class

Share this information with students.

The endocrine system is one of the most incredible and intricate systems in the body.

> "Men go abroad to wonder at the heights of mountains, at the huge waves of the sea, at the long courses of the rivers, at the vast compass of the ocean, at the circulation motions of the stars; and they pass by themselves without wondering."
>
> —St. Augustine

To most people, the endocrine system seems somewhat mysterious. So I want to give you an up close and personal encounter with your endocrine system. [Take a large book and quickly slam it against a table in the classroom. This is meant to really startle students.]

The shock you just felt was the release of epinephrine (Adrenalin) from your adrenal gland! It is your body's response to danger. The adrenal gland is one of the glands of the endocrine system. Now that you are all fully awake, alert, and oriented × 3, we will begin our study.

Are you ready to *regulate* your knowledge by exploring the endocrine system. You'll be in full *control* once you master the language of endocrinology!

Objective 1
Identify the anatomical structures of the endocrine system by correctly labeling them on anatomical illustrations

- Text page(s) 752–762

Teaching Strategies

1. Explain the importance of learning the parts of the endocrine system.
2. Using a diagram or model, identify each part of the endocrine system as it is discussed.
3. To learn the anatomy of the endocrine system, have the students label them on an anatomical diagram.

Content Abstract

Endocrinology is the study of the endocrine glands. It is the healthcare specialty that studies the anatomy and physiology of the endocrine system and uses diagnostic tests, medical and surgical procedures, and drugs to treat endocrine system diseases.

The anatomy of the endocrinology system includes:

1. hypothalamus
2. pituitary gland (anterior and posterior)
3. pineal body
4. thyroid gland
5. parathyroid glands
6. thymus gland
7. pancreas
8. adrenal glands (adrenal cortex and adrenal medulla)
9. ovaries
10. testes

Experience Multimedia	
See the PowerPoint presentation on the accompanying Instructor's Media Library for an animation showing the endocrine system.	

Objective 2
Describe the actions of hormones released by endocrine glands

- Text page(s) 762–763

Teaching Strategy

Explain the importance of learning the action of hormones released by the endocrine glands.

Content Abstract

The endocrine system uses hormones as chemical messengers. They are secreted into the blood and travel throughout the body to produce an action. The action of hormones can involve stimulation or inhibition, meaning that some hormones stimulate a gland or organ to release its hormones (stimulation); other hormones keep a gland or organ from releasing its hormones (inhibition).

Box 14-1: Classroom Activity

ENDOCRINE GLANDS

Create a table on the board while students create the same table in their notes, indicating each endocrine gland, where it is located in the body, and what hormone it secretes.

Box 14-2: Instructor Activity

MNEMONIC DEVICE

Share this information with students.

1. The many hormones of the endocrine system and their actions throughout the body can be confusing to students. To encourage students and inject a little humor into this otherwise complex and serious chapter, you can share the following observation with students. "Sixteen endocrine glands and 26 hormones coming right at you. Wow! Of course, this should pose no problem for someone as intelligent and incredibly talented as yourself. Did I mention how spiffy you look today?"

   Source: Adapted from a newspaper advertisement for Bell Atlantic Telephone.

2. Use this mnifty mnemonic device to help you remember all the hormones of the anterior pituitary gland.

   FLAGTOP   **FSH, LH, ACTH, GH, TSH, MSH, p**rolactin

3. A researcher at the Mayo Clinic was attempting to identify hormones secreted by the adrenal gland. He identified five substances that he called Substances A, B, C, D, and E. To obtain only 2 ounces of Substance E, he had to grind up 300,000 pounds of cattle adrenal glands. In 1941, the United States received an intelligence report that Germany was giving adrenal gland extract to its pilots to enable them to fly at high altitudes. Although this report was false, it stimulated financial backing for adrenal gland research. Substance E later became known as *cortisone*.

Objective 3
Build endocrine words from combining forms, prefixes and suffixes

• Text page(s) 769–770

Teaching Strategy

Create a PowerPoint presentation with combining forms, prefixes, and suffixes with their meanings. Use this presentation in class. All students participate in a "medical terminology bee." All students stand and take turns defining the combining form, prefix, or suffix displayed. If the student gets the answer right, the student remains standing and continues to play. If the student gets the answer wrong, the student will be seated and is out of the game. The last person standing is the winner. A prize could be given to the winner.

Objective 4
Describe common endocrine diseases

• Text page(s) 771–783

Content Abstract

Disease	Meaning
Hyperpituitarism	Hypersecretion of one or all of the hormones from the anterior pituitary gland
Hypopituitarism	Hyposecretion of one or all of the hormones from the anterior pituitary gland
Galactorrhea	Hypersecretion of prolactin
Failure of lactation	Hyposecretion of prolactin
Gigantism	Hypersecretion of growth hormone during childhood and puberty
Acromegaly	Hypersecretion of growth hormone during adulthood
Dwarfism	Hyposecretion of growth hormone during childhood and puberty (see Box 14-3)
Syndrome of inappropriate ADH	Hypersecretion of antidiuretic hormone (ADH)

Disease	Meaning
Diabetes insipidus	Hyposecretion of antidiuretic hormone (ADH)
Postpartum hemorrhage	Hyposecretion of oxytocin after delivery
Uterine inertia	Hyposecretion of oxytocin during labor
Seasonal affective disorder	Hypersecretion of melatonin
Goiter	Chronic and progressive enlargement of the thyroid gland (see Box 14-4)
Graves' disease	Autoimmune disease with hypersecretion of thyroid hormones
Hyperthyroidism	Hypersecretion of thyroid hormones
Hypothyroidism	Hyposecretion of thyroid hormones (see Box 14-5)
Thyroid carcinoma	Malignant tumor of the thyroid gland
Thyroid nodule	Small, usually benign, tumor of the thyroid gland
Thyroiditis	Inflammation and destruction of thyroid gland tissue
Hyperparathyroidism	Hypersecretion of parathyroid hormone
Hypoparathyroidism	Hyposecretion of parathyroid hormone
Hyperinsulinism	Hypersecretion of insulin
Diabetes mellitus	Hyposecretion of insulin (see Box 14-6)
Diabetic ketoacidosis	Excessive, acidic ketones in the blood because fat is metabolized instead of glucose when there is no insulin
Hypoglycemia	Low levels of glucose in the blood
Hyperaldosteronism	Hypersecretion of aldosterone
Cushing's syndrome	Hypersecretion of cortisol
Addison's disease	Hyposecretion of cortisol (see Box 14-8)
Adrenogenital syndrome	Hypersecretion of androgens
Pheochromocytoma	Hypersecretion of epinephrine and norepinephrine
Precocious puberty	Hypersecretion of estradiol (female) or testosterone (male)
Infertility	Imbalance or lack of estradiol or progesterone (female) or hyposecretion of testosterone (male)
Menopause	Hyposecretion of estradiol
Gynecomastia	Enlargement of the male breasts due to excessive levels of androgens and testosterone

Box 14-3: Instructor Activity

DWARFISM

Share this information with students.

The world's shortest woman is Madge Bester. She is from South Africa and is 26 inches tall. Dwarfism occurs in about 1 in 10,000 births. Most of these children are from parents with average stature. Historically, dwarfs such as Tom Thumb and Anita the Living Doll were employed in show business, carnivals, and circuses, as were extremely obese, extremely thin, and bearded ladies.

Box 14-4: Instructor Activity

GOITER

Share this information with students.

People living in the "Goiter Belt," composed of states that are located away from salt water, must obtain their source of iodine from iodized salt or seafood. People who live in states near salt water obtain iodine from seafood.

Box 14-5: Instructor Activity

HYPOTHYROIDISM

Hypothyroidism in an infant or child is called *cretinism,* but when it occurs in an adult, it is called *myxedema.*

Box 14-6: Instructor Activity

DIABETES MELLITUS

Share this information with students.

1. Susan Turley, the author, worked for many years in the neonatal intensive care unit (NICU). She routinely took care of extremely small premature infants, weighing less than 2 pounds. Occasionally the infant of a diabetic mother would be brought into the NICU to be observed. This baby, who weighed over 10 pounds, would be placed in an incubator, where it seemed like a whale in a jar compared to the tiny two pound babies. Why was it so big? Because the mother's gestational diabetes mellitus had not been controlled; her blood sugar had been high many times because of not watching her diet or taking antidiabetic medication. This high level of glucose in the blood was transmitted through the placenta to the baby, whose pancreas was just fine and had no trouble making large amounts of insulin to metabolize the large amounts of glucose it was receiving. However, after delivery, the baby who had been used to constant high levels of glucose, now had to exist on a first feeding of sterile water followed by a small amount of milk or breast milk. This caused the baby's blood sugar level to suddenly fall. This baby, who had been active and crying, would suddenly become floppy and cyanotic and could even stop breathing!

2. People who smoke have an increased risk of up to 50 percent for developing diabetes mellitus. Smoking lowers the production of insulin and increases the development of insulin resistance syndrome. Smoking also raises the blood sugar level.

   Source: National Institutes of Health.

Box 14-7: Instructor Activity

HIRSUTISM

Many endocrine disorders can be detected by visually examining the patient. For example, a woman with excessive, dark hair on the face and extremities (hirsutism) could be experiencing an excessive output of the adrenal androgens.

Box 14-8: Instructor Activity	

ADDISON'S DISEASE

Former President John F. Kennedy always had a tanned look. His skin color was not solely due to his young age and athleticism. It was also due to Addison's disease, an endocrine disorder in which the cortex of the adrenal gland is destroyed by the body's own antibodies. The skin takes on an unusual bronzed appearance, even in areas not exposed to the sun.

Box 14-9: Instructor Activity	

ADENOMAS

The majority of endocrine diseases are due to adenomas. An adenoma can grow in the pituitary gland and cause hypersecretion or hyposecretion of hormones that affect other endocrine glands in the body. Also, an adenoma can grow in endocrine glands other than the pituitary gland.

Experience Multimedia	

See the PowerPoint presentation on the accompanying Instructor's Media Library for videos on the following topics covered in this chapter:

- Diabetes
- Insulin

Objective 5
Describe common endocrine diagnostic laboratory and radiology tests

- Text page(s) 784-786

Content Abstract

Test	Definition
Cortisol level	Blood test that measures the level of cortisol
Fasting blood sugar	Blood test that measures the level of glucose after the patient has fasted (not eaten) for at least 12 hours
Glucose tolerance test	Blood and urine tests that measure the level of glucose
Thyroid scan	Nuclear medicine procedure that shows the size and shape of the thyroid gland

BLOOD SUGAR TEST

Share this information with students.

1. Only fifty-seven percent of diabetics monitor their blood sugar level daily.

2. In the past, a diabetic patient had to use a small metal lancet with a sharp tip to manually puncture the fingertip to obtain blood for a blood sugar test. It was emotionally difficult for some patients to use the lancet to deliberately inflict pain on themselves. Then blood sugar monitors were created that automatically made the small incision as soon as the finger was touched to the machine. Until recently, the only recommended site for doing a blood sugar test was in the fingertip. Because there are a large number of nerve endings in the fingertips, this daily testing was quite painful. Now, some blood glucose meters allow you to use the forearm, thigh, or the fleshy part of the hand. Blues guitarist B.B. King appears in TV ads for the OneTouch blood glucose meter. He says that it allows him to test on his forearm and keep his fingertips healthy for guitar playing.

Experience Multimedia

See the PowerPoint presentation on the accompanying Instructor's Media Library for videos on the topic of performing a blood glucose evaluation

Objective 6
Describe common endocrine medical and surgical procedures and drug categories

- Text page(s) 786-788

Content Abstract

Procedure	Definition
ADA diet	Special physician-prescribed diet for diabetic patients that follows the guidelines of the American Diabetes Association
Thymectomy	Surgical procedure to remove the thymus in patients with myasthenia gravis
Thyroidectomy	Surgical procedure to remove the thyroid gland

Drug Category	Description	Example
Antidiabetic drugs	Treat type 2 diabetes mellitus by stimulating the pancreas to produce more insulin	DiaBeta, Diabinese, Glucotrol
Growth hormone drugs	Provide growth hormone	Humatrope, Protropin

SYNTHROID

Share this information with students.

In a list of the drugs prescribed most frequently in 2004, Synthroid for hypothyroidism was #5, with 44,000,000 prescriptions written.

Source: www.rxlist.com

ANTIDIABETIC DRUGS

Share this information with students.

1. Twenty percent of diabetics skip their medication because they can't afford it.
2. In 1922, researchers Frederick Banting and Charles Best extracted insulin from ground-up animal pancreas glands and injected it into a patient with diabetes mellitus. Before this, patients with diabetes mellitus were kept on extremely low-calorie diets (often to the point of starvation); this was the only known treatment. The word *insulin* is derived from the Latin word *insula,* meaning *island,* a reference to the islands of Langerhans in the pancreas. The first insulin injections were thick and muddy brown in color due to impurities from their source: ground-up beef and pork pancreas.

   Source: Susan M. Turley, *Understanding Pharmacology for Health Professionals.* Prentice Hall.

Objective 7
Define common endocrine abbreviations

- Text page(s) 789

Teaching Strategies

1. Stress the importance of learning abbreviations and their full meanings.
2. Encourage students to make flashcards for abbreviations and their meanings as well as their usual flashcards for word parts and their meanings.

Content Abstract

ACTH	adrenocorticotropic hormone
ADA	American Diabetes Association or American Dietetic Association
ADH	antidiuretic hormone
Ca, Ca++	calcium
CDE	certified diabetes educator
DI	diabetes insipidus
DKA	diabetic ketoacidosis
DM	diabetes mellitus
FBS	fasting blood sugar
FSH	follicle-stimulating hormone
FTI	free thyroxine index
GH	growth hormone
GTT	glucose tolerance test
HbA$_{1c}$	hemoglobin A$_{1c}$
IDDM	insulin-dependent diabetes mellitus
IRS	insulin resistance syndrome
K, K+	potassium

LH	luteinizing hormone
MSH	melanocyte-stimulating hormone
Na, Na+	sodium
NIDDM	non–insulin-dependent diabetes mellitus
NPH	neutral protamine Hagedorn (type of insulin)
OGTT	oral glucose tolerance test
RAIU	radioactive iodine uptake
RIA	radioimmunoassay
SAD	seasonal affective disorder
SIADH	syndrome of inappropriate ADH
T$_3$	triiodothyronine
T$_4$	thyroxine
T$_7$	free thyroxine index (FTI)
TFTs	thyroid function tests
TSH	thyroid-stimulating hormone
VMA	vanillylmandelic acid

Objective 8
Correctly spell and pronounce endocrine words

- Text page(s) 801-802

Teaching Strategies

1. Impress upon the students that medical words that are mispronounced are also probably going to be misspelled.
2. Encourage students to work on both pronunciation and spelling when studying.

Chapter Spelling Test

The chapter spelling test is included with the weekly chapter test. Dictate and spell (or xerox a handout that contains) this list of 10 spelling words. Give the list to students the week before the test. For the chapter test, select just 10 of these words to test.

1. acromegaly
2. diabetes mellitus
3. glucosuria
4. gynecomastia
5. hirsutism
6. hyperthyroidism
7. pituitary gland
8. polydipsia
9. synergism
10. thyromegaly

Chapter Pronunciation Test

Have students mark these 10 words listed in the Pronunciation Checklist for the chapter. During the week, they will call your office or home answering machine and pronounce each word.

1. acromegaly
2. diabetes mellitus
3. euthyroidism
4. glucosuria
5. ketoacidosis
6. hirsutism
7. homeostasis
8. hyperpituitarism
9. hyperthyroidism
10. polydipsia

Objective 9
Apply your skills by analyzing an endocrinology report

- Text page(s) 799-800

Content Abstract

Read the physician's office note and answer questions provided.

Objective 10
Test your knowledge of endocrinology by completing review exercises in the textbook and the CD-ROM learning activities

- Text page(s) 791-798 (first complete all the in-chapter exercises on pp. 768-770)

Teaching Strategies

1. Assign the Chapter Review Exercises in the textbook for homework.
2. Remind students to refer to the Answer Key at the end of the textbook to check their answers.
3. Refer to the CD-ROM Learning Activities in this section for multimedia learning experiences.

Experience Multimedia
See PowerPoint presentation on the accompanying Instructor's Media Library for videos on the topic of a career as a diabetes educator.

Homework Activities

1. Complete all of the exercises in the chapter, finishing the Chapter Review Exercises at the end of the chapter. Write in your textbook so that your instructor can verify that you did this work. See the Answer Key at the end of the book to check your answers.

2. Make flashcards for all of the prefixes, suffixes, and combining forms in the chapter. An index card makes a good homemade flashcard. One side of the flashcard should contain the word part and the other side should contain the meaning of the word part. Flashcards can also be printed from the CD-ROM. Flashcards can be carried everywhere and reviewed while waiting for a doctor's appointment, waiting for the bus, etc. Recruit family members, especially children, to help you study with your flashcards.

    As an additional self-quiz, first look at the meaning of the word part and then remember what the word part is.

3. During class, your instructor assigned 10 words from the Pronunciation Checklist on pp. 801-802. Practice the pronunciation of those words and then call your instructor's office or home phone number some time during the week and leave a message as you give your name and then pronounce each of the words.

4. Complete the Word Search for Chapter 14.

5. Refer to the Experience Multimedia CD-ROM Learning Activities Checklist for a list of activities to complete on the interactive CD-ROM.

6. Create a "mnifty mnemonic device" memory aid in the form of a rhyme, a word, or an abbreviation that helps you remember something about this body system.

7. Research the secondary complications of uncontrolled diabetes mellitus. Write a one-page summary of the findings.

8. Use the Internet to locate medical photographs of people with endocrine disorders.

9. Research and write a one-page paper about the personal story, symptoms, diagnosis, treatment, and aftermath of an endocrine disease as it affected one of these famous people.

Barbara Bush, former first lady	Graves' disease
Gail Devers, Olympic runner	Graves' disease
John F. Kennedy, former president	Addison's disease
B.B. King, blues guitarist	Diabetes mellitus
Mary Tyler Moore, actress	Diabetes mellitus
Jackie Robinson, baseball player	Diabetes mellitus
Sugar Ray Robinson, boxer	Diabetes mellitus
Rod Stewart, singer	Graves' disease

10. Keep a running list in your notebook of sound-alike words or combining forms that have the same meanings. Title this list of challenging words and word parts as "Perplexing Pairs." Begin by writing down the words or word parts found in the Word Alert boxes in this chapter. Then add the word parts found in the It's Greek to Me box at the end of this chapter. Add any other words or word parts that you found particularly confusing. You will add to this list as you complete each chapter. Examples:

orth/o-	vs.	arthr/o-
myel/o-	vs.	my/o-
perine/o-	vs.	peritone/o-
cephal/o-	vs.	encephal/o-

Word Search

Complete this word search puzzle that contains Chapter 14 words. Look for the following words as given in the list below. The number in parentheses indicates how many times the word appears in the puzzle.

ACTH (2)
Addison
adenoma
Cushing
diabetes
dwarf
euthyroidism
FSH
glands
glucose
goiter

hormone
insulin
ketoacidosis
NIDDM
nodule
OGTT
pancreas
pituitary
RIA
SIADH
TSH

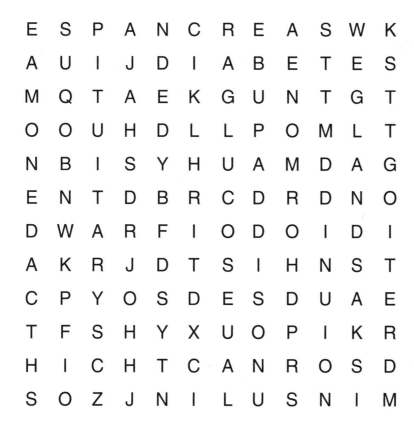

```
E  S  P  A  N  C  R  E  A  S  W  K
A  U  I  J  D  I  A  B  E  T  E  S
M  Q  T  A  E  K  G  U  N  T  G  T
O  O  U  H  D  L  L  P  O  M  L  T
N  B  I  S  Y  H  U  A  M  D  A  G
E  N  T  D  B  R  C  D  R  D  N  O
D  W  A  R  F  I  O  D  O  I  D  I
A  K  R  J  D  T  S  I  H  N  S  T
C  P  Y  O  S  D  E  S  D  U  A  E
T  F  S  H  Y  X  U  O  P  I  K  R
H  I  C  H  T  C  A  N  R  O  S  D
S  O  Z  J  N  I  L  U  S  N  I  M
```

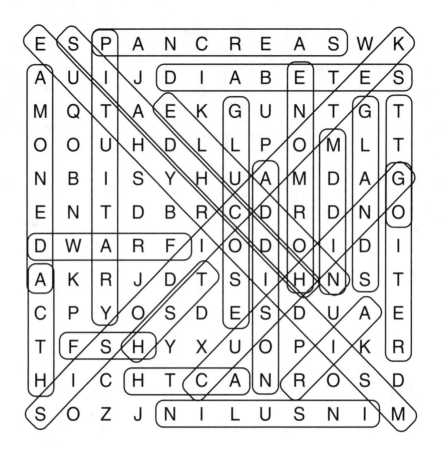

CHAPTER 15

Ophthalmology

Eyes

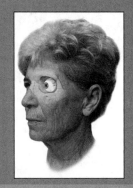

Instructor Activity for the Beginning of Class

Share this information with students.

1. Bulls are colorblind. The red cape in the bull ring appears gray to them. It is the motion that irritates them and causes them to charge.

   Source: Ask Yahoo, February 24, 2004.

2. Proportional to their size (up to 60 feet long), mysterious giant squids have the largest eyes of any animal in the world—each eye is as large as a human head.

   Source: David Grann, "The Squid Hunter," *New Yorker Magazine,* May 17, 2004.

Joke to tell at the beginning of class:

   Q: What famous dialogue line from the movies is the favorite of ophthalmologists?

   A: "Here's looking at you, kid" (Humphrey Bogart, from "Casablanca").

Set your *sights* on becoming a star *pupil.* You'll be *seeing* clearly once you master the medical language of ophthalmology.

Objective 1
Identify the anatomical structures of the eye by correctly labeling them on anatomical illustrations

- Text page(s) 806-815

Teaching Strategies

1. Explain the importance of learning the parts of the eye.
2. Use a visual aid (diagram) or model to show the parts of the eye as each is discussed.
3. To learn the anatomy of the eye, have the students label the parts of the eye on an anatomical diagram.

Content Abstract

Ophthalmology is the medical specialty that studies the anatomy and physiology of the eye and uses diagnostic tests, medical and surgical procedures, and drugs to treat eye diseases.

 The anatomy of the eye includes:

1. eyelid and conjunctiva
2. sclera and cornea
3. iris and pupil
4. lacrimal gland
5. choroid and ciliary body
6. lens
7. anterior and posterior chambers
8. posterior cavity
9. retina (rods and cones)
10. extraocular muscles
11. optic nerve

Box 15-1: Instructor Activity
INTERESTING FACTS
Share this information with students.

1. The eyes blink about 17,000 times each day and about 4,200,000 times per year. The muscles that turn the eye in all directions move about 100,000 times each day.

   Source: Fun Science Facts, www.hightechscience.org/funfacts.htm

2. How can two parents with brown eyes produce a child who has blue eyes? Brown is a dominant eye color. People with brown eyes can carry two brown genes, but they can also carry a brown and a blue gene. Blue is a recessive gene and is not expressed in the presence of the brown dominant gene. If both parents have a blue recessive gene, and both parents give that blue recessive gene to the child, then the child will have blue/blue genes and will have blue eyes.

3. All babies' eyes appear slate gray to blue at birth because of the lack of the brown pigment melanin in the iris. Exposure to light triggers the production of melanin by melanocytes. Babies who inherit a brown/brown or brown/blue gene have a large number of melanocytes in their iris and they develop dark brown or light brown eyes. Babies who inherit a blue/blue or blue/green gene have no melanocytes in the iris.

4. Word Alert

Macula	Dark, orange-yellow area with indistinct margins on the retina
Macule	Small, flat pigmented spot on the skin
Posterior chamber	Narrow space posterior to the iris
Posterior cavity	Largest open area in the eye; it lies between the lens and the retina

5. Note the interesting structure of the superior oblique muscle. It goes through a ligament that acts as a pulley, so that when the superior oblique muscle contracts, it does not pull the eyeball superiorly (as its name would imply). Instead, it pulls the eyeball inferiorly and medially.

6. To remember the function of the cones in the retina (as opposed to the rods) think "C" is for cones and for color.

Experience Multimedia

See the PowerPoint presentation on the accompanying Instructor's Media Library for an animation showing the eye.

Objective 2
Describe the process of vision

- Text page(s) 814-815

Teaching Strategy

Explain the importance of learning the process of vision.

Content Abstract

Light rays from an object pass through the cornea, which bends the rays to begin to focus them. The light rays enter the pupil and pass through the lens, which also bends the light rays to focus them on the retina. Light rays from objects directly in the line of vision fall on the macula, which produces an image. The retina contains special light-sensitive cells known as rods and cones. The image of the object is actually upside down and facing in the opposite direction when it touches the retina. A message is relayed via the optic nerve. The visual cortex of the brain turns the image right side up and faces it in its original direction so that it matches the object that was seen. It also creates three-dimensional, stereoscopic vision with a perception of depth or distance.

Objective 3
Build medical words from combining forms, prefixes, and suffixes

- Text page(s) 819-820

Teaching Strategy

Bring in a standard Scrabble game board set. The rules of the game are modified in that only medical words are allowed. Students must use words from the current body system or medical topic being studied. Students may use a medical dictionary (but only half of the points are awarded). Students can be required to define the words as they play them. At the conclusion of the game, students may take a quiz on the words that have been used.

Objective 4
Describe common eye diseases

- Text page(s) 821-828

Content Abstract

Disease	Meaning
Blepharitis	Inflammation or infection of the eyelid
Blepharoptosis	Drooping of the upper eyelid from excessive fat or sagging of the tissues due to old age
Ectropion	Weakening of connective tissue in the lower eyelid in older patients, allowing the lower edge to fall outward
Entropion	Weakening of the muscle in the lower eyelid in older patients, allowing the lower edge to fall inward
Hordeolum	Red, painful swelling or pimple containing pus near the edge of the eyelid
Dacryocystitis	Infection of the lacrimal sac
Xerophthalmia	Insufficient production of tears with eye irritation
Conjunctivitis	Inflamed, reddened, and swollen conjunctiva with dilated blood vessels on the sclera
Corneal abrasion	Trauma or irritation removes the superficial layers of the cornea
Exophthalmos	Pronounced outward bulging of the anterior surface of the eye with a startled, staring expression
Scleral icterus	Yellow coloration of the conjunctivae and sclerae from liver disease
Anisocoria	Unequal sizes of the pupils

Disease	Meaning
Glaucoma	Increased intraocular pressure because aqueous humor cannot circulate freely
Hyphema	Blood in the anterior chamber
Photophobia	Abnormal sensitivity to bright light
Uveitis	Inflammation or infection of the uveal tract
Aphakia	Absence of the lens due to surgical removal
Cataract	Clouding of the lens (see Box 15-2)
Presbyopia	Loss of flexibility of the lens with loss of accommodation
Color blindness	Genetic absence of certain cones in the retina, often green and red (see Box 15-3)
Diabetic retinopathy	Growth of new, fragile retinal blood vessels in diabetic patients
Macular degeneration	Chronic, progressive loss of central vision as the macula degenerates (see Box 15-4)
Night blindness	Decreased visual acuity at night (see Box 15-5)
Papilledema	Inflammation and edema of the optic disk
Retinal detachment	Separation of the retina from the choroid layer
Retinitis pigmentosa	Inherited condition of pigment deposits behind the rods and cones with loss of color vision and central vision
Retinoblastoma	Malignant tumor of the retina in children
Retinopathy of prematurity	Fibrous tissue in the retina due to high levels of oxygen needed by a premature baby
Nystagmus	Involuntary, rhythmic movements of the eye
Strabismus	Deviation of one or both eyes medially or laterally
Astigmatism	Surface of the cornea is curved more steeply on one side of the eye than on the other, so there is no single point of focus (see Box 15-6)
Hyperopia	Farsightedness
Myopia	Nearsightedness
Amblyopia	Brain ignores the visual image from the one eye that has strabismus
Blindness	Partial or complete lack of vision
Diplopia	Double vision
Scotoma	Temporary or permanent visual field defect

Box 15-2: Instructor Activity

CATARACT

The vision of a person with cataracts can be described like trying to look through a window that is fogged up with steam or covered with wax paper. More than half of all Americans will have a cataract by the age of 80. Prevent cataracts by wearing sunglasses and not smoking.

Source: American Academy of Ophthalmology.

Box 15-3: Instructor Activity

COLOR BLINDNESS

Share this information with students.

1. In 1798, John Dalton, an English physicist, first described the condition of color blindness.
2. Everyone is born color blind! An infant does not begin to see color until about 4 months of age when the cones begin to function. About 1 in every 40,000 babies does not develop cones in the retina and has no color vision; the most common color blindness is red-green, which affects 1 in every 25 people.

   Source: www.drgreene.com

Box 15-4: Instructor Activity

MACULAR DEGENERATION

Researchers have found that in about half the cases of age-related macular degeneration, the cause is a single gene that has undergone a mutation.

Source: ScienCentralNews at www.sciencentral.com

Box 15-5: Instructor Activity

NIGHT BLINDNESS

Share this information with students.

A deficiency of vitamin A can lead to night blindness.

Box 15-6: Instructor Activity

ASTIGMATISM

Astigmatism was first discovered and named in 1801.

Box 15-7: Classroom Activity

SURVEY

Draw these tables on the board. For each item, ask for a show of hands, and put a number in the number column. Stress that students do not need to participate if they choose not to reveal their medical history. Be sure to include yourself, the instructor, in the count.

Eye Disease	Number	Percentage of the Total
Myopia		
Hyperopia		
Astigmatism		
Presbyopia		
Total		100%

Corrected Vision	Number	Percentage of the Total
Glasses		
Bifocals		
Contact lens		
LASIK surgery		
Cataract surgery		
Other surgery		
Total		100%

Objective 5
Describe common eye diagnostic laboratory and radiology tests

- Text page(s) 829-831

Content Abstract

Test	Definition
Color blindness testing	Diagnostic procedure to determine the degree of red or green color blindness
Fluorescein angiography	Orange dye injected intravenously reveals microaneurysms and hemorrhages in the retina
Fluorescein staining	Orange dye is touched to the cornea to reveal corneal ulcers
Gonioscopy	Diagnostic procedure for glaucoma
Tonometry	Diagnostic procedure for increased intraocular pressure and glaucoma
Slit-lamp examination	Uses a slit-lamp and microscope to examine the cornea, anterior chamber, iris, and lens
Tonometry	Detects the increased intraocular pressure of glaucoma
Visual acuity testing	Diagnostic procedure to test near and distance vision
Ultrasonography	Radiologic procedure that uses high-frequency sound waves to create an image of the eye

Box 15-8: Instructor Activity

OPTHALMOLOGIST VS. OPTOMETRIST VS. OPTICIAN

Share this information with students.

An ophthalmologist is a medical doctor (M.D.) trained to treat eye diseases, and who can perform surgery. An optometrist (O.D.) is a doctor of optometry who can do everything an M.D. can do, except surgery. An optician is an allied health professional who grinds lenses according to a prescription from an M.D. or O.D..

CONTACT LENSES

Susan Turley, the author, wore contact lenses for many years. Once before inserting her contact lenses, she used a facial scrub that contained ground-up apricot pits. When she inserted her contact lenses, some of the granules got in her eye. She was in extreme pain because the sharp edges of the apricot pit granules were scraping her eye. She had to go to the emergency department. There, the emergency department doctor touched a thin paper impregnated with fluorescein dye to her eye. Her tears spread the dye across her eye. Then a slit-lamp exam caused the dye to turn bright green, revealing the scratched areas of the cornea. She was given an antibiotic ointment and instructed not to wear her contact lenses for 10 days.

Objective 6
Describe common eye medical and surgical procedures and drug categories

- Text page(s) 831-838

Content Abstract

Procedure	Definition
Dilated funduscopy	Medical procedure to examine the posterior cavity
Eye patching	Medical procedure in which the eye is covered with a soft bandage and a hard outer shield after eye trauma or eye surgery
Blepharoplasty	Plastic surgery procedure to the eyelids to remove fat and sagging skin
Cataract extraction	Surgical procedure to remove a lens affected by a cataract
Corneal transplantation	Surgical procedure to replace a damaged or diseased cornea
Enucleation	Surgical procedure to remove the eye from the orbit
Myopia surgery	Surgical procedure to correct nearsightedness
Strabismus surgery	Surgical procedure to correct esotropia or exotropia

Drug Category	Description	Example
Antibiotic drugs	Treat bacterial infections of the eye	Genoptic, Ocuflox
Antiviral drugs	Treat viral infections of the eye	Vira-A, Viroptic
Chemotherapy drugs	Kill rapidly dividing cancer cells in the eye	carboplatin, Vincristine
Mydriatic drugs	Dilate the pupil	atropine, Mydriacyl

Box 15-10: Instructor Activity

OPHTHALMOSCOPE

Share this information with students.

In 1851, Hermann von Helmholtz, a German physiologist, invented the ophthalmoscope.

Box 15-11: Instructor Activity

CONTACT LENS

Share this information with students.

In 1936, an optometrist in New York invented the hard contact lens.

Box 15-12: Instructor Activity

CATARACT SURGERY

Share this information with students.

1. In 1988, the first laser cataract surgery was performed by Dr. Patricia Bath. She is also the first African American female physician to receive a patent for a medical device.
2. During cataract surgery, the cloudy lens is broken up and removed in pieces and replaced by a rigid lens of plastic. This creates clear vision, but patients still need reading glasses for near vision. A new flexible Crystalens works with the eye's own muscles to naturally change focus from near to far effortlessly.

Source: Parade Magazine (Sunday newspaper supplement), July 18, 2004.

Box 15-13: Instructor Activity

LASIK

Share this information with students.

LASIK is an acronym meaning "laser-assisted *in situ* keratomileusis" (shaping the cornea).

Box 15-14: Instructor Activity

PRESBYOPIA

Share this information with students.

1. The FDA has approved a procedure to treat presbyopia. ViewPoint CK (conductive keratoplasty) uses radiowaves to tighten small areas of collagen to increase the curvature of the cornea and improve near vision.
2. A manuscript from 1299 read, "I find myself so oppressed by the years that I no longer have the strength to read or write without the glasses known as spectacles, lately invented for the comfort of the old souls who have become weaksighted."
3. By the 1350s, glasses were popular. Painters often put glasses on people in their paintings, even paintings of Biblical times; one painter even put glasses in a scene from the Garden of Eden. Spectacles were included by name in wills because they were so expensive.

   Benjamin Franklin (1706-1790) was nearsighted. Later in life, he also developed presbyopia. Because he became tired of changing from one pair of glasses to another, he cut the lenses from one pair of glasses in half and switched them with half of the lenses in the other pair, thus inventing bifocal glasses in 1760.
4. Early frames for glasses were secured to a hat. By the end of the 1700s, the earpieces were invented. In the 1850s, glasses were sold by traveling peddlers.
5. In 1862, Dutch physician Hermann Snellen invented the Snellen chart for testing distance vision.
6. Visual acuity is expressed as a ratio. The top number is the distance the patient is standing from the Snellen eye chart; this is always constant at 20 feet. The bottom number is the distance at which a person with normal vision could have read the same line on the chart. Therefore, if a person has 20/200 vision, this means that at 20 feet the patient can only see what a "healthy eye" sees at 200 feet.
7. The first glass eye was made in 1832 by Ludwig Müller-Uri, a glassblower in Lauscha, Germany. Today, even though artificial eyes can be manufactured from plastic, no other material is said to be equal to a glass eye created from a special blend of Cryolite glass.

Box 15-15: Instructor Activity

OPHTHALMIC DRUGS

Share this information with students.

Topical eyedrops and topical eye ointments are formulated differently than topical skin ointments. Ophthalmic drugs are specially prepared so that they do not irritate the delicate tissues of the eye. Regular antibiotic or anti-inflammatory drugs for the skin cannot be used in the eyes.

Experience Multimedia

See the PowerPoint presentation on the accompanying Instructor's Media Library for a video on the topic of administering ophthalmic medications.

Objective 7
Define common eye abbreviations

- Text page(s) 839

Teaching Strategies

1. Stress the importance of learning abbreviations and their full meanings.
2. Encourage students to make flashcards for abbreviations and their meanings as well as their usual flashcards for word parts and their meanings.

Content Abstract

ARMD	age-related macular degeneration		**O.D.**	Doctor of Optometry
CK	conductive keratoplasty		**OS, O.S.**	left eye (oculus sinister)
ECCE	extracapsular cataract extraction		**OU, O.U.**	each eye (oculus uterque), both eyes (oculus unitas)
EOM	extraocular movements			
EOMI	extraocular muscles intact		**PD**	prism diopter
HEENT	head, eyes, ears, nose, and throat		**PERRL**	pupils equal, round, and reactive to light
ICCE	intracapsular cataract extraction		**PERRLA**	pupils equal, round, reactive to light and accommodation
IOL	intraocular lens			
IOP	intraocular pressure		**PRK**	photorefractive keratectomy
LASIK	laser-assisted *in situ* keratomileusis		**ROP**	retinopathy of prematurity
LTK	laser thermal keratoplasty		**RP**	retinitis pigmentosa
OD, O.D.	right eye (oculus dexter)		**VF**	visual field

Objective 8
Correctly spell and pronounce eye words

- Text page(s) 849-850

Teaching Strategies

1. Impress upon the students that medical words that are mispronounced are also probably going to be misspelled.
2. Encourage students to work on both pronunciation and spelling when studying.

Chapter Spelling Test

The chapter spelling test is included with the weekly chapter test. Dictate and spell (or xerox a handout that contains) this list of 20 spelling words. Give the list to students the week before the test. For the chapter test, select just 10 of these words to test.

1. accommodation
2. aphakia
3. astigmatism
4. blepharitis
5. cataract
6. conjunctiva
7. funduscopy
8. glaucoma
9. macular degeneration
10. mydriasis
11. myopia
12. nystagmus
13. ophthalmologist
14. papilledema
15. phacoemulsification
16. presbyopia
17. retinoblastoma
18. scotoma
19. strabismus
20. ulcerative keratitis

Box 15-16: Classroom Activity

GAMES

1. From week to week, pick a different one of these spelling games to use during class. (The descriptions and instructions for the games are in the section "The Art and Craft of Teaching.")

   Beanbag Spelling Toss
   Scrabble
   Spelling Bee
   Gridlock
   Hangman

2. From week to week, pick a different one of these pronunciation games to use during class. (The descriptions and instructions for the games are in the section "The Art and Craft of Teaching.")

   Parroting
   Hieroglyphics
   Beach Ball Blast

Chapter Pronunciation Test

Have students mark these 20 words listed in the Pronunciation Checklist for the chapter. During the week, they will call your office or home answering machine and pronounce each word.

1. aphakia
2. aqueous humor
3. blepharoptosis
4. conjunctiva
5. exophthalmos
6. fluorescein angiography
7. glaucoma
8. hyphema
9. laser photocoagulation
10. macular degeneration
11. mydriasis
12. myopia
13. nystagmus
14. ophthalmologist
15. papilledema
16. presbyopia
17. retinoblastoma
18. tonometry
19. vitreous humor
20. xerophthalmia

Objective 9
Apply your skills by analyzing an ophthalmology report

- Text page(s) 847-848

Content Abstract

Read the Consultation Report and answer the questions provided.

Box 15-17: Classroom Activity

MEDICAL REPORT

Have students find and circle these words in the medical report: myopia, neurologist, migraine, scotoma, hemianopia, osteoarthritis, tonsillectomy, appendectomy, conjunctivae, sclerae, anicteric, exudates, exophthalmos, funduscopy, hemorrhage, tonometry. Have the students look in their book and write out a description or definition for each circled medical word. Then begin reading the report by having a student read the first header or sentence from the medical report on page 847. If one of the circled words occurs in that sentence, the student must also give their description or definition of that medical word. The next student reads the next header or sentence until the report is finished. This is to familiarize students with reading medical reports and analyzing words, while also gaining practice in pronouncing words.

Objective 10
Test your knowledge of ophthalmology by completing review exercises in the textbook and the CD-ROM learning activities

- Text page(s) 841-846 (first complete all the in-chapter exercises on pp. 818-819)

Teaching Strategies

1. Assign the Chapter Review Exercises in the textbook for homework.
2. Remind students to refer to the Answer Key at the end of the textbook to check their answers.
3. Refer to the CD-ROM Learning Activities in this section for multimedia learning experiences.

Experience Multimedia

See the PowerPoint presentation on the accompanying Instructor's Media Library for videos on the topic of a career as an optician.

Homework Activities

1. Complete all of the exercises in the chapter, finishing the Chapter Review Exercises at the end of the chapter. Write in your textbook so that your instructor can verify that you did this work. See the Answer Key at the end of the book to check your answers.

2. Make flashcards for all of the prefixes, suffixes, and combining forms in the chapter. An index card makes a good homemade flashcard. One side of the flashcard should contain the word part and the other side should contain the meaning of the word part. Flashcards can also be printed from the CD-ROM. Flashcards can be carried everywhere and reviewed while waiting for a doctor's appointment, waiting for the bus, etc. Recruit family members, especially children, to help you study with your flashcards.

   As an additional self-quiz, first look at the meaning of the word part and then remember what the word part is.

3. During class, your instructor assigned 20 words from the Pronunciation Checklist on pages 849-850. Practice the pronunciation of those words and then call your instructor's office or home phone number some time during the week and leave a message as you give your name and then pronounce each of the words.

4. Complete the Word Search for Chapter 15.

5. Refer to the Experience Multimedia CD-ROM Learning Activities Checklist for a list of activities to complete on the interactive CD-ROM.

6. Create a "mnifty mnemonic device" memory aid in the form of a rhyme, a word, or an abbreviation that helps you remember something about this body system.

7. Develop a crossword puzzle based on this chapter. Have some answers in the puzzle go from top to bottom (DOWN words) and others go from right to left (ACROSS words). The words should intersect with each other at several points. Make one list of clues for DOWN words and another list of clues for ACROSS words.

8. Keep a running list in your notebook of sound-alike words or combining forms that have the same meanings. Title this list of challenging words and word parts as "Perplexing Pairs." Begin by writing down the words or word parts found in the Word Alert boxes in this chapter. Then add the word parts found in the It's Greek to Me box at the end of this chapter. Add any other words or word parts that you found particularly confusing. You will add to this list as you complete each chapter. Examples:

orth/o-	vs.	arthr/o-
myel/o-	vs.	my/o-
perine/o-	vs.	peritone/o-
cephal/o-	vs.	encephal/o-

9. Investigate the U.S. Food and Drug Administration's site that answers consumers' questions about LASIK eye surgery: www.fda.gov/cdrh/lasik/.

10. Research and report on all the options that are available to correct the vision of a person who is nearsighted. Include details about each technique and its advantages and disadvantages.

11. If it is time for your regular eye examination, write a one-page summary of everything that was done. Think of questions ahead of time to ask the optometrist or ophthalmologist. Ask about all the different vision testing equipment that is used.

12. Take the complete Ishihara test for color blindness. Go to http://www.toledo-bend.com/colorblind/Ishihara.html.

13. Interview someone who has glaucoma or cataracts. Prepare a list of questions to be used during the interview.

Word Search

Complete this word search puzzle that contains Chapter 15 words. Look for the following words as given in the list below. The number in parentheses indicates how many times the word appears in the puzzle.

cataract
conjunctivae
cornea
EOMI
eye (3)
fundus
iris (2)
LASIK
lens
limbus
macular
myopia

ocular
ophthalmology
optic
PERRL
presbyopia
pupil
retina
retinopathy
rods
sclera
visual
vitreous

```
Y  H  T  A  P  O  N  I  T  E  R  C  F
W  G  C  A  T  A  R  A  C  T  Y  X  U
M  Y  O  P  I  A  R  E  L  C  S  E  N
A  T  R  L  E  L  C  E  M  O  R  R  D
C  F  N  Y  O  I  O  Y  D  N  O  E  U
U  L  E  N  S  M  Y  E  S  J  D  T  S
L  C  A  D  I  B  L  L  A  U  S  I  V
A  I  H  S  I  U  E  A  L  N  W  N  R
R  R  P  R  I  S  X  A  H  C  B  A  A
M  I  I  U  L  K  F  C  I  T  P  O  L
H  S  K  Y  P  E  R  R  L  I  H  Z  U
W  E  S  U  O  E  R  T  I  V  K  P  C
P  R  E  S  B  Y  O  P  I  A  F  U  O
```

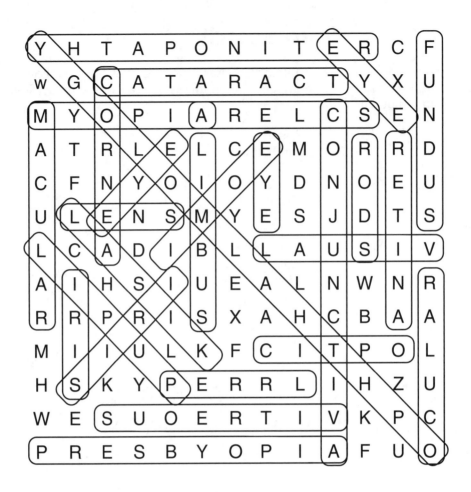

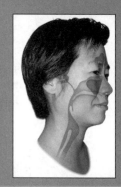

Otolaryngology

Ears, Nose, and Throat

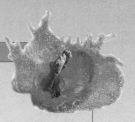

Objective 1
Identify the anatomical structures of the ears, nose, and throat (ENT) system by correctly labeling them on anatomical illustrations

- Text page(s) 854-863

Teaching Strategies

1. Explain the importance of learning the parts of the ENT (ears, nose, and throat) system.
2. Use a model of the ear to show the students the various parts.
3. To learn the anatomy of the ENT system, have the students label them on an anatomical diagram.

Content Abstract

Otolaryngology is the medical specialty that studies the anatomy and physiology of the ears, nose, mouth, and throat (ENT) and uses diagnostic tests, medical and surgical procedures, and drugs to treat ENT diseases.

The anatomy of the ENT system consists of:

1. external ear
2. middle ear
3. inner ear
4. nasal cavity
5. sinuses
6. oral cavity
7. pharynx
8. larynx

Box 16-1: Instructor Activity

INTERESTING FACTS

Share this information with students.

1. Word Alert
Malleus	First bone in the middle ear
Malleolus	Bony projection on each side of the leg near the ankle

2. The smallest bone in the body is the stapes in the middle ear. It is only 0.11 inches long.
   Source: Fun Science Facts, www.hightechscience.org/funfacts.htm

3. The middle ear cavity is only about as large as an aspirin tablet.

4. The ears of a cricket are located on its legs, just below the knees.
   Source: Fun Science Facts, www.hightechscience.org/funfacts.htm

5. Olfactory (smell) receptors in the nose can distinguish 10,000 different odors. They are also sensitive enough that they can detect a sulfur smell if it is only 1 part in 460 million parts of air.
   Source: The Human Body, TimeLife Books.

6. The highest recorded speed of a sneeze was 102 mph!
   Source: www.education-world.com

7. The hard palate is formed by the joining of the right and left halves of the maxillary and palatine bones. You can feel where the two sides of these bones join by running your tongue along the anterior-to-posterior ridge on the roof of your mouth. Going posteriorly, you move from the maxillary bone to the palatine bone. You can also feel where the hard palate transitions to the soft palate near the back of your throat. If you put your finger on your face in front of your ear and open and close your lower jaw, you can feel the posterior bony tip of the mandible moving.

Objective 2
Describe the process of hearing

- Text page(s) 864

Teaching Strategy

Explain the importance of learning the process of hearing.

Content Abstract

The external ear catches sound waves and funnels them toward the tympanic membrane. The sound waves are converted to mechanical motion as they cause the tympanic membrane to move the malleus, then the incus, then the stapes. The stapes transmits the motion to the oval window, which in turn causes the inner ear fluid on the other side of the oval window to vibrate. The vibration is transmitted to the cochlea, where there are tiny hairs that detect different frequencies of sound, sending nerve impulses through the cochlear branch of the auditory nerve to the auditory center of the brain. The number of hairs that are stimulated corresponds to the loudness of the sound.

Objective 3
Build ENT words from combining forms, prefixes, and suffixes

- Text page(s) 869-870

Teaching Strategy

Bring in a standard Scrabble game board set. The rules of the game are modified in that only medical words are allowed. Students must use words from the current body system or medical topic being studied. Students may use a medical dictionary (but only half of the points are awarded). Students can be required to define the words as they play them. At the end of the game, students may take a quiz on the words that have been used.

Objective 4
Describe common ENT diseases

- Text page(s) 871-878

Content Abstract

Disease	Meaning
Acoustic neuroma	Benign tumor of the auditory nerve
Cerumen impaction	Mass of earwax, epithelial cells, and hair that occludes the external auditory canal (see Box 16-3)
Cholesteatoma	Benign tumor of the middle ear
Hemotympanum	Blood in the middle ear
Labyrinthitis	Bacterial or viral infection of the semicircular canals of the inner ear, causing severe vertigo
Ménière's disease	Edema of the semicircular canals causing hearing loss and vertigo
Motion sickness	Dysequilibrium with headache, dizziness, nausea, and vomiting caused by riding in a car, boat, or airplane (see Box 16-4)
Otitis externa	Bacterial infection of the external auditory canal
Otitis media	Acute or chronic bacterial infection of the middle ear (see Box 16-5)
Otorrhea	Drainage of serous fluid or pus from the ear
Otosclerosis	Formation of bone between stapes and oval window, immobilizing the bones of the middle ear
Ruptured tympanic membrane	Tear in the tympanic membrane because of excessive pressure or infection
Tinnitus	Constant or intermittent buzzing, ringing sounds in the ear
Vertigo	Sensation of movement and dizziness when the body is not moving
Allergic rhinitis	Allergic symptoms in the nose
Anosmia	Loss of the sense of smell
Epistaxis	Sudden, sometime severe, bleeding from the nose
Polyp	Benign growth from the mucous membrane of the nose or sinus
Rhinophyma	Red, enlarged nose with lumps, due to acne rosacea
Septal deviation	Lateral displacement of the nasal septum
Sinusitis	Bacterial infection of one or all of the sinus cavities
Upper respiratory infection	Bacterial or viral infection of the nose or the nose, ears, and throat
Cancer of the mouth and neck	Malignant tumor of the mouth and neck
Cervical lymphadenopathy	Enlarged lymph nodes in the neck
Cleft lip and palate	Congenital lack of fusion of the maxilla and soft tissues of the upper lip

Disease	Meaning
Cold sores	Infection with herpes simplex virus, type 1
Glossitis	Inflammation of the tongue
Laryngitis	Inflammation or infection of the larynx
Leukoplakia	Thickened, white patch on the mucous membranes of the mouth, due to tobacco use
Pharyngitis	Infection of the throat
Temporomandibular joint syndrome	Clicking and pain on movement of the jaw joint
Thrush	Infection of the mouth due to the yeast *Candida albicans* (see Box 16-10)
Tonsillitis	Bacterial infection of the palatine tonsils
Vocal cord nodule or polyp	Benign growth on the surface of the vocal cord (see Box 16-11)

Box 16-2: Instructor Activity

SIGN LANGUAGE

Share this information with students.

In 1817, a French teacher, Laurent Clerc, founded the first school for the deaf in Hartford, Connecticut. He began teaching French Sign Language, though many of his students were already fluent in their own forms of local, natural sign language.

Box 16-3: Instructor Activity

CERUMEN IMPACTION

Share this information with students.

Some people form more earwax than others. In the elderly, generally dry skin and a lack of sebaceous gland secretion can create earwax that is thick. The growth of hair in the ears in middle age also blocks the removal of earwax.

Box 16-4: Instructor Activity

MOTION SICKNESS

Share this information with students.

Motion sickness is a common but extremely uncomfortable sensation that affects certain people riding in a car, boat, or airplane. The herb ginger, the antihistamine drugs Benadryl and Dramamine, and the transdermal patch TransdermScop can be used to prevent motion sickness, although, as the author found out, the transdermal patch can have the severe side effect of urinary retention and inability to void.

Box 16-5: Instructor Activity

OTITIS MEDIA

Share this information with students.

Otitis media is common in young children because the short eustachian tube is in a nearly horizontal position that allows bacteria to enter the middle ear from the nasopharynx. In addition, some children are put to bed with their bottles, and swallowing movements allow air and bacteria from the mouth to enter the eustachian tubes to the middle ear.

Box 16-6: Instructor Activity

COMMON COLD

Share this information with students.

Most people contract two or more colds per year. There are over 120 different viruses, not to mention bacteria, that cause colds. The common cold is considered the single most expensive illness in the United States in terms of time lost from work/school.

Source: Susan Turley, *Understanding Pharmacology for Health Professionals.* Prentice Hall.

Box 16-7: Instructor Activity

WORD ALERT

Share this information with students.

Mastoiditis	Infection of the air cells of the bone of the mastoid process
Mastitis	Infection of the mammary glands of the breast

Box 16-8: Instructor Activity

RESISTANT BACTERIA IN THE NOSE

Share this information with students.

1. Patients in a hospital run the risk of developing an infection with methicillin-resistant staphylococcus aureus (MRSA) (pronounced "mer-sah"). This bacterium has become resistant to penicillin-category antibiotics and an infection can be fatal.

2. A study published in the *Journal of Infectious Diseases* states that epidemiologists have found that more than two million people in the United States carry MRSA in their noses. Most of these people do not become sick, but can easily spread MRSA.

Source: *The Baltimore Sun,* January 27, 2006.

Box 16-9: Instructor Activity

TOPICAL LIQUID COCAINE

Share this information with students.

1. Susan Turley, the author, worked for an ENT physician. Patients came into the office, complaining of chronic nasal stuffiness. In order to examine the nasal passageways, the physician painted the muscoa with a few drops of topical liquid cocaine. This immediately opened up the nasal passageways and patients always remarked how wonderful this was and asked the physician to prescribe some of those nose drops for them. The physician would just smile and nod because cocaine is a powerful vasoconstrictor that shrinks the nasal mucosa, but it is also a controlled substance, a Schedule II drug under federal law with a high potential for abuse and could never be prescribed for nasal stuffiness.

   Another patient of this physician was a cocaine addict. He had used cocaine so many times that the blood vessels in his nasal mucosa had constricted to the point of killing the tissue. He now had a hole not only in his nasal mucosa but clear through his nasal septum.

2. Drugs with the potential for abuse and dependence were first regulated by the Harrison Narcotics Act of 1914. In 1970, The Comprehensive Drug Abuse Prevention and Control Act established five categories of schedule drugs (controlled substances) the Drug Enforcement Administration (DEA) to regulate controlled substances.

   Source: Susan Turley, *Understanding Pharmacology for Health Professionals.* Prentice Hall.

Box 16-10: Instructor Activity

THRUSH

Share this information with students.

At one time, thrush was almost exclusively seen in babies. The warm, moist environment of the mouth made a perfect growth medium for yeast. Now, thrush, also known as oral candidiasis, is often seen in AIDS patients, where it is an opportunistic infection that begins because of the patient's compromised immune system.

Box 16-11: Instructor Activity

VOCAL STRAIN

Share this information with students.

Vocal strain from constant singing can create vocal nodules or polyps, even in famous singers—from classically trained Julie Andrews to rock stars who then must be taught how to scream correctly.

Box 16-12: Instructor Activity

NOISE REDUCTION HEADSETS

Share this information with students.

Noise reduction headsets are sold for hearing protection from various causes: from snoring partners, loud music, and traffic noise to commercial earmuffs used in high noise areas of industrial construction and around aircraft.

Experience Multimedia

See the PowerPoint presentation on the accompanying Instructor's Media Library for videos on the following topics covered in this chapter:

- Otitis media
- Deafness
- Allergic rhinitis

Objective 5
Describe common ENT diagnostic laboratory and radiology tests

- Text page(s) 879-881

Content Abstract

Test	Definition
Audiometry	Hearing test that measures hearing acuity and documents hearing loss
Brainstem auditory evoked response	Analyzes the brain's response to sounds
Tympanometry	Hearing test that measures the ability of the tympanic membrane and the bones of the middle ear to move back and forth
Culture and sensitivity	Laboratory test of a swab of material from the nose, tonsils, or throat that is grown on culture medium in a Petri dish to identify the bacterium causing an infection and what antibiotic drugs it is sensitive to

Experience Multimedia

See the PowerPoint presentation on the accompanying Instructor's Media Library for videos on the topic of throat cultures.

Objective 6
Describe common ENT medical and surgical procedures and drug categories

- Text page(s) 882-886

Content Abstract

Procedure	Definition
Otoscopy	Medical procedure to examine the external auditory canals and tympanic membranes
Romberg's sign	Medical procedure to assess equilibrium
Cheiloplasty	Surgical procedure to repair the lip
Myringotomy	Surgical procedure whereby an incision is made in the tympanic membrane to drain fluid from the middle ear
Rhinoplasty	Surgical procedure that uses plastic surgery to change the size and shape of the nose

Drug Category	Description	Example
Antibiotic drugs	Treat bacterial infections of the ears, nose, sinuses, or throat	amoxicillin, Bactrim,Septra
Decongestant drugs	Constrict blood vessels and decrease swelling of the mucous membranes of the nose and sinuses due to colds and allergies	Afrin, Dristan, Drixoral, Sudafed
Corticosteroid drugs	Treat inflammation of the ears, nose, or mouth	Beconase, Flonase, Rhinocort

Box 16-13: Instructor Activity

FACE TRANSPLANT

Share this information with students.

A 38-year-old French woman whose face had been severely mauled by a dog received the world's first face transplant on November 30, 2005. The graft, from a brain-dead donor, contained a nose, lips, and chin. By the end of January 2006, it was reported that the woman was using her new lips to take up smoking again.

Source: BBC News at http://news.bbc.co.uk

Box 16-14: Instructor Activity

RHINOPLASTY

Share this information with students.

Susan Turley, the author, had a rhinoplasty some years ago. She wrote about this experience and entitled the article "Who Nose?"

Box 16-15: Instructor Activity

SINUSITIS

Share this information with students.

1. Chronic maxillary sinusitis that is not responsive to antibiotic drugs may be treated in the ENT physician's office with a sinus lavage. In this procedure, the nasal mucosa high in the nose is numbed with a topical anesthetic drug and then injected with an anesthetic drug. Then a large metal syringe with a pointed trocar tip is inserted through the mucosa. As the resistance of the bone around the sinus is encountered, a fair amount of pressure is used to push the tip through the bone and into the sinus cavity. This often causes a cracking sound. Once the tip is within the sinus, the pointed tip of the trocar is removed, leaving the open end of the syringe tube. The plunger of the syringe is pushed to inject sterile saline into the sinus cavity to flush out infection and debris. The infection and debris along with the saline solution flow out of the sinus and out of the mouth into an emesis basin held beneath the patient's chin.

2. Simple nasal irrigation has a long history of tradition in Oriental cultures, where the nose and sinuses are cleansed regularly by "sniffing" up salt water from the palm of the hand.

Box 16-16: Instructor and Classroom Activity

INTUBATION

1. Ask students to open their mouths as wide as they can and look around the room. They will notice that some students can open their mouths widely while others can only make a space of two inches between their teeth.
2. Susan Turley, the author, worked with Lynette Marks, M.D., an anesthesiologist in the Department of Anesthesiology at The Johns Hopkins Medical Institutions. They categorized the causes of difficult intubation and directed the Medic Alert National Difficult Airway Database.
3. The medical procedure of endotracheal intubation to establish an airway was presented in Chapter 4, Pulmonology, on page 183. Often, however, it is the anatomical structure of the mouth, throat, and larynx that creates difficulties during intubation. The following is a case history of a patient with difficult intubation.

> A 72–year-old male was admitted to the emergency department with pulmonary edema. As the staff was preparing to urgently intubate him for respiratory failure, he informed them that he was a Medic Alert member and that he knew he was a difficult airway/intubation (as identified during a prior surgery). The staff immediately paged the anesthesiology department and also attempted to retrieve his EPR (electronic patient record) as well as his old paper medical record. It was found that all documentation of his prior surgery was in his old paper medical record which was in off-site storage and not immediately available. The anesthesiologist then contacted the Medic Alert Foundation. They immediately faxed the difficult airway information containing the patient's specific successful airway algorithm.[*] In part, the information from Medic Alert read as follows: "Clinical airway algorithm: Unanticipated difficulty. Unsuccessful asleep direct laryngoscopy with a Mac #3, Miller #3 (on four attempts). Successful intubation using oral fiberoptic intubation. Primary difficulty encountered: Long epiglottis. Recommendation for future intubation: Fiberoptic intubation.

[*]An algorithm is a set of rules that can solve a problem in a limited number of steps.

Source: Case study from Lynette Marks, M.D., Chairman of the Anesthesia Advisory Council of the Medic Alert Foundation.

Box 16-17: Instructor Activity

DRUGS

Share this information with students.

1. When they were introduced, the antihistamine drugs Hismanal and Seldane were hailed as superior to Benadryl for treating allergy symptoms because they were less sedating. However, both of these drugs were later implicated in sudden cardiac arrest and were taken off the market. The molecular formula for Seldane was modified and the resulting new drug Allegra is still on the market.

   Source: Susan Turley, *Understanding Pharmacology for Health Professionals.* (Prentice Hall).

2. In 1979, Ciba-Geigy introduced the first transdermal patch drug delivery system. The drug was scopolamine for motion sickness.

   Source: Susan Turley, *Understanding Pharmacology for Health Professionals.* Prentice Hall.

Experience Multimedia

See the PowerPoint presentation on the accompanying Instructor's Media Library for a video on the topic of otic drops.

Objective 7
Define common ENT abbreviations

• Text page(s) 887

Teaching Strategies

1. Stress the importance of learning abbreviations and their full meanings.
2. Encourage students to make flashcards for abbreviations and their meanings as well as their usual flashcards for work parts and their meanings.

Content Abstract

ABR	auditory brainstem response
AD, A.D.	right ear (auris dextra)
AS, A.S.	left ear (auris sinister)
AU, A.U.	each ear (auris uterque), both ears (auris unitas)
BAER	brainstem auditory evoked response
BOM	bilateral otitis media
C&S	culture and sensitivity
dB, db	decibel
EAC	external auditory canal

ENT	ears, nose, and throat
HEENT	head, eyes, ears, nose, and throat
Hz	hertz
PE	polyethylene (tube)
PND	postnasal drip (or drainage)
SOM	serous otitis media
T&A	tonsillectomy and adenoidectomy
TM	tympanic membrane
TMJ	temporomandibular joint
URI	upper respiratory infection

Objective 8
Correctly spell and pronounce ENT words

- Text page(s) 897–898

Teaching Strategies

1. Impress upon the students that medical words that are mispronounced are also probably going to be misspelled.
2. Encourage students to work on both pronunciation and spelling when studying.

Chapter Spelling Test

The chapter spelling test is included with the weekly chapter test. Dictate and spell (or xerox a handout that contains) this list of 20 spelling words. Give the list to students the week before the test. For the chapter test, select just 10 of these words to test.

1. adenoids	11. otitis media
2. allergic rhinitis	12. pharynx
3. buccal mucosa	13. pharyngitis
4. cerumen	14. polypectomy
5. epistaxis	15. presbyacusis
6. eustachian tube	16. temporomandibular joint
7. laryngeal	17. tonsillar
8. larynx	18. turbinate
9. malleus	19. tympanoplasty
10. myringotomy	20. vertigo

GAMES

1. From week to week, pick a different one of these spelling games to use during class. (The descriptions and instructions for the games are in the section "The Art and Craft of Teaching.")

   Beanbag Spelling Toss
   Scrabble
   Spelling Bee
   Gridlock
   Hangman

2. From week to week, pick a different one of these pronunciation games to use during class. (The descriptions and instructions for the games are in the section "The Art and Craft of Teaching.")

   Parroting
   Hieroglyphics
   Beach Ball Blast

| Chapter Pronunciation Test |

Have students mark these 20 words listed in the Pronunciation Checklist for the chapter. During the week, they will call your office or home answering machine and pronounce each word.

1. adenoids	11. nasolabial
2. audiometry	12. otalgia
3. buccal mucosa	13. pharynx
4. candidiasis	14. pharyngeal
5. cholesteatoma	15. polypectomy
6. epistaxis	16. rhinophyma
7. larynx	17. Rinne test
8. laryngeal	18. sensorineural hearing loss
9. mucosal	19. tonsillectomy
10. myringotomy	20. vestibular

Objective 9
Apply your skills by analyzing an otolaryngology report

- Text page(s) 895-896

Content Abstract

Read the physician chart note and answer questions provided.

Objective 10
Test your knowledge of otolaryngology by completing review exercises in the textbook and the CD-ROM learning activities

- Text page(s) 889-894 (first complete all the in-chapter exercises on pp. 868-870)

Teaching Strategies

1. Assign the Chapter Review Exercises in the textbook for homework.
2. Remind students to refer to the Answer Key at the end of the textbook to check their answers.
3. Have the students complete the learning activities provided on the interactive CD-ROM.

Experience Multimedia
See the PowerPoint presentation on the accompanying Instructor's Media Library for videos on the topic of a career in audiology.

Homework Activities

1. Complete all of the exercises in the chapter, finishing the Chapter Review Exercises at the end of the chapter. Write in your textbook so that your instructor can verify that you did this work. See the Answer Key at the end of the book to check your answers.

2. Make flashcards for all of the prefixes, suffixes, and combining forms in the chapter. An index card makes a good homemade flashcard. One side of the flashcard should contain the word part and the other side should contain the meaning of the word part. Flashcards can also be printed from the CD-ROM. Flashcards can be carried everywhere and reviewed while waiting for a doctor's appointment, waiting for the bus, etc. Recruit family members, especially children, to help you study with your flashcards.

   As an additional self-quiz, first look at the meaning of the word part and then remember what the word part is.

3. During class, your instructor assigned 20 words from the Pronunciation Checklist on pp. 897-898. Practice the pronunciation of those words and then call your instructor's office or home phone number some time during the week and leave a message as you give your name and then pronounce each of the words.

4. Complete the Word Search for Chapter 16.

5. Refer to the Experience Multimedia CD-ROM Learning Activities Checklist for a list of activities to complete on the interactive CD-ROM.

6. Create a "mnifty mnemonic device" memory aid in the form of a rhyme, a word, or an abbreviation that helps you remember something about this body system.

7. Develop a crossword puzzle based on this chapter. Have some answers in the puzzle go from top to bottom (DOWN words) and others go from right to left (ACROSS Words). The words should intersect with each other at several points. Make one list of clues for DOWN words and another list of clues for ACROSS words.

8. Research and write a one-page paper about the personal story, symptoms, diagnosis, treatment, and aftermath of a hearing impairment as it affected one of these famous people.

Ludwig von Beethoven	Musician, composer
Lou Ferrigno	Actor
Marlee Matlin	Actress
Helen Keller	Spokesperson for the blind and deaf

9. Look at a decibel (dB) scale that lists the many levels of noise generated in different environments. See www.coolmath.com/decibels1.htm. Construct your own decibel scale. Include the items from the Web site. Also include these items: a whisper 30 dB, heavy rainfall 50 dB, the level at which damage to hearing can begin to occur 85 dB, lawn mower 90 dB, loud rock concert 115 dB, race car noise 130 dB, fireworks 150 dBb, shotgun blast 170 dB.

   Source: Parade Magazine (Sunday newspaper supplement), February 5, 2006.

10. Keep a running list in your notebook of sound-alike words or combining forms that have the same meanings. Title this list of challenging words and word parts as "Perplexing Pairs." Begin by writing down the words or word parts found in the Word Alert boxes in this chapter. Then add the word parts found in the It's Greek to Me box at the end of this chapter.) Add any other words or word parts that you found particularly confusing. You will add to this list as you complete each chapter. Examples:

orth/o-	vs.	arthr/o-
myel/o-	vs.	my/o-
perine/o-	vs.	peritone/o-
cephal/o-	vs.	encephal/o-

11. Look in your medicine cabinet. Find ENT prescription or over-the-counter drugs. List their drug names. Also look on the label and find any medical words. Write down these medical words and then look up and write their medical definitions.

12. Learn how to say your name using American Sign Language. Go to www.masterstech-home.com/ASLDict.html. Go to the bottom of the page and click on Here is the ASL Alphabet.

13. Interview someone who uses a hearing aid. Make up a list of questions beforehand, including how their hearing loss began, how they were diagnosed, what types of hearing aids there are, and how they care for their hearing aid.

14. Visit the Web site www.webwhispers.org to learn about the electronic speech devices used by patients who have had a laryngectomy.

Word Search

Complete this word search puzzle that contains Chapter 16 words. Look for the following words as given in the list below. The number in parentheses indicates how many times the word appears in the puzzle.

adenoids
auditory
aural
cerumen
cochlea
ears
ENT
epistaxis
ethmoid
helix
incus
larynx
malleus
mucosa

nasopharyngeal
nose (2)
oral
pharynx
rhinitis
Rinne
sinus (2)
throat
TMJ (2)
tonsil
tympanoplasty
URI
vertigo

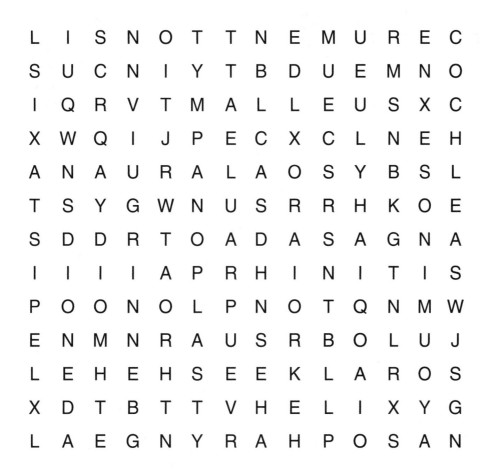

```
L  I  S  N  O  T  T  N  E  M  U  R  E  C
S  U  C  N  I  Y  T  B  D  U  E  M  N  O
I  Q  R  V  T  M  A  L  L  E  U  S  X  C
X  W  Q  I  J  P  E  C  X  C  L  N  E  H
A  N  A  U  R  A  L  A  O  S  Y  B  S  L
T  S  Y  G  W  N  U  S  R  R  H  K  O  E
S  D  D  R  T  O  A  D  A  S  A  G  N  A
I  I  I  I  A  P  R  H  I  N  I  T  I  S
P  O  O  N  O  L  P  N  O  T  Q  N  M  W
E  N  M  N  R  A  U  S  R  B  O  L  U  J
L  E  H  E  H  S  E  E  K  L  A  R  O  S
X  D  T  B  T  T  V  H  E  L  I  X  Y  G
L  A  E  G  N  Y  R  A  H  P  O  S  A  N
```

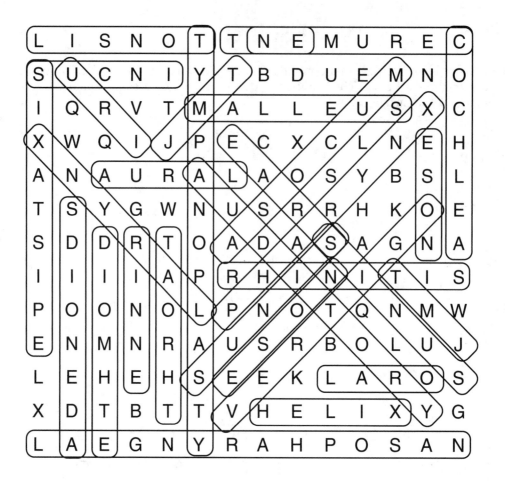

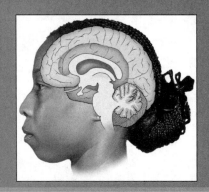

CHAPTER 17
Psychiatry

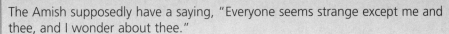

Instructor Activity for the Beginning of Class

The standard joke about mental illness: One out of every four people is mentally ill. Check three friends. If they seem okay, then you're it.

The Amish supposedly have a saying, "Everyone seems strange except me and thee, and I wonder about thee."

People joke about mental illness because it makes them uncomfortable. Those with mental illness often do unusual things that bring them to the attention of others and expose them to ridicule. Many people with social phobias, panic disorders, or obsessive-compulsive disorders try to hide their abnormal thoughts. One man successfully concealed his obsessive-compulsive disorder from his wife, only to have her discover him in their living at 2 a.m. carefully straightening the fringe on the edge of their area rug.

Today, we know that mental illness often is based on an imbalance of important hormones and neurotransmitters in the brain. In the past, that was not known and all sorts of remedies were used. Trephining was drilling a hole in the cranium to let out evil spirits. Patients were strapped to chairs. In the mid-1800s, patients with mental illness were housed in insane asylums, often with violent criminals. Social reformer Dorothea Dix advocated for better treatment of the mentally ill and improved conditions in mental hospitals. She was a schoolteacher and while teaching in a jail she happened to go to the basement and saw many insane people chained in cells without any food, clothing, or heat. She traveled through many states, addressing the state legislatures about the care of the mentally ill. Later she traveled to many foreign countries and did the same. When she was 60 years old, she served as the superintendent of female nurses during the Civil War for the Union Army.

Source: Biography of Dorothea Lynde Dix at Web site: www.dhhs.state.nc.us/mhddsas/DIX/dorothea.html

During the 1800s, the treatment for mental illness could include the use of the drugs digitalis, ipecac, alcohol, or opium. In 1903, barbiturates were synthesized and used as sedatives for agitated patients. Before World War II, schizophrenic patients were treated in several ways: They were exposed to malaria to produce a high fever and delirium, injected with enough insulin to cause convulsions and coma, or given electroshock therapy.

Source: Susan Turley, *Understanding Pharmacology for Health Professionals.* Prentice Hall.

Don't *panic.* It's time to get in the *mood* to learn about the mind. You'll be on your best *behavior* once you master the language of psychiatry.

Objective 1
Identify the anatomical structures
of the brain that are related to psychiatry

- Text page(s) 902-904

Teaching Strategy

Explain the importance of learning the parts of the brain that are related to psychiatry.

Content Abstract

Psychiatry is the medical specialty that studies the anatomy and physiology of the brain and the functioning of the mind and uses diagnostic tests, medical and psychiatric procedures, and drugs to treat psychiatric diseases.

The anatomy of the brain pertaining to psychiatry consists of:

1. thalamus
2. hypothalamus
3. hippocampus
4. amygdaloid bodies
5. fornix

Objective 2
Describe the process of an emotional response

- Text page(s) 905-906

Teaching Strategy

Explain the importance of learning the process of an emotional response.

Content Abstract

A current thought, sensory input from one of the five senses, a recalled memory, or a combination of all three can trigger an emotion. An emotion is an intense state of feelings. The presence of an emotion in the thoughts produces an outward display on the face, changes in behavior, and physical symptoms and signs in the body. The prevailing, predominant emotion is known as the person's mood.

Neurotransmitters are chemicals that relay messages from one neuron to the next. They play an important role in emotion and behavior. Neurotransmitters include epinephrine, norepinephrine, dopamine, serotonin, and gamma-amino butyric acid (GABA).

Objective 3
Build psychiatric words from combining forms, prefixes, and suffixes

- Text page(s) 907

Objective 4
Describe common psychiatric diseases

- Text page(s) 908-921

Content Abstract

Disease	Meaning
Generalized anxiety disorder	Dwelling on "What if . . ." questions
Obsessive-compulsive disorder	Constant, persistent, uncontrollable thoughts (obsessions) that occupy the mind, cause anxiety, and compel the patient to perform excessive, repetitive, meaningless activities for fear of what might happen if these are not done (see Box 17-1)
Panic disorder	Sudden attacks of severe, overwhelming anxiety without an identifiable cause
Phobia	Intense, unreasonable fear of a specific thing or situation (see Box 17-2)
Posttraumatic stress disorder	Disabling reaction to an excessively traumatic situation in the past
Amnesia	Partial or total loss of long-term memory
Delirium	Confusion and agitation due to toxic levels of chemicals, drugs, or alcohol in the blood
Dementia	Gradual, progressive loss of cognitive function
Attention-deficit hyperactivity disorder	Short attention span with distractability and acting out (see Box 17-3)
Autism	Inability to communicate or form significant relationships with others, and a lack of interest in doing so (see Box 17-4)
Encopresis	Passage of stool into clothing after age five
Oppositional defiant disorder	Aggressive behavior and refusal to obey rules
Reactive attachment disorder	Inability to bond emotionally
Tourette's syndrome	Frequent, spontaneous movements and vocal tics
Anorexia nervosa	Extreme, chronic fear of being fat and an obsession with becoming thinner (see Box 17-5)

(continued)

Disease	Meaning
Bulimia	Gorging with food and then vomiting for fear of weight gain
Depersonalization	Loss of connection between personal thoughts, self, and environment
Fugue	Impulsive flight away from one's life
Identity disorder	Loss of connection between thoughts, identity, memory, and environment
Malingering	Faking medical or psychiatric symptoms on purpose to get a reward
Munchausen syndrome	Faking medical or psychiatric symptoms to get attention but not being aware of one's motivation
Body dysmorphic syndrome	Overconcern with minor defects in body appearance
Conversion disorder	Sudden nonfunctioning of a body part without any physical illness
Hypochondriasis	Preoccupation with bodily sensations and fear of disease
Exhibitionism	Exposing the genitals to strangers to obtain power and arousal
Fetishism	Using an object to obtain sexual arousal
Masochism	Enduring pain and humiliation to obtain sexual arousal
Pedophilia	Sexual contact with children to obtain power and arousal
Rape	Forced sexual intercourse with a nonconsenting adult
Sadism	Using the pain and humiliation of others to obtain sexual arousal
Transsexualism	Belief that you have been assigned the wrong sexual identity
Transvestism	Wearing clothes belonging to the opposite sex
Voyeurism	Obtaining sexual arousal by secretively viewing other people who are naked or having sexual relations
Intermittent explosive disorder	Sudden, explosively violent outbursts unrelated to what is going on
Kleptomania	Overwhelming impulse to steal things that have little or no value
Pyromania	Setting fires for pleasure of watching people come to fight them
Trichotillomania	Pulling hair from out of the head
Bipolar disorder	Chronic mood swings between mania and depression (see Box 17-6).
Cyclothymia	Chronic, mild bipolar disorder
Major depression	Severe, chronic depression and apathy (see Box 17-7)
Premenstrual dysphoric disorder	Premenstrual syndrome symptoms plus depression and anxiety
Seasonal affective disorder	Depression and weight gain from too much melatonin
Delusional disorder	False beliefs concerning events of everyday life

Disease	Meaning
Schizophrenia	Chronic loss of touch with reality in most or all aspects of life with bizarre behavior and breakdown of thought processes, (see Box 17-8)
Antisocial personality	Disregard for written and unwritten rules and standards of conduct of society
Avoidant personality	Avoidance of social contact because of shyness
Borderline personality	Fear of abandonment, resulting in self-destructive relationships
Dependent personality	Wanting to be told what to do and think
Narcissistic personality	Exaggerated sense of self-worth and importance
Obsessive-compulsive personality	Perfectionistic; feels there is only one way to do things
Dissociative disorders	Characterized by a breakdown between the conscious mind and a person's identity, personality and memory

Box 17-1: Instructor Activity

OBSESSIVE-COMPULSIVE DISORDER

Share this information with students.

An elderly man had a compulsive disorder which led him to consume, in addition to regular meals, 25 soft-boiled eggs every day. He did this for at least 15 years.

Box 17-2: Instructor Activity

PHOBIAS

Share this information with students.

Millionaire Howard Hughes suffered from two phobias: agoraphobia (fear of crowds or public places) and microphobia (fear of germs). He always had all the windows blacked out in whatever hotel penthouse he was staying in, he never shook hands and always used paper towels to pick up objects. He suffered from obsessive-compulsive disorder his entire life. He was obsessed with the size of peas (his favorite food) and used a special fork to sort them by size before he ate them. In later years, he also obsessively kept all of his urine in glass jars.

Source: "Howard Hughes," Wikipedia, the Free Encyclopedia.

Box 17-3: Instructor Activity

ADHD

Share this information with students.

Video games are now being used for children with ADHD to train the network of the brain that is involved in attention. This area undergoes important development between ages three and seven. This training helps children to continue to focus on a particular task. Researchers found that the brain network develops a more mature response after just five training sessions. DNA shows that people have different versions of the dopamine transporter gene and that patients with one version of this gene tend to have more difficulty with attention span.

Source: ScienCentralNews at www.sciencentral.com for January 10, 2006.

Box 17-4: Instructor Activity

AUTISM

Share this information with students.

About two million people in the United States are afflicted with autism. Tristin is a 12-year-old child with mild autism. Many children with autism are unable to speak, but Tristin can and he has tried to express what his world is like: "When you're inside the autism, you just disconnect from everybody and everything. You don't feel anything. You just stop feeling. I think it kind of works like a tunnel, and you're inside, alone, all the time. It's like you're in a tiny little world somewhere else, and you can't really pay attention to anything outside of that little world anymore . . . [A person might] think going outside is a normal and easy experience, but there's color and sound and cars and that kind of stuff, which is very overstimulating. . . . There's so much to take in that you can't really process all of it . . . so you just get unconnected from the world and everybody."

Source: William Lychack, "When You're Inside the Autism, You Just Disconnect from Everything," *Life Magazine,* January 20, 2006.

Box 17-5: Instructor Activity

ANOREXIA NERVOSA

Share this information with students.

The mortality associated with anorexia nervosa is 6-20 percent, usually due to starvation or suicide.

Box 17-6: Instructor Activity

BIPOLAR DISORDER

Share this information with students.

A mother describes the bizarre behavior of her son, who suffers from manic-depressive disorder (bipolar disorder). During the manic phase, "He goes into a bank, seats himself at the desk of the vice president, expounds on the evil bond between banks and money, and demands immediate changes in the system . . . Worse things occur during the height of a mania-heightened frenzy: baseless accusations, verbal abuse, assaultive behavior ranging from spitting to a slap or a punch because someone expresses different political views. He burns with flaming energy and rage, consuming only himself until the illness causes the flagrant behavior to be subdued with neuroleptic medication."

Source: S. Garson, "The Sound and Fury of Mania," *Newsweek,* April 13, 1987.

Box 17-7: Instructor Activity

DEPRESSION

Share this information with students.

A study in 2004 showed that the level of the hormone serononin (which prevents depression) rose after petting a dog.

Source: University of Missouri at Columbia.

Box 17-8: Instructor Activity

SCHIZOPHRENIA

Share this information with students.

Studies published in two medical journals have concluded that heavy use of marijuana in some teenagers whose genetic/family history put them at added risk for mental health disorders increases their chances of developing psychosis or schizophrenia.

Source: The Baltimore Sun, January 27, 2006.

Box 17-9: Instructor Activity

ALCOHOL

Share this information with students.

1. A blackout is a period of time in which a person who has been drinking alcohol cannot remember anything. The alcohol stops their ability to form a memory. The person insists that everything is fine, does not lose consciousness, and appears to be functioning normally but is actually very impaired. These people appear normal because their pre-blackout memories are intact that allow them to walk, talk, drive, etc. A blackout can occur the very first time a person drinks, even without drinking a lot of alcohol, especially if the person is binge drinking. Try this simple memory test to determine if a person is experiencing blackout: Ask the person to remember three words that you pick yourself. Have the person repeat the words. Then continue the conversation about other things for five minutes. Then ask the person to repeat the three words. If they miss even one word, it is a sign they have lost short-term memory and are in a blackout. A person in a blackout should never be allowed to drive.

   Source: Donal Sweeney, *The Alcohol Blackout: Walking, Talking, Unconscious & Lethal.* Mnemosyne Press. The author is a physician and a member of the American Society of Addiction Medicine.

2. Women are more affected by drinking than men because overall their bodies contain less water and the alcohol that is consumed is dissolved in less water and therefore reaches a higher concentration.

   Source: National Institute on Alcohol Abuse and Alcoholism.

Experience Multimedia

See the PowerPoint presentation on the accompanying Instructor's Media Library for videos on the following topics covered in this chapter:

- Autism
- Eating disorders
- Panic attacks
- Obsessive-compulsive disorder
- Antisocial behavior
- Bipolar disorder
- Gender identity disorder
- Schizophrenia
- Sexual and physical abuse
- Dissociative disorders
- Drug and alcohol abuse

Objective 5
Describe common psychiatric diagnostic tests

- Text page(s) 922-923

Content Abstract

Test	Definition
Drug level	Blood test to determine the level of an antipsychotic drug in patients who are noncompliant with their medication schedule
Urine test for drugs	Urine test to detect illegal drugs
CT scan or MRI scan	Radiologic procedure used to document loss of brain tissue or structural abnormalities of the brain that might contribute to a psychiatric illness
Intelligence testing	Intelligence tests are administered if the patient is suspected of having any degree of mental impairment or retardation
Psychiatric interview	Provides the first insights into the patient's mental illness
Rorschach test	Uses cards with abstract shapes on them; also known as the inkblot test

---

Box 17-10: Instructor Activity

PSYCHOANALYSIS

Share this information with students.

In 1896, Sigmund Freud first uses the term *psychoanalysis.*

The following is an excerpt from a psychiatric report on a young, teenaged male with mild autism.

> There is a significant history of behavioral disorganization with the patient showing difficulties with behavioral and emotional control since kindergarten. His presentation is notable for clear signs of cognitive disorganization. He shows persistent rigidity in his thinking without the capacity to shift focus effectively and spontaneously. Results of psychological functioning tests are notable for signs of grandiosity in thinking and of making harsh judgments, either positive or negative. Responses for the Rorschach test indicate patterns seen in persons with bipolar disorder, including mildly paranoid ideation and perceptions of damaged or dying objects. Responses for the Roberts Apperception Test are similar. The content of his stories includes individuals dying. At other times, stories were finished in an immatune way with resolutions that were magical or illogical. This is usually seen in much younger children and suggests a fantasy basis for psychological coping with significant disorganization.

Box 17-11: Instructor Activity

IQ

Share this information with students.

There have been various classification systems for IQ. Terman's classification includes six categories:

IQ Range	Classification
140 and over	Genius or near genius
120-140	Very superior intelligence
110-120	Superior intelligence
90-110	Normal or average intelligence
80-90	Dullness
70-80	Borderline deficiency
Below 70	Definite feeble-mindedness

Objective 6
Identify common psychiatric procedures and drug categories

- Text page(s) 924-927

Content Abstract

Procedure	Definition
Art therapy	Drawing or creating other types of art while talking about it with an art therapist
Detoxication	Observation of an alcohol-addicted patient undergoing withdrawal
Electroconvulsive therapy	Uses an electrical current and electrodes on the head to produce seizures
Group therapy	Provides simultaneous therapy to several patients who have a similar mental illness like anxiety, depression, or being a victim of sexual abuse
Hypnosis	Places the patient in a sleeplike trance; used to treat anxiety and phobias and to help patients stop smoking or lose weight

Drug Category	Description	Example
Antianxiety drugs	Treat anxiety and neurosis	Tranxene, Valium, Xanax
Antidepressant drugs	Treat depression by prolonging the action of norepinephrine or serotonin	Elavil, Paxil, Zoloft
Drugs for alcoholism	Inhibit an enzyme that metabolizes the breakdown products of alcohol	Antabuse

Box 17-12: Instructor Activity

VALIUM

Share this information with students.

1. In 1945, researchers were looking for a new antibiotic to use against bacteria that were already becoming resistant to penicillin. One drug tested was found to produce muscle relaxation and exert a calming effect in animals. From this parent molecule, the first minor tranquilizer was developed in 1955 and marketed as meprobamate (Equanil, Miltown). In 1955, a researcher at Hoffman-La Roche laboratories was searching for a compound to make a commercial dye, but the chemicals tested were not useful as dyes. A year and a half of research yielded no usable products. As he was doing his final cleanup of the project, he noted a single sample that he had forgotten to send for testing. He noted, "We were under great pressure by this time because my boss told us to stop these foolish things and go back to more useful work. I submitted it [the sample] for animal testing . . . I thought myself that it was just to finish up." That last sample, which was nearly forgotten, turned out to be chlordiazepoxide (Librium). It was released for sale in 1960 and became the first of the benzodiazepine class of minor tranquilizers for the treatment of neurosis and anxiety. The same researcher continued to work on the basic molecular structure and, even before marketing of Librium had begun, he had synthesized the new drug diazepam (Valium). The trade name Valium is derived from the Latin word *valere*, which means *to be healthy*. The wild European plant valerian has been known since the time of Hippocrates to calm the nerves. In 1970, Valium became the number one prescription drug in the United States.
2. In 1951, while evaluating a drug for its effectiveness in treating tuberculosis, researchers noted that even seriously ill and dying patients developed a happy, optimistic attitude. This drug later became the first in the category of MAO inhibitors used to treat depression.

Source: Susan Turley, *Understanding Pharmacology for Health Professionals.* Prentice Hall.

Box 17-13: Instructor Activity

INTERESTING FACTS

Share this information with students.

1. In 1994, the book *Prozac Nation: Young and Depressed in America* was published.
2. Although Elvis Presley officially died of a heart attack in 1977, the State Board of Medical Examiners found that he had been prescribed some 12,000 pills—tranquilizers, stimulants, sedatives, and painkillers—in the last 18 months of his life.

Source: The Prudent Use of Medicines. TimeLife Books, 1981.

Objective 7
Define common psychiatric abbreviations

- Text page(s) 927

Teaching Strategies

1. Stress the importance of learning abbreviations and their full meanings.
2. Encourage students to make flashcards for abbreviations and their meanings as well as their usual flashcards for word parts and their meanings.

Content Abstract

ADD	attention deficit disorder	**OD**	overdose
ADHD	attention deficit hyperactivity disorder	**PCP**	phencyclidine (angel dust, a street drug)
BDI	Beck Depression Inventory	**PMDD**	premenstrual dysphoric disorder
CBT	cognitive behavioral therapy	**PTSD**	posttraumatic stress disorder
CNS	central nervous system	**Psy**	psychiatry, psychology
DT	delirium tremens	**Psych**	psychiatry, psychology
ECT	electroconvulsive therapy	**SAD**	seasonal affective disorder
ETOH	alcohol (liquor)	**SSRI**	selective serotonin reuptake inhibitor
LSD	lysergic acid diethylamide (a street drug)	**TAT**	Thematic Apperception Test
MAO	monoamine oxidase (inhibitor drug)		
OCD	obsessive-compulsive disorder		

Objective 8
Correctly spell and pronounce psychiatric words

- Text page(s) 939–940

Teaching Strategies

1. Impress upon the students that medical words that are mispronounced are also probably going to be misspelled.
2. Encourage students to work on both pronunciation and spelling when studying.

Chapter Spelling Test

The chapter spelling test is included with the weekly chapter test. Dictate and spell (or xerox a handout that contains) this list of 15 spelling words. Give the list to students the week before the test. For the chapter test, select just 10 of these words to test.

1. amnesia
2. anorexia nervosa
3. delirium tremens
4. delusion
5. dementia
6. euphoria
7. hallucination
8. homicidal ideation
9. hypnosis
10. paranoia
11. phobia
12. psychiatry
13. psychosis
14. schizophrenia
15. suicide

GAMES

1. From week to week, pick a different one of these spelling games to use during class. (The descriptions and instructions for the games are in the section "The Art and Craft of Teaching.")

   Beanbag Spelling Toss
   Scrabble
   Spelling Bee
   Gridlock
   Hangman

2. From week to week, pick a different one of these pronunciation games to use during class. (The descriptions and instructions for the games are in the section "The Art and Craft of Teaching.")

   Parroting
   Hieroglyphics
   Beach Ball Blast

| Chapter Pronunciation Test |

Have students mark these 15 words listed in the Pronunciation Checklist for the chapter. During the week, they will call your office or home answering machine and pronounce each word.

1. anorexia nervosa
2. autism
3. bulimia
4. delirium tremens
5. delusion
6. dementia
7. detoxification
8. electroconvulsive therapy
9. euphoria
10. homicidal ideation
11. milieu
12. obsessive-compulsive disorder
13. psychiatry
14. psychosis
15. schizophrenia

Objective 9
Apply your skills by analyzing a psychiatric report

- Text page(s) 937-938

Content Abstract

Read the medical letter and answer the questions provided.

Objective 10
Test your knowledge of psychiatry by completing review exercises in the textbook and the CD-ROM learning activities

- Text page(s) 929-936

Teaching Strategies

1. Assign the Chapter Review Exercises in the textbook for homework.
2. Remind students to refer to the Answer Key at the end of the textbook to check their answers.
3. Have the students complete the learning activities provided on the interactive CD-ROM.

Experience Multimedia	
See the PowerPoint presentation on the accompanying Instructor's Media Library for videos on the topic of a career as a social worker.	

Homework Activities

1. Complete all of the exercises in the chapter, finishing the Chapter Review Exercises at the end of the chapter. Write in your textbook so that your instructor can verify that you did this work. See the Answer Key at the end of the book to check your answers.

2. Make flashcards for all of the prefixes, suffixes, and combining forms in the chapter. An index card makes a good homemade flashcard. One side of the flashcard should contain the word part and the other side should contain the meaning of the word part. Flashcards can also be printed from the CD-ROM. Flashcards can be carried everywhere and reviewed while waiting for a doctor's appointment, waiting for the bus, etc. Recruit family members, especially children, to help you study with your flashcards.

   As an additional self-quiz, first look at the meaning of the word part and then remember what the word part is.

3. During class, your instructor assigned 20 words from the Pronunciation Checklist on pages 939-940. Practice the pronunciation of those words and then call your instructor's office or home phone number some time during the week and leave a message as you give your name and then pronounce each of the words.

4. Complete the Word Search for Chapter 17.

5. Refer to the Experience Multimedia CD-ROM Learning Activities Checklist for a list of activities to complete on the interactive CD-ROM.

6. Create a "mnifty mnemonic device" memory aid in the form of a rhyme, a word, or an abbreviation that helps you remember something about this body system.

7. Develop a crossword puzzle based on this chapter. Have some answers in the puzzle go from top to bottom (DOWN words) and others go from right to left (ACROSS Words). The words should intersect with each other at several points. Make one list of clues for DOWN words and another list of clues for ACROSS words.

8. Use a PDR (*Physician's Desk Reference*) to look up some of the drugs used to treat psychiatric diseases.

9. Take a test to see if you are a hypochondriac. The Whiteley Index is a widely used test for hypochondria; see http://www.uib.no/med/avd/med_a/gastro/wilhelms/whiteley.html.

10. Research and write a one-page paper about the personal story, symptoms, diagnosis, treatment, and aftermath of mental illness as it affected one of these famous people.

Art Buchwald, columnist	Depression
Ludwig von Beethoven, composer	Bipolar disorder
Drew Carey, actor	Depression
Karen Carpenter, singer	Anorexia nervosa
Winston Churchill, British statesman	Bipolar disorder
Patty Duke, actress	Bipolar disorder
Vincent van Gogh, artist	Bipolar disorder
George Frederick Handel, composer	Bipolar disorder
Abraham Lincoln, President	Depression
Mary Todd Lincoln, First Lady	Schizophrenia
John Nash, mathematician	Schizophrenia
Mary-Kate Olsen, actress	Anorexia nervosa
Sylvia Plath, author	Depression
Tracy Ullman, actress	Bipolar disorder
Mike Wallace, TV journalist	Depression
Tennesse Williams, playwright	Depression

11. Did you ever wonder what the Rorschach (inkblot) test is like? There are only 10 Rorschach inkblots. Psychologists want the inkblots to be kept from the general public, so that patients' reactions will be spontaneous. Therefore if you see an example of a Rorschach inkblot in an article or in a book, it is a fake. Explore this Web site and learn what the testing psychologist won't tell you! Go to http://www.deltabravo.net/custody/rorschach.php.

12. Search the Internet for stories about people who have unusual "phobias" and write a description of their plight.

13. Research the topic of suicide and compile statistics about suicide. Write a one-page summary of your findings.

14. Watch the movie *Patch Adams,* starring Robin Williams. It is about a physician in 1969 who worked in a psychiatric hospital.

15. Research the issues around attention-deficit hyperactivity disorder and the drugs used to treat it. Address the issue: Should schools recommend that certain children take those drugs?

Word Search

Complete this word search puzzle that contains Chapter 17 words. Look for the following words as given in the list below. The number in parentheses indicates how many times the word appears in the puzzle.

addict
ADHD
affect
anger
anorexia
anxiety
autism
CNS (2)
delusions
dementia
depression
drugs
ETOH
help
insane
limbic

LSD
manic
milieu
mood
OCD
panic
personality
phobia
SAD
sadism
sane
sanity
schizophrenia
suicide
therapy

```
N  J  P  E  R  S  O  N  A  L  I  T  Y
O  A  F  F  E  C  T  P  K  D  S  T  P
I  C  I  N  A  M  C  M  A  C  E  D  A
S  N  A  L  C  A  I  S  I  I  P  N  R
S  S  U  I  C  I  D  E  X  L  G  B  E
E  B  N  M  L  B  D  N  E  E  I  Y  H
R  A  D  B  J  O  A  H  R  Q  T  E  T
P  C  O  I  V  H  U  O  O  I  K  C  U
E  W  O  C  D  P  T  I  N  S  A  N  E
D  E  M  E  N  T  I  A  A  U  J  S  T
H  K  S  N  O  I  S  U  L  E  D  W  O
D  R  U  G  S  B  M  S  I  D  A  S  H
A  I  N  E  R  H  P  O  Z  I  H  C  S
```

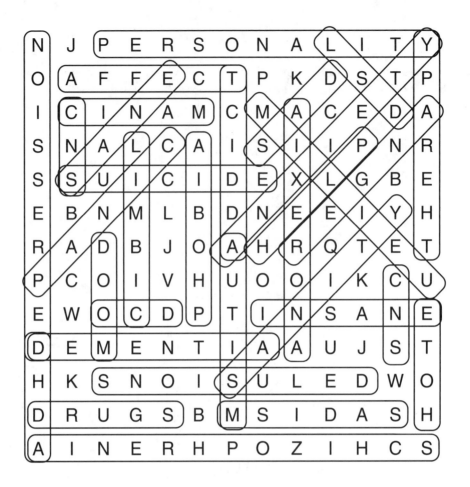

Oncology

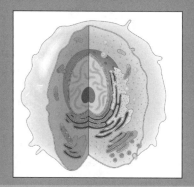

Instructor Activity for the Beginning of Class

Ask the students: "If you could think of one word that universally strikes fear in the hearts of everyone who hears it, what would that one word be?" [Answer: Cancer.]

Cancer cells are the anarchists of the body, for they know no law, pay no regard for the commonwealth, serve no useful function, and cause disharmony and death in their surrounds.

Source: Michael Gerald, *Pharmacology: An Introduction to Drugs.* Prentice Hall.

As bleak as that picture sounds, there is actually much hope for cancer patients, as new drugs and treatments are constantly being discovered.

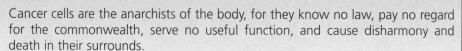

Objective 1
Identify the anatomical structures of a cell by correctly labeling them on an anatomical illustration

• Text page(s) 944-947

Teaching Strategy

Explain the importance of learning the parts of a cell relative to oncology.

Content Abstract

Cancer begins as a single normal cell that becomes abnormal. The anatomical structures of normal cell include:

1. cell membrane
2. cytoplasm
3. organelles (chromosomes, endoplasmic reticulum, golgi apparatus, lysosomes, messenger RNA, and mitochondria, nucleus, and ribosomes)

Box 18-1: Instructor Activity

INTERESTING FACTS

Share this information with students.

1. In 1962, researchers Watson and Crick received the Nobel Prize for identifying the double-helix structure of DNA in the nucleus of a cell.
2. If the spiral of DNA in the nucleus of just one human cell was stretched out in a single line, it would extend more than six feet.
   Source: The Human Body, TimeLife Books.
3. In 1996, Dolly the sheep became the first animal to be cloned from the cells of another animal. She died on February 14, 2003.
4. In 2000, the map of the human genome was completed.

Objective 2
Describe the process by which normal cells become cancerous cells

- Text page(s) 947-949

Teaching Strategies

1. Explain the importance of learning the process by which normal cells become cancerous cells.
2. Explain the causes of cancer.

Content Abstract

Mitosis is the process by which a cell divides. Mitosis begins in the nucleus. Normal body cells divide in an orderly fashion and in response to a particular need. The rate of mitosis is different for each type of cell. Skin cells have a high rate of mitosis because they are constantly being shed from the surface of the body. In contrast, muscle cells divide less frequently. Suppressor genes keep a cell from dividing excessively.

Damage to the DNA consists of genetic mutations that delete, reverse their normal order, or break off segments and insert them into other chromosomes (a process known as *translocation*). Damage to the DNA in the nucleus can be caused by a number of different factors: carcinogens, pathogens, or hereditary. Most of these factors do not immediately cause cancer. It is only after prolonged exposure that the cellular DNA is damaged beyond repair.

Objective 3
List the six characteristics of cancerous cells and tumors

- Text page(s) 949-950

Teaching Strategy

Explain the importance of learning the characteristics of cancerous cells and tumors.

Content Abstract

The characteristics of cancerous cells and tumors include:

1. Cancerous cells are not part of and do not contribute to the normal structure and function of the body. Once a single cancerous cell has been produced, it stops functioning as a normal cell and takes on the characteristics of a cancerous cell.
2. Cancerous cells lack differentiation and cannot perform the specialized functions of normal cells.
3. Cancerous cells are of varying size and are not arranged in an orderly fashion like normal cells.
4. Cancerous cells divide more rapidly than normal cells.
5. The growth of cancerous cells cannot be easily controlled by the body.
6. Cancerous cells form a tumor that is irregular in shape and is not encapsulated like a benign tumor.
7. Cancerous tumors release a substance that causes blood vessels in the surrounding tissues to grow into the tumor to provide it with nutrients. This process is known as *angiogenesis*. The tumor grows rapidly but often has a central core of tissue that is necrotic because the blood supply was inadequate.
8. Cancerous cells are invasive. They penetrate (infiltrate) normal tissues around them, hindering tissue function and destroying normal cells.
9. Cancerous tumors break off and move through the blood vessels and lymphatic vessels to other sites in the body. This process is known as *metastasis*. The cancerous cells are said to metastasize and are characterized as being metastatic.

NORMAL VS. ABNORMAL CELLS

Draw a table on the board like the one given below. Divide the students into two groups. Have each group get together, look at pages 949-950, and find the answers to fill in the blank rows under their assigned column. Then they should come to the board and fill in their column.

	Normal Cells	Cancerous Cells / Tumor
Relationship to the body		
Differentiation		
Size and arrangement		
Rate of division		
Control of growth		

Objective 4
Build oncologic words from combining forms, prefixes, and suffixes

- Text page(s) 953-954

Objective 5
Describe common oncologic diseases

- Text page(s) 955-963

Content Abstract

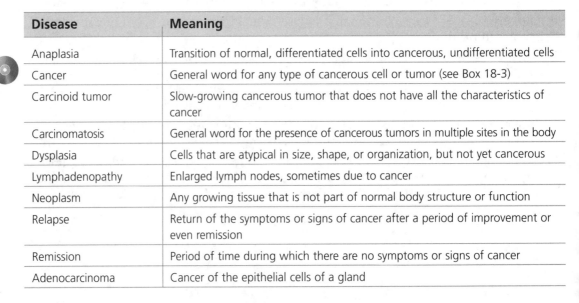

Disease	Meaning
Anaplasia	Transition of normal, differentiated cells into cancerous, undifferentiated cells
Cancer	General word for any type of cancerous cell or tumor (see Box 18-3)
Carcinoid tumor	Slow-growing cancerous tumor that does not have all the characteristics of cancer
Carcinomatosis	General word for the presence of cancerous tumors in multiple sites in the body
Dysplasia	Cells that are atypical in size, shape, or organization, but not yet cancerous
Lymphadenopathy	Enlarged lymph nodes, sometimes due to cancer
Neoplasm	Any growing tissue that is not part of normal body structure or function
Relapse	Return of the symptoms or signs of cancer after a period of improvement or even remission
Remission	Period of time during which there are no symptoms or signs of cancer
Adenocarcinoma	Cancer of the epithelial cells of a gland

Disease	Meaning
Carcinoma	Cancer of the epithelial cells of the skin and mucous membranes of organs
Malignant melanoma	Cancer of melanocytes of the skin
Angiosarcoma	Cancer of a blood vessel or lymphatic vessel
Astrocytoma	Cancer of an astrocyte in the brain
Chondrosarcoma	Cancer of cartilage
Ewing's sarcoma	Cancer of the growth zone at the end of a bone
Fibrosarcoma	Cancer of a tendon, ligament, aponeurosis, or scar tissue
Glioblastoma multiforme	Cancer of an immature astrocyte in the brain
Kaposi's sarcoma	Cancer of the skin and subcutaneous tissue
Leiomyosarcoma	Cancer of the smooth (involuntary) muscle of an organ or gland
Liposarcoma	Cancer of the fatty tissue
Myosarcoma	Cancer of a muscle
Neurofibrosarcoma	Cancer of cells around a nerve
Oligodendroglioma	Cancer of a myelin-forming cell around a nerve
Osteosarcoma	Cancer of a bone
Rhabdomyosarcoma	Cancer of a skeletal (voluntary) muscle
Sarcoma	Cancer of connective tissues
Leukemia	Cancer of leukocytes in the blood
Lymphoma	Cancer of a lymph node, lymphoid tissue, or lymphocytes
Multiple myeloma	Cancer of the bone marrow (see Box 18-4)
Choriocarcinoma	Cancer of the chorion around the embryo during pregnancy
Dysgerminoma	Cancer of an immature oocyte in the ovary
Embryonal cell cancer	Cancer of an embryonal cell
Germ cell tumor	Cancer of an immature oocyte or spermatoblast in the ovary or testis
Hepatoblastoma	Cancer of an embryonal cell in the liver
Neuroblastoma	Cancer of an embryonal cell in the autonomic nervous system
Retinoblastoma	Cancer of an embryonal cell in the retina
Seminoma	Cancer of an immature spermatoblast in the testis
Teratoma	Cancer of the ovary or testis that contains cells from other parts of the body
Wilm's tumor	Cancer of an embryonal cell of the kidney

Box 18-3: Instructor Activity

FACTS ABOUT CANCER

Share this information with students.

1. Lung cancer kills more people each year than breast, prostate, and colorectal cancer combined.

   Source: American Association of Retired People, www.aarp.org

2. According to the American Cancer Society, cancer kills more than 500,000 Americans each year.
3. There are more than 100 distinct types of cancer that each have their own unique symptoms and signs and require their own treatment modalities.
4. The most common causes of cancer death in men include lung cancer, colorectal cancer, then prostate cancer.

Box 18-4: Instructor Activity

MULTIPLE MYELOMA

Share this information with students.

Susan Turley's (the author's) mother died from multiple myeloma. The average life expectancy after diagnosis is just one to two years. Her mother lived a few weeks short of two years after having undergone chemotherapy. Amazingly, her mother's best friend also developed multiple myeloma the previous year and died in about two years. Although multiple myeloma is a rare cancer that affects just 1 in every 4,300 Americans each year, epidemiologists did not think these two cases were related or were statistically significant. In other words, the fact that two women who were best friends and former neighbors had both developed the rare cancer multiple myeloma within a year of each other was labeled as just a coincidence.

Box 18-5: Instructor Activity

BREAST CANCER

Share this information with students.

1. The average American woman has a one in seven chance of developing breast cancer during her lifetime. If she inherits the BRCA1 or BRCA2 gene, her risk increases to one in two chances. Annual mammography is recommended for all women with ultrasound followup of suspicious areas on mammography. However, magnetic resonance imaging (MRI) can spot nearly twice as many cancers as mammography, and so it is recommended for women in the high-risk category.

   Source: CBS News, "HealthWatch," July 28, 2004.

2. The American Cancer Society recommends that women in their 20s and 30s have a clinical breast examination (CBE) as part of a periodic (regular) health exam by a health professional, preferably every three years. After age 40, women should have a breast exam by a health professional every year.

3. Ask students: When a woman performs a self-examination of the breasts, the breast tissue is palpated for lumps. What other area is also felt? [Answer: under the arm, where the axillary lymph nodes are located.] Breast cancer cells that have spread or metastasized will become trapped in the axillary lymph nodes. In fact, the lymph nodes are often so full of cancer that they must be surgically removed along with the breast.

Box 18-6: Instructor Activity

LEUKEMIA

Share this information with students.

1. At the time of diagnosis of acute leukemia, one trillion cancer cells are generally present and widely distributed throughout the body of the patient. If an antileukemic drug were able to kill 99.9 percent of those cells, the patient would show symptomatic improvement even though he or she would still harbor one billion cancer cells.

   Source: Michael Gerald, *Pharmacology: An Introduction to Drugs.* Prentice Hall.

2. Survival rates for leukemia have increased from 14 percent in the year 1960 to more than 44 percent by the year 2000.

Experience Multimedia

See the PowerPoint presentation on the accompanying Instructor's Media Library for videos on the following topics covered in this chapter:

- Genetics of cancer
- Breast cancer
- Skin cancer
- Leukemia

Objective 6
Describe common oncologic diagnostic laboratory and radiology tests

- Text page(s) 963–967

Content Abstract

Test	Definition
Bone marrow aspiration	Cytology test on marrow removed from the bone
Exfoliative cytology	Cytology test on cells or secretions scraped or washed from the body
Frozen section	Cytology test that involves freezing a tissue specimen obtained from a biopsy
Karyotype	Cytology test used to examine the chromosome under the microscope
Receptor assays	Cytology test that measures the number of estrogen and progesterone receptors
BRCA1 or BRCA2 gene	Blood test for genetic mutation related to breast cancer
Carcinoembryonic antigen	Blood test that detects a protein that is normally present in an embryo but should be not present in an adult

(continued)

Test	Definition
Prostate-specific antigen	Blood test that measures a protein from the prostate gland that is elevated in cancer of the prostate
Tumor markers	Blood test for antigens on the surface of cancer cells
Urinalysis	Urine test that detects chemical compounds in the urine that are indicative of various types of cancers
Mammography	Radiologic procedure that uses x-rays to produce an image of the breast to detect tumors

Box 18-8: Instructor Activity

MAMMOGRAPHY

Share this information with students.

1. In 1969, the first mammography of the breast was performed.
2. Annual mammography is recommended for all women, with ultrasound follow-up of suspicious areas on mammography. However, magnetic resonance imaging (MRI) can spot nearly twice as many cancers as mammography, and so is recommended for women in the high-risk category.

Source: CBS News, "HealthWatch," July 28, 2004.

3. On regular mammography, an estimated 15-20 percent of cancers are missed. In a controversial move in 2003, the American Cancer Society (ACS) recommended stopping breast self-examination because research did not show that it saved lives. The ACS does recommend annual mammography for women over age 40. The National Cancer Institute and the Institute of Medicine recommend mammography every one to two years.

Source: Family Circle Magazine, October 19, 2004.

Box 18-9: Instructor Activity

PAP SMEAR AND CERVICAL CANCER

Share this information with students.

1. In 1943, the Pap test for cervical cancer was invented by George Papanicolaou.
2. The American Cancer Society recommends annual Pap smears (screening test for ovarian cancer) at ages 20 and 21, followed by tests at one-year or three-year intervals.
3. There are 50 million Pap smears performed annually in the United States. Of these, only about 4,000 detect new cases of cervical cancer. Cervical cancer is almost always caused by the sexually transmitted disease of human papillomavirus (HPV). There are more than 100 types of HPV, which fall into two main categories: HPV types that are a high risk for causing cervical cancer and HPV types that are a low risk for causing cervical cancer (but do cause genital warts). Now the DNA with Pap test can show whether the abnormal cells on a Pap smear belong to the high-risk catetory of HPV.

Source: Parade Magazine (Sunday newspaper supplement), October 10, 2004.

Objective 7
Describe common oncologic medical and surgical procedures and drug categories

- Text page(s) 967-975

Content Abstract

Procedure	Definition
Bone marrow transplantation	Medical treatment for patients with leukemia and lymphoma
Electrosurgery	Medical procedures that uses electrical current to remove small cancerous tumors on the skin
Staging	Medical and surgical procedures that classify cancer by how far it has spread in the body
Brachytherapy	Category that includes both interstitial and intracavitary radiotherapy
Intracavitary radiotherapy	Radioactive implants are inserted into a body cavity near the tumor
Biopsy	Surgical procedure to remove tissue from a suspected cancerous tumor
Lumpectomy	Excision of a small tumor, usually in the breast

Drug Category	Description	Example
Alkylating drugs	Break DNA strands in cancerous cell by substituting an alkyl group	Cytoxan, Emcyt
Antiemetic drugs	Not a chemotherapy drug; treat nausea and vomiting	Compazine, Phenergan
Antimetabolite drugs	Block folic acid required by the cancerous cell	fluorouracil, Gemzar, methotrexate
Chemotherapy antibiotic drugs	Inhibit an enzyme needed for cell division	Adriamycin, bleomycin
Chemotherapy enzyme drugs	Break down amino acid that cancerous cells needs	Elspar, Oncaspar
Hormonal drugs	Produce an opposite hormonal environment from the one that the cancer needs to reproduce	Arimidex, Femara Lupron, Megace, Nolvadex
Mitosis inhibitor drugs	Cause DNA strands in the cancerous cell to break	Camptosar, VePesid
Monoclonal antibodies	Bind to antigens on surface of cancerous cell and destroy it	Campath, Herceptin
Platinum drugs	Create crosslinks in the DNA strands that prevent the cancerous cell from dividing	cisplatin, Platinol-AQ

Box 18-10: Instructor Activity

CHEMOTHERAPY

Share this information with students.

1. Susan Gunn is a chef at a hospice. Her customers are the patients of the hospice who are there because they have less than 6 months to live. The hospice provides comfort and pain management, and food is considered an integral part of the comfort factor. Chef Susan honors her patients' requests for special foods: foods that bring back happy memories; foods that were their favorites. One former patient showed her his late mother's tin recipe file box. Using the handwritten bread pudding entry, Gunn took him back to his childhood. She notes," There are days when some patients can't tolerate the smell of food. But other times, a glorious resusgence of appetite is the benefit for patients who have discontinued treatment with chemotherapy. Those cravings can be fleeting, so we try to accommodate them promptly." At the hospice, comfort foods like meatloaf, macaroni and cheese, and chicken noodle soup are available every day, as well as ice cream and cookies.

   Source: Anne Haddad, "Offering Comfort From the Kitchen," *The Baltimore Sun,* February 7, 2001.

2. The discovery of the first chemotherapy drug happened as researchers reviewed records from World War I and noticed that soldiers who were exposed to the chemical weapon nitrogen mustard gas had decreased levels of white blood cells. It was thought that this effect could be used as a therapeutic effect to treat leukemia patients whose white blood cell counts are abnormally high.

3. New chemotherapy drugs have been discovered in Caribbean sea sponges, in the bark of the Pacific yew tree, and in the periwinkle plant.

   Source: Susan Turley, *Understanding Pharmacology for Health Professionals.* Prentice Hall.

Box 18-11: Instructor Activity

INTERESTING FACTS

Share this information with students.

1. The best "treatment" for cancer is preventing it in the first place, whenever possible. Two thirds (2/3) of cancer deaths can be prevented by healthy lifestyle **choices.** The American Cancer Society suggests:

   Cut out tobacco

   Hold the fat

   Opt for high fiber fruits, vegetables, and grains

   Intake of alcohol, only in moderation

   Call your doctor for regular checkups

   Exercise every day

   Safeguard your skin from the sun

2. Studies have shown that dosages of 1,000 international units of vitamin D may reduce the incidence of cancer of the ovary, breast, and colon by as much as 50 percent.

   Source: Parade Magazine (Sunday newspaper supplement), January 29, 2006.

3. Two out of three survivors of childhood cancer who received chemotherapy or radiation therapy develop health problems later in life and about one-third of these have life-threatening health problems. These problems include secondary cancers, heart disease, infertility, early menopause, cognitive defects, depression, and pain.

   Source: www.news-medical.net, July 29, 2004.

4. The *New England Journal of Medicine* reported a change in the treatment for ovarian cancer. Instead of just giving chemotherapy intravenously, researchers found that giving chemotherapy intravenously as well as into the abdomen through a catheter increased the length of life for women.

   Source: USA Today, January 5, 2006.

5. New procedure for treating lung, prostate, gastrointestinal, and head and neck cancers: intensity modulated radiation therapy (IMRT). A CAT scan is used to pinpoint the tumor and direct radiation therapy. It is possible to give four to eight times more radiation with less chance of damaging healthy, nearby cells.

   Source: American Association of Retired People at www.aarp.org

6. New procedure for treating lung, colon, breast, prostate, and pancreatic cancer: Monoclonal antibodies that seek out cancer cells and block their growth. Can also provide a target at which to direct radiation and chemotherapy that will kill the cancer cells. Examples: Iressa and Tarceva.

   Source: American Association of Retired People at www.aarp.org

7. Future procedure for treating lung cancer: inhaled cancer drugs. These are inhaled much like the drug in an asthma inhaler. The drug goes into the lungs and does not exert side effects in other parts of the body. Expected to be available in one to two years.

   Source: American Association of Retired People at www.aarp.org

8. In the late 1830s, ketchup was used as a medicine. It was sold as Dr. Miles' Compound Extract of Tomato. Recently, the antioxident lycopene in tomatoes has been found to reduce the risk of prostate cancer.

9. There has been a longstanding debate over whether marijuana (a Schedule I drug) should be legally available to treat patients with pain from advanced cancer. In 1996, the voters in California passed Proposition 215 to allow these patients to have marijuana if approved by their primary care physician. Eight other states passed similar laws. However, the federal law that prohibits the manufacture and distribution of marijuana takes precedence over any state laws. The American Medical Association (AMA) advised that marijuana does provide medical benefit to these patients, and many other groups also supported the legalization of marijuana to varying extents. In May 2001, however, the Supreme Court issued a decision that federal drug laws that ban marijuana have no exceptions, not even for medical necessity.

   Source: Susan Turley, *Understanding Pharmacology for Health Professionals.* Prentice Hall.

Objective 8
Define common oncologic abbreviations

- Text page(s) 976

Teaching Strategies

1. Stress the importance of learning abbreviations and their full meanings.
2. Encourage students to make flashcards for abbreviations and their meanings as well as their usual flashcards for word parts and their meanings.

Content Abstract

AFP	alpha fetoprotein
ALL	acute lymphocytic leukemia
AML	acute myelogenous leukemia
BMT	bone marrow transplantation
BRCA	breast cancer (gene)
Bx	biopsy
Ca	carcinoma, cancer
CEA	carcinoembryonic antigen
chemo	chemotherapy (slang)
CIN	cervical intraepithelial neoplasia
CLL	chronic lymphocytic leukemia
CML	chronic myelogenous leukemia
CRT	certified radiation therapist
CTR	certified tumor registrar
DNA	deoxyribonucleic acid

ER	estrogen receptor
FIGO	Federation Internationale de Gynécologie et Obstétrique
5-HIAA	5-hydroxyindoleacetic acid
HCG	human chorionic gonadotropin
mets	metastases (slang)
NK	natural killer (cells)
PICC	peripherally inserted central catheter
PR	progesterone receptor
PSA	prostate-specific antigen
RNA	ribonucleic acid
TACE	transarterial chemoembolization
TNM	tumor, nodes, metastases
VMA	vanillylmandelic acid

Objective 9
Correctly spell and pronounce oncologic words

- Text page(s) 987-988

Teaching Strategies

1. Impress upon the students that medical words that are mispronounced are also probably going to be misspelled.
2. Encourage students to work on both pronunciation and spelling when studying.

Chapter Spelling Test
The chapter spelling test is included with the weekly chapter test. Dictate and spell (or xerox a handout that contains) this list of 20 spelling words. Give the list to students the week before the test. For the chapter test, select just 10 of these words to test.

1. adenocarcinoma
2. benign
3. biopsy
4. cancerous
5. chemotherapy
6. chondrosarcoma
7. cytology
8. dysplastic
9. excisional biopsy
10. exploratory laparotomy
11. genetic
12. heredity
13. leukemia
14. lymphadenopathy
15. lymphoma
16. metastases
17. metastatic
18. neoplasm
19. oncologist
20. squamous cell carcinoma

Chapter Pronunciation Test

Have students mark these 20 words listed in the Pronunciation Checklist for the chapter. During the week, they will call your office or home answering machine and pronounce each word.

1. adenocarcinoma
2. benign
3. chemotherapy
4. chondrosarcoma
5. dysplastic
6. excisional biopsy
7. exfoliative cytology
8. exploratory laparotomy
9. genetic
10. heredity
11. Kaposi's sarcoma
12. karyotype
13. leukemia
14. lymphadenopathy
15. lymphoma
16. metastases
17. metastatic
18. neoplasm
19. oncologist
20. squamous cell carcinoma

Objective 10
Apply your skills by analyzing an oncology report

- Text page(s) 984-985

Content Abstract

Read the two Pathology Reports and answer questions provided.

Objective 11
Test your knowledge of oncology by completing the chapter review exercises in the textbook and the CD-ROM learning activities

- Text page(s) 978-984 (first complete all the in-chapter exercises on pp. 953–954)

Teaching Strategies

1. Assign the Chapter Review Exercises in the textbook for homework.

2. Remind students to refer to the Answer Key at the end of the textbook to check their answers.

3. Have the students complete the learning activities provided on the interactive CD-ROM.

Experience Multimedia

See the PowerPoint presentation on the accompanying Instructor's Media Library for videos on the topic of a career in surgical technology.

Homework Activities

1. Research and write a one-page paper about the personal story, symptoms, diagnosis, treatment, and aftermath of cancer as it affected one of these famous people.

Breast Cancer

Shirley Temple Black	Child actress, diplomat
Julia Child	TV chef
Betty Ford	Former First Lady
Peggy Fleming	Olympic ice skater and TV commentator
Linda Ellerbee	TV journalist
Olivia Newton-John	Singer, actress
Sandra Day O'Connor	Supreme Court Justice
Nancy Reagan	Former First Lady
Cokie Roberts	TV journalist
Carly Simon	Singer
Suzanne Somers	Actress

Lymphoma

Dick Gregory	Civil rights activist and comedian
King Hussein	King of Jordan
Charles Lindbergh	Aviator
Mickey Mantle, Jr.	Baseball player
Roger Maris	Baseball player
Jackie Kennedy Onassis	Former first lady
Mr. T	Actor

Prostate Cancer

Harry Bellafonte	Singer
Bob Dole	U.S. senator and presidential candidate
Robert Goulet	Singer
Rudy Giuliani	Major of New York City
Bob Kerry	U.S. senator and presidential candidate
Nelson Mandela	President of South Africa
Arnold Palmer	Golfer
Linus Pauling	Nobel Prize winner
Colin Powell	Former Secretary of State
Telly Savalas	Actor
Norman Schwarzkopf	Army general

Testicular Cancer

Lance Armstrong	Bicycle racer
Scott Hamilton	Olympic ice skater

2. Visit the Web site for the American Cancer Society at www.cancer.org and explore the various sections on the site. Write a one-page summary of at least three interesting facts that you learned.

3. Ben Dustin, a 9-year-old patient with leukemia that was in remission, asked the Make-a-Wish Foundation to help him develop a video game to help kids with cancer cope with their stress and pain. Read how Ben's Game was created by Ben and a famous movie studio. The video monsters are colds and side effects of chemotherapy. The ammunition is help you get from the hospital, pharmacy, and your family. Download this game for free and play it. Go to the Make-a-Wish Foundation's Web site at www.makewish.org and look for Ben's Game.

4. Call a local hospice and request a brief tour of the facility. Ask about the kind of patients who come to the hospice and the kind of healthcare workers who care for them. Write a one-page summary of your experience (remember to omit any patients' names). Alternatively, give a three-minute oral presentation of your experience to the class.

5. On Google, type in the phrase "Top 10 Cancer Hospitals" and do a search. Compare the different listings that come up and see which hospitals are mentioned more than once. Using the information you discover, rate the cancer hospitals and pick the ones you think are the best.

6. Locate a local cancer support group and attend a meeting. Write a one-page report on your experience (remember to omit any persons' names). Alternately, give a three-minute presentation of your experience to the class.

7. Research and write a short description of one of the following recommended cancer screening tests
   a. mammogram (breast cancer screening)
   b. prostate-specific antigen (prostate cancer screening)
   c. colonoscopy (colon cancer screening)

8. Go to the Web site for the National Cancer Institute (www.cancer.gov) and do a search on "clinical trials." Write a one-page summary about several interesting facts that you find.

9. The National Program of Cancer Registries (NPCR) recognizes that there is a shortage of Cancer Registrars. NPCR and the National Cancer Registrars Association (NCRA) developed a cancer registrar recruitment project to increase the number of trained professionals choosing a career as a cancer registrar. Health Information Management (HIM) students and other allied health professionals should be aware of this career option of cancer registrar. For more information, visit http://www.cdc.gov/cancer/npcr/training/QualityData/index.htm. If you are interested in this career, explore this Web site and view the PowerPoint slide program.

Word Search

Complete this word search puzzle that contains Chapter 18 words. Look for the following words as given in the list below. The number in parentheses indicates how many times the word is found in the puzzle.

adenocarcinoma
cancer
carcinogen
cell (2)
chemotherapy
chromosomes
debulk
DNA
excising
gene
genetic (2)

health
heredity
invade
malignant
metastasis
mutations
neoplasm
node
nucleus
TNM
tumor (2)

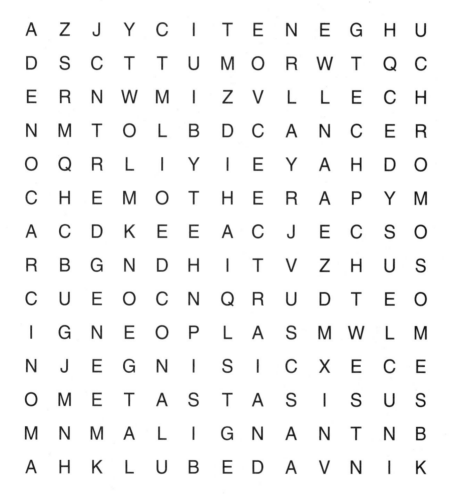

```
A  Z  J  Y  C  I  T  E  N  E  G  H  U
D  S  C  T  T  U  M  O  R  W  T  Q  C
E  R  N  W  M  I  Z  V  L  L  E  C  H
N  M  T  O  L  B  D  C  A  N  C  E  R
O  Q  R  L  I  Y  I  E  Y  A  H  D  O
C  H  E  M  O  T  H  E  R  A  P  Y  M
A  C  D  K  E  E  A  C  J  E  C  S  O
R  B  G  N  D  H  I  T  V  Z  H  U  S
C  U  E  O  C  N  Q  R  U  D  T  E  O
I  G  N  E  O  P  L  A  S  M  W  L  M
N  J  E  G  N  I  S  I  C  X  E  C  E
O  M  E  T  A  S  T  A  S  I  S  U  S
M  N  M  A  L  I  G  N  A  N  T  N  B
A  H  K  L  U  B  E  D  A  V  N  I  K
```

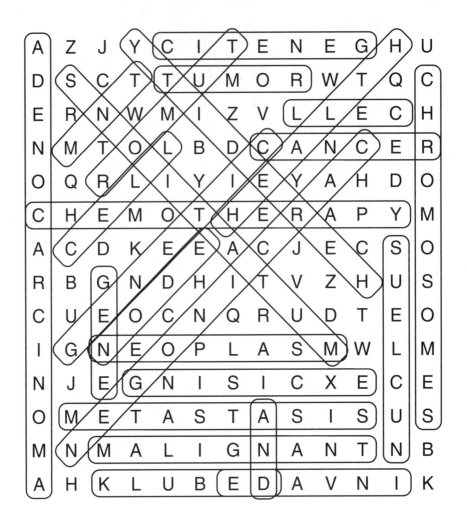

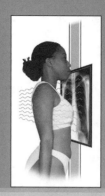

CHAPTER **19**

Radiology and Nuclear Medicine

Instructor Activity for the Beginning of Class

The first radiologists lacked protective clothing and often placed their own hand into the x-ray machine to make sure it was working properly. This led to radiation dermatitis and radiation-induced cancer. Susan Turley, the author, often heard family stories about her grandfather, who was a physician. Later in his career, he became a radiologist. During the Great Depression of 1930, the hospital where he had worked for many years laid him off and he went back to private practice. Years later he had to give up his practice because of fatigue and blood cell abnormalities, possibly due to the late effects of radiation poisoning.

Although there were relatively few women physicians in the early 1900s, a number of them entered the field of radiology when it first opened up as a medical specialty. One female physician, Alberta Lucille Hart, graduated at the top of her class from the University of Oregon Medical School. As she began to practice medicine, she encountered a great deal of discrimination, and so she changed her name to Alan Hart, became a radiologist, and wrote a popular book on radiology. She dressed in suits and smoked a pipe.

Source: Penn State University College of Medicine.

Scan this chapter until you see the whole *picture* of medical language used in radiology.

Objective 1
Describe five radiologic procedures that use x-rays

- Text page(s) 992–996

Teaching Strategy

Explain the importance of learning the radiologic procedures that use x-rays.

Content Abstract

Radiology is the medical specialty that studies anatomy and physiology, energy (x-rays, a magnetic field, sound waves), and radiation and uses technology to create images of the internal structures of the body. Nuclear medicine is the medical specialty that uses radioactive substances to create images of internal structures of the body.

 The five radiologic procedures that use x-rays are:

1. roentgenography
2. fluoroscopy
3. mammography
4. bone density tests
5. computerized axial tomography

Box 19-1: Instructor Activity

VIEW A RADIOGRAPH

If you have had an x-ray recently, you can obtain a copy of the actual film from the facility where it was taken. Just go to the facility and request the x-ray film. You will be asked to sign it out and take responsibility for bringing it back to the facility. Patients are often asked to go the radiology facility and obtain their x-ray and carry it themselves when they are referred to the office of a specialist. Obtain radiographs (x-rays) and use them as visual aids during class.

Box 19-2: Instructor Activity

X-RAYS

Share this information with students.

1. In 1913, the x-ray tube was invented by a researcher at General Electric.
2. In 1971, computerized axial tomography (CAT) was introduced.
3. Fetuses are more susceptible than adults to the damaging effects of x-rays, partly because their cells are rapidly dividing and growing into specialized cells and tissues.
4. Routine x-ray procedures represent about 70 percent of all diagnostic radiologic procedures performed each year. Traditionally, the x-ray image is captured on an x-ray film that is developed using liquid photographic chemicals. A newer technique, computed radiography (CR), uses an imaging plate that is scanned by a laser, and the image is converted to an electrical signal. The digital signal is sent to a computer where it can be stored or printed on laser film. This is known as dry imaging. Of note: Standard x-ray films contain a small amount of silver. When a film is to be destroyed, it must be sent to a silver reclaiming company that subjects the film to a solution that collects the silver content of the film.

Experience Multimedia

See the PowerPoint presentation on the accompanying Instructor's Media Library for videos on the following topics covered in this chapter:

- MRIs
- Ultrasounds
- Brain scans

Objective 2
Describe common roentgen views and patient positions

- Text page(s) 995

Teaching Strategy

Explain the importance of learning the common roentgen views and patient positions.

Content Abstract

During roentgenography, the patient is placed between the x-ray beam and an x-ray plate. The x-rays from the x-ray machine travel through the patient's body to the x-ray plate. The image is in various shades of black, white, and gray that correspond to the density of various tissues.

Some of the common roentgen views and patient positions are:

Exam	View (Projection)	Patient Position
PA chest x-ray	Posteroanterior	Standing or sitting
AP chest x-ray	Anteroposterior	Standing or sitting
Lateral chest x-ray	Lateral	Standing or sitting
Oblique x-ray	Oblique (midway between anterior and lateral)	Standing, sitting, or lying
Cross-table lateral x-ray	Lateral	Lying
Lateral decubitus x-ray	Lateral	Lying on the side
Flat plate of the abdomen	Anteroposterior	Lying
KUB (kidneys, ureters, bladder)	Anteroposterior	Lying

Objective 3
Identify common radiologic procedures that use iodinated contrast dye

- Text page(s) 997-1000

Teaching Strategies

1. Explain the importance of learning the common radiologic procedures that use iodinated contrast dye.
2. Obtain copies of radiologic films that use contrast dye to be used as visual aids for students.

Content Abstract

Contrast medium (barium) or iodinated contrast dyes can be used to enhance the details and outline anatomical structures on roentgenographic images and fluoroscopic images. Some of the procedures that use contrast medium or iodinated contrast dye include:

1. angiography
2. arthrography
3. barium enema
4. intravenous cholangiography
5. oral cholecystography

6. hysterosalpingography
7. lymphangiography
8. myelography
9. pyelography
10. upper gastrointestinal series

Box 19-3: Instructor Activity

INTERESTING INFORMATION

Share this information with students.

1. Barium sulfate is a chalky chemical that shows up as white on x-ray film. It is not an iodinated contrast dye.
2. Contrast medium or contrast dye is a substance that is used to make specific organs, blood vessels, or types of tissue (such as tumors) more visible during an x-ray, CT scan, ultrasound, or MRI.

Objective 4
Describe the radiologic procedure that uses a magnetic field

- Text page(s) 1003-1004

Teaching Strategies

1. Explain the importance of learning the radiologic procedure that uses a magnetic field and radiowaves.
2. Obtain copies of MRIs (magnetic resonance imaging) to be used as visual aids for students.

Content Abstract

Magnetic resonance imaging (MRI) uses a strong magnetic field inside a scanner to align protons in the atoms of the patient's body. Then high-frequency radiowaves are sent through the patient's body. The protons absorb the radiowaves and then emit signals. The signals, which vary according to the type of tissue, are used to construct an image. An MRI scan does not use x-rays so the patient is not exposed to any radiation.

Box 19-4: Instructor Activity

MAGNETIC RESONANCE IMAGING

Share this information with students.

1. After seven years of technical research, the first MRI machine performed on a human occurred on July 3, 1977. It took almost five hours to produce one image.
   Source: www.howstuffworks.com/mri.htm

2. Metal objects can become projectiles if they are taken into an MRI suite. Paper clips, pens, keys, and any other small metal objects can be pulled out of pockets without warning, at which point they fly toward the opening of the magnet (where the patient is placed) at very high speeds, posing a threat to everyone in the room.

3. Credit cards, bank cards, and anything else with magnetic encoding will be erased by most MRI systems.

Objective 5
Describe the radiologic procedure that uses an electron beam

- Text page(s) 1004

Teaching Strategy

Explain the importance of learning the radiologic procedure that uses an electronic beam.

Objective 6
Describe the radiologic procedures that use sound waves

- Text page(s) 1005-1006

Teaching Strategy

Explain the importance of learning the radiologic procedures that use sound waves.

Content Abstract

Ultrasonography or sonography uses pulses of inaudible, ultra high-frequency sound waves to create images of the internal structures of the body. A hand-held ultrasound transducer that emits sound waves is held against the skin over the organ or structure to be imaged. A conducting gel on the skin optimizes transmission of the sound waves. The transducer is moved back and forth to view the organ or structure from different angles.

Procedures that use sound wave technology include echocardiography and Doppler ultrasonography.

Box 19-5: Instructor Activity

ULTRASOUND

Print out the image below and pass it around the class. Tell students that this is what a state-of-the-art sonogram looked like in 1982. Ask students to see if they can identify the head, flexed arm, and abdomen of the fetus. Locate someone who has recently been pregnant and has had a now state-of-the-art three-dimensional ultrasonography done. Borrow the picture of that test or refer students to Figure 13-27 on page 719 to see the difference.

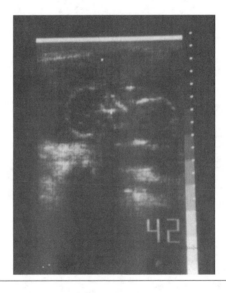

Objective 7
Describe five nuclear medicine procedures that use gamma rays or positrons

- Text page(s) 1007-1011

Teaching Strategy

Explain the importance of learning the nuclear medicine procedures that use gamma rays or positrons.

Content Abstract

Radiopharmaceuticals are manmade or naturally occurring radioactive substances (radionuclides) that have been processed and measured so that they can be given as a drug dose. They are administered intravenously, except for radioactive gases, which are administered by inhalation. Radiopharmaceuticals are also called tracers because their presence in areas of benign or cancerous tumors and areas of the body can be traced by the gamma rays they produce. The radiopharmaceuticals used in nuclear medicine imaging have short half-lives of a few hours to a few days, which means that the patient is only exposed to minimal amounts of radiation.

Nuclear medicine radiopharmaceuticals that emit gamma rays include

1. gallium-67
2. indium-111
3. iodine-123, iodine-131
4. krypton-81m
5. technetium-99m
6. thallium-201
7. xenon-133

A positron is a positively charged particle that has the same mass as an electron, but the opposite charge. Radioactive substances that emit positrons are used in positron emission tomography (PET). Like a CT scan or an MRI scan, a PET scan is a tomography that produces individual images of the body in "slices." However, it is different in that a PET scan produces images of the metabolism and physiology of an organ. PET scans are of particular value in identifying areas of cancer and areas of ischemia in the heart.

Box 19-6: Instructor Activity

PET SCAN

Share this information with students.

The first PET (positron emission tomography) scanner was introduced in 1975 and was mainly used for research.

Objective 8
Build radiology and nuclear medicine words from combining forms, prefixes, and suffixes

- Text page(s) 1017-1018

Objective 9

Describe common radiologic and nuclear medicine drug categories

- Text page(s) 1019

Teaching Strategy

Explain the various uses of barium, iodinated contrast dye, and other radiopharmaceutical drugs.

Content Abstract

Drug Category	Description	Example
Barium	An insoluble metallic element found in the earth	Baro-cat, Barosperse, Tomocat
Iodinated contrast dye	Contrast dye that contains iodine	Gastrografin, Hypaque, Isovue, Omnipaque
Other drugs	Radioactive substances that emit gamma rays	gallium-67, iodine-123, krypton-81m

Objective 10
Define common radiology and nuclear medicine abbreviations

- Text page(s) 1020

Teaching Strategies

1. Stress the importance of learning abbreviations and their full meanings.
2. Encourage students to make flashcards for abbreviations and their meanings as well as their usual flashcards for word parts and their meanings.

Content Abstract

AP	anteroposterior
Ba	barium
BE	barium enema
CAT	computerized axial tomography
CT	computerized tomography
CXR	chest x-ray
DEXA, DXA	dual energy x-ray absorptiometry
DSA	digital subtraction angiography
EBT	electron beam tomography
IVC	intravenous cholangiography
IVP	intravenous pyelography
KUB	kidneys, ureters, bladder
Lat	lateral
MRA	magnetic resonance angiography
MRI	magnetic resonance imaging

MUGA	multiple-gated acquisition (scan)
PA	posteroanterior
PET	positron emission tomography
QCT	quantitative computerized tomography
R, r	roentgen (unit of exposure to x-rays or gamma rays)
rad	radiation absorbed dose
RAIU	radioactive iodine uptake
rem	roentgen-equivalent man
RNV	radionuclide ventriculography
RRT	registered radiologic technologist
SPECT	single-photon emission computed tomography
TEE	transesophageal echocardiography
UGI	upper gastrointestinal (GI) series
US	ultrasound
V/Q	ventilation-perfusion scan

Objective 11
Correctly spell and pronounce radiology and nuclear medicine words

- Text page(s) 1029

Teaching Strategies

1. Impress upon the students that medical words that are mispronounced are also probably going to be misspelled.
2. Encourage students to work on both pronunciation and spelling when studying.

Chapter Spelling Test

The chapter spelling test is included with the weekly chapter test. Dictate and spell (or xerox a handout that contains) this list of 15 spelling words. Give the list to students the week before the test. For the chapter test, select just 10 of these words to test.

1. arteriography
2. anteroposterior
3. coronary angiography
4. decubitus position
5. echocardiogram
6. fluoroscopy
7. hysterosalpingogram
8. intravenous pyelography
9. lymphangiography
10. mammography
11. positron emission tomography
12. radionuclide
13. technetium
14. thallium
15. ultrasonography

Box 19-7: Classroom Activity

GAMES

1. From week to week, pick a different one of these spelling games to use during class. (The descriptions and instructions for the games are in the section "The Art and Craft of Teaching.")

   Beanbag Spelling Toss
   Scrabble
   Spelling Bee
   Gridlock
   Hangman

2. From week to week, pick a different one of these pronunciation games to use during class. (The descriptions and instructions for the games are in the section "The Art and Craft of Teaching.")

   Parroting
   Hieroglyphics
   Beach Ball Blast

Chapter Pronunciation Test

Have students mark these 15 words listed in the Pronunciation Checklist for the chapter. During the week, they will call your office or home answering machine and pronounce each word.

1. arteriography
2. anteroposterior
3. coronary angiography
4. decubitus position
5. echocardiogram
6. fluoroscopy
7. hysterosalpingogram
8. intravenous pyelography
9. lymphangiography
10. mammography
11. positron emission tomography
12. radionuclide
13. technetium
14. thallium
15. ultrasonography

Objective 12
Apply your skills by analyzing a radiology report

- Text page(s) 1026-1028

Content Abstract

Read the three Radiology Reports and answer the questions provided.

Box 19-8: Classroom Activity

MEDICAL REPORT

In the reports, circle all the medical words. Then list them and write their definitions. Rewrite the medical words in English as if you were explaining them to the patient.

Objective 13
Test your knowledge of radiology and nuclear medicine by completing review exercises in the textbook and the CD-ROM learning activities

- Text page(s) 1021-1025

Teaching Strategies

1. Assign the Chapter Review exercises in the textbook for homework. Remind students to refer to the Answer Key at the end of the textbook to check their answers.

2. Have the students complete the learning activities provided on the interactive CD-ROM.

Experience Multimedia

See the PowerPoint presentation on the accompanying Instructor's Media Library for videos on the topic of a career as a radiologic technologist.

Homework Activities

1. Investigate the Web site of Penn State University College of Medicine. It describes the first women physicians who entered the field of radiology when it first began as a medical specialty. See www.xray.hmc.psu.edu/rci/ss7/ss7_3.html.

2. Visit a local ambulatory radiology center. Interview a radiology (x-ray) technician. Prepare a list of questions to be used during the interview. Ask about working conditions and patient contact. Write a one-page summary of this.

3. If you are pregnant, obtain a copy of your prenatal ultrasound. Write a one-page summary describing the experience of having an ultrasound. If you have a close friend who is pregnant, ask permission to go with her when she has a prenatal ultrasound done.

4. The American Cancer Society has an on-line mammogram reminder. This interactive tool sends an e-mail message each year as a reminder to schedule your mammogram. To register yourself or someone you love, go to http://www.cancer.org/docroot/PED/content/PED_2_3x_Mammogram_Reminder.asp.

Word Search

Complete this word search puzzle that contains Chapter 19 words. Look for the following words as given in the list below. The number in parentheses indicates how many times the word appears in the puzzle.

apron
artifact
barium
DEXA
Doppler
dose
echo
fluoroscopy
KUB
MUGA
nuclear

PET scan
projection
rad (2)
radiation
scan
spiral
tomography
tracer
ultrasound
x-ray

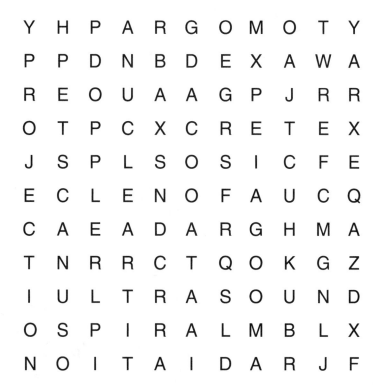

```
Y  H  P  A  R  G  O  M  O  T  Y
P  P  D  N  B  D  E  X  A  W  A
R  E  O  U  A  A  G  P  J  R  R
O  T  P  C  X  C  R  E  T  E  X
J  S  P  L  S  O  S  I  C  F  E
E  C  L  E  N  O  F  A  U  C  Q
C  A  E  A  D  A  R  G  H  M  A
T  N  R  R  C  T  Q  O  K  G  Z
I  U  L  T  R  A  S  O  U  N  D
O  S  P  I  R  A  L  M  B  L  X
N  O  I  T  A  I  D  A  R  J  F
```

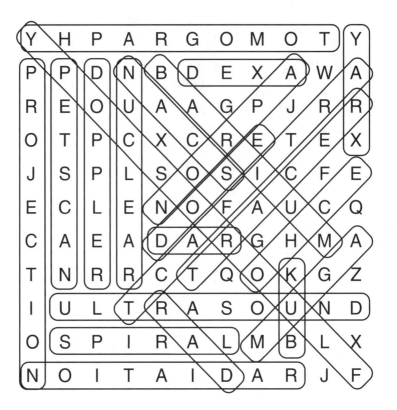

Test Bank

CHAPTER 1

Multiple Choice

Choose the one alternative that best completes the statement or answers the question.

1. Select the abbreviation that would NOT appear in a history and physical examination.
   a. ROS
   b. CC
   c. CPR
   d. HPI

2. Anesthesia is defined as:
   a. a state of unawareness.
   b. pertaining to the lack of breathing.
   c. condition of not feeling.
   d. without pain.

3. Bradycardia is defined as a:
   a. fast heart rate.
   b. reversal of abnormal heart rate.
   c. process of recording the heart rate.
   d. condition of a slow heart rate.

4. Which is the suffix for the process of using an instrument to examine a body part?
   a. -scopy
   b. -gram
   c. -oma
   d. -graphy

5. Which is true of a combining form?
   a. A medical word can have only one combining form.
   b. The combining form consists of a root and a prefix.
   c. The combining form shows a suffix attached to a root.
   d. A combining form has a hyphen after the last letter to show that it is only a part of a medical word.

6. The prefix that means after or behind is:
   a. poly-.
   b. post-.
   c. pre-.
   d. peri-.

7. Which word means inflammation of the lungs?
   a. neuritis
   b. retinitis
   c. pneumonitis
   d. mastitis

8. Vertebrae means:
   a. one bone of the spine.
   b. more than one bone of the spine.
   c. pertaining to the spine.
   d. in the direction toward the spine.

9. Which is the plural form of apex?
   a. apexs
   b. apices
   c. apis
   d. apae

10. For the word intrahepatic, the prefix intra- means _____ the liver.
    a. between
    b. below
    c. beside
    d. within

11. The physician performed a laryngectomy on the:
    a. skin.
    b. lungs.
    c. voicebox.
    d. nose.

12. Which of the following is true about a prefix?
    a. A medical word can have more than one prefix.
    b. Every medical word has a prefix.
    c. A prefix can mean a surgical procedure.
    d. There are several variations of the prefix that means pertaining to.

13. Peritonsillar means pertaining to _____ the tonsils.
    a. within
    b. below
    c. around
    d. in front of
14. Dysuria would be defined as pertaining to _____ urination.
    a. absence of
    b. excessive
    c. slow
    d. difficult
15. The plural of the word meaning the air tube leading to the lungs is:
    a. bronchi.
    b. bronchae.
    c. bronchus.
    d. broncha.
16. Which is true of a suffix in medical terminology?
    a. A suffix is never a single letter.
    b. Two suffixes may appear in a single medical word.
    c. A suffix by itself is sometimes used as a medical word.
    d. A suffix can begin a medical word.
17. A gastroscopy is the process of:
    a. examining the stomach with an instrument.
    b. recording the activity of the stomach.
    c. creating an image of the stomach using x-ray.
    d. removing a part of the stomach.
18. Tachycardia means:
    a. behind the heart.
    b. painful heart.
    c. within the heart.
    d. fast heart rate.
19. HIPAA assures the patient that his medical information is:
    a. legible.
    b. accurate.
    c. documented in a prescribed format.
    d. secure.
20. The word part sub- is a:
    a. root.
    b. suffix.
    c. prefix.
    d. combining form.
21. A commonly used abbreviation for the word diagnosis is:
    a. DS.
    b. DG.
    c. Dx.
    d. Dd.
22. Which suffix indicates a surgical procedure?
    a. -ist
    b. -osis
    c. -pathy
    d. -ectomy
23. Five separate language skills are critical to communication. Which skill involves the processing of medical language?
    a. thinking and analyzing
    b. reading
    c. listening
    d. speaking
24. Which of the following is the skill that involves relaying the medical language?
    a. thinking and analyzing
    b. reading
    c. speaking
    d. listening
25. The study of word origins and derivations is:
    a. etymology.
    b. medicology.
    c. eponymology.
    d. greekology.
26. Which is an optional word beginning?
    a. prefix
    b. combining vowel
    c. suffix
    d. combining form
27. Which is the foundation of a medical word?
    a. prefix
    b. combining vowel
    c. suffix
    d. combining form
28. The combining form arthr/o- means:
    a. bone.
    b. straight.
    c. joint.
    d. mouth.
29. The combining form mast/o- means:
    a. nose.
    b. retina.
    c. face.
    d. breast.
30. The combining form hepat/o- means:
    a. blood.
    b. liver.
    c. kidney.
    d. urine.
31. The suffix -al means:
    a. process.
    b. condition.
    c. pertaining to.
    d. state of.

32. The suffix -oma means:
    a. tumor, mass.
    b. enlargement.
    c. cancer.
    d. disease.
33. Which is the plural form for the word vertebra?
    a. vertebrices
    b. vertebrax
    c. vertebraes
    d. vertebrae
34. Which is the plural form for the word testis?
    a. testes
    b. testium
    c. testises
    d. testices
35. The abbreviation CPR means:
    a. computerized patient record.
    b. computerized patient report.
    c. computerized paper record.
    d. central paper repository.
36. Treatment of a person without consent is against the law and is considered to be:
    a. assault.
    b. molestation.
    c. battery.
    d. arson.
37. The abbreviation HIPAA means:
    a. Health Improvement for Pediatric and Adults Act.
    b. Healthcare Improvement for Performance, Accountability, and Assessment.
    c. Health Insurance Portability and Accountability Act.
    d. Health Insurance Performance and Accuracy Act.
38. A physician's office note may follow the SOAP format. SOAP stands for:
    a. subjective, objective, assessment, plan.
    b. symptoms, observations, assessment, performance.
    c. symptoms/signs, opinion, assessment, plan.
    d. subjective, objective, assessment, performance.
39. The abbreviation CC means:
    a. clinical copy.
    b. central complaint.
    c. chief complaint.
    d. computerized copy.
40. If a physician documented: "Lungs revealed no rales. Heart negative. Skin: no masses found," it would be found under the _____ section in a SOAP format.
    a. subjective
    b. objective

c. assessment
d. plan
41. If a physician documented: "Patient was given a prescription for Loritab. Have patient make an appointment to see me again in 2 weeks," it would be found under the _____ section in a SOAP format.
    a. subjective
    b. objective
    c. assessment
    d. plan
42. The plural form for the word phalanx is:
    a. phalanxs.
    b. phalanices.
    c. phalanges.
    d. phalanx.
43. The combining form ven/o- means:
    a. vein.
    b. artery.
    c. blood vessel.
    d. leg.
44. A medical word contains two combining forms in a row followed by a suffix. The second combining form begins with a vowel, and the suffix begins with a vowel. This word was formed by:
    a. dropping the combining vowel on the first combining form.
    b. keeping the combining vowel on the first combining form.
    c. keeping the combining vowel on the second combining form.
    d. keeping the combining vowel on the first and second combining forms.
45. The suffix -graphy means:
    a. process of recording.
    b. a record.
    c. x-ray.
    d. instrument.
46. The suffix -pathy means:
    a. disease.
    b. suffering.
    c. lab.
    d. disease, suffering.
47. Every medical word contains a:
    a. prefix.
    b. suffix.
    c. combining form.
    d. both b and c
48. The combining form pneumon/o- means:
    a. heart.
    b. lung.
    c. stomach.
    d. blood.

49. The suffix -ar means:
    a. condition, state, thing.
    b. a process; being or having.
    c. inflammation of.
    d. pertaining to.

50. The suffix -megaly means enlargement. Which word means enlargement of the liver?
    a. hepatomegaly
    b. cardiomegaly
    c. retinomegaly
    d. neuroma

51. The word endotracheal means within the:
    a. stomach.
    b. trachea.
    c. vein.
    d. vessel.

52. The prefix brady- means:
    a. fast.
    b. normal.
    c. average.
    d. slow.

53. The prefix dys- means:
    a. bad.
    b. good.
    c. painful, difficult, or abnormal.
    d. new.

54. What is the difference between the prefixes hyper- and hypo-?
    a. Hyper- means good and hypo- means excellent.
    b. Hyper- means bad and hypo- means very bad or critical.
    c. Hyper- means large and hypo- means small.
    d. Hyper- means more than normal and hypo- means below or deficient.

55. Which basic rule is CORRECT for building medical words?
    a. Join the prefix to the beginning of the combining form.
    b. Join the prefix to the end of the combining form.
    c. Join the suffix to the beginning of the combining form.
    d. Always add a hyphen along with the prefix.

56. What is the correct pronunciation of intra-nasal?
    a. IN-trah-NAY-zal
    b. in-TRAH-nay-zal
    c. IN-oh-nay-ZAL
    d. in-trah-NAY-aal

57. The origin of medical language is in:
    a. Latin.
    b. Greek.

    c. Latin and Greek.
    d. many languages, including Latin and Greek.

58. Which of the following are NOT characteristics of combining forms?
    a. Every medical word contains a combining form.
    b. Every combining form occurs at the end of a medical word.
    c. Prefixes and suffixes modify the meaning of the combining form.
    d. A medical word may contain more than one combining form.

59. The medical word part which gives a medical word its meaning is the:
    a. prefix.
    b. suffix.
    c. hyphen.
    d. combining form.

60. The combining form in the word appendicitis is:
    a. appendic/o-.
    b. -itis.
    c. appen-.
    d. -citis.

61. The combining form of the word pneumonia means:
    a. pneumon/o-.
    b. lung or air.
    c. condition or state of.
    d. infection.

62. Knowledge of medical language includes:
    a. spelling medical words.
    b. analyzing medical words.
    c. pronouncing medical words.
    d. all of the above.

63. The parts of a combining form include the:
    a. root and a suffix.
    b. prefix and a hyphen.
    c. root and the combining vowel.
    d. suffix and a combining vowel.

64. Which of the following is an example of a combining form?
    a. intra-
    b. -ectomy
    c. ven/o-
    d. poly-

65. Which of the following is an example of a suffix?
    a. -ia
    b. post-
    c. dys-
    d. nas/o-

66. Suffixes such as -iatry, -itian, and -logy describe:
    a. medical specialties or specialists.
    b. procedures or instruments.
    c. diseases.
    d. colors.
67. The parts of a medical word can include:
    a. combining forms.
    b. suffixes.
    c. prefixes.
    d. all of the above
68. Prefixes such as hypo- and poly- indicate:
    a. time or speed.
    b. a characteristic.
    c. amount or size.
    d. weight.
69. The prefixes anti- and dys- belong to a category that describes:
    a. a characteristic.
    b. amount or size.
    c. time or speed.
    d. all of the above.
70. In the medical word alcoholism, the suffix -ism means:
    a. condition, state, thing.
    b. pertaining to.
    c. disease from a specific cause.
    d. medical treatment.
71. Which suffix means process of recording?
    a. -pathy
    b. -graphy
    c. -ation
    d. -iatry
72. Medical words must be defined by analyzing them, beginning with the:
    a. prefix.
    b. combining form.
    c. suffix.
    d. Latin gender.
73. Medical words are derived from ancient languages such as:
    a. Greek and Latin.
    b. English.
    c. French and Dutch.
    d. all of the above
74. Form the plural of a Latin feminine noun by:
    a. changing -us to -i.
    b. adding an s.
    c. changing -a to -ae.
    d. changing -um to -a.
75. Which word is an example of a Latin masculine singular noun?
    a. bacterium
    b. phalanx

    c. carcinoma
    d. nucleus
76. Form the plural of a Latin neuter noun by changing -um to:
    a. -a.
    b. -ae.
    c. -oma.
    d. none of the above
77. Which word is an example of a Greek singular noun?
    a. ganglion
    b. atrium
    c. bronchi
    d. testis
78. The medical word diverticulum is a Latin neuter noun. You would make the plural form by changing the word ending -um to:
    a. -a.
    b. -ices.
    c. -us.
    d. -ae.
79. Which of the following is a disadvantage of the paper medical record?
    a. Only one person at a time can access information in it.
    b. It can become lost.
    c. It can take time to retrieve if it is stored in an off-site location.
    d. all of the above
80. Which abbreviation stands for the federal regulation that says that health information must be kept secure?
    a. CPR
    b. HIPAA
    c. SOAP
    d. HPI
81. The S in SOAP note format stands for:
    a. surgery.
    b. scope.
    c. severity.
    d. subjective.

Short Answer

Write the word or phrase that best completes each statement or answers the question.

82. Dermatology is the _____ of the skin.
83. The suffix -al means _____ _____.
84. Polyuria means a condition of _____ urine.
85. In the word intravenous, the prefix intra- means _____.
86. Cardiomegaly means _____ of the heart.
87. Myopathy is a _____ of a muscle.
88. Carcinoma is a cancerous _____.

89. The prefix that means slow is _____.

90. The plural of diagnosis is _____.

91. _____ is the study of word origins and derivations.

92. The _____ _____ of a medical word is the foundation of the word.

93. _____ is a combining form meaning lung or air.

94. _____ is a combining form meaning heart.

95. _____ is a combining form referring to a part of the eye.

96. A _____ appears at the end of a word and modifies the meaning of the combining form.

97. _____ is a suffix meaning the process of recording.

98. A _____ is a medical word part, which modifies the meaning of the combining form and always appears at the beginning of the word.

99. The prefix in the word bradycardia means _____.

100. A _____ attaches to the beginning of a combining form and modifies its meaning.

101. _____ is the study of word origins and derivations.

102. The _____ _____ is where healthcare professionals document all care provided to a patient.

103. When the patient signs a consent form for surgery, it is known as giving _____ _____.

104. Patient charting may be done in the SOAP format. What do these letters stand for?
   S _____
   O _____
   A _____
   P _____

105. The abbreviation CC stands for _____ _____.

106. The abbreviation HIPAA stands for
   _____ _____ _____
   _____ _____ _____.

107. The study of the heart is known as _____.

108. A _____ _____ contains two parts: a root and a combining vowel.

109. A _____ is always positioned at the end of a medical word.

110. The abbreviation Dx stands for _____.

111. The abbreviation PE stands for _____ _____.

112. The prefix _____ means after or behind.

113. The combining form _____ means stomach.

114. The combining form _____ means mind.

True/False

Write 'T' if the statement is true and 'F' if the statement is false.

_____115. Medical words are derived from several languages, including Latin and Greek.

_____116. There are only three word parts: combining forms, suffixes, and prefixes. These word parts always mean the same thing, no matter where they appear.

_____117. Not every medical word contains a combining form.

_____118. Prefixes and suffixes modify the meaning of a medical term.

_____119. Medical words may only contain one combining form.

_____120. Every medical word contains a suffix.

_____121. Every medical word contains a prefix.

_____122. A prefix can be as small as a single letter.

_____123. In order to define a medical word, you must first define the suffix, followed by the prefix, and finally, the combining form.

_____124. The patient's health record is considered a legal document.

_____125. The atria are the lower chambers of the heart.

_____126. The suffixes -ac, -ar, and -al, mean pertaining to.

_____127. In the SOAP format of documentation, the physician combines subjective (S) information gathered from the patient with objective (O) information from an exam to arrive at the assessment (A) and a plan (P) for treatment.

_____128. All medical and anatomical words have their origin in the Greek and Latin languages.

_____129. The term arthrosis means pertaining to a joint.

_____130. The suffix -scopy means the process of recording.

_____131. A neuroma is a tumor of a nerve.

_____132. The condition hypothyroidism refers to a disease caused by above-normal functioning of the thyroid gland.

_____133. The consent to treatment is a document signed by the patient that allows a physician to perform a surgical operation on the patient.

_____134. Volunteering to help in a medical setting is a good substitute for actually studying medical language.

_____135. Medical language is the key to a successful career in the healthcare field.

_____136. Healthcare professionals use medical language every day to communicate with patients, but not with other healthcare professionals.

_____137. The combining vowel gives meaning to the medical word.

_____138. The medical record is more accurately known as the health record.

_____139. A medical word always has a prefix, combining form, and a suffix.

Essay

Write your answer in the space provided or on a separate sheet of paper.

140. Describe the process of analysis that is used to define a medical word.

141. Why are so many medical words derived from Latin or Greek?

142. List the five separate language skills that are critical to communicate in medical language.

143. Briefly explain the origins of medical words.

144. List three characteristics of a combining form.

145. List three characteristics of a prefix.

146. List three characteristics of a suffix.

CHAPTER 2

Multiple Choice

Choose the one alternative that best completes the statement or answers the question.

1. The plane that divides the body into top and bottom sections is the _____ plane.
   a. frontal
   b. transverse
   c. coronal
   d. midsagittal

2. A patient with a cancerous tumor may seek treatment for his condition from a physician whose specialty is called:
   a. geriatrics.
   b. neonatology.
   c. radiology.
   d. oncology.

3. The integumentary system includes diseases of the:
   a. bones, cartilage, joints.
   b. ovaries, tubes, uterus.
   c. skin, nails, oil glands.
   d. gallbladder, liver, stomach.

4. The predicted outcome of a disease is the:
   a. prognosis.
   b. diagnosis.
   c. etiology.
   d. exacerbation.

5. The front of the body is known as the anterior or _____ section.
   a. dorsal
   b. supine

   c. prone
   d. ventral

6. The word lateral pertains to the _____ of a structure.
   a. front
   b. side
   c. back
   d. head or top

7. The part of anatomy that divides the thoracic cavity from the abdominal cavity is the
   a. mediastinum
   b. umbilicus
   c. viscera
   d. diaphragm

8. The region of the abdominopelvic area that is centered and inferior to the umbilical region is the _____ region.
   a. hypochondriac
   b. hypogastric
   c. inguinal
   d. epigastric

9. Lying on the posterior part of the body is known as:
   a. caudal.
   b. distal.
   c. supine.
   d. prone.

10. If medical science describes a disease (such as Alzheimer's disease) as etiology unknown, the disease is said to be:
    a. nosocomial.
    b. idiopathic.
    c. degenerative.
    d. iatrogenic.

11. If an infant is born with cerebral palsy from a decrease of oxygen to his brain in the uterus or during delivery, his disease is categorized as:
    a. hereditary.
    b. degenerative.
    c. congenital.
    d. environmental.

12. A stethoscope would perform a part of the physical examination known as:
    a. palpation.
    b. viewing.
    c. inspection.
    d. auscultation.

13. Which is an example of a physician extender?
    a. licensed practical nurse
    b. physical therapist
    c. nurse practitioner
    d. pharmacist

14. An example of a symptom would be:
    a. pain in the joints.
    b. an irregular heart beat.
    c. coughing up blood.
    d. a fever of 102 degrees.
15. Moving in a direction toward the lower part of the body, tail, or feet is known as:
    a. cephalad.
    b. coronal.
    c. caudad.
    d. cranial.
16. The directional opposite of distal is:
    a. superficial.
    b. deep.
    c. superior.
    d. proximal.
17. Otorhinolaryngology is a branch of medicine specializing in conditions of the:
    a. spinal cord, nerves, spinal fluid.
    b. ureters, urethra, bladder.
    c. testes, epididymus, penis.
    d. ears, nose, throat.
18. Palliative care would be a major goal of care in a/an:
    a. ambulatory surgery center.
    b. hospice.
    c. emergency department.
    d. clinic.
19. An example of viscera would be:
    a. bone.
    b. skin.
    c. intestines.
    d. teeth.
20. The patient had a mass in the inguinal area. In which part of the abdominopelvic region would this mass be found?
    a. in the groin
    b. at the navel
    c. directly above the stomach
    d. beneath the ribs
21. A temporary improvement in the symptoms and signs of a disease without a cure is:
    a. exacerbation.
    b. remission.
    c. relapse.
    d. sequela.
22. Which doctor's practice is limited to treating disorders of the feet?
    a. D.P.M.
    b. D.O.
    c. D.D.S.
    d. D.C.

23. The suffixes -ic and -al mean:
    a. study of.
    b. knowledge of.
    c. pertaining to.
    d. toward.
24. Which is a body cavity?
    a. thoracic
    b. umbilical
    c. epigastric
    d. iliac
25. The patient has had joint pain and skin lesions for the past three years without increasing in severity. Since these conditions are due to her lupus erythematosus, her disease course would be termed:
    a. chronic.
    b. acute.
    c. exacerbated.
    d. in remission.
26. All of the following are body planes, EXCEPT:
    a. coronal.
    b. supine.
    c. midsagittal.
    d. transverse.
27. Which body plane divides the body into right and left sections?
    a. coronal
    b. supine
    c. midsagittal
    d. transverse
28. Which body plane is also called the frontal plane?
    a. coronal
    b. supine
    c. midsagittal
    d. transverse
29. Which is the only horizontal plane that divides the body?
    a. coronal
    b. supine
    c. midsagittal
    d. transverse
30. Moving toward the head is known as the _____ direction.
    a. cephalad
    b. plantar
    c. caudad
    d. hyperextension
31. Moving from the body toward the end of a limb is moving in a _____ direction.
    a. inferior
    b. proximal
    c. distal
    d. superior

32. Which body cavity is a continuation of the cranial cavity as it travels down the midline of the back?
    a. spinal
    b. abdominal
    c. thoracic
    d. pelvic

33. The central area in the thoracic cavity located between the lungs is the:
    a. pleura.
    b. diaphragm.
    c. mediastinum.
    d. viscera.

34. The human body can be divided into _____ abdominopelvic quadrants and _____ abdominopelvic regions.
    a. four; nine
    b. ten; six
    c. nine; four
    d. six; ten

35. Which body system contains the nose, throat, larynx, trachea, bronchi, lungs, and alveoli?
    a. cardiovascular
    b. respiratory
    c. gastrointestinal
    d. hematology

36. The function of this body system is the distribution of blood throughout the body.
    a. cardiovascular
    b. respiratory
    c. gastrointestinal
    d. hematology

37. Which medical specialty involves the study of newborn infants?
    a. pediatrics
    b. geriatrics
    c. neonatology
    d. embryology

38. Which abdominopelvic region is located below the navel?
    a. hypochondriac region
    b. epigastric region
    c. hypogastric region
    d. lumbar region

39. Which medical specialty deals with the female reproductive system?
    a. hematology
    b. urology
    c. gynecology
    d. oncology

40. Which word describes a disease or condition caused by medicine or treatment given to a patient?
    a. congenital
    b. iatrogenic

    c. hereditary
    d. environmental

41. A surgical wound infection is an example of a/an:
    a. idiopathic infection.
    b. etiologic infection.
    c. nosocomial infection.
    d. exacerbated infection.

42. When a patient is asymptomatic, this means that the patient:
    a. shows no symptoms or signs.
    b. has a hospital-acquired infection.
    c. is a hypochondriac.
    d. shows severe symptoms or signs.

43. Listening to the sounds of the heart is:
    a. palpation.
    b. palpitation.
    c. auscultation.
    d. inspection.

44. An abnormal condition or complication that arises because of the original disease and remains after the original disease has resolved is a/an:
    a. remission.
    b. sequela.
    c. exacerbation.
    d. relapse.

45. All of the following procedures are therapeutic, EXCEPT:
    a. cardiac catheterization.
    b. angioplasty.
    c. colon resection.
    d. cataract extraction.

46. A physician who is on the medical staff of a hospital and admits a patient to the hospital is a/an:
    a. consulting physician.
    b. attending physician.
    c. physician advisor.
    d. primary care physician.

47. Which indicates a disease that does not respond well to treatment?
    a. remission
    b. sequela
    c. refractory
    d. recuperation

48. The abbreviation Sx means:
    a. symptoms.
    b. treatment.
    c. prescription.
    d. surgery.

49. The abbreviation PCP means:
    a. pharmacy care provider.
    b. primary care physician.
    c. physician case provider.
    d. physical certified practitioner.
50. Which word means receiving guests and strangers?
    a. hospice
    b. nursing home
    c. respite
    d. palliative
51. Which of the following is NOT an approach for studying the body as discussed in your textbook?
    a. diseases approach
    b. anatomy and physiology approach
    c. microscopic to macroscopic approach
    d. body systems approach
52. A plane divides the body in all of the following directions EXCEPT:
    a. right and left.
    b. top and bottom.
    c. front and back.
    d. inside to outside.
53. An imaginary vertical plane that divides the entire body into front and back sections is:
    a. midsagittal plane.
    b. coronal plane.
    c. transverse plane.
    d. sagittal plane.
54. The medical specialty that studies the pharynx and esophagus is:
    a. gastroenterology.
    b. pulmonology.
    c. dentistry.
    d. otolaryngology.
55. A category of diseases where there is progressive destruction of cells due to disease or the aging process is:
    a. idiopathic.
    b. iatrogenic.
    c. degenerative.
    d. environmental.
56. Sudden worsening of the severity of a patient's signs or symptoms is known as:
    a. subacute.
    b. remission.
    c. exacerbation.
    d. sequela.
57. A disease that does NOT respond well to treatment is said to be:
    a. refractory.
    b. prognosis.

c. therapeutic.
d. in remission.
58. What is the most frequently used healthcare setting?
    a. outpatient surgery center
    b. ambulatory care center
    c. doctor's office
    d. long-term care facility
59. When a physician attempts to diagnose a patient, the first thing he or she does is:
    a. perform an H & P.
    b. complete a CRNA.
    c. refer the patient to an ENT doctor.
    d. perform PT.
60. What types of professionals support the physicians and nurses and perform specific services ordered by the physician?
    a. chiropractors
    b. allied health professionals
    c. CRNAs
    d. gynecologists
61. Which is the study of the lungs and respiratory system?
    a. cardiology
    b. pulmonology
    c. gastroenterology
    d. immunology
62. Which is the correct combining form meaning the lower back?
    a. lumb/o-
    b. cephal/o-
    c. ur/o-
    d. intern/o-
63. The area that is surrounded by the breast bone (sternum), ribs, and spinal column is called the:
    a. viscera.
    b. supine.
    c. transverse plane.
    d. thoracic cavity.
64. The medical specialty that deals with the use of drugs as medicines is:
    a. pharmacology.
    b. dermatology.
    c. dietetics.
    d. oncology.
65. The use of x-rays and other forms of radiation to diagnose and treat disease is called:
    a. oncology.
    b. eietetics.
    c. geriatrics.
    d. radiology and nuclear medicine.

66. Otolaryngology is the medical specialty that studies:
    a. eyes.
    b. ears.
    c. ears, nose, and throat.
    d. mouth.

67. Endocrinology is the medical specialty that studies:
    a. ears, nose, and throat.
    b. testes, ovaries, adrenal glands, pancreas, thymus, thyroid, parathyroid, pituitary, and pineal glands.
    c. breasts, ovaries, fallopian tubes, uterus, vagina, and external genitalia.
    d. scrotum, testes, epididymus, vas deferens, seminal vesicles, prostate gland, urethra, and penis.

68. Dermatology is the medical specialty that studies the:
    a. respiratory system.
    b. integumentary system.
    c. lymph system.
    d. immune syste.

69. The function of the gastrointestinal system is to:
    a. digest food.
    b. circulate blood.
    c. inhale and circulate gases.
    d. recognize and destroy disease-causing organisms.

70. Oncology is the study of:
    a. genetics.
    b. the feet.
    c. cancer.
    d. the eyes.

71. The coronal plane is named for a:
    a. body system.
    b. quadrant.
    c. suture.
    d. none of the above

72. The word dorsal means:
    a. anterior.
    b. front.
    c. side.
    d. back.

73. Two of the imaginary planes that divide the body derive their names from:
    a. prefixes.
    b. suture lines on the skull.
    c. anatomic position.
    d. body cavities.

74. The orientation of the coronal suture of the cranium corresponds to the orientation of the:
    a. prone position.
    b. midsagittal plane.

c. medial direction.
    d. frontal plane.

75. Which word is misspelled?
    a. proximally
    b. posterioanterior
    c. midsagittal
    d. viscera

76. Which word means towards the side or away from the midline?
    a. medial
    b. sagittal
    c. lateral
    d. transverse

77. The midsagittal plane divides the body into:
    a. top and bottom.
    b. anterior and posterior.
    c. right and left.
    d. microscopic and macroscopic.

78. The humerus is the bone of the upper arm. The proximal end of humerus is located next to the:
    a. spine.
    b. elbow.
    c. wrist.
    d. shoulder.

79. To move from the body to the end of a limb is to move:
    a. distally.
    b. proximally.
    c. caudally.
    d. superiorly.

80. The trachea, lungs, heart, and esophagus are all found in the:
    a. cranial cavity.
    b. thoracic cavity.
    c. abdominal cavity.
    d. pelvic cavity.

81. The abdominal cavity is _____ to the thoracic cavity.
    a. lateral
    b. inferior
    c. superior
    d. posterior

82. The _____ cavity is a continuation of the cranial cavity.
    a. abdominal
    b. dorsal
    c. thoracic
    d. spinal

83. Cells and cellular structures are:
    a. body systems.
    b. quadrants.
    c. microscopic.
    d. medical specialties.

84. The internal organs of all body cavities are known as:
    a. systems.
    b. pediatrics.
    c. pathogens.
    d. viscera.
85. Which structure can only be seen through a microscope?
    a. quadrant
    b. cell
    c. cavity
    d. body system
86. Cardiology involves the study, diagnosis, and treatment of diseases of the:
    a. stomach and intestines.
    b. bones, cartilage, ligaments, and joints.
    c. skin, hair, and nails.
    d. heart, arteries, veins, and capillaries.
87. The combining form pulmon/o- means:
    a. heart.
    b. lungs.
    c. blood.
    d. skin.
88. The endocrine system is composed of various organs that all:
    a. form a covering for the body.
    b. stimulate the muscles of the body.
    c. produce hormones within the body.
    d. help produce urine.
89. Ophthalmology studies the:
    a. skin.
    b. eyes.
    c. ears.
    d. female reproductive organs.
90. The study of the medical care of the elderly is known as:
    a. pediatrics.
    b. psychiatry.
    c. neonatology.
    d. geriatrics.
91. The study and treatment of cancer is known as:
    a. pharmacology.
    b. geriatrics.
    c. oncology.
    d. dietetics.
92. Oncology is the:
    a. study of tumors.
    b. treatment of the mind.
    c. knowledge of foods and diet.
    d. study of drugs.

93. Any change in the normal structure or function of the body is:
    a. physiology.
    b. hereditary.
    c. disease.
    d. anatomy.
94. The cause or origin of a disease is the:
    a. etiology.
    b. symptom.
    c. pathogen.
    d. excerbation.
95. Disease caused by an abnormality in the fetus is:
    a. degenerative.
    b. neoplastic.
    c. congenital.
    d. infectious.
96. Health is:
    a. a state of optimum wellness.
    b. physical and spiritual wellness.
    c. mental and social wellness.
    d. all of the above.
97. A patient who is asymptomatic:
    a. shows no symptoms or signs.
    b. cannot recover.
    c. has a nutritional disease.
    d. has no disease.
98. Acute is the opposite of:
    a. terminal.
    b. refractory.
    c. chronic.
    d. therapeutic.
99. Which of the following is a desirable medical outcome?
    a. remission
    b. disability
    c. exacerbation
    d. diagnosis
100. A patient cannot recover from an illness that is:
    a. therapeutic.
    b. terminal.
    c. chronic.
    d. infectious.
101. Which healthcare professional treats diseases of the bones, muscles, and nerves?
    a. chiropractor
    b. optometrist
    c. dentist
    d. podiatrist

102. The _____ is the leader of the healthcare team.
   a. physician extender
   b. therapist
   c. physician
   d. nurse

103. All of the following are physician extenders EXCEPT:
   a. audiologists.
   b. nurse midwives.
   c. nurse anesthetists.
   d. physician's assistants.

104. The suffix -ician means:
   a. medical therapy.
   b. disease.
   c. skilled professional.
   d. present at birth.

105. Nurses can do all of the following EXCEPT:
   a. make nursing diagnoses.
   b. prescribe medications.
   c. give hands-on care.
   d. administer medications.

106. The traditional setting for providing care for acutely ill patients is the:
   a. hospital.
   b. physician's office.
   c. clinic.
   d. hospice.

107. Which of the following is true of hospice care?
   a. provide care for patients with terminal illnesses
   b. provide emotional support for patients and families
   c. provide palliative care and counseling
   d. all of the above

108. The combining form ambulat/o- means:
   a. disease.
   b. servant.
   c. again and again.
   d. walking.

109. Sick people who visit a clinic are known as:
   a. inpatients.
   b. clients.
   c. residents.
   d. outpatients.

Short Answer

Write the word or phrase that best completes each statement or answers the question.

110. The abdomen can be divided by imaginary lines into four parts called _____.

111. The _____ cavity contains the brain.

112. The word _____ means pertaining to viewing very small structures with the aid of a special instrument.

113. Hypogastric means pertaining to _____ the stomach.

114. An infection that a patient acquires while in the hospital is a _____ infection.

115. The suffix in the word psychiatry means _____ _____.

116. The combining form enter/o- in the word gastroenterology means _____.

117. The medical specialty _____ is concerned with disorders surrounding the transportation of oxygen and nutrients to the body.

118. Moving toward the back of the body is considered moving in a _____ direction.

119. The _____ plane is an imaginary plane that divided the entire body into top and bottom sections.

120. Distal and _____ are directional opposites.

121. The _____ cavity is a hollow space that is surrounded by the bones of the skull.

122. The terms respiratory system and _____ system both pertain to the structure and function of breathing.

123. The medical specialty that is involved with the study of bones, cartilage, ligaments, and joints is _____.

124. _____ means toward the head of the body.

125. The medical specialty that deals with blood is called _____.

126. The medical specialty that deals with the prevention, diagnosis, and treatment of cancer is _____.

127. _____ is the study of the function of the structures of the body.

128. The front of the body is known as the _____ or _____ section.

129. The back of the body is known as the _____ or _____ section.

130. The _____ plane divides the body into right and left sections.

131. The _____ plane is an imaginary plane that divides the entire body into top and bottom sections.

132. The upper half of the body is known as the _____ section, and the lower half is known as the _____ section.

133. Moving toward the head is moving in a superior direction or _____ direction.

134. Moving toward the tailbone or the feet is moving in an _____ direction.

135. Moving from the body toward the end of a limb (arm or leg) is moving in a _____ direction or _____.

136. Moving from the end of a limb toward where it is attached to the body is moving in a _____ direction or _____.

137. Structures on the surface of the body are _____ or _____ structures.

138. Structures below the surface and inside the body are deep or _____ structures.

139. A _____ is a hollow space that is surrounded by bone.

140. The Greeks considered the _____ regions to be the seat of melancholy (sad feelings) because they contained the liver and spleen, which they thought released humors that caused different moods.

141. Organs are _____; that is, they can be seen with the unaided eye.

142. _____ is the study of the structures of the human body. _____ is the study of the function and workings of those structures.

True/False

Write 'T' if the statement is true and 'F' if the statement is false.

_____143. Anteroposterior is moving from front to back and posteroanterior is moving from back to front.

_____144. SNF is an abbreviation for health care provided to someone in their own home.

_____145. Geriatrics involves medical care for the elderly.

_____146. An example of an iatrogenic condition would be an inadvertent puncture of the uterus during abdominal surgery.

_____147. The primary care physician is the title of the doctor who is on a medical staff and admits the patient to the hospital.

_____148. Ambulatory surgery center patients are referred to as clients.

_____149. Medial and lateral are directional opposites.

_____150. Immunology involves studying the patient's lymphatic system.

_____151. The mediastinum is a cavity surrounded by the pelvic bones and spinal column.

_____152. A disease that is refractory does not respond well to treatment.

_____153. Patients who are asymptomatic can still have a disease process.

_____154. A neoplastic disease is a disease caused by the growth of a benign or malignant tumor or mass.

_____155. Palliative care is supportive medical and nursing care that is given prior to curing the patient's disease.

_____156. In the microscopic-to-macroscopic approach to the study of the body, organs are considered microscopic.

_____157. In the body systems approach, the human body can be studied according to its various organs and how they function together in a system.

_____158. The medical specialty approach organizes information about the anatomy, physiology, diseases, diagnostic tests, medical and surgical procedures, and drugs for each body system.

_____159. Both gynecology and obstetrics study the female genital and reproductive system, although from different points of view.

_____160. The epigastric region is one of the nine regions of the abdominopelvic area, located below and to the right of the stomach.

_____161. The body system that includes the skin, hair, nails, sweat glands, and oil glands is the lymphatic system.

_____162. Neurology is the body system that includes the brain, cranial nerves, spinal cord, spinal nerves, and neurons.

_____163. The diaphragm separates the thoracic cavity from the pelvic cavity.

_____164. The internal organs within body cavities are known as viscera.

_____165. The opposite of internal is superficial.

_____166. A quadrant is a hollow space surrounded by bones or muscles.

_____167. The study of immunology includes the study of blood and the lymphatic system.

_____168. The abbreviation for dentist is D.P.M.

Essay

Write your answer in the space provided or on a separate sheet of paper.

169. List the four processes of physical examination that a physician uses to arrive at a diagnosis and use one word to describe each of them.

170. Name two of the seven ways mentioned in the textbook as methods that can be used to organize the study of the body.

171. The stomach is located anterior to the pancreas. How then would you describe the location of the pancreas with respect to the stomach?

172. Differentiate between the words infectious and communicable.

173. What is health?

174. What is the anatomical position?

175. Define ancillary department and give at least two examples.

176. What is meant by the word hospice?

CHAPTER 3

Multiple Choice

Choose the one alternative that best completes the statement or answers the question.

1. The part of the stomach that is superior to the pylorus is the:
   a. pyloric sphincter.
   b. antrum.
   c. fundus.
   d. cardiac sphincter.

2. Which word is misspelled?
   a. ascites (fluid accumulation in the abdomen)
   b. ilius (absence of peristalsis)
   c. cirrhosis (chronic irreversible degeneration of the liver)
   d. hemorrhoids (protruding anal or rectal veins)

3. Swallowing of food is known as:
   a. mastication.
   b. deglutition.
   c. ingestion.
   d. defecation.

4. The portion of the biliary tree that sends bile from the gallbladder into the common bile duct is the:
   a. hepatic duct.
   b. parotid duct.
   c. alimentary duct.
   d. cystic duct.

5. The word emesis means:
   a. loose stools.
   b. difficulty swallowing.
   c. vomiting.
   d. excessive gas.

6. Steatorrhea is a symptom of:
   a. gastritis.
   b. cholecystitis.
   c. pancreatitis.
   d. stomatitis.

7. A single hernia pouch in the muscular wall of the colon is spelled:
   a. diverticulum.
   b. diverticula.
   c. diverticuli.
   d. diverticulus.

8. When a physician palpates the abdomen and documents, "No hepatomegaly," this means that there is no:
   a. tenderness occurring over the area of the appendix.
   b. mass felt in the intestines.
   c. inguinal hernia present.
   d. liver enlargement.

9. An EGD would include viewing the:
   a. stomach.
   b. ileum.
   c. cecum.
   d. ascending colon.

10. A patient with a disease of which organ will have low levels of the protein albumin?
    a. liver
    b. gallbladder
    c. pancreas
    d. salivary gland

11. Which word describes a characteristic of some hepatomas?
    a. mesenteric
    b. metastatic
    c. mucosal
    d. malabsorption

12. An inguinal hernia would appear in the area of the:
    a. stomach.
    b. naval.
    c. ribs.
    d. groin.

13. Which is an appropriate drug to treat GERD?
    a. Nexium
    b. Colace
    c. Imodium
    d. Phenergan

14. Which is the abbreviation for a type of feeding tube?
    a. PUD
    b. PEG
    c. CBD
    d. LES

15. A patient had a colonoscopy for complaints of bouts of diarrhea, cramping, and abdominal pain. The colonoscopy revealed no visualized abnormalities. The most likely diagnosis for the patient is:
    a. diverticulosis.
    b. irritable bowel syndrome.
    c. Crohn's disease.
    d. inflammatory bowel syndrome.

16. Which of the following is a pre-cancerous condition?
    a. liver cirrhosis
    b. diverticulosis
    c. colonic polyps
    d. ulcerative colitis

17. Which of the following is a possible diagnosis for a patient with pain in the right lower quadrant of the abdomen?
    a. cholecystitis
    b. esophagitis
    c. appendicitis
    d. pancreatitis

18. When a patient has a hernia that is swollen and can no longer be pushed back into the abdominopelvic cavity, it is known as:
    a. incisional.
    b. incarcerated.
    c. sliding.
    d. reducible.

19. During surgery the patient was found to have choledocholithiasis. In the operative report describing what is seen during the surgery, which anatomical structure is certain to be mentioned?
    a. cardiac sphincter
    b. mesentery
    c. cecum
    d. common bile duct

20. Telescoping of the intestines is known as:
    a. colic.
    b. intussusceptio.
    c. ileus.
    d. volvulus.

21. The abbreviation BRBPR is synonymous with:
    a. hematochezia.
    b. mastication.
    c. obstipation.
    d. anorexia.

22. Twisting of the bowel causing obstruction is known as:
    a. volvulus.
    b. intussusception.
    c. postoperative ileus.
    d. hernia.

23. The patient had surgery to remove a part of his intestine and rejoin the cut ends of the intestine. The word for this surgical intestinal reconnection is:
    a. colostomy.
    b. endoscopy.
    c. anastomosis.
    d. laparotomy.

24. The outpouchings in the walls of the intestine are called:
    a. antrum.
    b. rugae.
    c. fundus.
    d. haustra.

25. Telescoping of one segment of the intestine into the lumen of an adjacent segment is:
    a. volvulus.
    b. diverticula.
    c. intussusception.
    d. ileus.

26. Twisting of a loop of intestine around itself or around another segment of intestine because of a structural abnormality of the mesentery is:
    a. volvulus.
    b. diverticula.
    c. ileus.
    d. ascites.

27. An area where the mucosa has been forced out through small defects in the wall of the colon is:
    a. caries.
    b. ulcers.
    c. dysentery.
    d. diverticulum.

28. The abbreviation IBD stands for:
    a. Inflammatory bowel disease.
    b. Irritable bowel disease.
    c. Intestinal bowel disease.
    d. Incisional bowel disease.

29. A small, fleshy, benign or precancerous growth that arises from the mucosa of the colon is a:
    a. polyp.
    b. papule.
    c. pustule.
    d. cyst.

30. The passage of blood in the stool is:
    a. flatus.
    b. eructation.
    c. hematochezia.
    d. varicose veins.

31. The abbreviation ERCP stands for:
    a. enteroscopic retrograde cholangiogram.
    b. endoscopic retrograde cholangiopancreatography.
    c. esophagorectocholangiopancreatogram.
    d. esophagoscopic retrograde cholangiopancreatography.

32. The abbreviation BE stands for:
    a. bilirubin exam.
    b. barium enema.
    c. bowel enema.
    d. bilirubin enzyme.

33. The medical word meaning chewing is:
    a. mastication.
    b. eructation.
    c. deglutition.
    d. micturition.

34. Hepatosplenomegaly refers to:
    a. enlargement of the gallbladder.
    b. enlargement of the liver and spleen.
    c. softening of the liver and spleen.
    d. hardening of the kidney and spleen.

35. Drugs used to treat nausea and vomiting and motion sickness are called:
    a. antiemetic drugs.
    b. laxative drugs.
    c. antacid drugs.
    d. antidiarrheal drugs.

36. A surgical procedure to remove part of the stomach because of a cancerous tumor is:
    a. gastrostomy.
    b. gastrectomy.
    c. gastrotomy.
    d. enterectomy.

37. Inflammation of the oral mucosa of the mouth is:
    a. cholangitis.
    b. odontitis.
    c. stomatitis.
    d. pyloritis.

38. Which test involves a needle passing through the abdominal wall, injecting contrast material into the liver?
    a. IVC
    b. ERCP
    c. CT
    d. PTC

39. Which type of hepatitis is also known as serum hepatitis?
    a. Hepatitis A
    b. Hepatitis B
    c. Hepatitis C
    d. Hepatitis D

40. Chronic, progressive inflammation and finally irreversible degeneration of liver tissue, characterized by nodules and scarring, is known as:
    a. jaundice.
    b. hepatoma.
    c. cirrhosis.
    d. hepatitis.

41. Swollen, protruding veins in the rectum or in the perianal area, also known as piles, are called:
    a. hemorrhoids.
    b. rectocele.
    c. fecalith.
    d. melena.

42. The inability to voluntarily control bowel movements is known as:
    a. diarrhea.
    b. constipation.
    c. incontinence.
    d. incarceration.

43. The medical word patent means:
    a. closed.
    b. irregular.
    c. open.
    d. regular.

44. Which type of polyp has a thin stalk that supports a ball-shaped, irregular top?
    a. pedunculated
    b. strangulated
    c. incarcerated
    d. sessile

45. Which is a bacterial infection caused by an unusual strain of *E. coli,* a common bacterium in the large intestine?
    a. lactose intolerance
    b. adenocarcinoma
    c. dysentery
    d. polyps

46. The abbreviation PUD stands for:
    a. pelvic ulcer disease.
    b. percutaneous ulcerative disease.
    c. purulent ulcerative disease.
    d. peptic ulcer disease.

47. The vomiting of new or old blood is known as:
    a. regurgitation.
    b. hematemesis.
    c. hemoptysis.
    d. reflux.

48. Which structure hangs in the posterior oral cavity?
    a. lunula
    b. uvea
    c. vulva
    d. uvula

49. The gastrointestinal system begins with which of the following structures?
    a. esophagus
    b. oral cavity
    c. colon
    d. large intestine

50. All of the following are a specific pair of glands EXCEPT:
    a. parotid glands.
    b. submandibular glands.
    c. sublingual glands.
    d. salivary glands.

51. If a patient presents to the emergency room with a severe sore throat, which of the following structures is inflamed?
    a. larynx
    b. esophagus
    c. pharynx
    d. lingula

52. All of the following are parts of the stomach EXCEPT:
    a. uvula.
    b. cardia.
    c. fundus.
    d. pylorus.
53. Which of the following is NOT an accessory organ of digestion?
    a. liver
    b. gallbladder
    c. pancreas
    d. stomach
54. Which of the following is a strong acid that kills microorganisms on ingested food?
    a. hydrochloric acid
    b. pepsinogen
    c. gastrin
    d. digestive enzymes
55. When bile breaks apart large globules of fat, the process is known as:
    a. cholecystokinin.
    b. absorption.
    c. emulsification.
    d. elimination.
56. Which of the following enzymes breaks down the sugar in milk?
    a. amylase
    b. lipase
    c. protease
    d. lactase
57. If a patient experiences difficulty eating, the patient is said to have:
    a. anorexia.
    b. dyspepsia.
    c. dysphagia.
    d. gastritis.
58. Which of the following phrases describes a procedure in which a needle is passed through the abdominal wall and contrast material is injected into the liver?
    a. endoscopic retrograde cholangiopancreatography
    b. percutaneous transhepatic cholangiography
    c. oral cholecystography
    d. gastric analysis
59. Cancerous tumors of the gastrointestinal system are treated medically by a/an:
    a. oncologist.
    b. surgeon.
    c. gastroenterologist.
    d. cardiologist.

60. An omphalocele is a/an:
    a. umbilical hernia present at birth.
    b. hernia that cannot be pushed back into the abdominopelvic cavity.
    c. adhesion.
    d. incisional hernia.
61. What is the treatment for adhesions?
    a. medications
    b. exercise
    c. surgery
    d. rest
62. Blood vessels to the intestines can become twisted, decreasing the blood supply, and leading to the death of the intestines. This condition is called:
    a. intussusception.
    b. Crohn's disease.
    c. appendicitis.
    d. malrotation.
63. Colic is a/an:
    a. twisting of a loop of intestine.
    b. overdeveloped muscle in the stomach.
    c. common malady in babie.
    d. precursor to cancer.
64. The word ulcer means:
    a. stomach.
    b. intestinal.
    c. gut.
    d. sore.
65. Gravidarum is a Latin word meaning:
    a. regurgitation.
    b. of pregnancy.
    c. emesis.
    d. nausea.
66. Excessive overeating is known as:
    a. anorexia.
    b. polyphagia.
    c. dysphagia.
    d. cheilitis.
67. Gloss/o- means:
    a. mouth.
    b. saliva.
    c. tongue.
    d. teeth.
68. The membrane that lines the abdominopelvic cavity and secretes peritoneal fluid to fill the spaces between the organs is called the:
    a. pepsinogen.
    b. pyloric sphincter.
    c. peristalsis.
    d. peritoneum.

69. The gastrointestinal system is an elongated system that:
    a. begins at the mouth.
    b. goes through the thoracic cavity.
    c. fills most of the abdominopelvic cavity.
    d. All of the above.
70. The gag reflex is initiated when food touches the:
    a. soft palate.
    b. mouth.
    c. uvula.
    d. lips.
71. The word glossal refers to the:
    a. tongue.
    b. stomach.
    c. salivary glands.
    d. None of the above.
72. The gustatory cortex in the brain processes information sent by the:
    a. intestinal mucosa.
    b. oral cavity.
    c. taste receptors.
    d. palate.
73. All of the following are salivary glands EXCEPT:
    a. pharynx.
    b. submandibular.
    c. parotid.
    d. sublingual.
74. The word deglutition refers to:
    a. chewing, grinding, and tearing food.
    b. swallowing food.
    c. contractions of the esophagus.
    d. partially undigested food.
75. Peristalsis occurs in all of the following gastrointestinal structures and organs EXCEPT the:
    a. stomach.
    b. small intestine.
    c. colon.
    d. oral cavity.
76. The stomach is able to accommodate large amounts of food due to its:
    a. haustra.
    b. peristalsis.
    c. rugae.
    d. antrum.
77. The word cardia refers to the:
    a. heart.
    b. pharynx.
    c. salivary glands.
    d. stomach.
78. What is the purpose of the villi in the small intestine?
    a. to move digested food along the small intestine.
    b. to make digestive juices.
    c. to absorb digested nutrients.
    d. all of the above
79. The large intestine includes the:
    a. cecum, ileum, colon, and rectum.
    b. cecum, appendix, rectum, and anus.
    c. duodenum, rectum, anus, and perirectal area.
    d. none of the above
80. Small areas on the intestinal walls that contain white blood cells to destroy microorganisms are called:
    a. Peyer's patches.
    b. haustra.
    c. villi.
    d. mucosa.
81. Vermiform means:
    a. pink.
    b. small.
    c. wormlike.
    d. all of the above
82. The gallbladder is responsible for:
    a. concentrating and storing bile from the liver.
    b. neutralizing acid from the stomach.
    c. digesting proteins in foods.
    d. releasing digestive enzymes made by the pancreas.
83. Chemical digestion includes:
    a. mastication, deglutition, and peristalsis.
    b. enzymes and acid.
    c. mastication and enzymes.
    d. enzymes, deglutition, and acid.
84. Emulsification is the process of:
    a. secreting cholecystokinin.
    b. secreting intrinsic factor.
    c. bile breaking down fats.
    d. vitamin B_{12} breaking down proteins.
85. Which of the following are involved in the digestion of fat?
    a. amylase and hydrochloric acid
    b. hydrochloric acid and mastication
    c. lipase and pepsinogen
    d. emulsification and lipase
86. The sugar in milk is broken down in the small intestine by the enzyme:
    a. amylase.
    b. protease.
    c. lactase.
    d. lipase.

87. Absorbed food nutrients are carried by the blood in the portal vein to the:
   a. liver.
   b. anus.
   c. duodenum.
   d. gallbladder.

88. The process of elimination is called:
   a. feces.
   b. defecation.
   c. meconium.
   d. all of the above

89. The muscular ring that keeps food in the stomach from going back into the esophagus is the:
   a. celiac.
   b. sphincter.
   c. chyme.
   d. peristalsis.

90. The combining form sial/o- means:
   a. saliva.
   b. eating.
   c. mouth.
   d. stomach.

91. Gastroenteritis is an inflammation of the:
   a. liver and gallbladder.
   b. stomach and duodenum.
   c. pharynx and esophagus.
   d. stomach and intestines.

92. Infection of the pouch that hangs from the cecum is known as:
   a. colic.
   b. diverticulitis.
   c. appendicitis.
   d. colon cancer.

93. Which kind of hernia occurs along a surgical suture line?
   a. incarcerated
   b. inguinal
   c. umbilical
   d. incisional

94. Ascites is a disease of the:
   a. stomach.
   b. intestines.
   c. liver.
   d. mouth.

95. The combining form hepat/o- means:
   a. liver.
   b. stomach.
   c. intestines.
   d. rectum.

96. Cholelithiasis affects the:
   a. intestines.
   b. pancreas.

   c. liver.
   d. gallbladder.

97. A barium enema uses dye to outline the:
   a. colon.
   b. stomach.
   c. pancreas.
   d. pharynx.

98. An exploratory laparotomy makes an incision in the:
   a. stomach.
   b. mouth.
   c. abdominal wall.
   d. colon.

99. All of these combining forms means abdomen EXCEPT:
   a. enter/o-.
   b. celi/o-.
   c. abdomin/o-.
   d. lapar/o-.

100. The combining form cholecyst/o- means:
   a. bile ducts.
   b. liver.
   c. gallbladder.
   d. intestine.

101. Which one of these surgeries is used to create a permanent opening in the abdomen in order to feed a patient through a feeding tube?
   a. cholecystectomy
   b. gastrostomy
   c. gastrectomy
   d. colonoscopy

102. Which of the following is true of the gallbladder?
   a. stores bile
   b. releases bile when there is a fatty meal in the small intestines
   c. can get stones inside it
   d. all of the above

103. Which of the following correctly separates the medical word colonoscopy into its component word parts?
   a. prefix col/o-, combining form noscop/o-, suffix -y
   b. prefix colon/o-, suffix -scopy
   c. combining form col/o-, suffix -noscopy
   d. combining form colon/o-, suffix -scopy

104. Vomiting blood is known as:
   a. emesis.
   b. GERD.
   c. anorexia nervosa.
   d. hematemesis.

105. Passing dark or black blood through the rectum is known as:
    a. incontinence.
    b. diarrhea.
    c. melena.
    d. GERD.

106. An upper GI series is also known as a/an:
    a. colostomy.
    b. esophagoscopy.
    c. hemoccult test.
    d. barium swallow.

107. Most stomach ulcers are caused by:
    a. *Helicobacter pylori.*
    b. stress.
    c. too much acid.
    d. digestive enzymes.

108. Hepatitis is an inflammation of the:
    a. colon.
    b. liver.
    c. gallbladder.
    d. rectum.

109. When the intestine twists, forming an obstruction that prevents the passage of food, it is known as:
    a. hernia.
    b. volvulus.
    c. emesis.
    d. hemorrhoid.

110. Which of the following suffixes means enzyme?
    a. -tion
    b. -ac
    c. -ive
    d. -ase

111. Which of the following lists the parts of the small intestine in the correct order?
    a. ileum, jejunum, duodenum
    b. duodenum, ileum, colon
    c. duodenum, jejunum, ileum
    d. colon, duodenum, cecum

112. The internal open area within the intestine is known as the:
    a. lumen.
    b. villi.
    c. perineum.
    d. sphincter.

113. Which of the following contributes to the formation of diverticula?
    a. irritable bowel syndrome
    b. colon cancer
    c. low-fiber diet
    d. incontinence

114. Severe constipation is known as:
    a. obstipation.
    b. hematochezia.
    c. fecalith.
    d. rectocele.

115. Which word is misspelled?
    a. hepatosplenomegaly (enlargement of the liver and spleen)
    b. choledocholithiasis (condition of stones in the gallbladder)
    c. cirrosis (chronic liver degeneration)
    d. jaundice (yellow discoloration of the skin from liver disease)

116. Obstructive jaundice occurs when:
    a. there is a postoperative ileus.
    b. the liver has cancer.
    c. there is an intestinal obstruction.
    d. a gallstone blocks the flow of bile in bile ducts.

117. Pancreatitis can be due to all of the following EXCEPT:
    a. bacterial infection.
    b. gallstones.
    c. chronic alcoholism.
    d. viral infection.

118. The guaiac test detects:
    a. *Helicobacter pylori* infection.
    b. elevated liver enzymes.
    c. gastric adenocarcinoma.
    d. blood in the stool.

119. Which of the following is true of a gallbladder ultrasound?
    a. uses sound waves to create an image of the gallbladder
    b. is also known as a gallbladder sonogram
    c. uses a contrast dye to outline the bladder
    d. both a and b

120. Which abbreviation is a test for parasites in the stool?
    a. O&P
    b. LFTs
    c. UGI
    d. N&V

121. To determine if a polyp in the colon was benign or malignant, the physician would do a:
    a. liver function test.
    b. colostomy.
    c. biopsy.
    d. cholecystectomy.

122. Which is the medical word for a surgically created opening?
    a. stomach
    b. cavity
    c. stomatitis
    d. stoma

123. Which surgery creates an abdominal incision to widely open the abdominopelvic cavity?
    a. hemorrhoidectomy
    b. endoscopy
    c. exploratory laparotomy
    d. polypectomy
124. Antiemetic drugs are used to treat:
    a. vomiting.
    b. diarrhea.
    c. peptic ulcers.
    d. gastric cancer.

Short Answer

Write the word or phrase that best completes each statement or answers the question.

125. The long pouch extending from the cecum is called the _____.
126. _____ is the first stool of the newborn.
127. The condition of stones found in the gallbladder is known as _____.
128. Crampy abdominal pain in infants that occurs shortly after eating is called _____.
129. The combining form for the mouth is _____.
130. A/an _____ hernia occurs when a portion of intestine travels into the _____ canal to follow the line of descent of the testes.
131. Elevated levels of ALT and AST would be suggestive of _____ disease.
132. _____ _____ is a radiological test for gallbladder disease that uses contrast dye injected into a vein to outline the bile ducts.
133. Indigestion or epigastric pain is known as _____.
134. The wavelike contractions that move substances through parts of the digestive system are called _____.
135. The gastrointestinal system begins in the mouth or _____ _____.
136. The sight, smell, and taste of food cause the salivary glands to release _____ into the mouth.
137. The teeth tear, chew, and grind the food, a process known as _____ .
138. The stomach is divided into five areas: _____, _____, _____, _____, and _____.
139. _____ is the semisolid mixture of partially digested food, saliva, and digestive juices in the stomach.
140. The _____ _____ or _____ _____ is a long, hollow tube that receives partially digested food from the stomach.
141. The _____ is a 10-inch, C-shaped segment that curves around the pancreas and connects with the jejunum.

142. Hanging from the external wall of the cecum is the _____, a thin tube that is closed at its distal end.
143. The peritoneum forms a thick, fan-shaped sheet known as the _____ that is attached to the posterior wall of the abdominal cavity and supports the jejunum and ileum.
144. Bile is a combination of bile acids, mucus, fluid, and two pigments: the green pigment biliverdin and the yellow pigment _____.
145. The _____ is an accessory organ of digestion. It is a teardrop-shaped, dark green sac posterior to the liver.
146. Chemical digestion consists of the actions of _____ and acids that break down foods into molecules of nutrients that can be absorbed and used by the body.
147. Amniotic fluid and shed skin cells, plus mucus and bile from the fetal gastrointestinal tract, form _____, a thick, sticky, green-to-black substance that is passed as the first stool.
148. _____ drugs treat nausea, vomiting, and motion sickness.
149. The abbreviation GERD stands for _____ _____.
150. _____ is the semisolid mixture of partially digested food, saliva, and digestive juices in the stomach.
151. The suffix in the word gastritis means _____.
152. _____ fluid is a watery fluid that fills the spaces between the organs in the abdominopelvic cavity.
153. Bacteria in the large intestine feed on undigested food fiber, producing the intestinal gas called _____.
154. The _____ is a lidlike structure that seals the larynx when food is swallowed and directs food into the esophagus.
155. Excessive vomiting during the first few months of pregnancy is known as _____.
156. _____ is the abnormal absence of peristalsis in the small and large intestines, caused by tumor, adhesions, hernia, or other causes.
157. Bright red blood in the stool, also known as _____, indicates active bleeding in the lower gastrointestinal system.
158. Another name for hepatitis A is _____ hepatitis.
159. The patient had surgery to remove an infected appendix. The medical word for this procedure is _____.
160. The combining form cholecyst/o- means _____.
161. Another name for the digestive system is _____ _____.

162. _____ is the medical specialty that studies the digestive system.

163. In the phrase vermiform appendix, the word vermiform means _____.

True/False

Write 'T' if the statement is true and 'F' if the statement is false.

_____164. The digestive enzymes amylase and lipase are produced by the liver.

_____165. If a patient had melena, his laboratory report would show the results of a guaiac- positive stool.

_____166. An example of a medication to treat emesis would be Compazine.

_____167. One knows that lipase is an enzyme because of the suffix -ase.

_____168. The patient complains of not having a desire to eat. This symptom is known as ascites.

_____169. The alimentary canal is also called the GI tract.

_____170. Lingu/o- and gloss/o- are combining forms for the salivary gland.

_____171. Bile is stored and released from the gallbladder to break down fats into fatty acids.

_____172. A gastroplasty is performed to treat severely obese patients.

_____173. A patient with ascites will show a yellow-orange discoloration of the skin.

_____174. The sublingual glands are located under the lower jaw bone.

_____175. The liver is an accessory organ of digestion and is not physically involved in the process of digestion.

_____176. The word polyphagia means difficult or painful eating.

_____177. A cholecystotomy is the surgical removal of the gallbladder.

_____178. Serum hepatitis is another name for Hepatitis A.

_____179. One of the word parts in hematemesis means blood.

_____180. High-fiber diets and laxatives are avoided in patients with irritable bowel syndrome.

_____181. Polyps are benign and never become cancerous.

_____182. A chronic, progressive inflammation and eventual irreversible degeneration of liver tissue characterized by nodules and scarring is called ascites.

_____183. In a polypectomy the polyps may be removed from the colon using forceps or a snare.

_____184. Difficult or painful eating is known as dysphagia.

_____185. The first part of the small intestine is the jejunum.

_____186. The liver has special cells known as hepatocytes that continuously produce bile.

_____187. Anorexia nervosa can cause a person to decrease food intake to the point of starvation.

_____188. The pancreas is an accessory organ of digestion.

_____189. Cholecystokinin is a hormone that stimulates the pancreas to release lipase.

_____190. A temporary stopping of peristalsis following surgery is known as a postoperative ileus.

_____191. Dysphagia is the medical word for indigestion.

_____192. Hemorrhoids are varicose veins of the rectum.

_____193. Polyps in the colon can be an inherited condition present in several members of the same family.

_____194. Emesis is another word for vomiting.

_____195. Hematochezia is the presence of blood in vomited stomach contents.

_____196. Both gloss/o- and lingu/o- mean mouth.

Essay

Write your answer in the space provided or on a separate sheet of paper.

197. Explain why the CLO test is done when a patient has gastric ulcers.

198. The newspaper reported an epidemic outbreak of viral hepatitis in a children's camp. Although you did not hear the type of hepatitis, you correctly assumed that it was hepatitis A. Explain your reasoning.

199. Briefly discuss esophageal varices.

200. What is the difference between mechanical digestion and chemical digestion?

201. What is a stool culture and sensitivity (C & S) test?

202. Define the word endoscopy.

203. What is a gastroplasty?

204. Define the medical word choledocholithotomy.

CHAPTER 4

Multiple Choice

Choose the one alternative that best completes the statement or answers the question.

1. Which word is misspelled?
   a. eupnea
   b. expectoration
   c. empyema
   d. exspiration

2. Which combining form means lung?
   a. alveol/o-
   b. pulmon/o-
   c. thorac/o-
   d. pleur/o-

3. Antibiotics are used to treat pneumococcal pneumonia because the condition is caused by a:
   a. virus.
   b. fungus.
   c. bacterium.
   d. dust particle.

4. Breathing that is easier in an upright position is called:
   a. bradypnea.
   b. tachypnea.
   c. orthopnea.
   d. dyspnea.

5. Which is a form of pneumoconiosis?
   a. tuberculosis
   b. anthracosis
   c. atelectasis
   d. bronchiectasis

6. Which is the name for the hollow spheres of cells within the lungs where oxygen and carbon dioxide are exchanged?
   a. alveoli
   b. bronchioles
   c. cilia
   d. parenchyma

7. Which patient would have an elevated serum carboxyhemoglobin?
   a. a premature newborn
   b. a man who attempted suicide by staying in a running car in a closed garage
   c. a former cigarette smoker with advanced emphysema
   d. an elderly woman with Legionnaires' disease with multiple organ involvement

8. For the patient's cough the physician prescribed the antitussive drug:
   a. albuterol (Proventil).
   b. cromolyn (Intal).
   c. hydrocodone (Hycodan).
   d. rifampin.

9. Which combining form means breast bone?
   a. stern/o-
   b. cost/o-
   c. mediastin/o-
   d. thorac/o-

10. The medical procedure performed with a stethoscope is called:
    a. aspiration.
    b. intubation.

    c. auscultation.
    d. expectoration.

11. An example of COPD would be:
    a. acute bronchitis.
    b. chronic bronchitis.
    c. bronchiectasis.
    d. bronchospasm.

12. Which is a condition that accompanies heart failure and is characterized by noninfectious fluid build-up in the alveoli and lung tissues?
    a. pulmonary edema
    b. empyema
    c. pneumonia
    d. pleural effusion

13. Which abbreviation does not stand for a type of dyspnea or difficulty breathing?
    a. SOB
    b. DOE
    c. PPD
    d. PND

14. An example of a URI would be:
    a. nasopharyngitis.
    b. acute bronchitis.
    c. pneumonitis.
    d. pleuritis.

15. Which finding would create an abnormal ABG result?
    a. rhonchi
    b. hemoptysis
    c. hypercapnia
    d. expectoration

16. Which sound will be heard on inspiration?
    a. clubbing
    b. rales
    c. sputum
    d. tubercles

17. The patient had a positive reaction to the Mantoux test. What would be the next test done on this patient?
    a. culture and sensitivity of his throat
    b. pulmonary function tests to measure breathing capacity
    c. arterial blood gases to determine the level of breathing impairment
    d. a chest x-ray to identify suspicious lesions

18. Reactive airway disease is also known as:
    a. asthma.
    b. atelectasis.
    c. asbestosis.
    d. aspiration.

19. Which device would indicate to a physician that the patient has hypoxemia?
   a. cannula
   b. ventilator
   c. pulse oximeter
   d. face mask

20. Patients on mechanical ventilation may also require a _____ to provide access to the lungs.
   a. tracheostomy
   b. bronchoscopy
   c. thoracotomy
   d. thoracentesis

21. Which drug is not used to treat asthma?
   a. salmeterol (Serevent)
   b. isoniazid (INH)
   c. cromolyn (Intal)
   d. triamcinolone (Azmacort)

22. Which is the medical word for voice box?
   a. pharynx
   b. trachea
   c. larynx
   d. epiglottis

23. The turbinates are located in the:
   a. hilum.
   b. thorax.
   c. pleural cavity.
   d. nasal cavity.

24. Which serious disease is genetically linked or inherited?
   a. cystic fibrosis
   b. respiratory distress syndrome
   c. chronic bronchitis
   d. sudden infant death syndrome

25. Pulmonology is the study of the:
   a. lungs.
   b. trachea.
   c. alveoli.
   d. sternum.

26. As the nasal cavity continues posteriorly, it merges with the upper part of the throat or:
   a. larynx.
   b. trachea.
   c. bronchus.
   d. pharynx.

27. The lidlike structure that seals off the larynx is called the:
   a. esophagus.
   b. pharynx.
   c. epiglottis.
   d. trachea.

28. Which structure is composed of smooth muscle rather than cartilage?
   a. bronchioles
   b. bronchi
   c. lumen
   d. bronchial tree

29. The irregularly shaped area between the two lungs that contains the trachea is called the:
   a. diaphragm.
   b. sternum.
   c. thorax.
   d. mediastinum.

30. Which is not a basic function of the respiratory system?
   a. warming and moistening incoming air
   b. exchanging carbon monoxide for oxygen
   c. mechanically causing air to flow into the lungs
   d. serving as a passageway through which air can enter and leave the body

31. A prolonged, extremely severe, life-threatening asthma attack is known as:
   a. bronchospasm.
   b. status asthmaticus.
   c. bronchitis.
   d. bronchiectasis.

32. The abbreviation COPD stands for:
   a. chronic obstructive pulmonary disease.
   b. chronic obstructive pulmonary distress.
   c. cardiopulmonary disease.
   d. cardiopulmonary distress.

33. Which is a high-pitched, harsh, crowing sound due to obstruction in the trachea or larynx?
   a. wheezes
   b. rales
   c. stridor
   d. rhonchi

34. A localized collection of pus in the thoracic cavity is:
   a. emphysema.
   b. influenza.
   c. empyema.
   d. asthma.

35. Which is a severe and sometimes fatal bacterial infection that begins with flu-like symptoms, body aches, and fever, followed by severe pneumonia with possible liver and kidney degeneration?
   a. influenza
   b. emphysema
   c. asthma
   d. Legionnaire's disease

36. Another name for anthracosis is:
    a. charcoal lung disease.
    b. black lung disease.
    c. gray lung disease.
    d. green lung disease.

37. Pneumonia that affects all the lobes of one lung is called:
    a. lobar.
    b. panlobar.
    c. double.
    d. single.

38. Coughing up blood-tinged sputum is known as:
    a. hematemesis.
    b. hemothorax.
    c. hemoptysis.
    d. expectoration.

39. The abbreviation AFB stands for:
    a. acid formed bacillus.
    b. acid-fast bacterium.
    c. acid formed bacteria.
    d. acid-fast bacillus.

40. The abbreviation PND stands for:
    a. pulmonary nocturnal disease.
    b. paroxysmal nocturnal disease.
    c. paroxysmal nocturnal dyspnea.
    d. pleural nocturnal dyspnea.

41. Which is a Greek word that means without a pulse?
    a. asphyxia
    b. anoxic
    c. anoxia
    d. tachypnea

42. An abnormally low level of oxygen at the cellular level is called:
    a. hypercapnia.
    b. cyanosis.
    c. hypoxemia.
    d. hypoxia.

43. In unventilated spaces, carbon monoxide from smoke or car exhaust builds up in the bloodstream, combining with hemoglobin in the blood to form:
    a. oxygen.
    b. carboxyhemoglobin.
    c. carbon dioxide.
    d. embolus.

44. The diagnostic procedure to measure the capacity of the lungs and the volume of air that the lungs can move during inhalation and exhalation is called:
    a. pulse oximetry.
    b. Heimlich maneuver.

c. pulmonary function test.
d. arterial blood gases.

45. Which is a handheld device that is used to manually breathe for the patient on a temporary basis?
    a. respirator
    b. Ambu bag
    c. ventilator
    d. nasal cannula

46. Which is a procedure that removes one entire lung?
    a. pneumonectomy
    b. thoracotomy
    c. lobectomy
    d. tracheostomy

47. Which drug is used to suppress the cough center in the brain?
    a. antitussive
    b. antibiotic
    c. antitubercular
    d. expectorant

48. The form in which oxygenated blood travels from the lungs to the heart is called:
    a. respiration.
    b. inhalation.
    c. deoxygenated blood.
    d. oxyhemoglobin.

49. The anatomical part of the lungs where oxygen and carbon dioxide are exchanged is the:
    a. trachea.
    b. alveoli.
    c. bronchiole.
    d. bronchi.

50. Which is a waste product of metabolism that is exhaled by the pulmonary system?
    a. carbon dioxide
    b. oxygen
    c. carbon monoxide
    d. oxyhemoglobin

51. Muscles that lie between the ribs are called the:
    a. diaphragm.
    b. thoracic muscles.
    c. pleura.
    d. intercostal muscles.

52. A patient comes into the hospital for treatment of an acute infection of the bronchi that he has had for two days. He has a fever of 104 degrees, and a productive cough. The most likely name of this condition is:
    a. chronic bronchitis.
    b. acute bronchitis.
    c. asthma.
    d. bronchiectasis.

53. Incomplete expansion or collapse of part or all of a lung due to mucus, tumor, or a foreign body that blocks the bronchus is called:
    a. atelectasis.
    b. bronchiectasis.
    c. adult respiratory distress syndrome.
    d. stridor.

54. Which is an inherited, eventually fatal disease of the exocrine cells that is carried by a recessive gene?
    a. atelectasis
    b. bronchiectasis
    c. emphysema
    d. cystic fibrosis

55. A localized collection of purulent material in the thoracic cavity is called:
    a. pneumonia.
    b. chronic bronchitis.
    c. empyema.
    d. pneumococcal pneumonia.

56. Which of the following types of pneumonia affects only one lobe of a lung?
    a. lobar pneumonia
    b. panlobar pneumonia
    c. double pneumonia
    d. bronchopneumonia

57. Which is the word for abnormally high levels of carbon dioxide in the arterial blood?
    a. cyanosis
    b. hypoxemia
    c. hypercapnia
    d. carboxyhemoglobin

58. The combining form mucos/o- means:
    a. lung.
    b. respiration.
    c. mucous membrane.
    d. nasal.

59. The combining form parenchym/o- means:
    a. mucosa.
    b. runctional cells of an organ.
    c. GI tract.
    d. wall of a cavity.

60. Which is true of the thoracic cavity?
    a. It is the cavity for the gastrointestinal system.
    b. It contains the lungs and structures in the mediastinum.
    c. It is inferior to the pelvic cavity.
    d. It is superior to the cranial cavity.

61. Irregular crackling or bubbling sounds during inspiration are called:
    a. rhonchi.
    b. stridor.

c. wheezes.
d. rales.

62. Which word means incomplete expansion or collapse of part or all of a lung due to mucus, tumor, trauma, or a foreign body that blocks the bronchus?
    a. ARDS
    b. atelectasis
    c. abnormal breath sounds
    d. stridor

63. Which is a Greek word that means inflation?
    a. emphysema
    b. bronchitis
    c. pneumonia
    d. sputum

64. Empyema means:
    a. chronic, irreversibly damaged alveoli that become large air spaces that trap air.
    b. localized collection of pus in the thoracic cavity.
    c. purulent.
    d. pneumophila.

65. Which is true about an opportunistic infection?
    a. The microorganism waits in the body for an opportunity to cause disease.
    b. It always occurs as a lung infection.
    c. It is seldom serious or critical.
    d. It is also called SARS.

66. Difficult, labored, or painful respiration due to lung disease is known as:
    a. cough.
    b. paroxysma.
    c. dyspnea.
    d. expectoration.

67. Emphysema is part of which disease?
    a. SIDS
    b. RDS
    c. COPD
    d. TB

68. Which respiratory disease is found almost exclusively in patients with AIDS?
    a. *pneumocystis carinii* pneumonia
    b. COPD
    c. anthracosis
    d. eupnea

69. Pulmonary edema (fluid in the lungs) is caused by:
    a. smoking.
    b. tuberculosis.
    c. left-sided congestive heart failure.
    d. obstructive sleep apnea.

70. Empyema is:
    a. extra air filling the alveoli.
    b. bluish discoloration of the skin.
    c. an occupational lung disease.
    d. Pus in the thoracic cavity.
71. A car accident patient with a hemothorax has _____ in the chest cavity.
    a. pus
    b. blood
    c. fluid
    d. air
72. Which of these healthcare professionals would perform endotracheal intubation?
    a. anesthesiologist in the operating room
    b. paramedic in an ambulance
    c. physician in the emergency department
    d. all of the above
73. The medical word for a collapsed lung is:
    a. aspiration pneumonia.
    b. cystic fibrosis.
    c. atelectasis.
    d. apnea.
74. Which instrument is used to visualize the area when endotracheal intubation is performed?
    a. bronchoscope
    b. laryngoscope
    c. lung scan
    d. nasal cannula
75. The medical abbreviation for shortness of breath (SOB) when exercising is:
    a. URI.
    b. DOE.
    c. CPR.
    d. CXR.
76. Which of these abbreviations stands for a device that delivers a premeasured dose of medication to the lungs when the patient inhales?
    a. TPR
    b. CPAP
    c. O_2
    d. MDI
77. A lobectomy is the surgical removal of:
    a. the trachea.
    b. the mediastinum.
    c. the larynx.
    d. a part of the lung.
78. The phrase "lobar pneumonia" indicates:
    a. what part of the lung is affected by pneumonia.
    b. that a bacteria caused the pneumonia.
    c. when the pneumonia occurred.
    d. that the patient aspirated food into the lungs.

79. Intercostal retractions in respiratory distress syndrome are visible:
    a. in the flaring nostrils.
    b. as bluish discoloration of the skin.
    c. between the ribs.
    d. none of the above
80. The Heimlich maneuver is performed for persons who:
    a. have stopped breathing.
    b. have carbon monoxide poisoning from a fire.
    c. are choking on food.
    d. are having an asthma attack.
81. Respiration consists of:
    a. breathing in and inhalation.
    b. breathing out and exhalation.
    c. inspiration and inhalation.
    d. inspiration and exhalation.
82. A normal depth and rate of respirations is known as:
    a. dyspnea.
    b. eupnea.
    c. tachypnea.
    d. apnea.
83. Patients who have to sit upright to sleep have:
    a. tuberculosis.
    b. pulmonary embolism.
    c. cyanosis.
    d. orthopnea.
84. Which of the following measure the oxygen level in the blood?
    a. chest x-ray and auscultation
    b. culture and sensitivity
    c. pulse oximeter and arterial blood gas
    d. spirometry and carboxyhemoglobin
85. All of the following combining forms mean breath or air EXCEPT:
    a. spir/o-.
    b. hal/o-.
    c. pne/o-.
    d. steth/o-.
86. Which is the misspelled word?
    a. pneumonectomy
    b. eupnea
    c. pnumonia
    d. tachypnea

Short Answer

Write the word or phrase that best completes each statement or answers the question.

87. A normal depth and rate of respiration is known as _____.
88. Mr. Smith's lung cancer was inoperable; therefore he was referred to a/an _____, a physician who treats cancers medically.

89. The physician suspected tuberculosis when George Richards complained of _____, or coughing up blood.

90. The patient had bluish-gray discoloration of his skin from abnormally low levels of oxygen and high levels of carbon dioxide in his body. His abnormal coloration is called _____.

91. To indicate that a surgical incision was made into the chest cavity to access the lung, the thoracic surgeon dictated: "A _____ was performed."

92. The medical word for a collapsed lung is _____.

93. A/an _____ _____ _____ automatically delivers a pre-measured dose or puffs of a bronchodilator or corticosteroid to a person who has asthma.

94. PCP or *Pneumocystis carinii* pneumonia is often a complication of an advanced stage of _____.

95. Blockage of one of the pulmonary arteries with a blood clot or fat globule is called a pulmonary _____.

96. Using aspirin to relieve symptoms of influenza in a child could cause _____ syndrome.

97. The medical word for the windpipe is the _____.

98. The _____ nerve causes the diaphragm to contract and initiate inhalation.

99. The protein-fat compound that creates surface tension and keeps the walls of the alveoli from collapsing is called _____.

100. The _____ are three long, bony projections in the nasal cavity that break up and slow down air as it is inhaled through the nose.

101. _____ means pertaining to a normal rate and rhythm of breathing.

102. Blood that contains low levels of oxygen and high levels of carbon dioxide is called _____ blood.

103. _____ is a high-pitched, harsh, crowing sound due to obstruction in the trachea or larynx.

104. _____ is an occupational lung disease also known as coal miner's lung.

105. _____ is a general word for any occupational lung disease caused by chronically inhaling some type of dust or particle.

106. Infection of some or all of the lobes of the lungs and the bronchi is called _____.

107. A pulmonary _____ is a blockage of one of the pulmonary arteries due to a blood clot or fat globule.

108. The nasal cavity is divided internally by the nasal _____ into right and left sides.

109. As the nasal cavity continues posteriorly, it merges with the upper part of the throat or _____.

110. During swallowing, muscles in the neck pull the larynx up to meet the _____, a lidlike structure that seals off the larynx, so food moves across the top of the epiglottis and into the esophagus, not into the larynx.

111. _____ is an adjective that refers to the bronchi and the lungs.

112. The _____ is a hollow sphere of cells that expands and contracts with each breath.

113. All the alveoli are collectively known as the pulmonary _____, the functional part of the lung, as opposed to the connective tissue framework that surrounds and supports the alveoli.

114. The _____ is a bony cage that consists of the _____ (breast bone) anteriorly, the ribs laterally, and the spinal column posteriorly.

115. The _____, an irregularly shaped area between the two lungs, contains the trachea.

116. The inferior aspect of the thoracic cavity is covered by the _____, a muscular sheet that contracts to enlarge the thoracic cavity and draw in air.

117. The respiratory control center sends nerve impulses to the _____ nerve, causing the diaphragm to contract and initiate inspiration.

118. _____ consists of breathing in and breathing out.

119. Breathing in is known as _____ or _____.

120. Breathing out is known as _____ or _____.

121. _____ is a hypersensitive reaction of the bronchioles to a triggering agent.

122. _____ is the medical word for the windpipe.

123. _____ is the medical word for the throat.

124. _____ is the unit of measurement that a physician uses to describe the amount and duration of cigarette smoking.

125. Exposure to _____ has been found to be the reason that inner-city poor children have high rates of asthma.

126. A nasal cannula provides the patient with the additional _____ that he or she needs.

127. The smallest air passageways to the lungs are called _____.

128. Cigarette smoking immobilizes and eventually destroys the _____, small hairs that line the respiratory tract.

129. The phrenic nerve stimulates the _____ to begin the process of inhalation.

130. The opposite of tachypnea is _____.

True/False

Write 'T' if the statement is true and 'F' if the statement is false.

_____131. Expiration can have two meanings: to breathe out and to die.

_____132. The purpose of an endotracheal intubation is to establish an airway in a patient.

_____133. A Heimlich bag is a handheld device to temporarily manually assist breathing in a patient.

_____134. The medical transcriptionist typed: "The patient's nasal mucus membranes were swollen and inflamed." The transcriptionist spelled all of the words in the sentence correctly.

_____135. Pulmon/o- and pne/o- are both combining forms meaning lung.

_____136. Hypoxemia is low oxygen in the blood; hypoxia is low oxygen at the cellular level.

_____137. PPD is an abbreviation for a chest x-ray view.

_____138. An incentive spirometer encourages deep breathing in a postsurgical patient.

_____139. The presence of AFB in sputum could indicate a tuberculosis infection.

_____140. A common cause of walking pneumonia would be *Streptococcus pneumoniae*.

_____141. An abnormally low levels of oxygen in the arterial blood is called oxyhemoglobin.

_____142. Asthma is characterized by the sudden onset of hyper-reactivity of the bronchioles.

_____143. The small tubular branches of airway that carry air into and out of the alveoli are called bronchi.

_____144. Oxygen is a waste product of aerobic metabolism.

_____145. Although the lungs are similar in size, the right lung is slightly larger and has three lobes, while the left lung only has two lobes.

_____146. A carboxyhemoglobin test is done to measure the level of carbon monoxide in the patient's blood when carbon monoxide poisoning is suspected.

_____147. An oximeter is a small, noninvasive device that measures the oxygen saturation in a patient's blood.

_____148. Supplemental oxygen is given to patients to raise their oxygen levels.

_____149. A bronchoscope is a surgical procedure that uses a flexible lighted tube to examine the trachea and bronchi.

_____150. The terms thoracentesis and thoracocentesis mean the same thing.

_____151. Endotracheal intubation is used to establish an airway for the patient who is not breathing.

_____152. The epiglottis is a lidlike structure that closes the larynx when food is swallowed and directs food into the esophagus.

_____153. A pneumonectomy is a surgery to treat patients with asthma.

_____154. The right lung has two lobes and the left lung has three lobes.

_____155. Chronic bronchitis plus emphysema equals chronic obstructive pulmonary disease.

_____156. Double pneumonia is pneumonia that is twice as severe as regular pneumonia.

_____157. Tuberculosis is caused by a virus.

_____158. The suffix -pnea means breathing.

Essay

Write your answer in the space provided or on a separate sheet of paper.

159. What role does surfactant play in respiratory distress syndrome?

160. Explain why a barrel chest is found in advanced emphysema.

161. Explain the differences between a tracheotomy and a tracheostomy and what they are used for.

162. What are bronchodilator drugs and what type of patient are they used for?

163. What are mast cell stabilizer drugs and what are they used for?

164. Trace the flow of air through the respiratory system.

165. What is the pleura?

CHAPTER 5

Multiple Choice

Choose the one alternative that best completes the statement or answers the question.

1. In a physical assessment, the heart rate is determined by palpating the pulse in the _____ artery in the wrist.
   a. axillary
   b. brachial
   c. radial
   d. ulnar

2. Acute coronary syndrome includes all of the following conditions except:
   a. unstable angina.
   b. acute endocarditis.
   c. acute myocardial ischemia.
   d. acute myocardial infarction.

3. The valve located between the right atrium and right ventricle is the:
   a. tricuspid valve.
   b. pulmonary valve.
   c. mitral valve.
   d. bicuspid valve.

4. When the levels are elevated, which lab test is not diagnostic of an acute myocardial infarction?
   a. CPK-MB
   b. LDH
   c. LDL
   d. troponin

5. Which surgical procedure is done to provide the myocardium with a new source of blood supply when a coronary artery is occluded?
   a. cardiopulmonary bypass
   b. cardioversion
   c. coronary artery bypass graft
   d. electrocardiography

6. Which is a chronic condition in which the enlarged heart cannot pump sufficient amounts of oxygenated blood to the body?
   a. arteriosclerotic heart disease
   b. orthostatic hypotension
   c. angina pectoris
   d. congestive heart failure

7. Which measurement is a reading from a sphygmomanometer?
   a. 120/80 mm Hg
   b. 200 mg/dl
   c. 80 BPM
   d. S1 and S2 normal

8. Tests revealed that Mrs. Roger's mitral valve does not close properly, causing a back flow of blood through it. The medical word to describe this valve problem is:
   a. extravasation.
   b. compensation.
   c. regurgitation.
   d. bruit.

9. In the pathway of the flow of blood through the heart, oxygenated blood returns from the lungs and enters the:
   a. right atrium.
   b. right ventricle.
   c. left atrium.
   d. left ventricle.

10. Myocardial ischemia from the coronary arteries being partially blocked with atherosclerosis will cause:
    a. elevated blood pressure readings.
    b. chest pain.
    c. slowed heart rate.
    d. shortness of breath.

11. The medical procedure sclerotherapy is performed to treat:
    a. varicose veins.
    b. coronary atherosclerosis.
    c. peripheral artery disease.
    d. thrombophlebitis.

12. A defibrillator would be used for which condition?
    a. sick sinus syndrome
    b. first-degree heart block
    c. mitral valve prolapse
    d. ventricular fibrillation

13. Pericarditis, an accumulation of fluid in the pericardial sac, can lead to cardiac _____, a condition in which the fluid presses on the heart and stops it from beating.
    a. bigeminy
    b. bruit
    c. diastole
    d. tamponade

14. Which is a very serious type of heart block in which no impulses are conducted to the ventricles?
    a. left bundle branch block
    b. sick sinus syndrome
    c. trigemy
    d. third-degree AV block

15. Which is a feature of rheumatic heart disease?
    a. cardiac arrest
    b. valve vegetations and stenosis
    c. tachycardia
    d. transposition of the great vessel

16. The patient with left-sided heart failure would most likely be treated with two types of drugs: diuretics to remove water accumulation in the tissues and _____ to strengthen heart contractions.
    a. antibiotic drugs
    b. aspirin
    c. digitalis drugs
    d. thrombolytic drugs

17. The patient had an aneurysmectomy with insertion of a graft for the condition described as a/an:
    a. artery occluded with plaque.
    b. area of weakness in the wall of an artery.
    c. diseased heart valve.
    d. incompetent valve of a large vein.

18. Which is a sign of peripheral artery disease?
    a. low blood pressure
    b. arrhythmia
    c. phlebitis
    d. intermittent claudication

19. The section of the electrical conduction system of the heart that is located just after the AV node is the:
    a. Purkinje fibers.
    b. sinoatrial node.
    c. bundle of His.
    d. bundle branches.
20. Which condition requires an insertion of a permanent cardiac pacemaker?
    a. murmur
    b. atrial septal defect
    c. sick sinus syndrome
    d. cor pulmonale
21. Mrs. Jean Bentley came to the doctor with jugular vein distention and peripheral edema. Her diagnosis most likely is:
    a. hypotension.
    b. arrhythmia.
    c. second-degree heart block.
    d. right-sided heart failure.
22. The patient is in the emergency department with an occluded coronary artery due to a thrombus. Which type of drug will be administered to break apart this clot and restore circulation in the artery?
    a. drug for hyperlipidemia
    b. aspirin
    c. thrombolytic drug
    d. digoxin (Lanoxin)
23. The tetralogy of Fallot is a set of four defects one of which is:
    a. a narrowed pulmonary valve.
    b. vegetations.
    c. heart block.
    d. edema.
24. Which test could provide information to determine the extent of coronary artery narrowing?
    a. cardiac catheterization
    b. lipid profile
    c. electrocardiogram
    d. electrophysiologic study
25. Telemetry alerts ICU nursing personnel of what event?
    a. prolapsed heart valve
    b. hypertensive crisis
    c. deep venous thrombosis
    d. cardiac arrest
26. The cardiovascular system consists of the heart and:
    a. lungs.
    b. brain.
    c. blood vessels.
    d. skin.

27. How many chambers are inside the heart?
    a. one
    b. two
    c. three
    d. four
28. The mitral valve is located between the:
    a. left atrium and the left ventricle.
    b. left ventricle and the aorta.
    c. right atrium and the right ventricle.
    d. right ventricle and the pulmonary artery.
29. Which layer of the heart is known as the muscular layer?
    a. myocardium
    b. epicardium
    c. pericardium
    d. endocardium
30. The largest artery in the body is the:
    a. coronary artery.
    b. aorta.
    c. carotid artery.
    d. pulmonary artery.
31. Where is the peroneal artery located?
    a. upper leg
    b. behind the knee
    c. front aspect of the lower arm
    d. lateral aspect of the lower leg
32. Which type of blood vessel carries blood back to the heart?
    a. artery
    b. arteriole
    c. vein
    d. capillary
33. The abbreviation SA stands for:
    a. systole node.
    b. sinoatrial node.
    c. sinus node.
    d. systemic node.
34. Which is a neurotransmitter for the sympathetic nervous system that increases the heart rate to prepare for exercise or the fight or flight response?
    a. potassium
    b. calcium
    c. epinephrine
    d. acetylcholine
35. Any disease condition of the heart muscle that includes heart enlargement and heart failure is called:
    a. angina pectoris.
    b. myocardial infarction.
    c. arrhythmia.
    d. cardiomyopathy.

36. The abbreviation MI stands for:
    a. myocardial infarction.
    b. myocardial ischemia.
    c. myocardial inflammation.
    d. myocardial injury.
37. Inflammation and bacterial infection of the inner lining of the heart and valves is called:
    a. pericarditis.
    b. endocarditis.
    c. necrosis.
    d. peripheral edema.
38. Which of the following is not a congenital abnormality that can occur in the fetal heart as it develops?
    a. foramen ovale
    b. atrial septal defect (ASD)
    c. ventricular septal defect (VSD)
    d. tetralogy of Fallot
39. Which word is derived from a Greek word meaning dilation?
    a. tachycardia
    b. arteriosclerosis
    c. aneurysm
    d. murmur
40. Which word means elevated blood pressure?
    a. hypercholesterolemia
    b. hypocholesterolemia
    c. hypertension
    d. hypotension
41. Which is a sudden, severe vasoconstriction and spasm of the arterioles in the fingers and toes, often triggered by cold or emotional upset?
    a. Raynaud's phenomenon
    b. phlebitis
    c. hypotension
    d. peripheral artery disease
42. The abbreviation CRP stands for:
    a. cardiac reactive protein.
    b. C-reactive protein.
    c. cardiopulmonary resuscitation.
    d. none of the above
43. The combing form tele/o- means:
    a. distant.
    b. destroy.
    c. separate.
    d. close.
44. Which is a radiologic procedure in which a catheter is placed in the femoral artery and threaded to the aorta, then into the heart?
    a. aortography
    b. echocardiography
    c. venography
    d. coronary angiography

45. Which nuclear medicine procedure is also known as a radionuclide ventriculography (RNV) or gated blood pool scan?
    a. echocardiography
    b. electrocardiography
    c. multiple-gated acquisition (MUGA) scan
    d. single-photon emission computed tomography (SPECT) scan
46. Which ultasonography images the flow of blood in the arteries?
    a. Doppler
    b. echocardiography
    c. thallium stress test
    d. ventriculography
47. Which is not a vital sign?
    a. temperature
    b. apex
    c. respirations
    d. pulse
48. The combining form transplant/o- means:
    a. to establish an opening.
    b. pertaining to.
    c. internal, within.
    d. to move something to another place.
49. What structure divides the heart into right and left halves?
    a. atria
    b. ventricle
    c. septum
    d. mediastinum
50. What are the ropelike structures at the bases of the tricuspid and aortic valves?
    a. pericardium
    b. chordae tendinae
    c. ventricles
    d. interventricular septum
51. The heart has several layers and membranes, each with its own specialized function. Which of the following is the muscular layer of the heart?
    a. myocardium
    b. endocardium
    c. epicardium
    d. pericardium
52. The first arteries to branch off of the aorta feed the heart muscle itself. These arteries are called:
    a. common carotid arteries.
    b. pulmonary arteries.
    c. subclavian arteries.
    d. coronary arteries.
53. The smallest blood vessel in the body is the:
    a. aorta.
    b. venule.
    c. arteriole.
    d. capillary.

54. Which is the area of specialized nervous tissue in the heart that is known as the pacemaker of the heart?
    a. Purkinje fibers
    b. sinoatrial node
    c. atrioventricular node
    d. bundle of His
55. A period of unresponsiveness during a normal heartbeat is called:
    a. refractory period.
    b. repolarization.
    c. asystole.
    d. heart block.
56. Which is a temporary small blood vessel that connects the pulmonary artery to the aorta in the fetal heart?
    a. foramen ovale
    b. mediastinum
    c. ductus arteriosus
    d. popliteal artery
57. Mild-to-severe chest pain caused by ischemia of the myocardium is called:
    a. cardiomegaly.
    b. cardiomyopathy.
    c. congestive heart failure.
    d. angina pectoris.
58. What is inflammation and bacterial infection of the inner lining of the heart and the valves called?
    a. pericarditis
    b. myocarditis
    c. endocarditis
    d. stenosis
59. Which term means located within the ventricle?
    a. cardiac
    b. interventricular
    c. intraventricular
    d. interatrial
60. Bicuspid means:
    a. 3 heads.
    b. 2 valves.
    c. 2 cusps.
    d. in the middle.
61. Which is the partitioning wall that divides the heart into right and left halves?
    a. septum
    b. valve
    c. apex
    d. chordae tendineae
62. Which serous membrane covers the outer surface of the myocardium?
    a. pericardium
    b. epicardium

c. endocardium
d. chordae tendineae
63. Which structure secretes pericardial fluid, a slippery, watery fluid that allows the two membranes of the pericardial sac to slide smoothly past one another?
    a. pericardial sac
    b. epicardial sac
    c. endocardium
    d. myocardium
64. Which word reflects the relationship of the heart and the chest cavity?
    a. thoracic
    b. cardiothoracic
    c. cardiac
    d. mediastinal
65. Which word means the central opening in a vessel through which fluid flows?
    a. vasculature
    b. lumen
    c. intima
    d. artery
66. Vasoconstriction causes the blood pressure to:
    a. go up.
    b. go down.
    c. remain the same.
    d. pulsate.
67. The femoral artery delivers blood to the:
    a. arm.
    b. head.
    c. trunk.
    d. leg.
68. Which artery is behind the knee?
    a. iliac
    b. renal
    c. brachial
    d. popliteal
69. All of the following structures are part of the electrical system of the heart EXCEPT:
    a. SA node.
    b. bundle of His.
    c. HDL.
    d. AV node.
70. The opening of a blood vessel through which the blood flows is a:
    a. lumen.
    b. capillary.
    c. Purkinje fiber.
    d. plaque.
71. Angina pectoris is to myocardial infarction as:
    a. plaque is to EKG.
    b. bradycardia is to cholesterol.
    c. varicose veins is to CABG.
    d. ischemia is to cell death.

72. Inflammation of the membrane surrounding the heart is known as:
    a. valvulitis.
    b. pericarditis.
    c. mitral stenosis.
    d. phlebitis.
73. The right side of the heart is divided from the left side of the heart by the:
    a. coronary arteries.
    b. valves.
    c. capillaries.
    d. septum.
74. The P wave or QRS complex are related to:
    a. the circulation of the blood.
    b. the diastolic pressure.
    c. an electrocardiogram.
    d. an aneurysm.
75. The cause of essential hypertension is:
    a. unknown.
    b. mitral stenosis.
    c. congestive heart failure.
    d. palpitation.
76. An aneurysm is:
    a. an embolus.
    b. a weak spot in the artery wall.
    c. an abnormally slow heart rate.
    d. bad cholesterol.
77. Congestive heart failure involving the right side of the heart would be evident in the body as:
    a. hypertension.
    b. tachycardia.
    c. hemostasis.
    d. edematous feet.
78. Which is the medical word that means pertaining to within the ventricle?
    a. interventricular
    b. intraventricular
    c. atrioventricular
    d. none of the above
79. Which is the PMI where auscultation of the heart is done?
    a. apex
    b. myocardium
    c. endocardium
    d. great vessels
80. The purpose of the coronary arteries is to bring oxygenated blood to the:
    a. aorta.
    b. heart.
    c. lungs.
    d. mediastinum.

81. Which artery brings oxygenated blood to the brain, head, and face?
    a. jugular
    b. coronary
    c. carotid
    d. pulmonary
82. All of the following arteries carry oxygenated blood to the arm EXCEPT the _____ artery.
    a. popliteal
    b. axillary
    c. radial
    d. brachial
83. The abdominal aorta divides into the:
    a. carotid arteries.
    b. peroneal arteries.
    c. brachial arteries.
    d. iliac arteries.
84. Systemic circulation refers to the flow of blood to the:
    a. body.
    b. heart.
    c. lungs.
    d. all of the above
85. The normal small opening in the fetal heart that closes at birth is known as the:
    a. sinoatrial node.
    b. bundle of His.
    c. foramen ovale.
    d. lumen.
86. Cardiomegaly is the medical word for:
    a. heart attack.
    b. heart enlargement.
    c. irregular heartbeat.
    d. heart failure.
87. Plaque on the arterial walls is characteristic of:
    a. varicose veins.
    b. atherosclerosis.
    c. hypertension.
    d. congestive heart failure.
88. Which of the following is commonly called "good cholesterol"?
    a. HDL
    b. CHF
    c. LDL
    d. ASCVD
89. Using sound waves to create an image of the heart is known as:
    a. electrocardiography.
    b. auscultation.
    c. Holter monitor.
    d. echocardiography.

90. The combining form ven/o- has the same meaning as the combining form:
    a. phleb/o-.
    b. cardi/o-.
    c. arteri/o-.
    d. valvul/o-.

91. In the medical word arteriosclerosis, the combining form scler/o- means:
    a. heart chamber.
    b. narrowness.
    c. hard.
    d. artery.

92. Defibrillation is a way to:
    a. listen to the heart sounds.
    b. open an artery narrowed with plaque.
    c. create an image of the heart.
    d. treat a serious arrhythmia.

93. All of the following combining forms means blood vessel EXCEPT:
    a. vas/o-.
    b. angi/o-.
    c. vascul/o-.
    d. ather/o-.

94. Which word is misspelled?
    a. hypertriglyceridemia
    b. arhythmia
    c. aneurysmectomy
    d. sphygmomanometer

95. All of the following abbreviations refer to diseases of the blood vessels EXCEPT:
    a. PVD.
    b. CAD.
    c. HTN.
    d. HDL.

96. The abbreviation for which surgery is pronounced as "cabbage"?
    a. coronary artery bypass graft
    b. heart transplantation
    c. aneurysmectomy
    d. anastomosis

Short Answer

Write the word or phrase that best completes each statement or answers the question.

97. Enlargement of the heart is known as _____.

98. The _____ arteries supply blood to the myocardium.

99. Complete absence of a heartbeat is called _____.

100. The largest artery in the body is the _____; the two largest veins are the _____.

101. The Holter monitor is a type of portable device used to assess heart activity on a 24-hour basis by performing continuous _____.

102. A heart rate in the adult that is under 60 beats per minute is known as _____.

103. In a coronary artery bypass graft a part of the _____ vein is harvested from the leg and inserted into the myocardial coronary system.

104. _____ phenomenon occurs when there is a severe spasm and vasoconstriction in the fingers and toes, causing them to appear blue.

105. The abbreviation ASHD stands for _____ _____ _____.

106. The common _____ arteries carry blood to the head, brain, and face.

107. Structures that help regulate the blood flow between the atria and the ventricles are called the heart _____.

108. _____ is the process of listening to heart sounds with a stethoscope.

109. The _____ contains the pericardial sac that contains the heart, the great vessels, the thymus, and the trachea.

110. The sinoatrial (SA) node is also known as the _____ of the heart.

111. A neurotransmitter called _____ overrides the normal sinus rhythm causing the heart to beat faster during the "fight or flight" response.

112. _____ is the general word that describes enlargement of the heart, usually due to congestive heart failure.

113. A baby with an atrial septal defect has a hole in the interatrial _____.

114. _____ is an arrhythmia in which the heart beats too slowly.

115. A _____ contraction is an arrhythmia in which there are one or more extra contractions before the regular contraction.

116. An area of dilation and weakness in the wall of an artery is called a/an _____.

117. _____ is the study of the heart.

118. The _____ valve is located between the right atrium and the right ventricle.

119. The _____ valve is located between the left atrium and the left ventricle.

120. The _____ is the muscular layer that makes up the bulk of the heart.

121. The _____ is the specialized smooth cellular layer that lines the chambers of the heart and the heart valves.

122. The thoracic cavity contains the lungs and the _____, an irregularly shaped central area between the lungs.

123. _____ refers to the network of blood vessels associated with a particular organ.

124. All blood vessels are lined with _____, a smooth inner layer that promotes the flow of blood.

125. The smallest branches of an artery are known as _____.

126. All arteries have smooth muscle in their walls. When this smooth muscle contracts, the lumen of the artery decreases in size. This process is called _____.

127. The _____ arteries are the first arteries to branch off from the aorta.

128. The cardiac cycle consists of a contraction, known as _____, and a rest phase while the heart fills, known as _____.

129. A _____ is a physician who specializes in diagnosing and treating diseases of the heart.

130. _____ _____ is the medical word for a heart attack.

131. _____ is the medical specialty that studies the heart and its diseases and treatments.

132. The suffix -plasty in the medical word valvoplasty means _____ _____ _____ _____ _____.

133. The painting "The Starry Night" by Vincent van Gogh shows yellow halos around the stars that might be evidence of toxicity from the drug _____.

134. Tachycardia is the opposite of _____.

135. The patient had surgery to excise or remove a weakness in the wall of an artery. This surgery is known as a/an _____.

True/False

Write 'T' if the statement is true and 'F' if the statement is false.

_____136. The cause of the most common type of hypertension, essential hypertension, is unknown.

_____137. The atrioventricular node, or pacemaker, initiates the electrical impulse that begins each heartbeat.

_____138. In a blood pressure reading, systole, the upper number, represents the force of contraction of the ventricles.

_____139. A Doppler test is performed to stress the heart when the patient cannot do a treadmill exercise stress test.

_____140. When a patient feels the uncomfortable sensation of his heart thumping, this condition is called palpations.

_____141. Paroxysmal means a sudden or sharp attack.

_____142. The epicardium is the innermost layer of the heart that lines the heart chambers and valves.

_____143. Beta blockers, calcium channel blockers, and ACE inhibitors are various types of medications that can be used to treat essential hypertension.

_____144. AMI stands for acute mitral insufficiency.

_____145. The MUGA is a nuclear medicine test that evaluates how well the ventricular wall of the heart moves when it contracts.

_____146. A heart murmur is a normal sound that the heart makes when it is contracting.

_____147. In a patient with mitral valve prolapse, blood flows backwards into the left atrium, known as regurgitation.

_____148. Bradycardia, tachycardia, heart block, and flutter are all considered cardiac arrhythmias.

_____149. A patient presents to the emergency department having an acute anxiety attack and headache. When she is examined, her blood pressure is found to be 166/100. It can be said the she is hypotensive.

_____150. An elevated cholesterol level is known as hyperlipidemia.

_____151. Cardiac enzymes are enzymes that are released into the blood when myocardial cells are damaged or die.

_____152. A cardiac catheterization can only be done to diagnose a problem with the left side of the heart.

_____153. During angiography, a radiopaque dye is injected into a blood vessel to coat and outline it and the other nearby blood vessels.

_____154. Sclerotherapy is a medical procedure in which a sclerosing drug is injected into a varicose vein.

_____155. Antihypertensive drugs are used to treat low blood pressure.

_____156. The serous membrane that folds back on itself to form a pouch around the heart is known as the bundle of His.

_____157. The endothelium is the smooth inner lining of the heart chambers.

_____158. All arteries carry blood that contains a high level of oxygen.

_____159. The largest artery in the body is the pulmonary artery.

_____160. The symptoms of angina pectoris can be different in men than in women.

_____161. A Holter monitor is used to check the patient's heart rate at home for 24 hours.

_____162. The heart muscle gets the oxygenated blood it needs from the blood within its four chambers.

_____163. Triglycerides are known as "good" cholesterol.

_____164. A prolapse of a heart valve occurs when it becomes thickened and hardened.

_____165. During angina pectoris, there is severe pain and the cells of the heart muscle die.

_____166. Auscultation is using a stethoscope to listen to heart sounds.

Essay

Write your answer in the space provided or on a separate sheet of paper.

167. Explain why ventricular fibrillation is life threatening.

168. How is myocardial blood flow improved with a PTCA?

169. Both HDL and LDH are abbreviations for cardiac laboratory tests, but they are ordered for different reasons. Why is each test ordered?

170. How does aspirin help heart patients?

171. What are calcium channel blocker drugs and what are they used for?

172. Briefly describe the pulmonary circulation.

173. Briefly describe the electrical pathway and the major parts of the electrical conduction system of the heart.

174. What is angina pectoris?

CHAPTER 6

Multiple Choice

Choose the one alternative that best completes the statement or answers the question.

1. Pancytopenia could be found in a patient with:
   a. septicemia.
   b. lymphadenopathy.
   c. aplastic anemia.
   d. iron deficiency anemia.

2. The Bence Jones protein is found in the blood or urine of a patient with:
   a. infectious mononucleosis.
   b. multiple myeloma.
   c. anemia.
   d. AIDS.

3. The patient with lymphoma or leukemia could receive which medical treatment with the intent to put this cancer into remission?
   a. bone marrow transplantation
   b. blood transfusion
   c. prothrombin time
   d. excisional biopsy

4. A patient is receiving cancer chemotherapy. To help to prevent her red blood cell count from decreasing as a result of the chemotherapy, she is taking:
   a. vitamin B_{12}.
   b. Procrit.
   c. Cytoxan.
   d. anticoagulant.

5. Which is a severe blood clotting disorder in which blood clots form, which consume the clotting substances so the patient also has bleeding from several body sites?
   a. hemophilia A
   b. AIDS
   c. disseminated intravascular coagulation
   d. mononucleosis

6. Heterophil antibody test can aid in the diagnosis of:
   a. infectious mononucleosis.
   b. HIV infection.
   c. septicemia.
   d. candidiasis.

7. A deficiency in which nutritional substances obtained from the diet can cause an anemia?
   a. calcium and vitamin K
   b. magnesium and vitamin C
   c. zinc and vitamin A
   d. folic acid and vitamin B_{12}

8. The physician ordered blood work for his patient to include red blood cell indices. This test would include determining the:
   a. WBC count.
   b. mean cell volume.
   c. clotting time.
   d. blood type.

9. The patient who has _____ will be taking medications such as Invirase and Retrovir.
   a. PTT
   b. CBC
   c. PMN
   d. AIDS

10. One of the most abundant plasma proteins that keeps water from flowing into surrounding tissues of the body is:
    a. albumin.
    b. ferritin.
    c. bilirubin.
    d. bicarbonate.

11. John has classic hemophilia or hemophilia A. He requires treatment with factor _____ to avert abnormal bleeding.
    a. I
    b. II
    c. VIII
    d. X

12. If a person has had a splenectomy, he has lost an organ that:
    a. produces lymphocytes.
    b. stores whole blood.
    c. manufactures blood proteins.
    d. releases histamine.

13. The patient appeared pale and complained of being tired. Examination of her blood showed microcytic, hypochromic red blood cells. Her condition most likely is:
   a. pernicious anemia.
   b. leukemia.
   c. hemorrhage.
   d. iron deficiency anemia.

14. A patient with type B blood was accidentally given a transfusion of type A blood. Red blood cells were destroyed as a result. This is known as:
   a. hemolysis.
   b. hemostasis.
   c. homeostasis.
   d. coagulation.

15. The source of passive immunity that a mother gives to her infant through breast milk is known as:
   a. IgA.
   b. IgD.
   c. IgM.
   d. IgE.

16. The virus that causes AIDS invades the _____ and uses them for replication.
   a. CD4 cells
   b. T cell lymphocytes
   c. helper T cells
   d. all of the above

17. Patients on heparin will have a higher than normal value for _____ in their blood.
   a. thrombocytes
   b. partial thromboplastin
   c. hemoglobin
   d. mean cell volume

18. The patient came to the clinic with a sore throat and a fever. If he has a bacterial infection, which cell in his body would perform phagocytosis to engulf and destroy the bacteria?
   a. myelocytes
   b. eosinophils
   c. neutrophils
   d. thrombocytes

19. Select the lab test that reports the percentage of red blood cells in a sample of blood.
   a. HCT
   b. HLA
   c. PTT
   d. PMN

20. Post-surgical patients may be given heparin because they run the risk of developing:
   a. lymphadenopathy.
   b. thrombocytopenia.
   c. infection.
   d. deep vein thrombosis.

21. The Shilling test is done to diagnose:
   a. sickle cell anemia.
   b. pernicious anemia.
   c. AIDS.
   d. mononucleosis.

22. Which is a type of anemia with a genetic problem in the structure of hemoglobin that causes abnormally shaped red blood cells?
   a. polycythemia vera
   b. erythroblastosis fetalis
   c. sickle cell anemia
   d. pernicious anemia

23. Which is the medical word for the process of separating out one specific type of blood cell from donated blood?
   a. aggregation
   b. apheresis
   c. cross matching
   d. transfusion

24. The physician ordered the blood test ferritin to assist in making the diagnosis of:
   a. AIDS.
   b. pernicious anemia.
   c. iron deficiency anemia.
   d. septicemia.

25. Sickle cells belong to which red blood cell morphology category?
   a. anisocytosis
   b. thrombocytes
   c. pancytopenia
   d. poikilocytosis

26. Which is the process that occurs in the red marrow of long or flat bones by which all blood cells are formed?
   a. hematopoiesis
   b. erythogenesis
   c. metabolism
   d. hemostasis

27. Which is the fluid portion of the plasma that remains when clotting factors in the plasma are activated to form a blood clot?
   a. hemoglobin
   b. serum
   c. hemoglobulin
   d. heparin

28. Which is the most common leukocyte, comprising 40% to 60% of the leukocytes in the blood?
   a. neutrophils
   b. eosinophils
   c. basophils
   d. monocytes

29. Which cells are active in the blood clotting process?
    a. leukocytes
    b. erythrocytes
    c. thrombocytes
    d. white blood cells

30. A person with type A blood has:
    a. both A and B antigens on their erythrocytes.
    b. neither A nor B antigens on their erythrocytes.
    c. B antigens on their erythrocytes.
    d. A antigens on their erythrocytes

31. Which blood type is known as the universal donor?
    a. type A
    b. type B
    c. type AB
    d. type O

32. The combining form aggreg/o- means:
    a. clotting.
    b. fiber.
    c. crowding together.
    d. release.

33. Microorganisms, such as bacteria, viruses, protozoa, fungi, or yeast that invade the body are known as:
    a. tumors.
    b. pathogens.
    c. interferon.
    d. immunoglobins.

34. The body's continuing immune response and defense against pathogens it has seen before is known as:
    a. active immunity.
    b. passive immunity.
    c. immunoglobins.
    d. toxic immunity.

35. Which antibody is found in B cells?
    a. IgA
    b. IgD
    c. IgE
    d. IgG

36. There are _____ different classes of immunoglobins.
    a. seven
    b. ten
    c. four
    d. five

37. Which is a very large cell whose cytoplasm breaks away at the edges to form individual thrombocytes?
    a. megakaryoblast
    b. macrophage
    c. megakaryocyte
    d. monocyte

38. Which is a condition in which the number of erythrocytes in the blood is decreased?
    a. poikilocytosis
    b. Hodgkins' disease
    c. leukemia
    d. anemia

39. Which type of anemia is caused by failure of the bone marrow to produce erythrocytes?
    a. iron deficiency anemia
    b. aplastic anemia
    c. pernicious anemia
    d. sickle cell anemia

40. An increase in the number of erythrocytes is known as:
    a. polycythemia vera.
    b. leukemia.
    c. anemia.
    d. embolism.

41. Which medical word is used to refer to cancer of the white blood cells?
    a. leukemia
    b. anemia
    c. multiple myeloma
    d. adenocarcinoma

42. Which infectious disease is caused by the Epstein-Barr virus (EBV)?
    a. multiple myeloma
    b. AIDS
    c. mononucleosis
    d. hemophilia

43. Which is a blood test performed to monitor the effectiveness of the anticoagulant heparin when it is given in high doses to cardiac surgery patients?
    a. total prothrombin time (TPT)
    b. prothrombin time (PT)
    c. partial thromboplastin time (PTT)
    d. activated clotting time (ACT)

44. Which medical procedure involves the separation of plasma from the blood cells in whole blood?
    a. stem cell transplantation
    b. plasmapheresis
    c. blood donation
    d. blood transfusion

45. Which type of drug is given to suppress the immune response and decrease inflammation?
    a. chemotherapy drug
    b. immunosuppressant drug
    c. anticoagulant drug
    d. corticosteroid drug

46. The process by which all blood cells are formed is:
    a. hematology.
    b. erythrocyte.
    c. hemoglobin.
    d. hematopoiesis.

47. The fluid portion of the blood is the:
    a. plasma.
    b. lymphocyte.
    c. thymus.
    d. erythroblast.

48. Which is the most numerous type of blood cell?
    a. erythrocyte
    b. plasma cell
    c. leukocyte
    d. macrophage

49. Which of the following is not a type of leukocyte?
    a. erythrocyte
    b. neutrophil
    c. eosinophil
    d. basophil

50. Thrombocytes or platelets are active in which process?
    a. carrying oxygen
    b. fighting infection
    c. immune response
    d. blood clotting

51. Which plasma protein is too large to pass through the wall of the blood vessel and helps keep water from moving out of the plasma into the surrounding tissues?
    a. electrolytes
    b. antigens
    c. albumin
    d. heparin

52. When an injury occurs, thrombocytes stick to the damaged area of the blood vessel wall and form clumps to block the blood flow. This process is known as:
    a. fibrin.
    b. thrombus.
    c. blood clot.
    d. aggregation.

53. The immune response can detect and destroy which of the following?
    a. bacteria, viruses, protozoa, and other microorganisms
    b. disease-causing fungi or yeasts
    c. cancer cells
    d. all of the above

54. Any disease condition involving the cells in the blood is called:
    a. pancytopenia.
    b. septicemia.
    c. blood dyscrasia.
    d. anisocytosis.

55. What blood test shows the abnormal blood cells of anemia?
    a. electrophoresis
    b. peripheral blood smear
    c. white blood count
    d. blood chemistries

56. A DVT is a/an:
    a. blood clot.
    b. lymph node.
    c. anemia.
    d. blood cell.

57. A deficiency in the number of thrombocytes due to exposure of the bone marrow to radiation, chemicals, or drugs is called:
    a. hemophilia.
    b. thrombocytopenia.
    c. anemia.
    d. ecchymosis.

58. A generalized swelling of an arm or a leg that occurs after surgical removal of a chain of lymph nodes is known as:
    a. swollen glands.
    b. anemia.
    c. lymphedema.
    d. lymphoma.

59. Agglutination means:
    a. swelling.
    b. painful.
    c. clumping together.
    d. diseased.

60. Which filters the lymph?
    a. lymph nodes
    b. heart valves
    c. lymph vessels
    d. thymus

61. Which is the clotting factor that is activated just before a thrombus is formed?
    a. prothrombin
    b. fibrinogen
    c. lymph
    d. ferritin

62. Thrombocytes stick to a damaged area of the blood vessel wall and form clumps to block the blood flow. What is this process called?
    a. platelet aggregation
    b. typing
    c. clotting
    d. homeostasis

63. Which are the smallest leukocytes?
    a. WBCs
    b. lymphocytes
    c. monocytes
    d. basophils
64. All of the following are true of the spleen EXCEPT:
    a. produces red blood cells.
    b. stores supplies of blood.
    c. recycles old red blood cells.
    d. contains lymphocytes.
65. Where do all lymphatic vessels end?
    a. at one main lymph node
    b. in the aorta
    c. in large veins in the neck
    d. in the heart
66. Where is the thymus located?
    a. posterior to the stomach
    b. superior to the heart
    c. near lymphatic capillaries
    d. posterior to the sternum
67. All of the following are specialized types of lymphocytes EXCEPT:
    a. natural killer (NK) cells.
    b. helper T cells.
    c. interleukin.
    d. suppressor T cells.
68. A red blood cell that is very small and abnormal is said to be:
    a. normocytic.
    b. microcytic.
    c. hypochromic.
    d. sickled.
69. The medical word hemolysis is associated with:
    a. AIDS.
    b. leukemia.
    c. transfusion reaction.
    d. thrombosis.
70. Leukemia is named according to the type of leukocyte that is most prevalent in the blood and whether:
    a. it is malignant or not.
    b. infection is also present.
    c. the onset was acute or chronic.
    d. there is also lymphadenopathy.
71. Hemophilia is caused by an abnormal gene on:
    a. chromosome Y carried by the father.
    b. factor VIII in the blood.
    c. chromosome X carried by the mother.
    d. malignant lymphocytes in the blood.

72. Blood that is collected, filtered, and returned to the patient during surgery is known as _____ blood.
    a. sickle cell
    b. plasma
    c. clotted
    d. autologous
73. Which word is misspelled?
    a. spleen
    b. spleenectomy
    c. splenic
    d. splenomegaly
74. Viscosity refers to the _____ of the blood.
    a. color
    b. pH
    c. thickness
    d. clotting time
75. Which word is misspelled?
    a. albumin
    b. hematopoiesis
    c. antiarrhythmic drug
    d. hematacrit
76. All of the following are electrolytes EXCEPT:
    a. bicarbonate.
    b. Rh factor.
    c. sodium.
    d. potassium.
77. All of the following are laboratory tests to detect HIV EXCEPT:
    a. WBC differential.
    b. CD4 count.
    c. ELISA.
    d. viral load test.
78. All of the following are types of leukemia EXCEPT:
    a. AML.
    b. PRBC.
    c. CLL.
    d. ALL.
79. Which of the following contains hemoglobin that transports oxygen to the cells?
    a. plasma
    b. blood type
    c. erythrocyte
    d. lymph
80. All of these help form a clot EXCEPT:
    a. thrombocytes.
    b. clotting factors.
    c. leukocytes.
    d. fibrin.

81. The combining form erythr/o- means:
  a. inflammation.
  b. red.
  c. cancer.
  d. white.
82. Leukemia is a/an:
  a. bacterial infection of the blood.
  b. enlargement of the spleen.
  c. cancer with too many white blood cells.
  d. type of parasite.
83. A pathogenic organism is one that causes:
  a. disease.
  b. allergy.
  c. lymph.
  d. anemia.
84. Anemia is characterized by:
  a. blood clots.
  b. bacterial infection of the blood.
  c. too few red blood cells.
  d. too many white blood cells.
85. Which type of anemia is due to genetics?
  a. sickle cell anemia
  b. pernicious anemia
  c. iron-deficient anemia
  d. thrombocytopenia
86. If you have a bad sore throat, the physician might find _____ on your physical exam.
  a. metastasis
  b. splenomegaly
  c. leukemia
  d. cervical lymphadenopathy
87. Enlargement of the axillary lymph nodes could be caused by:
  a. breast cancer.
  b. pernicious anemia.
  c. thrombus.
  d. hematoma.
88. A malignant tumor of the lymph nodes is known as:
  a. lymphoma.
  b. sarcoma.
  c. metastasis.
  d. melanoma.
89. T lymphocytes mature in the:
  a. spleen.
  b. liver.
  c. plasma.
  d. thymus.
90. A _____ is a very large cell with a great deal of cytoplasm that breaks into cell fragments called thrombocytes.
  a. megakaryoblast
  b. platelet

  c. megakaryocyte
  d. lymphocyte
91. The protein in plasma is known as:
  a. ferritin.
  b. sodium.
  c. albumin.
  d. potassium.
92. The antigens that express blood groups are surface proteins found on the cell membranes of:
  a. leukocytes.
  b. blood factors.
  c. thrombocytes.
  d. erythrocytes.
93. Anemia is a decrease in the number of:
  a. platelets.
  b. serum
  c. lymphocytes.
  d. erythrocytes.
94. Which of these blood disorders is inherited?
  a. AIDS
  b. sickle cell anemia
  c. hemophilia
  d. both B and C
95. The common name is the "kissing disease," but healthcare professionals know it as:
  a. iron deficiency anemia.
  b. mononucleosis.
  c. transfusion reaction.
  d. AIDS.
96. All of these are laboratory tests that measure how quickly the blood clots EXCEPT:
  a. PT.
  b. PTT.
  c. CD4 count.
  d. ACT.
97. You can obtain a sample of blood from patient by doing:
  a. phlebotomy.
  b. venipuncture.
  c. bone marrow aspiration.
  d. Both A and B

Short Answer

Write the word or phrase that best completes each statement or answers the question.

98. Alice has infectious mononucleosis. Her physician palpated the left upper quadrant of her abdomen to determine if she had enlargement of the spleen, which is also called _____ .

99. It is necessary to perform a _____ , also known as a venipuncture, to draw a sample of venous blood from a patient.

100. The fluid portion of blood is called _____ .

101. The extremely immature cell found in the red marrow that is the precursor to all types of blood cells is called a _____ cell.

102. Infectious mononucleosis is caused by the _____ virus.

103. Petechiae are small, pinpoint _____ seen under the skin.

104. The abbreviations CML and CLL stand for chronic myelogenous _____ and chronic lymphocytic _____ .

105. The molecules within the erythrocytes that bind to oxygen are known as _____ .

106. Diseases such as rheumatoid arthritis and type 1 diabetes mellitus are classified as _____ because these diseases are characterized by antibodies that the body makes against its own tissues.

107. _____ is the healthcare specialty that studies the anatomy and physiology of the blood.

108. The process by which all blood cells are formed is _____.

109. An immature erythrocyte is called a/an _____.

110. The most common type of leukocyte is a _____.

111. Because they are able to engulf large numbers of cells and cellular debris, monocytes are also known as _____.

112. Strong elastic strands of _____ trap erythrocytes and form a thrombus.

113. Nine proteins in the plasma that may be activated by the presence of bacteria, viruses, or parasites are known as _____ proteins.

114. _____ immunity is the type of immunity that is conveyed by the mother's antibodies to the fetus via the placenta by colostrum (first breast milk).

115. _____ means the study of the blood.

116. _____ is the study of the immune response.

117. The fluid portion of blood, _____, is a clear, straw-colored liquid that makes up about 55% of the total volume of blood.

118. When clotting factors in the plasma are activated to form a blood clot, the fluid portion of plasma that remains is known as _____ .

119. _____ are the most numerous type of blood cell.

120. _____ is a red, iron-containing molecule.

121. _____, the process by which all blood cells are formed, occurs in the red marrow of long or flat bones (such as the sternum, ribs, hip bones, bones of the spinal column, and the long bones of the legs).

122. Any time the body experiences a significant blood loss, the kidneys secrete _____ , a hormone that dramatically increases the speed at which erythrocytes are produced and become mature.

123. _____ are cells that engulf microorganisms and destroy them with enzymes.

124. _____ are the least common leukocyte.

125. _____ are the largest leukocytes.

126. Chemical elements in the blood that carry a positive or negative electrical charge are called _____.

127. Losing a large amount of blood is known as a _____.

128. A _____ is a type of white blood cell that is a granulocyte and has three or more lobes.

129. A _____ is a type of white blood cell that has very little cytoplasm and is an agranulocyte with a round nucleus.

130. _____ and _____ are the two structures that are shared by the blood and the lymphatic system.

131. The _____ is the organ that serves as a storage area for reserve supplies of blood.

True/False

Write 'T' if the statement is true and 'F' if the statement is false.

_____132. The process of forming red blood cells in the bone marrow is called hematopoiesis.

_____133. Mature neutrophils are also known as bands or stabs.

_____134. The person with type O blood is known as a universal blood donor because the erythrocytes do not have antigens against type A or B blood.

_____135. Reed-Sternberg cells are found in patients with multiple myeloma.

_____136. Immature erythrocytes found in small numbers in a sample of blood are called reticulocytes.

_____137. Mr. Smith had a myocardial infarction a few years ago. He now takes aspirin daily to dissolve any new blood clots that may have formed.

_____138. Hemostasis is the stopping of bleeding after the formation of a blood clot.

_____139. Lymphedema of the arm is a common complaint of patients after surgery for breast cancer.

_____140. Donated blood is tested with a MonoSpot test to prevent passing the AIDS virus on to the recipient of a blood transfusion.

_____141. Immunology is the medical specialty that studies the anatomy and physiology of the blood.

_____142. Hematopoiesis occurs in the red bone marrow of the long or flat bones.

_____143. The amount of plasma in the blood is not related to how much water is taken into the body.

_____144. When erythrocytes are mature, they do not have a nucleus.

_____145. Eosinophils are active in allergic reactions to pollen, insect bites, animal dander, and other allergens.

_____146. Monocytes are the largest of the leukocytes, but they can only handle small amounts of cellular debris.

_____147. An anticoagulant drug prevents the blood from clotting.

_____148. Thrombolytic enzyme drugs dissolve blood clots by inhibiting the production of vitamin K.

_____149. Immunosuppressant drugs are given to suppress the immune response.

_____150. Both protease inhibitors and reverse transcriptase inhibitors are antiviral drugs used to combat HIV infection or AIDS.

_____151. Lymphatic capillaries have large openings in their walls that allow microorganisms or cancerous cells to enter.

_____152. The lymphatic circulation follows a continuous, circular path like that of the circulatory system of the blood.

_____153. Lymphatic tissue includes the tonsils and adenoids in the posterior oral cavity.

_____154. Cytokines are chemicals released by damaged body tissues that summon white blood cells to the area of injury.

_____155. Tumor necrosis factor destroys cancerous cells and endotoxins produced by certain bacteria.

_____156. The hematocrit laboratory test measures the total number of white blood cells in a blood sample.

_____157. An example of passive immunity is an immunization or a vaccination.

_____158. White blood cells are the most numerous cells in the blood.

_____159. Another name for a platelet is a thrombocyte.

_____160. Hemorrhage is the loss of a small amount of blood over time.

_____161. Leukemia is a cancer of the thrombocytes.

_____162. A, B, AB, BA, and O are blood types.

Essay

Write your answer in the space provided or on a separate sheet of paper.

163. What accounts for the episodes of severe pain in the extremities and abdomen in a patient with sickle cell anemia?

164. Why would a periodic phlebotomy be beneficial to the patient with polycythemia vera?

165. Describe what a phlebotomist does.

166. Briefly describe how the blood forms a clot.

167. Describe how a lymphangiography is performed.

168. What is a bone marrow aspiration test and why is it done?

169. What is a vaccination and why is it done?

170. What is the difference between a blood donation and a blood transfusion?

CHAPTER 7

Multiple Choice

Choose the one alternative that best completes the statement or answers the question.

1. The thick, crusty scar of necrotic tissue from a third-degree burn is called a/an:
   a. bulla.
   b. keloid.
   c. eschar.
   d. comedo.

2. Basal cell carcinoma arises from which type of tissue?
   a. squamous
   b. connective
   c. melanocytes
   d. epidermis

3. Which is the medical word for baldness?
   a. alopecia
   b. vitiligo
   c. folliculitis
   d. hirsutism

4. Which is a type of electrosurgery using a wire loop electrode to cut tissue?
   a. incision and drainage
   b. electrosection
   c. fulguration
   d. electrocoagulation

5. PUVA is used to treat:
   a. acne rosacea.
   b. acne vulgaris.
   c. psoriasis.
   d. vitiligo.

6. Which is the common term for a herpes simplex 1 infection?
   a. scabies
   b. cold sores
   c. blisters
   d. shingles

7. Which is not an allergic reaction?
   a. urticaria
   b. eczema
   c. scleroderma
   d. wheal

8. An I & D might be done to treat:
   a. laceration.
   b. shingles.
   c. psoriasis.
   d. furuncle.

9. A superficial skin wound such as a scratch would be a/an:
   a. excoriation.
   b. contusion.
   c. decubitus.
   d. cellulitis.

10. Sweat glands are also known as _____ glands.
   a. sebaceous
   b. adipose
   c. endocrine
   d. sudoriferous

11. Verrucae are caused by:
   a. viruses.
   b. bacteria.
   c. parasites.
   d. fungi.

12. The medical word for jock itch is tinea:
   a. corporis.
   b. pedis.
   c. cruris.
   d. capitus.

13. Dry skin is known as:
   a. eczema.
   b. keratosis.
   c. anhidrosis.
   d. xeroderma.

14. Acne vulgaris is characterized by papules, pustules, and:
   a. comedos.
   b. lipomas.
   c. bullae.
   d. macules.

15. An area of bleeding that occurs under the skin is known as:
   a. diaphoresis.
   b. ecchymosis.
   c. exudate.
   d. seborrhea.

16. The physician ordered a Tzanck test to aid in making the diagnosis of:
   a. squamos cell carcinoma.
   b. shingles.
   c. pediculosis.
   d. lupus erythematosus.

17. A keloid is an abnormally large scar due to excess:
   a. keratin.
   b. elastin.
   c. sebum.
   d. collagen.

18. When Mr. Smith was in the shower the hot water ran out. As the cold water poured on his body, the hairs on his skin stood up. This body response to cold is known as:
   a. exfoliation.
   b. piloerection.
   c. perspiration.
   d. anhidrosis.

19. If a patient has poor skin turgor, he has:
   a. a vitamin deficiency.
   b. dehydration.
   c. a lack of oxygen.
   d. jaundice.

20. Freckles or age spots are:
   a. furuncles.
   b. vesicles.
   c. macules.
   d. pustules.

21. The patient required _____ for the removal of his necrotic tissue from a wound.
   a. debridement
   b. dermabrasion
   c. Moh's surgery
   d. xenograft

22. Which surgical procedure is done for a cosmetic improvement to the aging face?
   a. autograft
   b. rhytidectomy
   c. dermabrasion
   d. curettage

23. White, depigmented areas of skin are called:
   a. albinism.
   b. pustules.
   c. pallor.
   d. vitiligo.

24. Pediculosis would be treated with:
   a. Accutane.
   b. Lotrimin.
   c. Zovirax.
   d. Nix.

25. Which healthcare specialty studies the anatomy and physiology of the integumentary system and uses diagnostic tests, medical and surgical procedures, and drugs to treat the integumentary diseases?
    a. neurology
    b. dermatology
    c. psychology
    d. oncology

26. The integumentary system covers the entire surface of the body and consists of the skin, hair, and:
    a. nails.
    b. eyes.
    c. ears.
    d. fingers.

27. The epidermis contains melanocytes, pigment cells that produce:
    a. keratin.
    b. melanin.
    c. collagen.
    d. elastin.

28. Which of the following does the dermis not contain?
    a. sweat glands
    b. nerves
    c. arteries
    d. keratin

29. The subcutaneous tissue is a loose, connective tissue located directly beneath the:
    a. epidermis.
    b. basal layer.
    c. dermis.
    d. adipose tissue.

30. Sebaceous glands are to oil glands as sudoriferous glands are to:
    a. sweat glands.
    b. endocrine glands.
    c. salivary glands.
    d. adrenal glands.

31. The combining form pil/o- means:
    a. sweat.
    b. sebum.
    c. skin.
    d. hair.

32. Which is a severe systemic allergic reaction that can be life threatening?
    a. local reaction
    b. allergen
    c. anaphylaxis
    d. allergy

33. Macule is derived from a Latin word that means a:
    a. dot.
    b. pimple.

c. spot.
d. nail.

34. Which is a general category for any type of skin lesion that is pink to red, flat or raised, pruritic or nonpruritic?
    a. neoplasm
    b. rash
    c. wound
    d. growth

35. A genetic mutation that results in nonfunctioning melanocytes that do not produce melanin is known as:
    a. albinism.
    b. cyanosis.
    c. jaundice.
    d. necrosis.

36. Irregular, reddened lines that become lighter and shiny as they heal and become scar tissue are called:
    a. linea nigra.
    b. vitiligo.
    c. keloids.
    d. striae.

37. Which of the following is not a type of burn?
    a. fourth degree
    b. third degree
    c. second degree
    d. first degree

38. An excessive, abnormally large scar is a:
    a. callus.
    b. corn.
    c. cicatrix.
    d. keloid.

39. Which is known as genital herpes?
    a. herpes whitlow
    b. herpes varicella-zoster.
    c. herpes simplex virus type 2
    d. herpes simplex virus type 1

40. Tinea, also known as ringworm, is named according to where it occurs on the body. Which one occurs in the groin and perineum?
    a. tinea pedis
    b. tinea corporis
    c. tinea cruris
    d. tinea capitis

41. Which is a benign, pigmented, flat macule that develops after sun exposure?
    a. freckle
    b. hives
    c. eschar
    d. lipoma

42. Which is a congenital abnormality in which there are extra fingers or toes?
    a. syndactyly
    b. polydactyly
    c. senile lentigo
    d. papilloma

43. Which one is not one of the four characteristics of a malignant melanoma?
    a. Border or edge is irregular and ragged.
    b. Color varies from black to brown to red in different patients.
    c. Diameter is variable and is growing.
    d. Each side of the lesion has a different shape (asymmetry).

44. The abbreviation SLE stands for:
    a. systemic lupus erythematosus.
    b. skin lesion enlargement.
    c. severe lupus erythematosus.
    d. senile lentigo eruption.

45. The medical name for split hair ends is:
    a. folliculitis.
    b. male pattern baldness.
    c. alopecia.
    d. schizotrichia.

46. Skin scraping is done to obtain fluid from within a vesicle and make a diagnosis. In which of the following is the smear made on a slide and then stained?
    a. Wood's lamp
    b. allergy skin testing
    c. Tzanck test
    d. C & S

47. Which process uses a chemical to remove the epidermis?
    a. dermabrasion
    b. microdermabrasion
    c. chemical peel
    d. laser skin resurfacing

48. Which surgical procedure uses a scalpel to remove an entire lesion?
    a. excisional biopsy
    b. incisional biopsy
    c. punch biopsy
    d. shave biopsy

49. Benadryl is a type of:
    a. antiviral drug.
    b. antipruritic drug.
    c. vitamin A-type drug.
    d. antifungal drug.

50. The healthcare specialty that studies the anatomy and physiology of the integumentary system is called:
    a. immunology.
    b. hematology.

51. The integumentary system consists of all of the following EXCEPT:
    a. skin.
    b. hair.
    c. nails.
    d. muscles.

52. The outermost layer of the skin is the:
    a. epidermis.
    b. dermis.
    c. collagen.
    d. subcutaneous.

53. The sebaceous glands are which type of gland?
    a. endocrine glands
    b. adipose glands
    c. exocrine glands
    d. keratin glands

54. Which is a life-threatening allergic reaction?
    a. local reaction
    b. systemic reaction
    c. hypersensitivity reaction
    d. anaphylaxis

55. A general word for any area of visible damage to the skin is:
    a. lesion.
    b. benign.
    c. malignant.
    d. dermatitis.

56. A patient was recently in contact with poison ivy. He is now experiencing severe itching. Another word for itching is:
    a. rash.
    b. pruritus.
    c. xeroderma.
    d. dermatitis.

57. Allergy skin testing is accomplished by what test?
    a. intradermal injection
    b. blood test
    c. culture and sensitivity
    d. skin scraping

58. A medical procedure that involves using a curette to scrape off the superficial part of a skin lesion is:
    a. cryosurgery.
    b. debridement.
    c. biopsy.
    d. curettage.

c. gastroenterology.
d. dermatology.

59. The use of a rapidly spinning wire brush or diamond surface to mechanically scrape the epidermis is:
    a. microdermabrasion.
    b. chemical peel.
    c. laser skin resurfacing.
    d. dermabrasion.

60. A biopsy which uses a small circular metal cutter to remove a plug-shaped core of skin is called:
    a. excisional biopsy.
    b. incisional biopsy.
    c. shave biopsy.
    d. punch biopsy.

61. An autoimmune disorder characterized by the production of excessive amounts of epidermal cells is known as:
    a. psoriasis.
    b. sarcoma.
    c. lupus.
    d. malignant melanoma.

62. An autoimmune disorder that causes the skin and internal organs to become progressively hardened is called:
    a. comedo.
    b. acne vulgaris.
    c. scleroderma.
    d. acne rosacea.

63. In _____, oily areas are interspersed with patches of dry, scaly skin and dandruff.
    a. seborrheic dermatitis
    b. anhidrosis
    c. diaphoresis
    d. alopecia

64. Schizotrichia is:
    a. malignancy.
    b. benign tumor.
    c. extra long nails.
    d. split ends on hair.

65. Onychomycosis is a:
    a. fungal infection of fingernails or toenails.
    b. bacterial infection of fingernails or toenails.
    c. loss of fingernails or toenails.
    d. fistula.

66. Abnormally curved fingernails and stunted growth of the fingers associated with a chronic lack of oxygen in patients with cystic fibrosis is known as:
    a. arthritis.
    b. curettage.
    c. clubbing.
    d. dermabrasion.

67. Removal of superficial and deep acne scars, fine or deep wrinkles, or tattoos, by means of topical chemicals, abrasion, or laser treatments is called:
    a. skin resurfacing.
    b. suturing.
    c. biopsy.
    d. skin graft.

68. A surgical procedure to remove all or part of a skin lesion for the purpose of diagnosis is called:
    a. biopsy.
    b. dermatoplasty.
    c. rhytidectomy.
    d. skin grafting.

69. What type of drug is used to treat ringworm?
    a. antiviral
    b. antibiotic
    c. antipruritic
    d. antifungal

70. The _____ route of medication administration uses a needle inserted just beneath the epidermis. This is used for the Mantoux tuberculosis test and allergy testing.
    a. intramuscular
    b. IV
    c. intradermal
    d. transdermal

71. Which type of burn does not cause blisters?
    a. first degree.
    b. second degree.
    c. third degree.
    d. All burns cause blisters.

72. Normal flora present on the skin are:
    a. areas of pigment variation due to melanocytes.
    b. present just in the hair follicles.
    c. bacteria that do not cause disease.
    d. none of the above

73. White hair in older people occurs because:
    a. melanin changes its pigment color.
    b. the hair follicles die.
    c. the skin becomes albino.
    d. melanocytes produce no melanin.

74. All of these patterns can be found on a fingerprint EXCEPT:
    a. follicles.
    b. loops.
    c. arches.
    d. whorls.

75. Adipocere is formed in:
    a. lipocytes in the fat.
    b. a dead body.
    c. the ridges of a fingerprint.
    d. the subcutaneous tissues.

76. Any inflammation of the skin is known as:
    a. a lesion
    b. edema.
    c. infection.
    d. dermatitis.
77. Which skin lesion is elevated and is semisolid or contains some fluid?
    a. pustule
    b. macule
    c. cyst
    d. fissure
78. A scale would be found in:
    a. acne.
    b. psoriasis.
    c. tinea pedis.
    d. shingles.
79. A sliding injury that pulls off the epidermis is known as a/an:
    a. abrasion.
    b. callus.
    c. hemorrhage.
    d. abscess.
80. Larger blisters that occur after a burn are:
    a. wheals.
    b. lacerations.
    c. bullae.
    d. ulcers.
81. In the phrase decubitus ulcer, decubitus means:
    a. tumor.
    b. deep sore.
    c. skin layer.
    d. lying down.
82. Large abscesses with connecting tunnels under the skin form a/an:
    a. caruncle.
    b. ulcer.
    c. laceration.
    d. lipoma.
83. Which herpes causes chickenpox?
    a. herpes simplex type 1
    b. herpes varicella-zoster
    c. herpes simplex type 2
    d. herpes whitlow
84. The same virus that causes chickenpox in children also causes this disease in older people.
    a. veruca
    b. xeroderma
    c. shingles
    d. basal cell carcinoma
85. Spandex, soaps, and detergents all can produce:
    a. actinic keratoses.
    b. contact dermatitis.

    c. squamous cell carcinoma.
    d. alopecia.
86. A congenital skin tumor composed of dilated blood vessels is known as a/an:
    a. hemorrhage.
    b. hematoma.
    c. hemangioma.
    d. malignant melanoma.
87. Examples of a nevus are:
    a. hemangioma and lipoma.
    b. freckle and macule.
    c. tinea corpora and warts.
    d. port-wine stain and moles.
88. AIDS patients often develop which skin malignancy?
    a. scleroderma
    b. Kaposi's sarcoma
    c. basal cell carcinoma
    d. malignant melanoma
89. A comedo is a:
    a. whitehead.
    b. wart.
    c. blackhead.
    d. freckle.
90. Severe acne rosacea that enlarges the nose is called:
    a. rhinophyma.
    b. alopecia.
    c. psoriasis.
    d. lipoma.
91. The medical word for the infant disease cradle cap is:
    a. alopecia.
    b. Kaposi's sarcoma
    c. eczema.
    d. onychomycosis.
92. Excessive sweating (due to a serious medical disease such as myocardial infarction) is known as:
    a. lipoma.
    b. diaphoresis.
    c. psoriasis.
    d. cellulitis.
93. A lipoma is a tumor composed of:
    a. fat.
    b. keratin.
    c. blood vessels.
    d. dermis.
94. Male pattern baldness is a type of:
    a. acne rosacea.
    b. dermatitis.
    c. lesion.
    d. alopecia.

95. Cryosurgery uses _____ to remove skin lesions.
    a. cold
    b. heat
    c. chemicals
    d. all of the above
96. A deep skin laceration is treated with:
    a. vitamin A-type drugs.
    b. liposuction.
    c. antiviral drugs.
    d. suturing.
97. A dermatome is:
    a. used to make a cut to form a skin graft.
    b. a skin area that sends sensory information to a spinal nerve.
    c. a surgical instrument.
    d. all of the above
98. Select the misspelled word.
    a. curettage
    b. eskar
    c. pruritus
    d. intradermal
99. Select the misspelled word.
    a. rytidectomy.
    b. vitiligo.
    c. wheal.
    d. cicatrix.
100. Which two combining forms mean nail?
    a. ungu/o- and onych/o-
    b. lip/o- and adip/o-
    c. pil/o- and trich/o-
    d. derm/o- and diaphor/o-
101. All of these combining forms means skin EXCEPT:
    a. cutane/o-.
    b. dermat/o-.
    c. adip/o-.
    d. integument/o-.
102. The epidermis is located _____ the dermis.
    a. below
    b. around
    c. within
    d. above
103. The constant shedding of dead skin cells is known as:
    a. subcutaneous.
    b. exfoliation.
    c. diaphoresis.
    d. shingles.
104. Alopecia is the opposite of:
    a. jaundice.
    b. an ulcer.
    c. hirsutism.
    d. anesthesia.
105. When oil secreted by the skin becomes hardened and dark it is known as:
    a. a follicle.
    b. a comedo.
    c. sebum.
    d. the lunula.
106. A disease of the skin in which the blood vessels of the face are dilated, the skin is very reddened, and the nose can become enlarged and knobby is called:
    a. acne vulgaris.
    b. diaphoresis.
    c. basal cell carcinoma.
    d. acne rosacea.
107. Which of these combining forms means dead?
    a. cutane/o-
    b. necr/o-
    c. seb/o-
    d. ungu/o-
108. Infestation with lice is known as:
    a. pediculosis.
    b. eschar.
    c. pruritus.
    d. cyanosis.
109. The loss of skin pigment in large patches is known as:
    a. cyanosis.
    b. ecchymosis.
    c. vitiligo.
    d. albinism.
110. A _____ is a regular scar, but a _____ is an excessive, overgrown scar.
    a. cicatrix; keloid
    b. blister; vesicle
    c. lipoma; carcinoma
    d. ulcer; nevus
111. Using a cannula to remove excess fatty tissue is known as:
    a. liposuction.
    b. cryosurgery.
    c. frozen section.
    d. skin graft.
112. Which of the following is true of the epithelium?
    a. It covers the external surface of the body as the skin
    b. It includes mucous membranes
    c. It lines body cavities
    d. all of the above

113. The hard, fibrous protein that fills epidermal cells is called:
   a. melanin.
   b. keratin.
   c. basal.
   d. sebum.

114. The thickest layer of the skin is the:
   a. epidermis.
   b. dermis.
   c. subcutaneous.
   d. none of the above

115. The dermis contains:
   a. melanin and keratin.
   b. arteries and veins.
   c. nerves.
   d. both b and c.

116. The layer of dead skin cells that arises from the epidermis around the base of the nail is called the:
   a. lunula.
   b. elastin.
   c. follicle.
   d. cuticle.

117. Cells from plants and animals can act as _____ to sensitive individuals.
   a. allergens
   b. dermatomes
   c. adipocere
   d. lesions

118. The definition of guarding or protecting refers to the combining form:
   a. phylact/o-.
   b. sensitive/o-.
   c. cutane/o-.
   d. lip/o-.

119. The combining form ungu/o- means:
   a. skin.
   b. oil gland.
   c. dermis.
   d. nail.

120. Which of these is a flat, pigmented spot?
   a. cyst
   b. scale
   c. pustule
   d. macule

121. A deep, penetrating skin wound is a/an:
   a. abscess.
   b. cicatrix.
   c. laceration.
   d. lipoma.

Short Answer

Write the word or phrase that best completes each statement or answers the question.

122. A xanthoma is a benign tumor that is the color _____.

123. The combining forms pertaining to the skin are derm/o- and _____.

124. Erythema is a word used to describe tissues that are _____ in color.

125. Onychomycosis is a fungal infection of the _____.

126. A general word for any visible disease or injury to the skin is called a skin _____.

127. Urticaria can also be called _____.

128. Cyanosis, icterus, and port wine stains all refer to _____ changes in the skin of the patient.

129. _____ is a complication of a superficial wound that becomes infected, presenting extensive involvement of skin and underlying connective tissues.

130. The patient's skin laceration healed nicely, leaving a _____ or scar.

131. The skin cancer that is assessed using the four characteristics, ABCD, is called _____ _____.

132. A/an _____ biopsy uses a scalpel to make an incision into part of a large lesion to remove a wedge of it.

133. _____ is a surgical procedure for any type of plastic surgery of the skin.

134. A/an _____ is a skin graft taken from another part of the patient's body.

135. Coal tar drugs are used to treat _____.

136. The _____ is the thin, outermost layer of the skin.

137. _____ are pigmented epidermal cells that contain a dark brown or black pigment.

138. The _____ contains both collagen and elastin fibers.

139. The sebaceous glands are _____ glands that secrete sebum.

140. The _____ is the body's first line of defense.

141. _____ is a severe systemic allergic reaction characterized by bronchoconstriction, hypotension, and shock.

142. The _____ _____ is an extremely large, flat, flexible body system that covers the entire surface of the body.

143. The _____ covers the external surface of the body (in the form of the skin), but also includes the mucous membranes that line the walls of internal cavities that connect to the outside of the body.

144. The _____ is a thicker layer beneath the epidermis.

145. The _____ is a loose, connective tissue directly beneath the dermis of the skin.

146. The sweat glands are also known as the _____ glands.

147. Each hair forms in a hair _____ in the dermis.

148. The _____ is the whitish half moon under the proximal nail plate, or the tip of the nail root.

149. A/an _____ is a hypersensitivity response to certain types of antigens known as allergens.

150. Eating peanuts, being stung by a bee, taking a drug they are already allergic to, or being exposed to latex gloves are all common causes of _____ in hypersensitive individuals.

151. A _____ is an area of any size of hemorrhage under the skin.

152. The level of hydration of the body can be determined by assessing the _____.

153. A bluish-purple discoloration of the skin and nails due to decreased oxygen levels in the blood is called _____.

154. _____ is a congenital abnormality in which there are extra fingers or toes.

155. _____ _____ _____ arises from the basal layer of the epidermis. It is the most common type of skin cancer.

156. _____ is the medical specialty that studies the skin.

157. The patient had a facelift to remove wrinkles. The medical word for this procedure is _____.

158. Melanocytes in the epidermis produce a black pigment known as _____.

159. A _____ is a specific area of skin that sends information about pain, temperature, and touch to one spinal nerve.

160. _____ _____ is the common name for tinea pedis.

161. The herpes-varicella zoster virus causes the itching and scabs of chickenpox in children. Then later in life, during times of stress, it can come back as the skin condition known as _____.

162. _____ _____ is the medical phrase for the common word bedsore.

True/False

Write 'T' if the statement is true and 'F' if the statement is false.

_____163. The skin is comprised of the epidermis, dermis, and subcutaneous tissue.

_____164. A person with dark skin has a greater production of melanin than someone with fair skin.

_____165. Sunlight exposure to the skin is important to the body's production of vitamin D.

_____166. Pil/o- is a combining form that refers to the nails.

_____167. The medical word for itching is pruritis.

_____168. A bedsore is also known as a decubitus ulcer.

_____169. A pilonidal sinus is found in the sacral area of the back.

_____170. A mole is known as a verruca.

_____171. Acne vulgaris is a condition found in middle-aged people and is characterized by facial redness, edema, and dilated blood vessels.

_____172. Paronchyia is an inflammation and infection of the skin along the nail cuticle.

_____173. The integumentary system covers the entire surface of the body and consists of the skin, hair, and the nails.

_____174. The process of dead skin cells being sloughed off is called epidermolytis.

_____175. The subcutaneous tissue is a type of nervous tissue beneath the dermis.

_____176. Sweating helps cool the body by the process of evaporation.

_____177. Hair cells are filled with follicles, which make the hair shaft strong.

_____178. Keratin in the epidermis absorbs ultraviolet light to protect the DNA in skin cells from undergoing genetic mutation.

_____179. All allergic reactions are hypersensitivity responses to allergens.

_____180. The skin of an infant has very few wrinkles because of the large amount of elastin in the dermis and a thick layer of fat in the subcutaneous tissue.

_____181. A neoplasm is a malignant growth that occurs in or on the skin.

_____182. Debridement is the removal of dead tissue from a wound, burn, or ulcer.

_____183. Liposuction is a surgical procedure to remove fat deposits and reshape the body.

_____184. The skin presents a moist and alkaline environment that discourages the growth of microorganisms.

_____185. Horizontal white bands on the nails indicate arsenic poisoning.

_____186. Acne rosacea occurs most often in adolescence.

_____187. Actinic keratoses caused by the sun are also known as solar keratoses.

_____188. The inability to sweat because of congenital absence of the sweat glands is known as diaphoresis.

_____189. Hirsutism is the medical word for male pattern baldness.

_____190. When the skin along the cuticle is infected with bacteria and pus, this is known as onychomycosis.

_____191. Transdermal drugs are administered by a needle into the subcutaneous tissue.

_____192. Coal tar drugs are used to treat psoriasis.

_____193. Botox injections are used to relax wrinkles.

_____194. The skin is the body's first line of defense against disease.

_____195. The deepest part of the epidermis is called the basal layer.

_____196. Neoplasms are tumors that can be either benign or malignant.

_____197. The outermost layer of the skin is the dermis.

_____198. Sunburn is the result of excessive melanin absorption of ultraviolet light.

_____199. The subcutaneous tissue acts as a layer of insulation to conserve body heat.

_____200. An elevated collection of blood under the skin is petechiae.

Essay

Write your answer in the space provided or on a separate sheet of paper.

201. Lisa developed anaphylaxis after being stung by a bee. Define anaphylaxis and list three symptoms of this condition that could be life threatening.

202. What is the reason for Moh's surgery? Describe the process of this surgery.

203. Briefly describe the structures and the function of the integumentary system.

204. What is the difference between a local allergic reaction and a systemic allergic reaction?

205. What is anaphylaxis?

206. What is the difference between necrosis and gangrene?

207. What is the difference between second- and third-degree burns?

CHAPTER 8

Multiple Choice

Choose the one alternative that best completes the statement or answers the question.

1. Which is a congenital deformity of one or both of the feet in which the foot is turned both inwardly and downwardly?
   a. hallux valgus
   b. genu varum
   c. genu valgus
   d. talipes equinovarus

2. Which is the misspelled word?
   a. mandible
   b. humorous
   c. coccyx
   d. ilium

3. Which is a fracture in which the bone is crushed into several pieces?
   a. comminuted
   b. depressed
   c. oblique
   d. compression

4. The patient had arthroscopic surgery of the knee joint to repair a torn:
   a. diaphysis.
   b. fontanel.
   c. meniscus.
   d. nucleus pulposus.

5. Gold compounds are used as medications to inhibit the immune system; therefore, they are useful in treating:
   a. rheumatoid arthritis.
   b. osteoporosis.
   c. osteoarthritis.
   d. muscles and strains.

6. AKA or BKA are abbreviations for which type of surgery?
   a. arthroplasty
   b. amputation
   c. arthrodesis
   d. autograft

7. If a patient had a fracture of the zygomatic arch, it would involve:
   a. a cervical vertebra.
   b. the pelvic girdle.
   c. one of the facial bones.
   d. the bones of the feet.

8. Which fracture would be found in children, because a child's bones are still flexible?
   a. depressed
   b. open
   c. compression
   d. greenstick

9. Which condition would most likely require an ORIF?
   a. hairline fracture
   b. nondisplaced fracture
   c. compound fracture
   d. simple fracture

10. The patient had an arthroplasty of his hip. Which is an abbreviation for this surgery?
    a. CDH
    b. MCP
    c. THR
    d. RUE

11. The deep socket in the hip bone where the femur is attached is known as the:
    a. acetabulum.
    b. glenoid fossa.
    c. calcaneus.
    d. foramen magnum.
12. The common term for kyphosis is:
    a. club foot.
    b. humpback.
    c. swayback.
    d. bowleg.
13. The results of the bone densitometry shows that Alaina Smith has abnormal thinning of bone due to postmenopausal:
    a. osteomyelitis.
    b. osteoporosis.
    c. osteomalacia.
    d. osteoarthritis.
14. Swayback, or an anterior curvature of the lumbar spine, is known as:
    a. scoliosis.
    b. ankylosis.
    c. kyphosis.
    d. lordosis.
15. The patient with gout will show elevated levels of _____ in his body.
    a. calcium
    b. vitamin D
    c. uric acid
    d. phosphorus
16. Crepitus is a/an:
    a. grinding noise heard as bone ends rub together.
    b. congenital hollow depression in the chest.
    c. condition in which the great toe is angled laterally toward the other toes.
    d. infection of bone and bone marrow.
17. Bone cells that eat away old or damaged bone, releasing calcium into the bloodstream, are called:
    a. osteoblasts.
    b. osteoclasts.
    c. osteocytes.
    d. osteophytes.
18. Ankylosing spondylitis is a chronic inflammation of the:
    a. hip.
    b. foot.
    c. hand.
    d. spine.
19. Which is a treatment for severe scoliosis of the spine?
    a. spinal fusion
    b. open reduction and internal fixation

    c. traction
    d. articulation
20. Which is a degenerative condition of the spine in which one vertebra moves anteriorly over another vertebra?
    a. kyphosis
    b. slipped disk
    c. spondylolisthesis
    d. ankylosing spondylitis
21. The patient was diagnosed with avascular necrosis of the _____ epiphysis.
    a. periosteal
    b. synovial
    c. femoral
    d. popliteal
22. The part of the skull that forms the back of the head is the _____ bone.
    a. occipital
    b. temporal
    c. frontal
    d. parietal
23. Osteotome and rongeur are:
    a. bone markings.
    b. orthopedic prosthetic devices.
    c. bony malalignments.
    d. orthopedic surgical instruments.
24. DJD is also known as:
    a. osteoporosis.
    b. osteopathy.
    c. osteoarthritis.
    d. osteomyelitis.
25. All of the following are facial bones EXCEPT:
    a. sphenoid.
    b. lacrimal.
    c. zygomatic.
    d. mandibular.
26. Ribs 8-10 are referred to as:
    a. floating ribs.
    b. false ribs.
    c. stationary ribs.
    d. true ribs.
27. Which section of the vertebrae is located in the lower back?
    a. lumbar
    b. cervical
    c. thoracic
    d. ventral
28. Which is the medical word for collarbone?
    a. malleolus
    b. scapula
    c. clavicle
    d. sternum

29. Which is the medical word for the lower arm bone that lies on the thumb side of the forearm?
    a. tibia
    b. ulna
    c. radius
    d. humerus
30. Which is the name for the bony prominence on the inside and outside of the ankle area?
    a. tarsal
    b. malleolus
    c. acromion
    d. calcaneus
31. The eight small bones of the wrist joint are known as the:
    a. tarsal bones.
    b. cancellous bones.
    c. carpal bones.
    d. phalanges.
32. Which is the medical word for the tailbone?
    a. clavicle
    b. coccyx
    c. lumbar
    d. sacrum
33. Which is the medical word for the thigh bone?
    a. femur
    b. fibula
    c. ulna
    d. ilium
34. Which type of fracture involves a bone that is crushed into several pieces?
    a. displaced fracture
    b. compression fracture
    c. comminuted fracture
    d. nondisplaced fracture
35. Infection in the bone and bone marrow is known as:
    a. osteomyelitis.
    b. osteomalacia.
    c. osteospondylitis.
    d. osteoporosis.
36. Which is the medical word for humpback?
    a. scoliosis
    b. lordosis
    c. kyphosis
    d. ankylosis
37. Which is a congenital deformity in which the lower legs are bent outward beginning at the knees?
    a. genu varum
    b. genu valgum
    c. hallux valgus
    d. talipes equinovarus

38. What medical procedure uses a protractor-like device to measure the angle and degrees of range of movement?
    a. physical therapy
    b. gonimetry
    c. closed reduction
    d. traction
39. Which is a surgical procedure performed to fuse the bones in a degenerated, unstable joint?
    a. arthrodesis
    b. amputation
    c. arthrocentesis
    d. joint replacement surgery
40. Which drugs inhibit bone from being broken down?
    a. gold compound drugs
    b. bone resorption inhibitor drugs
    c. corticosteroid drugs
    d. analgesic drugs
41. The abbreviation DIP means:
    a. distal iliac process.
    b. degenerative iliac pain.
    c. diaphyseal ipiphyseal process.
    d. distal interphalangeal joint.
42. The abbreviation BMD means:
    a. bone malalignment disorder.
    b. bone malunion disorder.
    c. bone mineral density.
    d. basal metabolic disease.
43. Pain in the joints is known as:
    a. arthralgia.
    b. osteoarthralgia.
    c. orthalgia.
    d. ostealgia.
44. An open fracture is also known as a _____ fracture.
    a. compound
    b. closed
    c. displaced
    d. comminuted
45. Which is a benign tumor of the cartilage?
    a. osteoma
    b. sarcoma
    c. chondroma
    d. malacoma
46. Which is the vertical bone of the anterior thorax to which the clavicle and the ribs are attached?
    a. sphenoid bone
    b. sternum
    c. scapula
    d. maxilla

47. The hinge-type and ball-and-socket joints are examples of _____ joints.
    a. synovial
    b. cartilage
    c. suture
    d. osseous

48. Which is the largest of the ankle bones?
    a. malleolus
    b. calcaneus
    c. hallux
    d. tarsal

49. Which skeletal type forms the central bony structure of the body around which other parts move?
    a. axial
    b. appendicular
    c. appendage
    d. sagittal

50. Which of the following is not a part of the skeletal structure of the head?
    a. frontal bone
    b. parietal bones
    c. sagittal suture
    d. sacrum

51. Which of the following bones of the chest is also known as the breast bone?
    a. rib
    b. clavicle
    c. sternum
    d. thorax

52. How many pairs of ribs are there?
    a. 14
    b. 12
    c. 10
    d. 8

53. Which bone is also known as the collarbone?
    a. clavicle
    b. scapula
    c. acromion
    d. glenoid fossa

54. Each wrist contains eight small, individual bones arranged in two rows. They are called the:
    a. metacarpal bones.
    b. phalangeal bones.
    c. carpal bones.
    d. metatarsals.

55. Bone is classified as what type of tissue?
    a. epithelial tissue
    b. connective tissue
    c. adipose tissue
    d. hematological tissue

56. During childhood, cartilaginous tissue is gradually replaced by bone in a process known as:
    a. suture synthesis.
    b. osteoclastic flow.
    c. periosteum.
    d. ossification.

57. The type of fracture in which the bone breaks into several pieces is called:
    a. displaced fracture.
    b. closed fracture.
    c. nondisplaced fracture.
    d. comminuted fracture.

58. Which is an example of a hinge-type joint?
    a. elbow
    b. shoulder
    c. hip
    d. toe

59. Which statement is true of synovial joints?
    a. frozen joints that have a joint capsule and a synovial membrane that makes synovial fluid
    b. fully moveable joints that have a joint capsule and a synovial membrane that makes synovial fluid
    c. partially moveable joints that have a joint capsule and a synovial membrane that makes synovial fluid
    d. fully moveable joints that have no joint capsule but do have a synovial membrane that makes synovial fluid

60. Osseous tissue pertains to:
    a. blood.
    b. muscle.
    c. bone.
    d. tissue.

61. The shaft of a long bone is called the:
    a. epiphysis.
    b. medullary process.
    c. diaphysis.
    d. periosteum.

62. During childhood, cartilaginous tissue is gradually replaced by bony tissue in a process known as:
    a. ossification.
    b. osteoblasting.
    c. osteoclasting.
    d. calcification.

63. The humerus is the:
    a. bone in the upper leg.
    b. bone in the upper arm.
    c. smaller of the two bones in the lower leg.
    d. larger of the two bones in the lower leg.

64. The meniscus is the:
    a. distal bony projection of the tibia.
    b. facial bone that forms the lower jaw.
    c. five long bones of the hand.
    d. crescent-shaped cartilage pad.

65. The ulna is the:
    a. forearm bone located along the thumb side of the lower arm.
    b. larger of the two bones of the lower leg.
    c. forearm bone located along the little finger side of the lower arm.
    d. inferior pointed tip of the sternum.

66. Facial bones that form the lateral edges of the eye sockets and the cheek bones are called:
    a. zygomatic bones.
    b. xiphoid process.
    c. turbinates.
    d. occipital.

67. Which is a benign tumor of the cartilage?
    a. osteosarcoma
    b. sarcoma
    c. osteoma
    d. chondroma

68. A transverse fracture is:
    a. fractured at an angle.
    b. when the bone has broken the skin.
    c. perpendicular to the long axis of the bone.
    d. the same as a greenstick fracture in children.

69. The long shaft of a bone is known as the:
    a. femur.
    b. medullary cavity.
    c. symphysis.
    d. diaphysis.

70. Which combining form means cartilage?
    a. osse/o-
    b. chondr/o-
    c. myel/o-
    d. arthr/o-

71. The combining form spondyl/o- has the same medical meaning as which combining form?
    a. oste/o-
    b. arthr/o-
    c. crani/o-
    d. vertebr/o-

72. The pubic _____ is a type of joint that has a cartilage pad and is nearly immovable.
    a. suture
    b. synovium
    c. bursa
    d. symphysis

73. Pain in a joint from any cause is known as:
    a. arthritis.
    b. arthrodesis.
    c. arthralgia.
    d. articulation.

74. The hip joint is replaced in a surgery called a total hip _____, and the artificial replacement hip is known as a _____.
    a. arthrodesis; bone scan
    b. arthroplasty; radiograph
    c. arthroscopy, internal fixation
    d. arthroplasty; prosthesis

75. A torn ligament is known as:
    a. a sprain.
    b. chondromalacia.
    c. spina bifida.
    d. a herniated disk.

76. _____ is when one lumbar vertebra slips forward out of alignment onto the vertebra below it.
    a. Osteitis
    b. Rheumatoid arthritis
    c. Spondylolisthesis
    d. Malalignment

77. The bones that form a synovial joint are held together by:
    a. ligaments.
    b. synovial fluid.
    c. red marrow.
    d. a symphysis.

78. Which is the combining form for the tailbone?
    a. coccyg/o-
    b. cost/o-
    c. calcane/o-
    d. crani/o-

79. Osteoarthritis is also known as:
    a. talipes.
    b. degenerative joint disease.
    c. rheumatoid arthritis.
    d. kyphosis.

80. Osseous tissue refers to:
    a. joint.
    b. cartilage.
    c. bone.
    d. vertebra.

81. Crepitus is a sound you would hear in a joint afflicted by:
    a. knock-knee.
    b. scoliosis.
    c. a bone tumor.
    d. degenerative joint disease.

82. Which condition is treated with a drug that contains real gold?
   a. osteoarthritis
   b. rheumatoid arthritis
   c. kyphosis
   d. Lyme disease

83. The adjective form of fibula is:
   a. fibulal.
   b. peroneal.
   c. fibular.
   d. osteal.

84. The anatomical name for the shin bone is the:
   a. tibia.
   b. humerus.
   c. illium.
   d. glenoid fossa.

85. Which of these is the combining form for rib?
   a. arthr/o-
   b. myel/o-
   c. cost/o-
   d. oste/o-

86. What disease can be described as a softening of the cartilage of the kneecap?
   a. bone tumor
   b. pectus excavatum
   c. hemarthrosis
   d. chondromalacia patellae

87. The abbreviation that describes a joint in the finger is:
   a. NSAID.
   b. DIP.
   c. AKA.
   d. BKA.

88. Mr. Rodriguez had osteoarthritis so badly that his hip joint had to be replaced. Which two abbreviations correspond to his disease and his surgery?
   a. DJD, BKA
   b. RA, NSAID
   c. ROM, LLE
   d. DJD, THR

89. Select the misspelled word.
   a. rheumatologist
   b. ankylosing spondylitis
   c. pectus excurvatum
   d. osteomyelitis

90. The abbreviations AKA and BKA both describe a/an:
   a. type of fracture.
   b. surgery to remove a leg.
   c. thinning of the bones.
   d. abnormality of the spinal column.

91. In hemarthrosis, the combining form hem/o- means:
   a. blood.
   b. joint.
   c. bone.
   d. skull.

92. The suffix -ics in orthopedics means:
   a. knowledge or practice.
   b. the study of.
   c. inflammation of.
   d. action or condition.

93. In an operative report for a patient with chondromalacia patellae, which anatomical structure is sure to be mentioned?
   a. cranium
   b. humerus
   c. kneecap
   d. elbow

94. In an operative report for a patient with pectus excavatum, what anatomical structure is sure to be mentioned?
   a. sternum
   b. cranium
   c. heelbone
   d. synovial joint

95. Genu varum (bowleg) is the opposite of:
   a. hallux valgus.
   b. pectus excavatum.
   c. rheumatoid arthritis.
   d. genu valgum.

96. The nucleus pulposis is located:
   a. in the bone marrow.
   b. within a joint.
   c. inside an intervertebral disk.
   d. around the glenoid fossa of the shoulder.

97. All of these are anatomical structures of a vertebra EXCEPT:
   a. spinous process.
   b. transverse process.
   c. olecranon process.
   d. foramen.

98. The spongy bone at the end of a long bone is also known as:
   a. bone marrow.
   b. cancellous bone.
   c. diaphysis.
   d. none of the above

99. A pediatric growth chart tracks:
   a. height.
   b. percentiles.
   c. weight.
   d. all of the above

100. Osteocytes is a general category that includes:
    a. osteoclasts.
    b. bone marrow.
    c. osteoblasts.
    d. a and c

101. Fractures that are allowed to heal without treatment might show:
    a. displacement.
    b. malalignment.
    c. bone tumor.
    d. osteoporosis.

102. The physician would order a blood test for uric acid levels if the patient were suspected of having:
    a. gout.
    b. rheumatoid arthritits.
    c. osteoporosis.
    d. degenerative joint disease.

103. Intra-articular means:
    a. around the bone.
    b. around the joint.
    c. within the bone.
    d. within the joint.

104. A bone spur might be treated with:
    a. closed reduction.
    b. extracorporeal shock wave therapy.
    c. goniometry.
    d. prosthesis.

105. Which surgical procedure might be performed to correct a deformity associated with hallux valgus?
    a. external fixation
    b. bunionectomy
    c. arthrocentesis
    d. amputation

106. The opening between cranial sutures in an infant is known as a:
    a. fontanel.
    b. foramen.
    c. suture.
    d. pubis.

107. Which cranial bone contains a bony cup that holds the pituitary gland?
    a. frontal
    b. temporal
    c. occipital
    d. sphenoid

108. The U-shaped bone in the neck that does not connect to any other bones is known as the:
    a. vertebra.
    b. hyoid.
    c. cervical.
    d. cranium.

109. A pathological fracture can be caused by:
    a. osteoporosis.
    b. a bone tumor.
    c. metastases to the bone.
    d. all of the above

110. School children are routinely tested for signs of:
    a. gout.
    b. scoliosis.
    c. fracture.
    d. rheumatoid arthritis.

111. The primary way to diagnose fractures and dislocations is by a/an:
    a. blood test for uric acid.
    b. bone density test.
    c. visual inspection.
    d. x-ray.

Short Answer

Write the word or phrase that best completes each statement or answers the question.

112. A benign tumor of cartilage is known as a _____.

113. Abnormal, excessive C-shaped or S-shaped lateral curvature of the spine is known as _____.

114. The surgical procedure done to remove a prominent part of a metatarsal bone of the foot is called a _____.

115. The medical word for pain in the joint is _____.

116. Blood in a joint cavity is called _____.

117. A fracture in the area of the wrist at the distal radius is known by the eponym _____ fracture.

118. The two combining forms meaning joint are arthr/o- and _____.

119. Abnormal softening of bones is known as _____.

120. Orth/o- means _____.

121. The anatomical name for the shin bone is the _____.

122. _____ sarcoma is a malignant tumor of the bone that occurs mainly in young men.

123. A fracture caused by a disease process such as osteoporosis, bone cancer, or metastasis to the bone is called a _____ fracture

124. Pain in the joint from injury, inflammation, or infection is called _____.

125. Displacement of the end of a bone from its normal position within a joint is called _____.

126. A bone _____ is a nuclear medicine procedure in which phosphate compounds are tagged with the radioactive tracer technetium-99m and injected intravenously.

127. A non-surgical procedure in which manual manipulation of a displaced fracture moves bone ends into normal alignment is called a closed _____.

128. _____ is a surgical procedure to remove all or part of an extremity because of trauma or circulatory disease, or infection.

129. _____ is a surgical procedure that uses an arthroscope inserted into the joint to visualize the inside of a joint and its structures.

130. A general word for the category of drugs used to suppress inflammation and decrease pain is _____.

131. The _____ skeleton consists of bones of the shoulders, arms, hips, and legs.

132. The _____ skeleton forms the central bony structure of the body around which other parts move. It consists of the bones of the head, chest, and spine.

133. The _____ bone forms the forehead and top of the cranium and ends at the coronal suture.

134. The _____ _____ is a large, round opening through which the spinal cord passes to join the brain.

135. The _____ bone forms the anterior base of the cranium.

136. When the fetus is in the uterus, the bones of the skull have large spaces between them called _____ or soft spots.

137. The _____ is a narrow wall of bone that forms the inferior part of the nasal septum and continues posteriorly to the cranium where it joins the sphenoid bone.

138. The _____ is a large, irregularly shaped-bone, known as the lower jaw.

139. The _____ is the triangular, most superior part of the sternum.

140. The area where the cartilage meets the rib is known as the _____ joint.

141. The _____ vertebrae (C1–C7) are located in the neck.

142. The _____ vertebrae (L1–L5) are located in the lower back.

143. Between the vertebrae (beginning with C2 and ending with S1) are the _____ _____, circular disks with two flat surfaces.

144. The _____ or collarbone is a thin, rodlike bone on each side of the anterior neck.

145. The _____ or shoulder blade is a triangular-shaped bone on either side of the vertebral column in the upper back. It has a long, bladelike spine along its upper half.

146. Each wrist contains eight small, individual _____ bones arranged in two rows.

147. The two ball-and-socket synovial joints in the body are the _____ and _____.

148. The two bones of the lower arm are the _____ and _____.

149. The two bones of the lower leg are the _____ and _____.

150. A person who has had an amputation is known as a/an _____.

151. The mature human skeletal system contains _____ bones.

True/False

Write 'T' if the statement is true and 'F' if the statement is false.

_____152. Bone breakdown is termed reabsorption.

_____153. The olecranon is the heel bone.

_____154. A DEXA scan is done to determine the extent of osteomyelitis in a patient.

_____155. An orthosis is a device that takes the place of a body part that has been removed.

_____156. Prednisone is an over-the-counter medication used to treat minor musculoskeletal injuries.

_____157. Hallux valgum is a disease of the hand.

_____158. A fracture in which cranial bones are pressed down inwardly toward the brain is called a depressed fracture.

_____159. Genu valgum is known as knock knee.

_____160. Arthrocentesis is done by removing fluid from the joint with an osteotome.

_____161. The skeletal system consists of 198 bones and other structures that are found throughout the body.

_____162. The axial skeleton forms the central bony structure of the body.

_____163. The facial bones protect the eyes and internal structures of the nose, mouth, and upper throat.

_____164. The bony edges of the fontanels fuse together to become immobile in early adulthood.

_____165. Foramen is derived from a Latin word that means opening.

_____166. The humerus, radius, and ulna are the three long bones in the arms.

_____167. Avascular necrosis is gangrene of the big toes due to exposure to extreme cold.

_____168. Osteomyelitis is cancer of the bone.

_____169. Arthrography is a radiologic procedure that uses a radiopaque contrast dye injected into a joint.

_____170. The bone marrow forms red blood cells, white blood cells, and platelets.

_____171. A joint is also known as a meniscus.

_____172. The medical word for a finger or a toe is phalanx.

_____173. The medical word for the kneecap is the olecranon.

_____174. A physical therapist is a physician who develops treatment and rehabilitation plans for a patient.

_____175. The cranium and facial bones make up the bony structure of the skull.

_____176. The bones of the ankle are called the carpal bones.

_____177. The deep bony socket in the hip joint is called the glenoid fossa.

_____178. A hairline fracture is one that occurs in the cranium along the hair line and scalp.

_____179. A prosthesis is a cast of fiberglass put around a fractured bone.

_____180. Goniometry is used to measure range of motion.

Essay

Write your answer in the space provided or on a separate sheet of paper.

181. Name the five regions of the spinal column.

182. The physician dictated, "The patient had a displaced fracture of the fibula that required a closed reduction and casting." Rewrite this sentence using non-medical words.

183. List three contributing factors to the development of osteoporosis in postmenopausal women.

184. What is the difference between lordosis and scoliosis?

185. What is gout?

186. What are bone density tests and how are they done?

187. What is a bone graft?

188. How does bone growth occur?

CHAPTER 9

Multiple Choice

Choose the one alternative that best completes the statement or answers the question.

1. The muscle that runs on a diagonal from the lower ribs to the iliac crest is the:
   a. latissimus dorsi muscle.
   b. rectus femoris muscle.
   c. rectus abdominis muscle.
   d. external abdominal oblique muscle.

2. The patient with cerebral palsy was described as having ataxia. This means that the patient:
   a. has slow skeletal muscle movements of his upper extremities.
   b. walks with an uncoordinated gait.
   c. has muscle jerking and spasms when he attempts movement.
   d. has slow, purposeless writhing of his hands.

3. The patient was in a coma for a long time in a nursing home. He eventually developed _____ or abnormal, fixed positions in which his muscles were permanently flexed.
   a. contractures
   b. contusions
   c. constrictions
   d. conductions

4. Torticollis is a condition that occurs in the muscles of the:
   a. hand.
   b. back.
   c. neck.
   d. shoulder.

5. A rhabdomyosarcoma is a malignancy of _____ tissue.
   a. involuntary muscle
   b. striated muscle
   c. tendon
   d. fascicle muscle

6. The large muscle of the buttocks that one sits on is the:
   a. rectus femoris.
   b. peroneal longus.
   c. gastrocnemius.
   d. gluteus maximus.

7. A physiatrist is a _____ who gains further specialized training that encompasses treatment for sports injuries.
   a. physical therapist
   b. physician
   c. chiropractor
   d. massage therapist

8. A podiatrist would treat an injury of which muscle?
   a. temporalis
   b. brachioradialis
   c. deltoiod
   d. flexor hallucis brevis

9. When a muscle tears away from a tendon or a tendon tears away from a bone it is known as:
   a. spasm.
   b. contusion.
   c. avulsion.
   d. contracture.

10. Myoclonus is characterized by muscle:
    a. inflammation.
    b. jerking.
    c. contractures.
    d. wasting.

11. Inflammation of a cordlike band of connective tissue that attaches a muscle to a bone is known as:
    a. bursitis.
    b. myositis.
    c. fascitis.
    d. tendonitis.

12. Acetylcholine receptor antibodies are found in patients with:
    a. myasthenia gravis.
    b. muscle contractures.
    c. fibromyalgia.
    d. muscular dystrophy.

13. Which is an incision into the thin connective tissue sheet that wraps around each individual muscle or a group of muscles?
    a. tenotomy
    b. myotomy
    c. bursotomy
    d. fasciotomy

14. Moving a body part away from the midline is known as:
    a. adduction.
    b. eversion.
    c. abduction.
    d. flexion.

15. A disorder of the hand that creates a flexion deformity of the fingers is called:
    a. a ganglion.
    b. Dupuytren's contracture.
    c. pronation.
    d. repetitive strain disorder.

16. An athletic injury with pain and inflammation of the flexor muscles over the anterior tibia would be found in the:
    a. elbow.
    b. wrist.
    c. neck.
    d. lower leg.

17. Trigger points, areas on a patient's body that are tender to touch and feel firm, are indicative of which condition?
    a. fibromyalgia
    b. rhabdomyoma
    c. muscular dystrophy
    d. restless leg syndrome

18. Abnormally slow skeletal muscle movements associated with Parkinson's disease are known as:
    a. dyskinesia.
    b. ataxia.
    c. hyperkinesias.
    d. bradykinesia.

19. A rotator cuff tear occurs at the:
    a. hip.
    b. knee.
    c. shoulder.
    d. wrist.

20. An EMG is a:
    a. diagnostic procedure used to diagnose nerve damage or muscle disease.
    b. laboratory test of enzymes that, when elevated, point to muscle damage.
    c. test that measures motor muscle strength.
    d. series of rehabilitation exercises following a musculoskeletal injury.

21. Surgical removal of the _____ gland is sometimes done to alleviate the symptoms of myasthenia gravis.
    a. pituitary
    b. thymus
    c. adrenal
    d. thyroid

22. A contusion due to a blunt injury to a muscle causes a condition commonly known as:
    a. strain.
    b. shin splint.
    c. bruise.
    d. whiplash.

23. Which is the characteristic symptom of myasthenia gravis?
    a. gradual paralysis
    b. sudden, temporary muscle spasms
    c. abnormal fatigue involving skeletal muscles
    d. widespread stiffness and internal pain over certain muscles

24. Which one is not one of the three types of muscles in the body?
    a. skeletal
    b. triceps
    c. smooth
    d. cardiac

25. Which type of muscle is involuntary and nonstriated?
    a. skeletal
    b. respiratory
    c. smooth
    d. cardiac

26. Which is a cordlike, nonelastic, white fibrous band of connective tissue?
    a. tendon
    b. muscle
    c. bursa
    d. joint

27. Which is the large muscle in the buttocks?
    a. rectus abdominis
    b. brachioradialis
    c. gluteus maximus
    d. temporalis
28. Which is the short muscle that flexes the big toe?
    a. flexor hallucis brevis
    b. brachioradialis
    c. gluteus maximus
    d. extensor digitorum
29. Bending a joint to decrease the angle between two bones or two body parts is known as:
    a. extension.
    b. abduction.
    c. flexion.
    d. adduction.
30. Which muscle moves the forehead skin to elevate the eyebrows or wrinkle the forehead?
    a. temporalis
    b. frontalis
    c. masseter
    d. orbicularis oris
31. Which muscle bends the lower arm toward the upper arm?
    a. triceps brachii
    b. thenar
    c. biceps brachii
    d. rectus abdominis
32. The gastrocnemius muscle:
    a. bends the foot downward.
    b. moves the food into the stomach.
    c. bends the upper body forward.
    d. straightens the lower arm.
33. The loss of muscle bulk in one or more muscles is known as:
    a. avulsion.
    b. hypertrophy.
    c. atrophy.
    d. contracture.
34. Painful contracture of the muscles on one side of the neck is known as:
    a. rotator cuff tear.
    b. repetitive strain injury.
    c. torticollis.
    d. myalgia.
35. Incoordination of the muscles during movement is known as:
    a. bradykinesia.
    b. ataxia.
    c. dyskinesia.
    d. hyperkinesis.

36. Which is an uncomfortable twitching of the muscles of the legs, particularly the calf muscles, along with an indescribable tingling, aching, or crawling-insect sensation?
    a. muscular dystrophy
    b. restless leg syndrome
    c. myalgia
    d. chronic fatigue syndrome
37. Inflammation and pain of the flexor and pronator muscles of the forearm where their tendons originate on the medial epicondyle of the humerus by the elbow joint is known as:
    a. golfer's elbow.
    b. medial epicondylitis.
    c. pitcher's elbow.
    d. all of the above
38. Which diagnostic procedure is performed to diagnose muscle disease or nerve damage?
    a. Tensilon test
    b. myelogram
    c. electromyography
    d. myoneurogram
39. During a muscle strength test, grip strength measures _____ strength.
    a. hand
    b. bone
    c. muscle
    d. back
40. During a muscle strength test, _____ strength is measured.
    a. extension
    b. adaptive
    c. motor
    d. reflex
41. Which condition is known as housemaid's knee?
    a. bursitis
    b. tremor
    c. shin splints
    d. tendonitis
42. A small, involuntary, sometimes jerky back-and-forth movement of the hands, neck, jaw, or extremities is known as:
    a. contracture.
    b. tremor.
    c. dyskinesia.
    d. ataxia.
43. Abnormal motions due to difficulty controlling the voluntary muscles are known as:
    a. contracture.
    b. hyperkinesis.
    c. dyskinesia
    d. ataxia.

44. Which is a normal condition of the muscles that occurs several hours after death?
    a. cardiac arrest
    b. rigor mortis
    c. bradykinesis
    d. atrophy

45. Which is another name for repetitive strain injury (RSI)?
    a. cumulative trauma disorder (CTD)
    b. polymyositis
    c. bursitis
    d. restless leg syndrome

46. Which is a painful, but temporary, condition characterized by a sudden, severe, involuntary, and prolonged contracture of a muscle, usually in the legs?
    a. muscle sprain
    b. tendonitis
    c. muscle spasm
    d. fibromyalgia

47. Which medical word means muscle wasting?
    a. hypertrophy
    b. atrophy
    c. ataxia
    d. dyskinesia

48. Which combining form means triangle?
    a. flex/o-
    b. maxim/o-
    c. delt/o-
    d. fasci/o-

49. There are approximately how many skeletal muscles in the body?
    a. 400
    b. 500
    c. 600
    d. 700

50. Which of the following is NOT a type of muscle in the body?
    a. skeletal
    b. cardiac
    c. polystriated
    d. smooth

51. Bending a joint to decrease the angle between two bones or two body parts is known as:
    a. flexion.
    b. extension.
    c. abduction.
    d. adduction.

52. Moving a body part around on its axis is known as:
    a. supination.
    b. eversion.

    c. adduction.
    d. rotation.

53. The intercostal muscles assist what functions?
    a. raising the shoulder
    b. moving the arm
    c. coughing and sneezing
    d. moving the neck

54. Maximus is a word that means:
    a. fastest.
    b. pertaining to.
    c. the largest one of a group.
    d. front or front part.

55. The neurotransmitter that initiates muscle contraction is:
    a. acetylcholine.
    b. aponeurosis.
    c. buccinator.
    d. fascicle.

56. A fluid-filled sac that decreases friction where a tendon rubs against a bone near a synovial joint is a/an:
    a. evertor.
    b. extensor.
    c. bursa.
    d. platysma.

57. A crushing injury to the muscles of the leg causes compartment syndrome, which in turn causes all of the following EXCEPT:
    a. pressure within the compartment of the leg.
    b. accumulation of blood in the compartment.
    c. cellular death and nerve damage.
    d. cardiac arrhythmias.

58. What type of drug is used to relieve muscle spasm and stiffness?
    a. corticosteroid drugs
    b. muscle relaxant drugs
    c. nonsteroidal anti-inflammatory drugs
    d. analgesic drugs

59. Which word means front?
    a. posterior
    b. anterior
    c. lateral
    d. dorsal

60. Which word means inactivity or paralysis coupled with continuing nerve impulses, causing a muscle to be progressively flexed and drawn into a position where becomes nearly immovable?
    a. fibromyalgia
    b. contracture
    c. atrophy
    d. avulsion

61. Which word means pain in several muscle groups?
    a. polymyalgia
    b. RSI
    c. myopathy
    d. myasthenia gravis

62. Abnormally slow muscle movements or a decrease in the number of spontaneous muscle movements is called:
    a. dyskinesia.
    b. myoclonus.
    c. bradykinesia.
    d. ataxic.

63. Inflammation of the bursal sac because of repetitive muscular activity or pressure on the bone underneath the bursa is called:
    a. restless leg syndrome.
    b. ganglion.
    c. bursitis.
    d. Dupuytren's contracture.

64. Which diagnostic procedure is used to diagnose muscle disease or nerve damage?
    a. tensilon
    b. EMG
    c. CPK-MM
    d. DTR

65. A muscle biopsy is a surgical procedure to:
    a. cut the fascia and release pressure from built up blood and tissue fluid in patients with compartment syndrome.
    b. suture together the torn ends of a muscle following an injury.
    c. make a definitive diagnosis when muscle weakness could be caused by many different muscular diseases.
    d. suture together the torn ends of a tendon following an injury.

66. NSAIDs are drugs used to:
    a. decrease inflammation.
    b. kill bacteria.
    c. kill viruses.
    d. relax muscles.

67. The abbreviation ROM means:
    a. range of motion.
    b. range of muscle mass.
    c. rate of measure.
    d. rate of myalgia.

68. Which statement is true about abbreviations?
    a. Abbreviations are commonly used in all types of medical documentation.
    b. Each abbreviation can only have one meaning.

c. There are no standard abbreviations for medical documentation.
    d. It is acceptable medical practice to use any abbreviation in medical documentation.

69. Movement around a central point or axis is known as:
    a. abduction.
    b. inversion.
    c. extension.
    d. rotation.

70. All of the following suffixes mean pertaining to EXCEPT:
    a. -ous.
    b. -or.
    c. -ary.
    d. -al.

71. The combining form muscul/o- has the same meaning as which combining form?
    a. ten/o-
    b. malign/o-
    c. contract/o-
    d. my/o-

72. The suffix -oma means:
    a. muscle.
    b. tumor or mass.
    c. contraction.
    d. weakness.

73. The suffix -ics in orthopedics means:
    a. knowledge or practice.
    b. the study of.
    c. inflammation of.
    d. action or condition.

74. The neck muscle that goes from the ear to the collarbone and sternum is the:
    a. aponeurosis.
    b. sternocleidomastoid.
    c. brachioradialis.
    d. gluteus maximus.

75. Which of the following is classified as a repetitive stress disorder?
    a. tennis elbow
    b. rhabdomyoma
    c. rotator cuff tear
    d. myasthenia gravis

76. Which is the abbreviation for the government organization that educates healthcare professionals about workplace-related injuries?
    a. NSAID
    b. PM&R
    c. OSHA
    d. COTA

77. The latissimus dorsi is a muscle of the:
    a. back.
    b. abdomen.
    c. upper leg.
    d. chest.
78. When your outstretched arm has the palm down, this is known as:
    a. rotation.
    b. insertion.
    c. pronation.
    d. flexion.
79. Skeletal muscles are also known as _____ muscles.
    a. rascial
    b. cardiac
    c. involuntary
    d. voluntary
80. Patients with Parkinson's disease who move with slow, shuffling movements have the muscle condition known as:
    a. restless legs syndrome.
    b. myalgia.
    c. contracture.
    d. bradykinesia.
81. Moving your head to indicate "yes" and then to indicate "no" would correspond to which two movements?
    a. contraction and relaxation
    b. flexion and rotation
    c. elevation and circumduction
    d. supination and extension
82. If you point your toe like a ballet dancer, you would be doing which movement?
    a. rotation
    b. abduction
    c. plantar flexion
    d. inversion
83. The pectoralis major muscle is located in the:
    a. buttocks.
    b. chest.
    c. forearm.
    d. thigh.
84. Lateral epicondylitis is a repetitive strain injury known as:
    a. myositis.
    b. myasthenia gravis.
    c. deep tendon reflex.
    d. tennis elbow.
85. Suturing of a cut tendon is a surgical procedure known as:
    a. electromyography.
    b. range of motion.
    c. tenorrhaphy.
    d. myorrhaphy.

86. The inability to coordinate voluntary movements, as found in someone with cerebral palsy, is known as:
    a. polymyositis.
    b. ataxia.
    c. fascia.
    d. supination.
87. A genetic disorder that causes progressive weakness as the muscle tissue turns to fat is known as:
    a. muscular dystrophy.
    b. myalgia.
    c. contracture.
    d. dyskinesia.
88. The intercostal muscles are:
    a. around the femur.
    b. between the ribs.
    c. across the chest.
    d. in the arm.
89. The masseter muscle is used for:
    a. arm movements.
    b. breathing.
    c. leg movements.
    d. chewing.
90. Select the misspelled word.
    a. rhabdomyosarcoma
    b. ganglian
    c. dyskinesia
    d. tremor
91. Hyperkinesia is the opposite of:
    a. tremor.
    b. ataxia.
    c. bursitis.
    d. bradykinesia.
92. An assistive device is one that can help a patient:
    a. perform ADLs.
    b. meet the requirements of ADA.
    c. have a positive DTR.
    d. decrease ROM.
93. A slender, elongated pocket of synovial membrane that contains synovial fluid is known as a/an:
    a. fascicle.
    b. bursa.
    c. tendon.
    d. fascia.
94. A flat, wide, white fibrous sheet of connective tissue that attaches a flat muscle to a bone or to deep muscles is known as a/an:
    a. tendon.
    b. ligament.
    c. bursa.
    d. aponeurosis.

95. Muscles get their names from their:
   a. shape.
   b. size.
   c. location.
   d. all of the above

96. A flexed and nearly immovable position of a muscle is known as a/an:
   a. contusion.
   b. contracture.
   c. avulsion.
   d. strain.

97. A percussion hammer is used to test:
   a. muscle strength.
   b. the presence of a contraction.
   c. muscle size.
   d. deep tendon reflexes.

Short Answer

Write the word or phrase that best completes each statement or answers the question.

98. Suturing the torn ends of a muscle after an injury is termed _____.

99. A general word for muscle pain is _____.

100. Bridget's housemaid's knee came from prolonged kneeling, causing _____, an inflammation of a pocket of synovial fluid near her knee joint.

101. A pulled muscle or muscle _____ is caused by overstretching a muscle to cause inflammation, pain, and swelling.

102. Loss of muscle bulk is known as muscle wasting or _____.

103. The medical word for muscle disease is _____.

104. Because of periodic, involuntary jerking movement of his hands and head, Mr. Jones is being treated with beta blocker for his essential familial _____.

105. Drugs such as Motrin and Feldene that are used to suppress inflammation and decrease pain are collectively known by the abbreviation _____.

106. During a car accident when a person's head snaps backward and forward, causing damage to the structures in the neck, the result is known as hyperextension-hyperflexion. The common term for this condition is _____.

107. Inflammation of a skeletal muscle with localized tenderness and swelling is known as _____.

108. All of the muscles of the body or in one part of the body are referred to as the _____.

109. The _____ is the beginning of a muscle where it is attached to a stationary or nearly stationary bone of the skeleton.

110. A muscle is attached to a bone at its origin or insertion by a _____.

111. Straightening and extending a joint to increase the angle between two bones or two body parts is known as _____.

112. Each muscle _____ is a bundle of individual muscle fibers.

113. When the electrical impulse reaches the end of the nerve cell, the nerve cell releases a neurotransmitter called _____.

114. A flat, white sheet of fibrous connective tissue that attaches a muscle to a bone or other structure is called a/an _____.

115. A/an _____ is a fluid-filled sac that decreases friction where a tendon rubs against a bone near a synovial joint.

116. The _____ _____ muscle is the largest muscle in the buttocks that moves the upper leg posteriorly and rotates it laterally.

117. A muscle _____ is a painful but temporary condition characterized by a sudden severe, involuntary and prolonged contraction of a muscle, usually in the legs.

118. Skeletal muscles are _____ muscles that contract and relax in response to conscious thought.

119. Skeletal muscles are _____, showing bands of color when examined under the microscope.

120. The _____ or beginning of a muscle is where it is attached to a stationary or nearly stationary bone of the skeleton.

121. The _____ or ending point is where the muscle attaches to the bone that it moves when it contracts and relaxes.

122. The muscle is attached to the bone at its origin and at its insertion by a _____.

123. Moving a body part away from the midline of the body is called _____.

124. Turning the palm of the hand upward is called _____.

125. Straightening and extending a joint to increase the angle between two bones or two body parts is called _____.

126. The muscle in the front shoulder, which is shaped like a triangle and raises and lowers the arm is called the _____.

127. The _____ muscle bends the lower arm toward the upper arm (flexion).

128. Each muscle _____ is a bundle of individual muscle fibers.

129. _____ is a chemical messenger that moves across the neuromuscular junction and acts as a key to unlock receptors on the muscle fiber.

130. Vigorous weight training can increase the size of a muscle, which is called muscle _____.

131. The group of muscles in the anterior and lateral thigh that straightens the lower leg (extension) is called the _____ _____ group. This group of muscle includes the rectus femoris, vastus lateralis, vastus intermedius, and vastus medialis muscles.

132. A muscle that produces extension is part of a muscle pair in which the other muscle produces _____.

133. A muscle that produces eversion is part of a muscle pair in which the other muscle produces _____.

134. In dorsiflexion, the toes are pointing _____ , and in plantar flexion, the toes are pointing _____.

135. The Achilles tendon is located in the _____.

136. The two muscles of the upper arm that flex and extend the arm are the _____ brachii and the _____ brachii.

137. _____ is the medical specialty that studies the anatomy, diseases, and treatment of the bones and muscles.

138. _____ is the common word for torticollis.

True/False

Write 'T' if the statement is true and 'F' if the statement is false.

_____139. Pronation means to turn the palm of the hand upward; supination means to turn the palm of the hand down.

_____140. A rhabdomyoma is a benign tumor that arises from striated or skeletal muscle.

_____141. Rigor mortis is a reversible condition if it is caught in time.

_____142. The electromyography is a test done to confirm myasthenia gravis.

_____143. The beginning of a skeletal muscle where it is attached is known as its origin and the ending point of attachment is known as the inversion.

_____144. Hamstrings is a collective name for the four muscles on the anterior and lateral aspect of the upper leg.

_____145. The word used to describe a site for the injection of a drug is intermuscular.

_____146. Muscular dystrophy is a genetic inherited disease due to a mutation of the gene that makes a muscle protein.

_____147. The masseter muscle is found in the area of the face.

_____148. Insertion of a needle to aspirate muscle tissue is known as a closed biopsy.

_____149. The combining form orth/o- in the word orthopedics means bone.

_____150. Skeletal muscles are voluntary muscles.

_____151. The flexor hallucis brevis muscle is a muscle of the hand.

_____152. The word part brachi/o- means arm and is found in words related to the arm.

_____153. The word pronation means turning the palm of the hand upward.

_____154. The orbicularis oculi muscle is a muscle of the head and neck that closes the eyelids.

_____155. The word hamstrings is a collective name for two muscles on the posterior aspect of the thigh.

_____156. Muscle fibers contain hundreds of nuclei scattered throughout the length of each fiber.

_____157. Each muscle fiber contains many muscle cells.

_____158. Polymyalgia is pain in several muscle groups.

_____159. When the deep tendon reflexes are tested, the impulse from tapping the patellar tendon goes to the brain and the brain makes a conscious decision to extend the leg.

_____160. The word rectus in the muscle name rectus abdominis means oblique.

_____161. Thenar is an adjective that refers to the leg.

_____162. The suffix -ceps means head.

_____163. A rhabdomyoma is a benign tumor of the muscle and a rhabdomyosarcoma is a malignant tumor of the tendon.

_____164. The Tensilon test is used to diagnose Dupuytren's contracture.

_____165. The size and strength of muscles decrease in older patients.

_____166. The gastrocnemius muscle propels food through the stomach.

_____167. Rigor mortis is the medical name for muscle atrophy.

_____168. Tremors are tiny, involuntary, back-and-forth movements that the patient cannot stop.

Essay

Write your answer in the space provided or on a separate sheet of paper.

169. What is the definition of a ganglionectomy?

170. Explain how the physician would use the results of the lab test CPK-MM to aid in making a diagnosis for a patient.

171. The patient was in an automobile accident and sustained severe crushing injuries and fractures in her right foot. She developed compartment syndrome. How could this condition lead to a loss of the use of her foot?

172. Describe how a contraction differs from a contracture.

173. List and describe the three types of muscles in the human body.

174. Explain how muscle pairs produce movement.

175. Explain how a muscle fiber contracts.

176. Briefly describe the disease muscular dystrophy, including symptoms and signs.

177. What is an electromyography?

CHAPTER 10

Multiple Choice

Choose the one alternative that best completes the statement or answers the question.

1. Cognex and Aricept are drugs used to treat:
   a. Alzheimer's disease.
   b. Bell's palsy.
   c. Guillain-Barré syndrome.
   d. Parkinson's disease.

2. Which condition occurs when a herniated intervertebral disk compresses a spinal nerve root?
   a. paraplegia
   b. causalgia
   c. spina bifida
   d. radiculopathy

3. Which condition commonly accompanies migraine headaches?
   a. narcolepsy
   b. seizures
   c. photophobia
   d. syncope

4. The autopsy report read, "Numerous neurofibrillary tangles and senile plaques are seen in the brain tissue." The diagnosis for this patient would be:
   a. stroke.
   b. glioma.
   c. Alzheimer's disease.
   d. epilepsy.

5. Some patients with epilepsy experience an _____ or forewarning of an impending seizure.
   a. automatism
   b. aura
   c. amnesia
   d. aphasia

6. In the later stages of Parkinson's disease the patient showed:
   a. jerking muscle contractions and incontinence.
   b. a mask-like facial expression and shuffling gait.
   c. stiff neck and lethargy.
   d. paralysis on one half of the body and difficulty speaking.

7. When the patient experienced trauma to the occipital lobe of the brain, his sense of _____ was affected.
   a. smell
   b. hearing
   c. vision
   d. taste

8. Spinal bifida may result in the protrusion of the spinal cord and its lining. This condition is known as:
   a. meningomyelosis.
   b. meningomyelocele.
   c. meningomyeloptosis.
   d. meningomyeloma.

9. Which neurotransmitter is the body's own natural pain reliever?
   a. acetylcholine
   b. serotonin
   c. dopamine
   d. endorphins

10. Grand mal seizures with unconsciousness and excessive motor activity are also known as:
    a. complex partial.
    b. tonic-clonic.
    c. focal motor.
    d. petit mal.

11. Mrs. Lynn had a stroke that left her with the inability to understand spoken or written words. This is known as:
    a. expressive aphasia.
    b. amnesia.
    c. epilepsy.
    d. receptive aphasia.

12. The cells of the nervous system that form the blood–brain barrier that keeps certain substances from gaining access to the brain are called:
    a. astrocytes.
    b. Schwann cells.
    c. ependymal cells.
    d. dendrites.

13. Which condition, with its lack of oxygenated blood to brain tissues, causes signs and symptoms of a stroke lasting only 24 hours?
    a. CTS
    b. TIA
    c. CSF
    d. TENS

14. Mrs. Sweet has diabetic neuropathy with tingling or pinprick sensations on her skin called:
    a. paraesthesia.
    b. neuralgia.
    c. causalgia.
    d. polyneuritis.

15. Which radiologic procedure uses several x-rays and sometimes an opaque dye to give multiple three-dimensional views of the brain or spinal cord?

    a. LP

    b. CT scan

    c. PET scan

    d. ICP

16. Which condition of the motor nerves of the spinal column is sometimes called Lou Gehrig's disease and has no known cause? It is characterized by muscle wasting, spasms, and eventual paralysis.

    a. multiple sclerosis

    b. von Recklinghausen disease

    c. amyotrophic lateral sclerosis

    d. neurofibromatosis

17. The numerical scale that measures the depth of a coma is known as the _____ Coma Scale.

    a. Babinski

    b. Glasgow

    c. Romberg

    d. Huntington

18. Cerebral palsy is caused by:

    a. a lack of oxygen to the infant's brain before or during delivery.

    b. vigorously shaking an infant.

    c. a genetic defect.

    d. a virus transmitted to the infant before or during birth.

19. In this condition, excessive cerebrospinal fluid causes intracranial pressure to increase, distending the ventricles of the brain and compressing brain tissue.

    a. anencephaly

    b. subdural hematoma

    c. Down syndrome

    d. hydrocephalus

20. Nuchal rigidity is an important sign of:

    a. postictal state.

    b. Bell's palsy.

    c. meningitis.

    d. migraine.

21. The patient sustained a gunshot wound in the upper lumbar area of his back that severed the spinal cord. This resulted in:

    a. hemiparesis.

    b. hemiplegia.

    c. paraplegia.

    d. quadriplegia.

22. Mrs. Sands was given a polysomnography to find out the underlying cause of her:

    a. epilepsy.

    b. dyslexia.

    c. cephalalgia.

    d. narcolepsy.

23. A syncopal episode would consist of all signs listed below EXCEPT:

    a. seizure.

    b. fainting.

    c. lightheadedness.

    d. brief loss of consciousness.

24. The middle layer of the meninges that surround the brain and the spinal cord is known as the:

    a. dura mater.

    b. pia mater.

    c. arachnoid.

    d. gyrus.

25. Which part of the brain regulates body temperature, sensations of hunger and thirst, and the circadian (24-hour) rhythm of the body?

    a. hypothalamus

    b. cerebrum

    c. ventricles

    d. cerebellum

26. Which cranial nerve controls swallowing?

    a. glossopharyngeal

    b. accessory

    c. vagus

    d. oculomotor

27. Which nerves carry nerve impulses away from the spinal cord?

    a. afferent nerves

    b. inferior nerves

    c. efferent nerves

    d. superior nerves

28. The cell body of a neuron sends the electrical impulse to the:

    a. synapse.

    b. myelin sheath.

    c. axon.

    d. dendrites.

29. The many pairs of cranial nerves are numbered as follows:

    a. 1 through 10.

    b. 1 through 12.

    c. I through XII.

    d. I through X.

30. The loss of the ability to communicate verbally or in writing is known as:

    a. amnesia.

    b. aphasia.

    c. dysphagia.

    d. ataxia.

31. The abbreviation AVM means:

   a. arteriovenous multiforme.

   b. atrioventricular multiforme.

   c. atrioventricular malformation.

   d. arteriovenous malformation.

32. Which is the medical word for headache?

   a. encephalitis

   b. cranialgia

   c. cephalalgia

   d. encephalodynia

33. Which condition is caused by a lack of oxygen to parts of the baby's brain during birth?

   a. muscular dystrophy

   b. cerebral palsy

   c. coma

   d. cerebrovascular accident

34. Paralysis on one side of the body is known as:

   a. quadriplegia.

   b. hemiplegia.

   c. paraplegia.

   d. duoplegia.

35. The effects of a _____ last 24 hours and are due to a temporary lack of oxygenated blood to an area of the brain.

   a. TIA

   b. CVA

   c. CNS

   d. CP

36. Which word describes a traumatic injury to the brain with no loss of consciousness, but there is some bruising with some bleeding in the tissues?

   a. coma

   b. convulsion

   c. contusion

   d. hemorrhaging

37. Which is another name for tonic-clonic seizures?

   a. petit mal seizures

   b. focal motor seizures

   c. absence seizures

   d. grand mal seizures

38. Which is a chronic, degenerative disease due to an imbalance in the levels of the neurotransmitters dopamine and acetylcholine in the brain?

   a. Huntington's chorea

   b. Parkinson's disease

   c. Alzheimer's disease

   d. dementia

39. Which condition is also known as Lou Gehrig's disease?

   a. amyotrophic lateral sclerosis

   b. muscular dystrophy

   c. carpal tunnel syndrome

   d. multiple sclerosis

40. Which condition is also known as tic douloreux?

   a. neurofibromytosis

   b. neuroma

   c. epilepsy

   d. trigeminal neuralgia

41. Which nuclear medicine procedure uses a radioactive substance that emits positrons?

   a. ultrasound

   b. MRI

   c. CT scan

   d. PET scan

42. The abbreviations VEP, VER, BAEP, BAER describe:

   a. evoked potentials.

   b. sleep study testing.

   c. nerve conduction studies.

   d. bone density test.

43. Which is a neurologic test in which the end of the metal handle of the percussion hammer is used to firmly stroke the outside of the foot from the heel to the toes?

   a. Glasgow scale

   b. mini status exam

   c. Babinski's sign

   d. verbal response test

44. Which medical procedure uses an electrical device to control chronic pain?

   a. GCS scale

   b. TENS unit

   c. LP

   d. MMSE

45. Which type of drug is used to treat Parkinson's disease?

   a. COMT inhibitor drugs

   b. corticosteroid drugs

   c. antiepileptic drugs

   d. analgesic drugs

46. The abbreviation CVA means:

   a. carpovascular accident.

   b. cardiovascular accident.

   c. cerebrovascular accident.

   d. cardiovascular atrophy.

47. Which is another name for the abbreviation LP?

   a. spinal tap

   b. local anesthetic

   c. epidural

   d. cerebrospinal fluid

48. Which of the following is NOT part of the central nervous system?
   a. cerebrum
   b. brain
   c. cranial nerves
   d. spinal cord

49. The brain is housed within what bony structure?
   a. cranium
   b. cranial cavity
   c. cerebrum
   d. ventricles

50. A very deep, anterior-to-posterior fissure divides the cerebrum into what right and left structures?
   a. corpus callosum
   b. meninges
   c. arachnoids
   d. hemispheres

51. Which of the following lobes coordinates and analyzes information received by the other lobes and uses it to predict future events and the benefits or consequences of actions taken?
   a. parietal lobe
   b. frontal lobe
   c. occipital lobe
   d. temporal lobe

52. The olfactory nerve controls what function?
   a. vision
   b. smell
   c. hearing
   d. breathing

53. The posterior or dorsal nerve roots of the spinal cord are categorized as what type of nerves?
   a. afferent nerves
   b. ventral nerves
   c. efferent nerves
   d. cranial nerves

54. Which nervous system cells form the blood–brain barrier?
   a. ependymal cell
   b. microglia
   c. Schwann's cell
   d. astrocyte

55. Neurotransmitters located between neurons in the hypothalamus, thalamus, and brainstem and that are the body's own natural pain relievers are called:
   a. acetylcholine.
   b. astrocytes.
   c. dopamine.
   d. endorphins.

56. The inability to verbally express thoughts is called:
   a. global aphasia.
   b. expressive aphasia.
   c. dysphasia.
   d. receptive aphasia.

57. Which hemisphere of the brain performs mathematical and logical reasoning and problem-solving?
   a. left
   b. right
   c. both
   d. neither. The brain stem is responsible for this brain function.

58. Which part of the brain acts as a relay station, sending sensory nerve impulses like pain and touch from the body to the cerebrum?
   a. hypothalamus
   b. thalamus
   c. pons
   d. brainstem

59. Which part of the brain is the most superior part of the brainstem and keeps the mind conscious?
   a. cerebellum
   b. pons
   c. midbrain
   d. medulla oblongata

60. What is the word for the multiple branches found at the beginning of a neuron that receive neurotransmitters from the previous neuron, convert it to an electrical impulse, and send it to the cell body?
   a. myelin sheaths
   b. synapses
   c. axons
   d. dendrites

61. In which type of seizure is there impaired consciousness with slight or no muscle activity?
   a. grand mal
   b. petit mal
   c. psychomotor
   d. focal

62. A collection of blood, which is a result of trauma to the head and forms in the tissue between the dura matter and the arachnoid, is called:
   a. hydrocephalus.
   b. Huntington's chorea.
   c. subdural hematoma.
   d. intraventricular hematoma.

63. A certain type of recurring, one sided-headache, which is often accompanied by nausea and/or vomiting and extreme sensitivity to light, is called:
    a. narcolepsy.
    b. migraine.
    c. meningitis.
    d. photophobia.

64. Which word is a general category for any type of disease or injury to a nerve?
    a. neuropathy
    b. neuroma
    c. neurofibromatosis
    d. neurofibroma

65. Which radiological procedure uses a magnetic field and radio waves to make a picture?
    a. CT scan
    b. MRI
    c. x-ray
    d. myelography

66. Which word means a surgical incision into the cranium to expose the brain tissue?
    a. craniotomy
    b. rhizotomy
    c. laminectomy
    d. biopsy

67. The combining form myel/o- means:
    a. nerve.
    b. spinal cord.
    c. vertebra.
    d. meninges.

68. Because of close living quarters in a dormitory, lack of sleep, and other factors, this infection can spread rapidly among college students.
    a. meningitis
    b. epilepsy
    c. multiple sclerosis
    d. Alzheimer's disease

69. A traumatic injury to the skull can cause a:
    a. brain tumor.
    b. migraine headache.
    c. radiculopathy.
    d. subdural hematoma.

70. A traumatic injury to the neck and spinal cord can result in:
    a. subdural hematoma.
    b. quadriplegia.
    c. stroke.
    d. Alzheimer's disease.

71. The _____ is the functional unit of the nervous system.
    a. nephron
    b. reflex
    c. neuron
    d. meninges

72. Which brain structure resembles a spider web?
    a. ventricle
    b. arachnoid
    c. vertebra
    d. cerebellum

73. Which types of activities are processed in the temporal lobe of the brain?
    a. conscious control of muscle movements
    b. vision
    c. emotion and personality
    d. hearing and smelling

74. Syncope is also known as:
    a. fainting.
    b. hydrocephalus.
    c. coma.
    d. epilepsy.

75. All of the following are congenital problems that are present at birth EXCEPT:
    a. multiple sclerosis.
    b. myelomeningocele.
    c. cerebral palsy.
    d. hydrocephalus.

76. Which is true of an EEG?
    a. It records electrical impulse of a reflex.
    b. It images the brain with contrast material.
    c. It determines nerve strength and deep tendon reflexes.
    d. It records brain wave patterns.

77. All of the following are types of epilepsy EXCEPT:
    a. grand mal.
    b. radiculopathy.
    c. absense.
    d. petit mal.

78. Which of the following is a surgical procedure to treat a herniated disk?
    a. craniotomy
    b. laminectomy
    c. neurorrhaphy
    d. ventriculoperitoneal shunt

79. People who use computers extensively are prone to get which of these diseases?
    a. herniated nucleus pulposus
    b. carpal tunnel syndrome
    c. dementia
    d. hyperesthesia

80. Which is the only cranial nerve that travels outside of the area of the head and neck?
    a. vagus
    b. auditory
    c. facial
    d. optic

81. The epidural space:
    a. is found in the spinal cord area.
    b. lies between the dura mater and the vertebra.
    c. is filled with fatty tissue and blood vessels.
    d. all of the above

82. All of the following are functions of the parasympathetic nervous system EXCEPT:
    a. producing peristalsis in the GI tract.
    b. stimulating the salivary glands during eating.
    c. constricting smooth muscles around arteries to raise blood pressure.
    d. preparing the body for sexual activity.

83. Which abbreviation stands for the fluid that circulates around the brain and spinal cord?
    a. ICP
    b. CSF
    c. HNP
    d. CNS

84. All of the following are types of brain tumors EXCEPT:
    a. glioblastoma multiforme.
    b. meningioma.
    c. Schwannoma.
    d. neurofibroma.

85. All of the following are associated with pain EXCEPT:
    a. causalgia.
    b. anesthesia.
    c. neuralgia.
    d. CRPS.

86. Which abbreviation is associated with a test to measure the metabolism in areas of the brain?
    a. MRI
    b. PET
    c. SCI
    d. CAT

87. Which two combining forms mean nerve root?
    a. neur/o- and nerv/o-
    b. myel/o- and spin/o-
    c. esthes/o- and sens/o-
    d. rhiz/o- and radicul/o-

88. A rhizotomy is performed to cut the:
    a. spinal nerves.
    b. ventricles.
    c. neurons.
    d. cerebellum.

89. Proprioception is the process of having:
    a. pain.
    b. nerve damage.
    c. body position.
    d. sensation.

90. Select the misspelled word.
    a. myelography
    b. paresthesia
    c. meninjitis
    d. syncope

91. During stereotactic neurosurgery, the surgeon is certain to encounter the:
    a. meninges.
    b. vertebra.
    c. spinal cord.
    d. nerve roots.

92. The largest part of the brain is the:
    a. cerebrum.
    b. cerebellum.
    c. thalamus.
    d. gyri and sulci.

93. Which type of cell produces the myelin covering around the axon of a neuron?
    a. oligodendroglia
    b. astrocyte
    c. microglia
    d. none of the above

94. The part of the nervous system that is active when the body is at rest is the:
    a. sympathetic nervous system.
    b. parasympathetic nervous system.
    c. somatic nervous system.
    d. all of the above

95. Shaken baby syndrome can cause:
    a. mental retardation.
    b. concussion.
    c. brain hemorrhage.
    d. all of the above

96. All of the following combining forms refer to a seizure EXCEPT:
    a. epilept/o-.
    b. convuls/o-.
    c. spin/o-.
    d. ict/o-.

97. All of the following are types of aphasia EXCEPT:
    a. amnesia.
    b. receptive.
    c. global.
    d. expressive.

98. Which medical word means water on the brain?
    a. epilepsy
    b. meningitis
    c. hydrocephalus
    d. dementia

99. Photophobia is associated with:
   a. migraine headaches.
   b. carpal tunnel syndrome.
   c. myelomeningocele.
   d. Parkinson's disease.

100. Cerebrospinal fluid can be examined by first doing a/an:
   a. EEG.
   b. skull x-ray.
   c. lumbar puncture.
   d. CT scan.

Short Answer

Write the word or phrase that best completes each statement or answers the question.

101. A spinal tap is also known as a _____ _____.

102. A chronic neurological disease that involves an imbalance of the levels of neurotransmitters, dopamine, and acetylocholine, is called _____.

103. The full name of a medical procedure to record the electrical activity of the brain is an _____.

104. James put his hand on a hot iron. An involuntary muscle reaction controlled by the spinal cord and called a _____ allowed him to remove his hand quickly from the heat before sustaining further tissue damage.

105. Convulsions are also called _____.

106. Difficulty speaking or understanding words is termed _____

107. Compression of the median nerve in the wrist from repetitive motions leads to _____ _____ _____.

108. In a diving accident the patient severely injured his cervical spinal cord at the level of C2. As a result he became a _____ and was paralyzed from the neck down, to include all four extremities.

109. A patient with a herniated _____ disk might benefit from surgery such as a diskectomy or laminectomy.

110. _____ is a radiologic procedure in which a radiopaque contrast dye is injected into the subarachnoid space at the level of the L3 and L4 vertebrae, which in turn outlines the spinal cavity.

111. _____ _____ is a diagnostic procedure in which an EEG is used to record changes in brain waves that occur following various stimuli.

112. _____ is a multifaceted test used to diagnose the many underlying conditions that can cause insomnia, sleep disruption, sleep apnea, or narcolepsy.

113. _____ sign is a result of a neurologic test in which the end of the metal handle of the percussion hammer is used to firmly stroke the outside of the foot from the heel to the toes.

114. A carotid _____ is a surgical procedure done to remove plaque from the carotid artery.

115. The surgical procedure, which inserts a plastic tube from the ventricles of the brain to the peritoneal cavity, and which continuously removes excess cerebrospinal fluid, is called a _____ shunt.

116. Also known as antiepileptic drugs, _____ drugs are given to prevent the seizures of epilepsy.

117. The brain and its surrounding structures fill the _____ cavity.

118. An involuntary muscle reaction that is controlled by the spinal cord is called a/an _____.

119. The _____ are four hollow chambers in the brain.

120. The _____ nervous system consists of the brain and the spinal cord.

121. The largest part of the brain is the _____.

122. The cerebral _____ or gray matter is the narrow outermost layer of the cerebrum that follows the curves of the gyri and sulci.

123. A very deep _____ that runs anterior to posterior divides the cerebrum into right and left hemispheres.

124. The two hemispheres are physically separate and their only connection is through the _____ _____, a thick, white band of nerves deep within the brain.

125. The _____ oblongata joins the pons to the spinal cord.

126. The entire brain and spinal cord are surrounded by three separate membrane layers that are collectively known as the _____.

127. A _____ is an involuntary muscle reaction that is controlled by the spinal cord.

128. A _____, an individual nerve cell, is the functional unit of the nervous system.

129. If the brain or spinal cord wants a voluntary skeletal muscle to move, this command is transmitted to the muscle by the _____ nervous system.

130. The _____ nervous system is active when the body is confronted with danger or during times of stress or anxiety.

131. _____ is brief, involuntary episodes of falling asleep during the daytime while engaged in activity.

132. An abnormal opening in the vertebral column through which the spinal cord and nerves may protrude to the outside of the body is called _____ _____.

133. A chronic, progressive, degenerative autoimmune disease in which the body makes antibodies against myelin is called _____ _____.

134. _____ _____ is a nutrient found in prenatal vitamins and fortified cereals that helps prevent the occurrence of myelomeningocele in infants.

135. A _____ unit is a device used to control chronic pain by stimulating the nerve endings.

136. The study of the anatomy, physiology, diseases, and tests of the nervous system is known as _____.

137. High folds or _____ and deep grooves or _____ are present on the surface of the cerebrum.

138. The olfactory nerve, cranial nerve I, sends information to the brain about the sense of _____.

139. The adjective form of coma is _____.

140. Mental retardation caused by a defect in chromosome 21 is known as _____ syndrome.

141. _____ is a skin condition caused by a herpes virus infection that causes painful eruptions along the course of a nerve in adults.

142. _____ _____ is the connecting tissue between the two hemispheres of the brain.

143. There are _____ pairs of cranial nerves and _____ pairs of spinal nerves.

True/False

Write 'T' if the statement is true and 'F' if the statement is false.

_____144. Guillain-Barré is a condition in which there is a paralysis with drooping of one side of the face due to inflammation of the facial cranial nerve.

_____145. Polyneuritis is defined as a severe burning sensation under the skin along a nerve branch.

_____146. A carotid endarterectomy removes plaque from the inner lining of the carotid artery to restore blood flow to the brain and decrease the possibility of a stroke.

_____147. A myography is an x-ray that uses dye to produce an image of the spinal anatomy.

_____148. Sciatica is pain and numbness of the lower back and below from compression of the lumbar nerve roots from L-4–L-5.

_____149. Patients with multiple sclerosis will have an abnormal MRI of the brain and spinal cord showing plaques or scarring of nerves in the spinal cord and brain.

_____150. A Romberg's neuroma causes damage to the nerve around the metatarsophalangeal joint between the ball of the foot and the toes.

_____151. The TENS unit is a device that is used to control chronic pain.

_____152. A ventriculoperitoneal shunt would be performed to remove excess cerebrospinal fluid associated with hydrocephalus.

_____153. A subdural hematoma would be located below the medulla oblongata

_____154. Patients with both expressive and receptive aphasia are said to have global aphasia.

_____155. An arteriovenous malformation is an abnormality in which arteries in the brain connect to other arteries, forming a twisted nest of blood vessels.

_____156. It is possible for lymphoma to arise in the brain.

_____157. A cerebrovascular accident is an automobile accident caused by a stroke.

_____158. Coma is defined as an irreversible loss of all brain function as confirmed by an electroencephalogram.

_____159. An autopsy of a patient who died of Alzheimer's disease will show classic neurofibrillary tangles and senile plaques.

_____160. An alpha fetoprotein test is conducted to diagnose muscular dystrophy in a fetus before birth.

_____161. The Glasgow Coma Scale is used to help diagnose the type of aphasia that a stroke patient may have.

_____162. A mini mental status examination (MMSE) is done to test a patient's concrete and abstract thought processes and long- and short-term memory.

_____163. A craniotomy is a surgical incision into the skull to expose the brain tissue, and is only done to diagnose brain tumors.

_____164. Epilepsy is diagnosed based on the characteristics of the seizure and the results of an MRI scan of the brain.

_____165. Tardive dyskinesia is a late effect of blinking and tongue movements seen with certain drugs that are used to treat Parkinson's disease.

_____166. The gray matter of the brain and spinal cord contains myelin.

_____167. Cerebrospinal fluid is formed in the ventricles of the brain.

_____168. A nerve impulse travels electrically across a synapse.

_____169. A herniated intravertebral disk is known as a slipped disk.

_____170. The suffix -cele means hernia.

_____171. A neurotransmitter is a chemical messenger that travels between nerve cells.

_____172. A reflex is a purposeful, voluntary muscle response to a stimulus.

_____173. A blood clot in an artery on the left side of the brain can cause symptoms of paralysis on the right side of the body.

_____174. The pons is the area where nerves from one side of the brain cross over to the other side of the body.

_____175. Cauda equina is the medical phrase that describes the nerve roots at the end of the spinal cord.

_____176. The proximal end of the spinal cord attaches to the cerebellum of the brain.

_____177. Mad cow disease is related to the human disease known as Creutzfeldt-Jakob disease.

_____178. Down syndrome is a congenital defect caused by an infection before the baby was born.

_____179. Complex partial seizures are also known as psychomotor seizures.

Essay

Write your answer in the space provided or on a separate sheet of paper.

180. Explain how a cerebrovascular accident leads to death of brain tissue.

181. Why is an electroencephalography used to diagnose epilepsy?

182. Name the three layers of the meninges, beginning with the outermost layer next to the cranial bones.

183. Describe the process of nerve transmission.

184. Briefly discuss the purpose of the parasympathetic nervous system.

185. Discuss the meaning of the phrase cerebrovascular accident.

186. What is dementia?

187. What is cerebral angiography and what is its purpose?

CHAPTER 11

Multiple Choice

Choose the one alternative that best completes the statement or answers the question.

1. The meatus of the urethra is a/an:
   a. muscle.
   b. gland.
   c. opening.
   d. sphincter.

2. The inability to voluntarily retain urine is:
   a. incontinence.
   b. hesitancy.
   c. micturition.
   d. retention.

3. Antispasmodic drugs such as Cystospaz are helpful in treating:
   a. overactive bladder.
   b. neurogenic bladder.
   c. cystocele.
   d. interstitial cystitis.

4. Which is an x-ray of urinary organs that does not use contrast dye?
   a. IVP
   b. BUN
   c. KUB
   d. CAPD

5. A nephropexy is done to correct:
   a. nephrolithiasis.
   b. nephropathy.
   c. nephrosclerosis.
   d. nephroptosis.

6. Which finding in a urinalysis would indicate the presence of a urinary tract infection?
   a. ketonuria
   b. pyuria
   c. polyuria
   d. oliguria

7. The plural of glomerulus is:
   a. glomeruli.
   b. glomerulices.
   c. glomerula.
   d. glomerulae.

8. If a patient is taking a diuretic such as Lasix, it will be necessary to replace the potassium lost in the urine with the medication:
   a. Proscar.
   b. Urispas.
   c. K-Dur.
   d. Pyridium.

9. Mr. Jones has a large kidney stone that is obstructing the flow of urine in his left kidney, resulting in kidney enlargement and backing up of urine into his ureter. This is known as:
   a. hydroureter.
   b. hypernephroma.
   c. incontinence.
   d. enuresis.

10. The condition _____ may be found in a diabetic patient who metabolizes fats instead of glucose for energy.
    a. oliguria
    b. polyuria
    c. ketonuria
    d. dysuria

11. Which is the abbreviation for the nursing procedure that documents the amount of fluids taken in and eliminated by a patient?
    a. CAPD
    b. cc
    c. I&O
    d. UA

12. The trigone is part of the:
    a. renal pelvis.
    b. bladder.
    c. prostate.
    d. urethra.

13. Stress _____ occurs in a woman when she laughs, coughs, or sneezes causing her to involuntary pass some urine.
    a. hesitancy
    b. retention
    c. dysuria
    d. incontinence

14. Which would be a normal finding in a urinalysis?
    a. casts
    b. albumin
    c. creatinine
    d. glucose

15. Which is a urinary radiological procedure in which x-rays are taken as the patient expels dye that was previously inserted into the bladder?
    a. voiding cystourethrography
    b. retrograde pyelography
    c. urinalysis
    d. intravenous pyelography

16. The urinary catheter that is inserted through the urethra to the bladder to remain for a period of time is a:
    a. suprapubic catheter.
    b. Foley catheter.
    c. straight catheter.
    d. condom catheter.

17. An ongoing life-saving procedure that is used to treat ESRD is:
    a. catheterization.
    b. percutaneous ultrasonic lithotripsy.
    c. hemodialysis.
    d. radiation.

18. Which are examples of drugs that would be prescribed to treat a urinary tract infection?
    a. Detrol and Urispas
    b. Esidrix and Lasix
    c. K-Lyte
    d. Macrobid and Gantrisin

19. A person with uremia would have elevated results for which of these laboratory tests?
    a. BUN
    b. C&S
    c. PSA
    d. I&O

20. Which is an eponym for the cancer of the kidney found in children?
    a. Wilms'
    b. Henle's
    c. Bowman's
    d. Foley's

21. In addition to creating and excreting urine in order to rid the body of wastes, the kidney also functions to influence:
    a. red blood cell production.
    b. blood pressure.
    c. the pH balance of the blood.
    d. all of the above

22. Two medical terminology combining forms meaning the urinary bladder are cyst/o- and:
    a. pyel/o-.
    b. cortic/o-.
    c. ur/o-.
    d. vesic/o-.

23. Which is a renal disease in which substances from the immune response to the streptococcus bacterium collect in the capillary network of the nephron?
    a. nephrotic syndrome
    b. pyelonephritis
    c. glomerulonephritis
    d. acute renal failure

24. The urinometer and refractometer are used to measure the _____ of urine.
    a. sediments
    b. specific gravity
    c. pH
    d. color

25. Epispadias or hypospadias would be corrected surgically with a:
    a. lithotripsy.
    b. cystectomy.
    c. urethroplasty.
    d. nephropexy.

26. Where does the renal artery enter and the renal vein and ureter exit the kidney?
    a. mediastinum
    b. urethra
    c. hilum
    d. glomerulus

27. What tube connects the bladder to the outside of the body?
    a. ureter
    b. vas deferens
    c. urethra
    d. vesicle
28. Which is the area of the kidney that includes the cortex and medulla?
    a. parenchyma
    b. glomerulus
    c. mucosa
    d. hilum
29. Which process involves the contractions of smooth muscle that propel urine through the ureter?
    a. reabsorption
    b. peristalsis
    c. filtration
    d. micturition
30. Which word means pertaining to the bladder?
    a. renal
    b. nephric
    c. urinary
    d. vesical
31. A kidney stone is also called a/an:
    a. calculus.
    b. calyx.
    c. vegetation.
    d. embolism.
32. Damage to the pores of the glomeruli that allows large amounts of albumin (protein) to leak into the urine, decreasing the amount of blood proteins, is known as:
    a. nephrotic syndrome.
    b. nephrolithiasis.
    c. nephroptosis.
    d. cystitis.
33. The abbreviation ARF means:
    a. acid resistant factor.
    b. acute renal factor.
    c. acute renal failure.
    d. acute renal focus.
34. An excessive amount of urea in the blood because of renal failure is known as:
    a. nephritis.
    b. urethritis.
    c. uremia.
    d. ureteritis.
35. Which is another name for nephroblastoma?
    a. bladder cancer
    b. cystitis
    c. Wilms' tumor
    d. uremia
36. A hernia in which the bladder bulges through a weakness in the muscular wall of the vagina or rectum is known as:
    a. neurogenic bladder.
    b. overactive bladder.
    c. cystocele.
    d. cystitis.
37. The formation of an abnormal passageway connecting the bladder to the vagina is known as:
    a. urinary retention.
    b. vesicovaginal fistula.
    c. vesicovaginal fissure.
    d. vesicovaginostomy.
38. Which is a congenital condition in which the female urethral meatus is incorrectly located near the clitoris or the male urethral meatus is incorrectly located on the upper surface of the shaft of the penis?
    a. epispadias
    b. hyperspadias
    c. hypospadias
    d. subspadias
39. Involuntary urination during sleep is known as:
    a. urinary incontinence.
    b. urinary retention.
    c. enuresis.
    d. urinary frequency.
40. Absence of urine production by the kidney is known as:
    a. anuria.
    b. bacteriuria.
    c. dysuria.
    d. pyuria.
41. Difficult or painful urination is known as:
    a. anuria.
    b. bacteriuria.
    c. dysuria.
    d. pyuria.
42. Blood in the urine is known as:
    a. anuria.
    b. bacteriuria.
    c. dysuria.
    d. hematuria.
43. Glucose in the urine is known as:
    a. anuria.
    b. bacteriuria.
    c. dysuria.
    d. glycosuria.
44. A decreased amount of potassium in the blood is known as:
    a. hypokalemia.
    b. hyperbilirubinemia.
    c. hyperkalemia.
    d. hypocalcemia.

45. Which is a blood test that measures the amount of urea?
    a. BUN
    b. UA
    c. C & S
    d. SG

46. Which radiologic procedure uses x-rays and radiopaque contrast dye that is inserted into the bladder through a cystoscope? The x-ray image is taken while the patient is urinating.
    a. cystometry
    b. renal angiography
    c. voiding cystourethrography
    d. nephrotomography

47. Which type of hemodialysis allows the patient to be ambulatory?
    a. CAPD
    b. Foley catheter
    c. hemodialysis
    d. CMG

48. Which type of drug blocks sodium from being absorbed from the tubule back into the blood?
    a. diuretic drugs
    b. antispasmodic drugs
    c. urinary analgesic drugs
    d. chemotherapy drugs

49. The abbreviation UTI means:
    a. urethral tract inflammation.
    b. urinary tomography intravenous.
    c. urinary tract infection.
    d. urethral and transurethral incision.

50. The urinary system does NOT include which of the following?
    a. pulmonary parenchyma
    b. kidney
    c. ureter
    d. bladder

51. Which of the following words cannot be paired with the word renal to indicate a part of the urinary system?
    a. capsule
    b. trigone
    c. pyramids
    d. medulla

52. Waste products excreted by the kidney include all of the following EXCEPT:
    a. urea.
    b. creatinine.
    c. uric acid.
    d. nephron.

53. Which of the following are NOT filtered out in the kidney?
    a. red blood cells
    b. electrolytes

c. water
d. glucose

54. Which of the following words does NOT refer to the process of eliminating urine from the body?
    a. urination
    b. micturition
    c. voiding
    d. reabsorption

55. Enlargement of the kidney due to constant pressure from backed up urine is called:
    a. hydronephrosis.
    b. glomerulonephritis.
    c. nephrolithiasis.
    d. polycystic kidney disease.

56. Inflammation and infection of the pelves of the kidneys is known as:
    a. cystitis.
    b. renal cell carcinoma.
    c. uremia.
    d. pyelonephritis.

57. Which of the following is NOT true regarding chronic renal failure?
    a. It begins with renal insufficiency.
    b. There is gradual worsening and progressive damage to the kidneys.
    c. It may lead to end-stage renal disease.
    d. It develops rapidly, sometimes due to trauma.

58. Which type of cancer occurs in children and arises from residual embryonic or fetal tissue?
    a. Wilms' tumor
    b. renal cell cancer
    c. bladder cancer
    d. uremia

59. A urinometer is used to measure which of the following?
    a. specific gravity
    b. blood in the urine
    c. pH of the urine.
    d. presence of glucose in the urine

60. Micturition means the process of:
    a. perspiring.
    b. voiding.
    c. creating urine in the kidney.
    d. creating urine in the bladder.

61. If the blood pressure decreases, the kidneys produce:
    a. concentrated urine with less water in it.
    b. diluted urine with more water in it.
    c. urine with blood in it
    d. electrolytes

62. Congenital means:
    a. inherited.
    b. present at birth.
    c. damaged.
    d. deformed.

63. Which word means having the function of or being able to walk?
    a. dilate
    b. profuse
    c. ambulate
    d. dialysate

64. Which is a flexible tube to drain urine that is inserted through the abdominal wall just above the pubic bone?
    a. catheter
    b. suprapubic catheter
    c. Foley
    d. condom

65. What is the process called when a nurse measures the amount of fluid produced by the body and the amount of fluid ingested by a patient?
    a. urinary in and out
    b. fluid measurement
    c. I&O (intake and output)
    d. urine specimen

66. Which is a surgical procedure to remove a severely damaged kidney from a patient with end-stage kidney failure and insert a new kidney from a donor?
    a. transplantation
    b. cystoscopy
    c. lithotripsy
    d. nephrectomy

67. Which word means the functional or working area of any organ (as opposed to the organ's structural framework)?
    a. glomerulus
    b. parenchyma
    c. nephron
    d. urea

68. Which is the correct order for the process of producing urine?
    a. filtration, collection of filtrate, reabsorption, collection of urine
    b. collection of filtrate, filtration, reabsorption, collection of urine
    c. reabsorption, filtration, collection of filtrate, collection of urine
    d. collection of urine, filtration, collection of filtrate, reabsorption

69. Which is a common passageway that collects fluid from many nephrons?
    a. cortex
    b. renal pelvis

c. distal convoluted tubule
    d. collecting duct

70. *E. coli* is the most common cause of:
    a. kidney stones.
    b. hypospadias.
    c. renal failure.
    d. urinary tract infections.

71. The functional unit of the kidney is known as the:
    a. collecting tubule.
    b. cortex.
    c. nephron.
    d. pelvis.

72. Hydroureter is most often caused by a:
    a. diuretic drug.
    b. kidney stone.
    c. urinary tract infection.
    d. all of the above

73. Placing a tube into the bladder in order to drain the urine is called:
    a. cystoscopy.
    b. dialysis.
    c. KUB.
    d. catheterization.

74. For a patient in end-stage renal failure, what are two of the three things that can take the place of the nonfunctioning kidneys?
    a. hemodialysis or renal transplantation
    b. peritoneal dialysis or catheterization
    c. diuresis or catheterization
    d. cystoscopy or hemodialysis

75. Another name for a KUB is a:
    a. flat plate of the abdomen.
    b. cystoscopy.
    c. catheterization.
    d. cystocele.

76. Involuntarily passing urine while sneezing, coughing, or laughing is called:
    a. urinary retention.
    b. stress incontinence.
    c. cystitis.
    d. nocturia.

77. A patient with hematuria would have _____ in the urine.
    a. casts
    b. protein
    c. glucose
    d. blood

78. A urine culture and sensitivity is done to identify the:
    a. bacteria causing a kidney stone.
    b. bacteria causing a UTI.
    c. antibiotics that would be effective against the bacteria.
    d. b and c

79. A small area behind the abdominal cavity that is filled with fatty tissues around the kidney is known as the:
    a. peritoneal cavity.
    b. abdominopelvic cavity.
    c. retroperitoneal space.
    d. flank.
80. An empty bladder collapses into folds called:
    a. mucosa.
    b. trigones.
    c. rugae.
    d. sphincters.
81. Waste products of metabolism that are excreted in the urine include:
    a. urea.
    b. creatinine.
    c. uric acid.
    d. all of the above.
82. The pH of the urine is related to the:
    a. amount of blood in it.
    b. color and odor.
    c. amount of protein in it.
    d. acidity or alkalinity.
83. Cystoscopy is a procedure to visualize the:
    a. bladder.
    b. abdominal cavity.
    c. retroperitoneal space
    d. kidney
84. Both ren/o- and nephr/o- mean:
    a. kidney.
    b. bladder.
    c. urine.
    d. nephron.
85. The suffix -scope means:
    a. process of using an instrument to examine.
    b. stone.
    c. laboratory procedure.
    d. instrument used to examine.
86. All of these are laboratory tests performed on a urine specimen EXCEPT:
    a. C & S.
    b. WBC.
    c. CAPD.
    d. UA.
87. The word pyelonephritis can be separated into:
    a. prefix, combining form, suffix.
    b. prefix, combining form, combining form.
    c. combining form, suffix, suffix.
    d. combining form, combining form, suffix.
88. A urinometer is a/an:
    a. procedure.
    b. disease condition.

c. measuring device.
d. type of surgery.
89. Which of the following is a disease that affects the kidneys?
    a. ESRD
    b. BUN
    c. GU
    d. KUB

Short Answer

Write the word or phrase that best completes each statement or answers the question.

90. A surgical procedure using a cystoscope and an instrument with interwoven wires to grasp and remove a calculus would be termed _____ basketing.
91. The word for urinary frequency and increased voluntary urination at night is called _____.
92. Formation of kidney stones is termed _____.
93. A diagnostic procedure done by inserting an instrument through the urethra to view the bladder is called a/an _____.
94. The absence of the production of urine is called _____.
95. Bacterial infection of the kidney that involves the renal pelvis is termed _____.
96. Uremic _____ occurs when excess urea is excreted through the sweat glands creating a white, powdery deposit on the skin.
97. The words micturition and voiding both mean the process of _____.
98. The word _____ is used to describe painful or difficulty urinating.
99. Because Mary was donating her left kidney to her twin sister, she was prepared for the surgery called a/an _____.
100. The _____ is a 12-inch tube that extends from the renal pelvis of the kidney to the bladder. There are two of them in every human.
101. The wall of the ureter contracts every 30 seconds to propel urine into the bladder in a process known as _____.
102. When the bladder is empty, the mucosa collapses into folds called _____.
103. In the male, as the urethra leaves the bladder, it travels through the _____ gland.
104. _____ is the process through which blood in the capillary pushes water, waste products, electrolytes, glucose, and other substances through pores in the glomerulus and out into Bowman's capsule.
105. The loop of Henle widens to become the _____ convoluted tubule.

106. If the pH of the blood decreases, this causes _____ to be reabsorbed, increasing the pH of the blood.

107. _____ is a complication that develops following an acute infection with streptococcus bacteria or with viruses.

108. In the word nephrolithiasis the combining form lith/o- means _____.

109. _____ means blood in the urine.

110. The _____ is a 12-inch tube that extends from the renal pelvis of the kidney to the bladder.

111. The _____ is an indentation in the medial surface of the kidney.

112. The renal _____ is the thin layer of tissue just beneath the renal capsule.

113. The _____ is a reservoir for storing urine.

114. The _____ is a tube that carries urine from the bladder to the outside of the body.

115. In men, as the urethra leaves the bladder, it travels though the _____ gland, a spherical gland at the base of the bladder.

116. The GU system means the _____ system.

117. The _____, a microscopic structure, is the functional unit of the kidney and the site of urine production.

118. If the number of red blood cells decreases, the kidneys secrete the hormone _____ to stimulate the bone marrow to produce more red blood cells.

119. _____ is a general word for any disease process involving the kidney.

120. A cancerous tumor of the kidney that occurs in children and arises from residual embryonic or fetal tissue is known as a/an _____.

121. The procedure of cleansing of the blood through the use of a machine instead of the kidney is called _____.

122. A _____ is a flexible tube used in medical procedures.

123. A graphic recording of the amount of urine and the amount of pressure within the bladder is called a _____.

124. _____ is a medical or surgical procedure that uses sound waves to break up a kidney stone.

125. The abbreviation KUB means _____, _____, and _____.

126. The _____ _____ sits like a cap on top of the kidney.

127. The prefix poly- in polycystic kidney disease means _____.

128. Anuria is the opposite of _____.

129. The study of the anatomy and physiology of the urine system plus related diseases and procedures is known as _____.

True/False

Write 'T' if the statement is true and 'F' if the statement is false.

_____130. Enuresis is the medical word for bedwetting.

_____131. Hematuria is the presence of excessive urea in the blood.

_____132. The renal cortex and medulla are the parenchyma of the renal organs.

_____133. The urethra is the tube that connects the kidney to the bladder.

_____134. Polyuria is always an indication of the presence of a urinary tract infection.

_____135. Bacterial urinary tract infections are most often caused by streptococcus.

_____136. ESWL is a procedure done to break up a urinary stone.

_____137. Renal colic is the pain and spasm of urinary organs associated with passage of a kidney stone.

_____138. A cystocele is an abnormal passageway connecting the bladder to the vagina.

_____139. The medical word for any disease process involving the kidney is nephrosis.

_____140. The word retroperitoneal means literally behind the peritoneum.

_____141. Electrolytes and glucose molecules are too large to pass through the pores in the glomerulus and thus remain in the blood.

_____142. The network of capillaries that makes up the glomerulus combines into a single arteriole that leaves Bowman's capsule and travels along the tubular parts of the nephron.

_____143. The proximal convoluted tubule of the nephron is a symptom of an abnormal condition.

_____144. If the blood is low in glucose, the body reacts by reabsorbing almost all of the glucose in the tubules to preserve blood glucose.

_____145. The total number of nephrons in the kidneys continues to decline with age and kidney capacity decreases proportionately.

_____146. The kidneys have a role in the maintenance of blood pressure by controlling the concentration of urine.

_____147. Calculogenesis is the process of forming stones.

_____148. Nephroptosis is a general word for any disease process involving the kidney.

_____149. A leukocyte esterase test is a test done to describe the characteristics of the urine.

_____150. The kidneys excrete urea, a waste product from protein metabolism.

_____151. A diuretic drug is one that decreases the amount of urine produced by the kidneys.

_____152. Nephrolithotomy is a surgical incision into the kidney to remove a stone.

_____153. In hemodialysis, a shunt is placed into the patient's abdominal cavity to insert fluid and remove waste products.

_____154. A dipstick can be used to do a routine urinalysis.

_____155. The prostate gland is part of the urinary system.

_____156. The urethras of men and women are the same length.

_____157. A BUN tests the urine for the presence of urea.

_____158. The suffix -ptosis means a state of prolapse or drooping.

_____159. A biopsy of the kidney is done to test for kidney stones.

Essay

Write your answer in the space provided or on a separate sheet of paper.

160. Why are women more prone to urinary tract infections than men?

161. Why would a culture and sensitivity test be done on a sample of urine?

162. What is blood urea nitrogen?

163. What is a culture and sensitivity test and what is it used for?

164. What is polycystic kidney disease?

165. What is renal failure?

166. What is erythropoietin and what is its function?

CHAPTER 12

Multiple Choice

Choose the one alternative that best completes the statement or answers the question.

1. The congenital condition in which the foreskin of the penis is too tight is known as:
   a. epispadias.
   b. hypospadias
   c. priapism
   d. phimosis

2. Balanitis is an inflammation of the:
   a. prostate.
   b. bladder.
   c. urethra.
   d. glans penis.

3. A TURP would be performed for:
   a. DRE.
   b. BPH.
   c. STD.
   d. TRUS.

4. For his genital herpes the patient takes:
   a. Cialis.
   b. Vibramycin.
   c. Estrace.
   d. Zovirax.

5. Inflammation of the anatomical structure that stores mature spermatozoa is called:
   a. orchitis.
   b. epididymitis.
   c. urethritis.
   d. prostatitis.

6. Which abbreviation indicates impotence in the male?
   a. VD
   b. DRE
   c. ED
   d. STD

7. The organism that causes genital warts is abbreviated as:
   a. HSV.
   b. HPV.
   c. HIV.
   d. FSH.

8. A man who has had a vasectomy will not be able to:
   a. get an erection.
   b. produce spermatozoa.
   c. impregnate a woman.
   d. produce ejaculate fluid.

9. An orchiopexy would be done for:
   a. cryptorchism.
   b. chordee.
   c. priapsm.
   d. varicocele.

10. If a man has had his prostate removed, which will occur?
    a. There will be a decrease in the volume of semen produced.
    b. There will be less testosterone secreted.
    c. Spermatogenesis will diminish.
    d. There will be less capacity for storage of spermatozoa.

11. Which lab test is done to screen for prostate cancer?
    a. FSH
    b. RPR
    c. TURP
    d. PSA

12. Which is the most common sexually transmitted disease? It is caused by a bacterium and sometimes causes painful urination in the male.
    a. genital herpes
    b. chlamydia
    c. genital warts
    d. AIDS

13. A varicocele can be the cause of:
    a. impotence.
    b. infertility.
    c. urinary hesitancy and dribbling.
    d. premature ejaculation.

14. Priapism creates pain and tenderness of the:
    a. scrotal sac.
    b. groin.
    c. male breast.
    d. penis.

15. Which anatomical word is misspelled?
    a. prostrate
    b. testis
    c. seminiferous tubules
    d. perineum

16. A medical procedure used to feel the prostate gland to detect enlargement or tenderness is abbreviated as:
    a. TSE.
    b. TUR.
    c. DRE.
    d. RPR.

17. The penile drainage from Mr. Miller was examined under a microscope and showed gram-negative diplococci that confirmed the diagnosis of:
    a. syphilis.
    b. gonorrhea.
    c. herpes simplex type 2.
    d. condylomata acuminata.

18. Spermatozoa and testosterone production take place in the:
    a. epididymis.
    b. inguinal canal.
    c. seminiferous tubules.
    d. ductus deferens.

19. Semen is produced in the:
    a. bulbourethral glands.
    b. prostate.
    c. seminal vesicles.
    d. all of the above

20. The location of the corpora cavernosa is the:
    a. upper surface of the penis.
    b. underside of the penis.
    c. base of the penis.
    d. tip of the penis.

21. After Mr. Parker's physical exam the physician noticed the laboratory report for levels of acid phosphatase were elevated. Therefore the physician ordered further tests to determine if Mr. Parker has:
    a. infertility problems.
    b. a urinary tract infection.
    c. prostate cancer.
    d. low male hormone production.

22. Mr. Grey had a routine semen analysis for infertility. His semen was evaluated for all of the following EXCEPT:
    a. DNA analysis of the spermatozoa.
    b. spermatozoa motility.
    c. spermatozoa morphology.
    d. sperm count.

23. The patient came to the physician's office complaining of a rash and swollen glands. The patient admitted to being sexually active without using a condom. The physician ordered lab work to include a VDRL to determine if the patient had:
    a. seminoma.
    b. syphilis.
    c. infertility.
    d. premature ejaculation.

24. Which condition could be relieved by insertion of a penile implant?
    a. dyspareunia
    b. premature ejaculation
    c. erectile dysfunction
    d. priapism

25. Each spermatozoon contains a head containing chromosomes and a tail or _____ that propels it.
    a. gamete
    b. gonad
    c. flagellum
    d. meiosis

26. The function of which of these is to display the male secondary sex characteristics, produce sperm, and, when appropriate, deposit sperm inside the female?
    a. external genitalia
    b. internal genitalia
    c. male genitourinary system
    d. endocrine system

27. Which includes the scrotum, testes, epididymis, penis, and urethra?
    a. internal genitalia
    b. vas deferens
    c. inguinal canal
    d. external genitalia

28. The soft pouch of skin behind the penis and in front of the legs is known as the:
    a. scrotum.
    b. gonads.
    c. testis.
    d. perineum.
29. Which is the most abundant and biologically active of all the male sex hormones?
    a. testosterone
    b. estrogen
    c. progesterone
    d. follicle stimulating
30. The bulbourethral glands are also known as the:
    a. prostate glands.
    b. Cowper's glands.
    c. adrenal glands.
    d. pituitary glands.
31. The foreskin of the penis is called:
    a. corpora cavernosa.
    b. corpus spongiosum.
    c. erectile tissue.
    d. prepuce.
32. Most cells in the body divide by the process of:
    a. meiosis.
    b. osmosis.
    c. mitosis.
    d. spermatogenesis.
33. An individual mature sperm is known as:
    a. spermatozoon.
    b. spermatocyte.
    c. gonad.
    d. spermatozoa.
34. The combining form crypt/o- means:
    a. obvious.
    b. hormone.
    c. liquid.
    d. hidden.
35. Inflammation or infection of the testes is called:
    a. oligospermia.
    b. orchitis.
    c. epididymitis.
    d. cryptorchism.
36. Another name for a seminoma is:
    a. prostate cancer.
    b. undescended testicle.
    c. testicular cancer.
    d. benign prostatic hypertrophy.
37. Downward curvature of the penis is known as:
    a. dyspareunia.
    b. chordee.
    c. balanitis.
    d. postcoital.

38. The abbreviation ED stands for:
    a. erection distress.
    b. erectile disease.
    c. erectile dysfunction.
    d. erectile drug.
39. Which is another name for venereal disease?
    a. sexually transmitted disease
    b. AIDS
    c. dyspareunia
    d. precoital disease
40. A gram-negative diplococcus or double sphere bacterium describes:
    a. *Neisseria gonorrhoeae.*
    b. *Chlamydia trachomatis.*
    c. Herpes simplex.
    d. *Treponema pallidum.*
41. Which is a lesion on the penis that ulcerates, forms a crust, and then heals?
    a. rash
    b. inflammation
    c. blister
    d. chancre
42. What is the Latin phrase that means knoblike tumors with sharp points?
    a. chlamydia
    b. *Condylomata acuminata*
    c. genital herpes
    d. gonorrhea
43. A patient with gynecomastia is said to have:
    a. an enlarged penis.
    b. an enlarged prostate.
    c. enlargement of the male breast.
    d. enlarged testicles.
44. Which blood test is used to diagnose infertility problems?
    a. hormone testing
    b. semen analysis
    c. DNA testing
    d. prostate-specific antigen
45. The abbreviation PSA stands for:
    a. Prostascint antibody.
    b. prostatic-specific acid.
    c. prostate-specific androgen.
    d. prostate-specific antigen.
46. The forward movement of spermatozoa is called:
    a. mobility.
    b. motility.
    c. morphology.
    d. fertility.

47. Which is used in nuclear medicine to detect areas of metastasis from a primary site of prostate cancer?
   a. ultrasonography
   b. x-ray
   c. testicular self-examination
   d. ProstaScint scan

48. Which is a surgical procedure to reposition an undescended testicle and fix it within the scrotum?
   a. orchiopexy
   b. orchiectomy
   c. prostatectomy
   d. vasectomy

49. Which word refers to testosterone produced by the testes, other testosterone-like hormones, or manufactured testosterone used in drugs?
   a. antibiotic
   b. antiviral
   c. androgen
   d. antibacterial

50. Proscar is a drug used to treat:
   a. cancer of the prostate gland.
   b. cancer of the testes.
   c. benign prostatic hypertrophy.
   d. sexually transmitted diseases.

51. Which of the following male genitourinary organs is not an external organ?
   a. scrotum
   b. testes
   c. vas deferens
   d. urethra

52. The suffix in the word genitourinary means:
   a. pertaining to.
   b. around.
   c. urine.
   d. genital.

53. The scrotum contains what organs?
   a. perineum
   b. penis
   c. ureter
   d. testes

54. The suffix in the word testicle means:
   a. small.
   b. witness.
   c. bag.
   d. gonad.

55. The singular form of the word spermatozoa is:
   a. spermatii.
   b. sperms.
   c. spermatozoon.
   d. spermatazoon.

56. The prefix in the word interstitial means:
   a. between.
   b. space.
   c. pertaining to.
   d. tissue.

57. The suffix in the word ejaculatory means:
   a. to expel suddenly.
   b. semen.
   c. pertaining to.
   d. having the function of.

58. The bulbourethral glands are also known as:
   a. Cowper's glands.
   b. urethral glands.
   c. prostate glands.
   d. Glans penis.

59. At birth, the male urethral meatus is covered by tissue known as the:
   a. prepuce.
   b. prostate gland.
   c. penis.
   d. corpora cavernosa.

60. Failure of one or both of the testicles to descend through the inguinal canal into the scrotum is:
   a. epididymitis.
   b. oligospermia.
   c. cryptorchism.
   d. orchitis.

61. The prefix in the word dyspareunia means:
   a. sexual intercourse.
   b. condition, state.
   c. pertaining to.
   d. painful, difficult, or abnormal.

62. The long tail on a spermatozoon that propels it and makes it motile is called the:
   a. flagellum.
   b. whip.
   c. gamete.
   d. gonad.

63. Which causes the interstitial cells of the testes to secrete testosterone?
   a. FSH
   b. LH
   c. contractions
   d. pressure within the cells

64. What is the process by which a spermatocyte reduces the number of chromosomes in its nucleus to 23 or half the normal number, to create a gamete?
   a. mitosis
   b. meiosis
   c. spermatogenesis
   d. corpora cavernosa

65. Which is NOT involved in the process of erection in the penis?
    a. corpora cavernosa
    b. corpus spongiosum
    c. prepuce
    d. erectile tissue

66. The process of producing a mature spermatozoon through the processes of mitosis and meiosis is called:
    a. spermatogenesis.
    b. ejaculation.
    c. spermatozoon.
    d. spermatocyte.

67. Which class of drugs treats a lack of production of testosterone by the testes because of cryptorchidism?
    a. antiviral drugs
    b. antibiotic drugs
    c. drugs for benign prostatic hypertrophy
    d. androgen drugs

68. Which surgical procedure in the male is done to prevent pregnancy in the female?
    a. resection
    b. dissection
    c. vasectomy
    d. prostatectomy

69. Which surgical procedure is performed on the male to remove the prepuce?
    a. orchiectomy
    b. circumcision
    c. orchiopexy
    d. biopsy

70. Morphology evaluation of spermatozoa means evaluation of the:
    a. number of sperm.
    b. motility of sperm.
    c. shape of sperm.
    d. size of sperm.

71. Undescended testicles are known as:
    a. enuresis.
    b. cryptorchism.
    c. BPH.
    d. balanitis.

72. Painful intercourse is known as:
    a. dysmenorrhea.
    b. penalgia.
    c. abstinence.
    d. dyspareunia.

73. Human immunodeficiency virus causes:
    a. testicular cancer.
    b. syphilis.
    c. acquired immunodeficiency syndrome.
    d. infertility.

74. The other name for the foreskin is the:
    a. glans penis.
    b. scrotum.
    c. prepuce.
    d. prostate gland.

75. Male infertility can be due to all of the following EXCEPT:
    a. erectile dysfunction.
    b. oligospermia.
    c. abnormal morphology of the sperm.
    d. circumcision.

76. Which abbreviation means a disease contracted through sexual contact?
    a. PSA
    b. STD
    c. BPH
    d. TURP

77. Surgical removal of the testis because of cancer is known as:
    a. orchiectomy.
    b. vasectomy.
    c. herniorrhaphy.
    d. TURP.

78. The external male genitalia includes which of the following structures?
    a. seminal vesicles
    b. prostate gland.
    c. ejaculatory duct.
    d. none of the above.

79. Stimulation of the testes in preparation to begin producing spermatozoa is the function of the:
    a. thyroid gland.
    b. adrenal glands.
    c. pituitary gland.
    d. thymus.

80. Balanitis is an inflammation and infection of the:
    a. testis.
    b. penis.
    c. scrotum.
    d. urethra.

81. TURP is a surgical procedure performed on the:
    a. testes.
    b. prostate gland.
    c. rectum.
    d. urinary bladder.

82. All of these combining forms mean sexual intercourse EXCEPT:
    a. pareun/o-.
    b. coit/o-.
    c. orchi/o-.
    d. venere/o-.

83. The suffix -ile in penile and erectile means:
    a. resembling.
    b. hernia.
    c. pertaining to
    d. action; condition.

Short Answer

Write the word or phrase that best completes each statement or answers the question.

84. The gonads or sex glands in the male are the _____.

85. The patient had a chancre on his penis from an infection by the organism *Treponema pallidum,* confirming the diagnosis of _____.

86. A seminoma is a malignancy of the _____.

87. Gynecomastia is an enlarged male _____.

88. In the medical word oligospermia the combining form olig/o- means _____.

89. Dyspareunia is painful or difficult _____.

90. The process of forming mature spermatozoa is called _____.

91. The patient complained of a mass in his left testis. The physician cut into and removed a small portion of the mass and sent this to the laboratory to be examined for cancer under the microscope. The surgical procedure done on this patient is called a/an _____ biopsy.

92. Surgical removal of a testis is a/an _____.

93. The radiologic procedure that uses high-frequency sound waves to produce an image is a/an _____.

94. The male genitourinary system shares the _____ with the urinary system.

95. A long coiled tube that is attached to the outer wall of each testis is called the _____.

96. The penis contains two columns of erectile tissue. The column of paired erectile tissue is called the _____ _____.

97. Immature sperm cells found in children are known as _____.

98. The process of forming mature spermatozoa is known as _____.

99. The passageway in the groin through which the testes travel as they descend from the abdomen to the scrotum is called the _____ canal.

100. The most abundant and most biologically active of the male sex hormones secreted by the testes is _____.

101. The suffix in the word phimosis means _____ or _____ _____.

102. The pathogen that causes genital herpes is herpes simplex type _____.

103. The pathogenic organism that causes genital warts (condylomata acuminata) is _____ _____.

104. The _____ is a soft pouch of skin behind the penis and in front of the legs.

105. The testes are the male _____ or sex glands.

106. The hormone _____ is the most abundant and biologically active of all the male sex hormones.

107. As part of the male genitourinary system, the testes contain the _____ tubules, a series of compartmentalized, tightly coiled tubules that produce spermatozoa or sperm.

108. The _____ is a long, coiled tube (over 20 feet in length) that is attached to the outer wall of each testis.

109. The _____ cord is a muscular tube that contains arteries, veins, nerves, and the vas deferens.

110. The _____ is a round gland at the base of the bladder in men.

111. The _____ glands are small, bulblike glands about the size of peas that are located on either side of the urethra just below the prostate gland.

112. Three columns of _____ tissue run the length of the penis. When they fill with blood during sexual arousal, they cause the penis to become firm and erect (an erection).

113. _____-stimulating hormone (FSH) causes the seminiferous tubules to enlarge.

114. The onset of _____ is also called adolescence.

115. Most cells in the body divide by the process of _____, in which the 46 chromosomes in the nucleus duplicate and then split, creating two identical cells each with 46 chromosomes.

116. Spermatozoa (and ova from the female) that have only half of the usual number of chromosomes are known as _____.

117. During childhood, the outer walls of the seminiferous tubules contain immature cells known as _____.

118. The _____ _____, also known as the ductus deferens, is a very long, narrow tube that receives spermatozoa from the epididymis.

True/False

Write 'T' if the statement is true and 'F' if the statement is false.

_____119. A circumcision is done to correct phimosis.

_____120. A varicocele is the downward curvature of the penis during erection.

_____121. The prepuce is another name for the scrotum.

_____122. An antibiotic drug is not effective against viral infections therefore an antibiotic would not be used to treat genital warts.

_____123. The scrotum is always a few degrees cooler than the core body temperature so that spermatozoa can develop properly.

_____124. A vasovasostomy is the word for the reversal of a vasectomy.

_____125. Postcoital pain occurs after sexual intercourse.

_____126. Drugs such as Cialis and Levitra produce a penile erection by boosting the production of testosterone.

_____127. Oligospermia is one of the causes of male infertility.

_____128. The male genitourinary (GU) system is composed of the external and internal genitalia.

_____129. The scrotum is always a few degrees warmer than the core body temperature.

_____130. The epididymis destroys defective spermatozoa.

_____131. Prostatic fluid and urine both use the urethra to the outside of the body.

_____132. BPH or benign prostatic hypertrophy is a cancerous condition of the prostate gland.

_____133. The suffix in the word prostatitis indicates that there is an inflammation in the prostate gland.

_____134. The word aspermia means high sperm count.

_____135. Transrectal ultrasonography is achieved by using an ultrasound probe inserted into the rectum to obtain an image of the scrotum.

_____136. A surgical procedure to remove a testis is called an orchiectomy.

_____137. Prostatectomy is a surgical procedure to reposition an undescended testicle.

_____138. A spermatocyte has 23 chromosomes.

_____139. Treponema pallidum is the bacterium that causes gonorrhea.

_____140. Syphilis can be detected by the VDRL test.

_____141. The word testis has a different meaning from the word testicle.

_____142. A vasovasostomy is used to reconstruct the vas in a patient who has previously had an orchiectomy and now wishes to have more children.

_____143. Testicular self-examination is a way to find cancer in its early stages.

_____144. A gamete has only 23 chromosomes.

_____145. In an uncircumcised male, the urethral meatus is covered by the prepuce.

_____146. Semen is a combination of spermatozoa and fluids from the seminal vesicles, prostate gland, and penis.

_____147. Testicular cancer usually arises from abnormally formed sperm.

Essay

Write your answer in the space provided or on a separate sheet of paper.

148. What importance is attached to the proper closing of the inguinal canal in the male infant?

149. Explain how a vasectomy, surgical removal of a portion of the vas deferens, would prevent the male from impregnating a female.

150. Why must the testes be located outside the body in the scrotum?

151. What is testosterone and what is its function?

152. What is the prostate gland and what is its function?

153. What is cryptorchism?

154. What is gynecomastia?

155. What is the digital rectal exam and how often should it be done?

CHAPTER 13

Multiple Choice

Choose the one alternative that best completes the statement or answers the question.

1. Uterine descensus is also known as uterine:
   a. inflammation.
   b. herniation.
   c. prolapse.
   d. malposition.

2. The neonate born at _____ weeks would be considered a term newborn.
   a. 30
   b. 35
   c. 40
   d. 45

3. Cryosurgery would be an option to remove _____ lesions after these lesions are identified on colposcopy.
   a. cervical
   b. uterine
   c. ovarian
   d. fallopian tube

4. Which is a surgical incision into the posterior edge of the vagina to prevent the tissue from tearing during delivery of the baby?
   a. episiotomy
   b. perineotomy
   c. laparotomy
   d. cervicotomy

5. A cesarean section would be performed for:
   a. placenta previa.
   b. hyperemesis gravidarum.
   c. ectopic or tubal pregnancy.
   d. incomplete abortion.

6. Which is a test done to determine if the fallopian tubes are open and unobstructed?
   a. pelvic ultrasound
   b. pelvimetry
   c. biparietal diameter
   d. hysterosalpingography

7. The opening for the cervical canal is the cervical:
   a. fundus.
   b. corpus.
   c. lumen.
   d. os.

8. How could a woman know that she was ovulating?
   a. She feels a dull backache.
   b. She becomes irritable.
   c. She notices a thick, white vaginal discharge of mucus.
   d. She has a rise of body temperature.

9. A myomectomy is done to remove:
   a. endometrial implants.
   b. ovarian cysts.
   c. excess breast tissue.
   d. uterine fibroid tumors.

10. HRT is treatment for:
    a. premenstrual syndrome.
    b. infertility to encourage ovulation.
    c. replacement of hormones during menopause.
    d. contraception.

11. The normal position of the uterus is:
    a. anteflexion.
    b. retroversion.
    c. anteversion.
    d. retroflexion.

12. Leukorrhea as a sign of a possible yeast infection is known as:
    a. pyometritis.
    b. candidiasis.
    c. pyosalpinx.
    d. genital herpes.

13. When a pregnant woman develops preeclampsia, she shows:
    a. weight loss, excessive thirst, glycosuria.
    b. abdominal pain, excessive bouts of vomiting, constipation.
    c. increased blood pressure, fluid retention, protein in the urine.
    d. abdominal swelling, dysuria, uterine bleeding.

14. A pregnant woman with _____ is more likely to carry a fetus that is large for its developmental age.
    a. essential hypertension
    b. gestational diabetes mellitus
    c. Rh negative blood type
    d. dietary deficiency of vitamin B_{12}

15. The abbreviation BUS refers to which type of tissue in the female reproductive system?
    a. adipose
    b. muscle
    c. glandular
    d. epithelial

16. Peau d'orange is a sign of possible breast cancer and appears as a:
    a. large mass felt in the upper outer quadrant of the breast.
    b. retracted nipple.
    c. yellow-orange fluid aspirated from the breast nipple.
    d. dimpling of the skin of the breast.

17. PID is:
    a. abnormal uterine bleeding.
    b. an infection of internal female reproductive organs.
    c. premenstrual alteration of the mood with depression and anxiety.
    d. descent of the uterus from its normal position.

18. Which is a risk factor for the genetic related type of breast or ovarian cancer?
    a. BRCA 1
    b. HRT
    c. DUB
    d. HSIL

19. Which is a drug that is used to induce labor?
    a. Ortho-Novum
    b. Ritodrine
    c. Clomid
    d. Pitocin

20. The eponym Braxton Hicks refers to:
    a. dilation of the cervix during labor.
    b. false labor pains.
    c. rupturing of the membranes during labor.
    d. the head as the presenting part during delivery.

21. The substance surfactant is present in the fetus from the seventh month of gestation and beyond. When surfactant is missing in an infant born prematurely, the child has problems:
    a. swallowing.
    b. producing urine.
    c. digesting.
    d. breathing.

22. During a delivery when the fetal scalp is visible at the vaginal introitus, it is called:
    a. effacement.
    b. ripening.
    c. crowning.
    d. dilation.
23. The first stool of the newborn is a greenish-black waste called:
    a. colostrum.
    b. meconium.
    c. lochia.
    d. molding.
24. Difficult or prolonged labor is known as:
    a. dystocia.
    b. involution.
    c. chloasma.
    d. dyspareunia.
25. After four days of development, the fertilized ovum is known as:
    a. female gonad.
    b. female gamete.
    c. embryo.
    d. fertilized eg.
26. Which is a synonym for the word menopause?
    a. menarche
    b. menorrhagia
    c. climacteric
    d. menses
27. Galactorrhea means a flow or discharge of:
    a. protein.
    b. urine.
    c. milk.
    d. blood.
28. The abnormal placement of the placenta with its edge partially or completely covering the cervical canal is known as:
    a. placenta previa.
    b. placenta separation.
    c. abruptio placentae.
    d. ectopic pregnancy.
29. A woman who has given birth to two or more children may be called:
    a. nulliparous.
    b. multiparous.
    c. nullgravida.
    d. biparous.
30. Which describes a woman who has had three spontaneous abortions and two live births?
    a. G3, P2, Ab0
    b. G3, P5, Ab0
    c. G5, P2, Ab3
    d. G2, P5, Ab3
31. The abbreviation LMP means:
    a. licensed medical practitioner.
    b. last menstrual period.
    c. last menstral period.
    d. late menstral period.
32. The abbreviation D & C means:
    a. dilate and currettage.
    b. dilitation and currettage.
    c. dilatation and currettage.
    d. dilation and curettage.
33. The abbreviation PMS means:
    a. premenstrual syndrome.
    b. postmenstral syndrome.
    c. postmenopausal syndrome.
    d. premenopausal syndrome.
34. The abbreviation CS means:
    a. caesarean section.
    b. cesarium section.
    c. cesarian section.
    d. cesarean section.
35. The first period of menstruation at the onset of puberty is known as:
    a. menarche.
    b. parturition.
    c. climacteric.
    d. ovulation.
36. Inflammation or infection of the fallopian tube is called:
    a. cervicitis.
    b. salpingitis.
    c. vaginitis.
    d. vulvitis.
37. Any type of difficult or abnormal labor and delivery is known as:
    a. eclampsia.
    b. dystocia.
    c. dyspareunia.
    d. gestation.
38. Which combining form means vagina?
    a. colp/o-
    b. metr/o-
    c. salping/o-
    d. episi/o-
39. Which procedure removes the uterine tubes and ovaries?
    a. total hysterectomy
    b. partial hysterectomy
    c. bilateral salpingo-oophorectomy
    d. salpingectomy

40. The abbreviation TAH-BSO means:
    a. total abdominal hysterectomy with bilateral salpingo-oophorectomy.
    b. transabdominal hysterectomy with bilateral salpingo-orchiectomy.
    c. total abdominal hysterectomy with bilateral salpingostomy.
    d. transabdominal hysterectomy with bilateral salpingo-ophorectomy.

41. The abbreviation PID means:
    a. peptic inflammatory disease.
    b. perineal inflammatory disease.
    c. pelvic inflammatory disease.
    d. pulmonary inflammatory disease.

42. A pregnancy test is a blood test performed to detect the presence of:
    a. HGC.
    b. LH.
    c. HCG.
    d. FSH.

43. Which is a system of assessing a newborn's well-being as calculated at 1, 5, and 10 minutes after birth?
    a. L/S ratio
    b. BPD
    c. Pap test
    d. Apgar score

44. Which drugs treat the symptoms of menopause caused by decreased levels of estradiol?
    a. hormonal chemotherapy drugs
    b. oral contraceptive pills
    c. hormone replacement therapy
    d. ovulation-stimulating drug

45. Which surgical procedure involves placing sutures fashioned into a loop around the cervix?
    a. episiotomy
    b. cerclage
    c. pelvimetry
    d. fundoplasty

46. In this surgical procedure, the entire breast is removed, as well as the overlying skin, the nipple, axillary nodes, and the pectoralis major and minor muscles.
    a. simple mastectomy
    b. total mastectomy
    c. radical mastectomy
    d. prophylactic mastectomy

47. The combining form hystero- means:
    a. ovary.
    b. uterus.
    c. vagina.
    d. fallopian tube.

48. Which procedure is done as part of a fertility workup?
    a. hysterosalpingography
    b. salpingectomy
    c. mammogram
    d. tubal ligation

49. A nuchal cord refers to an umbilical cord that is:
    a. wrapped around the neck of the fetus.
    b. separated from the fetus.
    c. diseased.
    d. not providing sufficient nourishment to the fetus.

50. Which of the following hormones is NOT one typically secreted by the ovaries?
    a. epinephrine
    b. estradiol
    c. progesterone
    d. androgen

51. All of the following are parts of the female external genitalia EXCEPT:
    a. labia majora.
    b. clitoris.
    c. vaginal introitus.
    d. ovary.

52. During which of the following phases is a woman most likely to lose a small amount of blood?
    a. proliferative phase
    b. secretory phase
    c. ischemic phase
    d. menstrual phase

53. Which of the following conditions is a cancerous condition?
    a. adenocarcinoma of the breasts
    b. galactorrhea
    c. fibrocystic disease
    d. cervical dysplasia

54. A patient with urinary incontinence receives a thorough examination by her physician. Of the following diagnoses, which one is the most likely cause?
    a. genital warts
    b. cervical dysplasia
    c. oligomenorrhea
    d. cystocele

55. Discharge of milk from the breasts when the patient is not pregnant or breastfeeding is called:
    a. galactorrhea
    b. fibrocystic disease
    c. mastitis
    d. pelvimetry

56. Oligohydramnios is:
   a. increased volume of amniotic fluid.
   b. decreased volume of amniotic fluid.
   c. incorrect placement of the placenta.
   d. dystocia.

57. An infant is stillborn. The Apgar score of the infant would likely be:
   a. 0.
   b. 3.
   c. 6.
   d. 9.

58. An infant that is not breathing is said to be:
   a. in fetal distress.
   b. apneic.
   c. bradycardic.
   d. jaundiced.

59. A medical procedure in which a hook is inserted into the cervix to catch and rupture the amniotic sac is called:
   a. amniotomy.
   b. assisted delivery.
   c. amniocentesis.
   d. version.

60. Which is a Latin word meaning pertaining to generation and birth?
   a. genitalia
   b. reproduction
   c. ovary
   d. gonad

61. This is the most abundant and most biologically active of the female hormones.
   a. progesterone
   b. oxytocin
   c. testosterone
   d. estradiol

62. The neonate's head, hands, and feet are often bluish, a temporary condition known as:
   a. vernix caseosa.
   b. scrocyanosis.
   c. ischemic phase.
   d. oogenesis.

63. On the anterior part of the newborn's head is a soft spot, also called the:
   a. meconium.
   b. molding.
   c. lochia.
   d. fontanel.

64. Crowning occurs in which stage of labor?
   a. Stage 1
   b. Stage 2
   c. Stage 3
   d. Stage 4

65. How long is the average menstrual cycle?
   a. 30 days
   b. 29 days
   c. 28 days
   d. 27 days

66. Pregnancy begins:
   a. at the moment of conception.
   b. in the ischemic phase.
   c. in the secretory phase.
   d. at ovulation.

67. Fraternal twins occur when:
   a. a single fertilized ova splits.
   b. two ova are fertilized.
   c. the father only carries X chromosomes.
   d. the father only carries Y chromosomes.

68. The process of labor and childbirth is known as:
   a. parturition.
   b. antepartum.
   c. prenatal.
   d. gestation.

69. The first thick, yellowish fluid produced by the breast after childbirth is called:
   a. lochia.
   b. milk.
   c. colostrum.
   d. meconium.

70. The ovaries are held in place by the:
   a. omentum.
   b. broad ligament.
   c. fallopian tubes.
   d. abdominal wall muscles.

71. A normal presentation of the fetus at the time of delivery would be:
   a. transverse.
   b. vertex.
   c. footling.
   d. breech.

72. All of these are complications of labor and delivery EXCEPT:
   a. effacement.
   b. nuchal cord.
   c. placenta previa.
   d. preeclampsia.

73. The medical word neonatologist can be separated into the component word parts of:
   a. prefix, combining form, combining form, suffix.
   b. combining form, combining form, combining form, suffix.
   c. prefix, combining form, suffix, suffix.
   d. combining form, combining form, suffix, suffix.

74. The medical word amenorrhea can be divided into the component word parts of:
    a. prefix, combining form, suffix.
    b. prefix, prefix, combining form, suffix.
    c. combining form, combining form, suffix.
    d. combining form, suffix, suffix.

75. A leiomyoma is a/an:
    a. type of uterine cancer.
    b. tumor of the smooth muscle of the uterus
    c. absence of menstrual periods.
    d. type of cervical dysplasia.

76. The beginning of menstruation at puberty is known as:
    a. anovulation.
    b. salpingitis.
    c. menses.
    d. menarche.

77. Which test involves looking at the cervix with a magnifying, lighted scope?
    a. mammography
    b. colposcopy
    c. Pap smear
    d. D&C

78. A Pap smear is used to detect:
    a. cervical dysplasia.
    b. hormone replacement therapy.
    c. amenorrhea.
    d. uterine fibroids.

79. A plastic surgery procedure to enlarge small breasts is known as:
    a. reduction mammoplasty.
    b. mastectomy.
    c. mammography.
    d. augmentation mammoplasty.

80. When the placenta prematurely separates from the uterine wall before the baby has been born, this is known as:
    a. crowning.
    b. ectopic pregnancy.
    c. lochia.
    d. abruptio placentae.

81. A mother who has had one cesarean section may be able to have this when she has her second baby.
    a. episiotomy
    b. HRT
    c. hysterosalpingogram
    d. VBAC

82. The test that uses sound waves to form an image of a body part is known as:
    a. mammography.
    b. x-ray.

    c. MRI.
    d. ultrasonography.

83. The ruptured follicle that secretes estradiol and progesterone is known as the:
    a. ovum.
    b. oocyte.
    c. corpus luteum.
    d. fallopian tube.

84. In fertilized ovum, the outer layer of cells or chorion develops into the:
    a. placenta.
    b. amniotic fluid.
    c. fetus.
    d. all of the above

85. Which combining form means ovary?
    a. oophor/o-
    b. uter/o-
    c. o/o-
    d. nat/o-

86. All of the following combining forms mean uterus EXCEPT:
    a. uter/o-.
    b. hyster/o-.
    c. metri/o-.
    d. lact/o-.

87. A woman with anovulation has:
    a. uterine prolapse.
    b. infertility.
    c. excessive menstruation.
    d. mastitis.

88. Infection of the fallopian tubes is known as:
    a. salpingitis.
    b. myometritis.
    c. cervical cancer.
    d. mastitis.

89. Infection of the breast is known as:
    a. endometriosis.
    b. mammitis
    c. preeclampsia.
    d. mastitis.

90. Nuchal cord refers to the umbilical cord being:
    a. abnormally long.
    b. prolapsed through the cervix.
    c. abnormally short.
    d. around the neck of the fetus.

91. All of the following tests can be performed on amniotic fluid EXCEPT:
    a. chromosome studies.
    b. Pap smear.
    c. L/S ratio.
    d. alpha fetoprotein.

92. The biparietal diameter is:
   a. the distance from the placenta to the fetus.
   b. used to measure breast cysts on mammography.
   c. checked often during labor and delivery.
   d. used to calculate gestational age.
93. An Apgar score is done on a:
   a. pregnant woman before delivery.
   b. newborn after delivery.
   c. pregnant woman after delivery.
   d. fetus of at least 30 weeks' gestation.
94. All of the following are types of assisted reproduction EXCEPT:
   a. GIFT
   b. IVF
   c. EGA
   d. ZIFT
95. A woman who has never been pregnant is:
   a. multiparous.
   b. nulligravida.
   c. infertile.
   d. all of the above

Short Answer

Write the word or phrase that best completes each statement or answers the question.

96. A cystocele is the herniation of the _____ into the vagina.
97. The patient required the surgical procedure of a _____ to remove the retained tissues from an incomplete abortion.
98. The developing human is called a/an _____ from day four of development through the eighth week of gestation.
99. The spontaneous loss of a pregnancy prior to 20 weeks gestation is called spontaneous _____.
100. A nuchal cord is one that is wrapped around the _____ of the fetus.
101. Inserting a needle into the pregnant uterus, aspirating and testing the fluid withdrawn is an _____.
102. Fallopian tubes or uterine tubes are also called the _____.
103. Colporrhaphy means suture of the _____.
104. The condition _____ is tissue from the lining of the uterus that becomes implanted on organs in the pelvic cavity such as the ovaries or the outer wall of the uterus.
105. A _____ biopsy uses three different angles of mammography to precisely locate the mass in the breast.
106. A Pap smear is known as _____ cytology because it examines cells that have been scraped from the cervix.

107. _____ is a diagnostic test that examines the fluid in the amniotic sac.
108. Failure of the ovaries to release a mature ovum at the time of ovulation is called _____.
109. The term endometrial contains a word part, which means internal or within. This word part is _____.
110. The process of forming a mature ovum is known as _____.
111. A head-down presentation of a baby in the birth canal is called a _____ presentation.
112. A mother's first milk is known as _____.
113. The skin of a newborn is covered with a thick, white, cheesy substance called _____ _____.
114. The study of women is called _____.
115. The _____ tubes connect the ovaries with the uterus.
116. The _____ of the uterus is the round, dome-like part.
117. The _____ is the body of the uterus.
118. The external _____ include the labia majora, labia minora, clitoris, vaginal introitus, and several glands that provide lubricating secretions.
119. The _____ _____ is a rounded, fleshy pad that overlies the pubic bone in women.
120. _____ hormone stimulates a single follicle each month in the female to rupture and release its mature ovum.
121. For the fetus, the period of time from conception to birth is known as the _____ period.
122. Another name for false labor is _____ _____ contractions.
123. The hormone _____ causes the uterus to begin to contract regularly in labor.
124. The thinning of the cervical wall during labor is called _____.
125. The moment of conception to the moment of birth is known as the period of _____.
126. After four days of development, the fertilized ovum is known as a/an _____.
127. The chorion develops into the _____, a pancake-like structure that is attached to the endometrium and is about 7 inches in diameter and 1 to 2 inches thick.
128. The first stool is a greenish-black, thick, sticky substance known as _____.
129. Eating nonfood items like clay, erasers, and chalk is known by the medical name of _____.
130. Tiny fingers or _____ on the end of the fallopian tube create currents that bring the ovum into the tube, where tiny hairs or _____ beat in waves to propel the ovum toward the uterus.

131. The release of _____ triggers the onset of labor.

132. _____ is the abbreviation for a surgical procedure in which the uterus, fallopian tubes, and ovaries are removed through an abdominal incision.

True/False

Write 'T' if the statement is true and 'F' if the statement is false.

____133. The small amount of blood coming from the uterus following childbirth is called colostrum.

____134. Drugs used to treat premature uterine contractions during pregnancy are tocolytics.

____135. Menarche is the first menses.

____136. A fertilized ovum begins to produce human chorionic gonadotropin (HCG) in the earliest stages of pregnancy.

____137. In the normal vaginal delivery, the placenta is expelled during the second stage of labor before delivery of the infant.

____138. Effacement is the thinning of the cervical wall during labor.

____139. Complete or partial separation of the placenta from the uterine wall during labor or delivery is an abruptio placenta.

____140. The human papillomavirus infection predisposes to the development of ovarian cancer.

____141. Gynecology is the medical specialty that studies the anatomy and physiology of the female reproductive system during pregnancy and childbirth.

____142. The ovaries are the female gonads or sex glands, which function as part of both the female reproductive system and the endocrine system.

____143. The myometrium is the inner layer of the uterus and is a specialized mucous membrane.

____144. Even before birth, female ovaries contain immature eggs.

____145. Unlike the male spermatozoon, the mature ovum is created ONLY by meiosis.

____146. During the secretory phase of the menstrual cycle, the corpus luteum degenerates into scar tissue and stops making progesterone and estradiol.

____147. During fertilization, many spermatozoa may attach to an ovum, but only one penetrates the ovum.

____148. Pelvic inflammatory disease (PID) is an infection that is often caused by a sexually transmitted disease.

____149. Fibrocystic disease of the breasts is a cancerous condition.

____150. The word vulva describes the external reproductive organs of either the male or the female.

____151. The ovaries function as part of the female reproductive system and the endocrine system.

____152. The breasts are part of the female reproductive system and the integumentary system.

____153. Pregnancy begins at the moment of gestation.

____154. Braxton Hicks contractions are a sign of impending labor.

____155. Menopause is also known as climacteric.

____156. An ectopic pregnancy occurs in the uterus.

____157. Uterine inertia normally occurs during the third stage of labor.

____158. BRCA1 is a genetic mutation that increases the risk of cervical cancer.

____159. A TRAM flap is a type of mastectomy performed for breast cancer.

____160. Leukorrhea describes a symptom of vaginal yeast infection caused by *Candida albicans*.

Essay

Write your answer in the space provided or on a separate sheet of paper.

161. How does a tubal ligation prevent conception?

162. Why would the obstetrician perform a pelvimetry on a pregnant woman?

163. Describe what is meant by the phrase completely dilated and 100% effaced.

164. Discuss the significance of lecithin and sphingomyelin levels in fetal lungs.

165. Describe three types of breast biopsy.

166. Discuss the differences between leiomyoma and leiomyosarcoma.

167. Briefly discuss the events that occur during the first stage of labor.

CHAPTER 14

Multiple Choice

Choose the one alternative that best completes the statement or answers the question.

1. Sustained muscle spasms from hypocalcemia is known as:
   a. virilism.
   b. synergism.
   c. tetany.
   d. lactation.

2. Insulin is secreted by the _____ cells in the islets of Langerhans of the pancreas.
   a. alpha
   b. beta
   c. gamma
   d. delta

3. A physical characteristic of Addison's disease is:
   a. abnormal fat distribution in the back and face called the buffalo hump and moon face.
   b. fatigue, weight loss, bronze skin pigmentation.
   c. severe headaches and hypertension.
   d. excessive body hair growth and deepening of the voice.

4. The master gland of the body is the:
   a. pituitary.
   b. pineal.
   c. adrenal.
   d. testes.

5. Which symptom is common to a patient with diabetes mellitus as well as diabetes insipidus?
   a. polyphagia
   b. glycosuria
   c. hyperglycemia
   d. polydipsia

6. Which is a lab test done to help diagnose diabetes insipidus?
   a. glucose tolerance test
   b. ADH stimulation test
   c. FSH assay
   d. glycosylated hemoglobin

7. Which is a treatment option for hyperthyroidism?
   a. thymectomy
   b. vanillymandelic acid
   c. radioactive sodium iodide (I^{131})
   d. radioimmunoassay

8. Which is the eponym for a form of thyroiditis classified as autoimmune?
   a. Hashimoto
   b. Cushing
   c. Addison
   d. Langerhans

9. Which is often a precipitating factor to the onset of type 2 diabetes mellitus?
   a. infertility
   b. skeletal muscle weakness
   c. vision changes
   d. obesity

10. Which hormone is secreted by alpha cells of the islets of Langerhans of the pancreas?
    a. glucose
    b. glucagon
    c. glucocorticoids
    d. glycogen

11. One of the neurotransmitters of the sympathetic nervous system that increases the heart rate and constricts smooth muscle in blood vessels to raise blood pressure in the "fight or flight" response is called:
    a. epinephrine.
    b. aldosterone.
    c. melatonin.
    d. prolactin.

12. Hypoglycemia can cause:
    a. elevated blood pressure, flushing of the skin, increased sensitivity to pain.
    b. slow heart rate, dry skin, constipation.
    c. headache, sweating, shakiness.
    d. decreased thirst, urination, and appetite.

13. A lab test for a patient showed low calcium levels in the blood. The physician would consider doing further testing on which endocrine gland to evaluate the cause of this hypocalcemia?
    a. thymus
    b. parathyroid
    c. adrenal medulla
    d. pineal

14. Thyromegaly is a sign of a:
    a. goiter.
    b. dwarfism.
    c. virilism.
    d. hypogonadism.

15. Increased cortisol levels would be found in patients with:
    a. Addison's disease.
    b. Graves' disease.
    c. Hashimoto's disease.
    d. Cushing's syndrome.

16. Abnormal levels of FSH point to improper functioning of the:
    a. adrenal medulla.
    b. pineal gland.
    c. thyroid.
    d. anterior pituitary gland.

17. It was in the middle of winter when the patient came to the doctor's office complaining of depression, weight gain, and problems with sleep. He was told that he had a condition related to hypersecretion of melatonin plus the lack of exposure to sunlight. He was diagnosed with:
    a. SAD.
    b. DKA.
    c. ADA.
    d. MSH.

18. A type 1 diabetic would be treated with:
    a. Humulin R.
    b. glyburide (DiaBeta).
    c. glipizide (Glucotrol).
    d. all of the above.

19. The transphenoidal hypophysectomy is done to remove the:
    a. pineal gland.
    b. thymus gland.
    c. pancreas.
    d. pituitary gland.

20. In order to see if the prescribed treatment was effective for diabetes mellitus in his patient, the physician ordered a:
    a. FSH assay.
    b. vanillylmandelic acid test.
    c. hemoglobin A1C.
    d. radioactive iodine uptake test.

21. Which is a dangerous complication associated with diabetes mellitus when the byproduct of imperfect fat combustion occurs in the patient?
    a. ketoacidosis
    b. aldosteronism
    c. myxedema
    d. hyperinsulinism

22. An endemic goiter is related to a deficiency of:
    a. calcium.
    b. sodium chloride.
    c. potassium.
    d. iodine.

23. A pregnant woman may be given the hormone _____ to stimulate her uterus to contract and begin labor.
    a. somastatin
    b. prolactin
    c. oxytocin
    d. progesterone

24. Hyposecretion of cortisol from the adrenal cortex is known as:
    a. Addison's disease.
    b. Cushing's syndrome.
    c. Graves' disease.
    d. gynecomastia.

25. The pineal body secretes which hormone that maintains the body's internal clock, the 24-hour wake-sleep cycle, and regulates the onset and duration of sleep?
    a. oxytocin
    b. calcitonin
    c. melatonin
    d. cortisol

26. The best definition of parathyroid is:
    a. abnormal thyroid.
    b. above the thyroid.

c. beside the thyroid.
    d. two parts of a pair of thyroid.

27. Hyposecretion of antidiuretic hormone is known as:
    a. hypoglycemia.
    b. diabetes insipidus.
    c. diabetes mellitus.
    d. panhypopituitarism.

28. Cushing's syndrome is due to:
    a. hyposecretion of cortisol in the adrenal medulla.
    b. hypersecretion of cortisol in the adrenal medulla.
    c. hypersecretion of cortisol in the adrenal cortex.
    d. hyposecretion of cortisol in the adrenal cortex.

29. Chronic and progressive enlargement of the thyroid gland is known as:
    a. hypergonadism.
    b. euthyroid.
    c. goiter.
    d. hypothyroidism.

30. Severe hypothyroidism in adults is known as:
    a. acromegaly.
    b. Graves' disease.
    c. myxedema.
    d. Cushing's syndrome.

31. Which is the process where two hormones work together to achieve a result?
    a. activation
    b. stimulation
    c. synergism
    d. tolerance

32. The abbreviation NIDDM means the same as:
    a. type 2 diabetes mellitus.
    b. non-insulin-dependent diabetes mellitus.
    c. adult-onset diabetes melitus.
    d. all of the above.

33. Which endocrine gland is known as the master gland of the body?
    a. parathyroid
    b. pituitary
    c. pancreas
    d. adrenal

34. The suffix -physis means:
    a. state of growing.
    b. abnormal condition.
    c. deficient.
    d. destruction.

35. The abbreviation GH means:
    a. glucose hemoglobin.
    b. gonad hormone.
    c. genital herpes.
    d. growth hormone.
36. Which type of drug is used to treat type 1 and type 2 diabetes mellitus?
    a. growth hormone drugs
    b. insulin
    c. antithyroid drugs
    d. corticosteroid drugs
37. Which gland is also called the neurohypophysis?
    a. thyroid gland
    b. parathyroid gland
    c. posterior pituitary gland
    d. anterior pituitary gland
38. Which blood test is performed to measure the level of glucose after the patient has not eaten for at least 12 hours?
    a. fasting blood sugar
    b. cortisol level
    c. glucose tolerance test
    d. glucose self-testing
39. The process by which two hormones exert opposite effects is known as:
    a. stimulation.
    b. inhibition.
    c. synergism.
    d. antagonism.
40. The combining form adren/o- means:
    a. kidney.
    b. gland.
    c. adrenal gland.
    d. urinary.
41. Hypersecretion of the growth hormone during adulthood causes:
    a. goiter.
    b. Cushing's syndrome.
    c. myxedema.
    d. acromegaly.
42. Excessive amounts of calcium in the blood is known as:
    a. hypocalcemia.
    b. hyperkalemia.
    c. hyperbilirubemina.
    d. hypercalcemia.
43. Which word is used to describe sustained muscle spasms?
    a. circadian
    b. tetany
    c. ergyism
    d. receptor

44. Glycosuria means that there is _____ in the urine.
    a. iron
    b. calcium
    c. blood
    d. glucose
45. Which type of diabetes begins in childhood or adolescence?
    a. adult-onset
    b. type 1
    c. non-insulin-dependent
    d. type 2
46. The hypersecretion of oxytocin causes:
    a. uterine inertia.
    b. goiter.
    c. dysparenuia.
    d. Graves' disease.
47. Hyposecretion of the growth hormone during childhood and puberty is:
    a. acromegaly.
    b. dwarfism.
    c. gigantism.
    d. diabetes insipidus.
48. Which of the following is not true regarding the endocrine system?
    a. All of the organs and glands of the endocrine system are influenced by the pituitary gland.
    b. They release substances called hormones.
    c. They release their hormones directly into the blood.
    d. Their hormones regulate specific body functions.
49. A gland which secretes a hormone which stimulates the ovaries to develop follicles is the:
    a. hypothalamus.
    b. pituitary gland.
    c. pineal body.
    d. thyroid gland.
50. What endocrine gland is also known as the master gland?
    a. hypothalamus
    b. thyroid gland
    c. pancreas
    d. pituitary gland
51. The parathyroid glands secrete a hormone which regulates the level of what substance in the blood?
    a. calcium
    b. insulin
    c. melanin
    d. melatonin

52. Which of the following endocrine glands contains structures known as the islets of Langerhans?
    a. thymus gland
    b. hypothalamus
    c. pituitary gland
    d. pancreas

53. The hormone which regulates electrolyte balance, and sodium and potassium balance is:
    a. aldosterone.
    b. glucagon.
    c. androgens.
    d. epinephrine.

54. What is the most abundant and biologically active female hormone?
    a. progesterone
    b. estradiol
    c. ovaries
    d. testosterone

55. The testes produce sperm when stimulated by FSH released by what gland?
    a. posterior pituitary gland
    b. hypothalamus
    c. androgen
    d. anterior pituitary gland

56. The action of hormones working together to accomplish the same result, is called:
    a. synergism.
    b. antagonism.
    c. stimulation.
    d. inhibition.

57. The form that sugar takes when it is stored in the liver and the skeletal muscles is called:
    a. glucose.
    b. insulin.
    c. estradiol.
    d. glycogen.

58. Another name for the pituitary gland is:
    a. hypothalamus.
    b. thalamus.
    c. hypophysis.
    d. thymus.

59. The pituitary gland has two main parts, the adenohypophysis and the:
    a. posterior pituitary gland.
    b. anterior pituitary gland.
    c. thymus.
    d. thyroid.

60. Together FSH and LH are known as:
    a. pineal bodies.
    b. gonadotropins.
    c. lobes.
    d. endocrine glands.

61. As part of the endocrine system, the pancreas secretes three hormones directly into the blood. They are:
    a. glucagon, insulin, and FSH.
    b. FSH, LH, and insulin.
    c. glucagon, insulin, and somatostatin.
    d. somatostatin, glycogen, and aldosterone.

62. The most common form of hyperthyroidism is:
    a. diabetes.
    b. Graves' disease.
    c. SAD.
    d. goiter.

63. Which disease is the result of a hypersecretion of cortisol?
    a. Cushing syndrome
    b. polyphagia
    c. polydipsia
    d. diabetes

64. A blood glucose monitor is an important tool for use in which disease?
    a. acromegaly
    b. diabetes
    c. precocious puberty
    d. infertility

65. Which is a urine test that measures glucose, ketones, and other substances in the urine?
    a. urine dipstick
    b. RAIU
    c. fine needle biopsy
    d. VMA

66. Which is a surgical procedure that removes the thyroid?
    a. transsphenoidal hypophysectomy
    b. thymectomy
    c. thyroidectomy
    d. parathyroidectomy

67. Which hormone stimulates the thyroid gland to secrete the thyroid hormones T3 and T4?
    a. TSH
    b. FSH
    c. LH
    d. aldosterone

68. The combining form pituit/o- and _____ both mean pituitary gland.
    a. adren/o-
    b. hypophys/o
    c. andr/o-
    d. secret/o-

69. A benign tumor of an endocrine gland is known as a/an:
    a. carcinoma.
    b. lipoma.
    c. diabetes mellitus.
    d. adenoma.

70. All of the following are diagnostic tests for diabetes EXCEPT:
    a. fasting blood sugar (FBS).
    b. blood level of growth hormone.
    c. glucose tolerance test.
    d. hemoglobin A1c.

71. Type 2 diabetes mellitus is:
    a. also known as adult-onset diabetes.
    b. treated with weight loss, exercise, and diet.
    c. treated with oral antidiabetic drugs.
    d. all of the above.

72. Infertility may have a hormonal cause due to a lack of:
    a. FSH.
    b. TFT.
    c. GTT.
    d. NPH.

73. NPH refers to a/an:
    a. organ.
    b. disease.
    c. drug.
    d. hormone.

74. ADA refers to a diet that would be prescribed for a patient with:
    a. anemia.
    b. diabetes.
    c. thyroid disease.
    d. precocious puberty.

75. A transsphenoidal hypophysectomy is a surgical procedure to remove an adenoma from the:
    a. thyroid gland.
    b. adrenal gland.
    c. pituitary gland.
    d. thymus.

76. The thyroid gland:
    a. regulates cellular metabolism.
    b. regulates potassium levels in the blood.
    c. stimulates the uterus to contract in labor.
    d. secretes insulin.

77. Excessive amounts of growth hormone after puberty result in:
    a. hyperthyroidism.
    b. stunted growth.
    c. acromegaly.
    d. diabetic complications.

78. Too little ADH from the posterior pituitary gland causes:
    a. gigantism.
    b. diabetes insipidus.
    c. thyroid cancer.
    d. hyperglycemia.

79. A congenital lack of thyroid hormone from birth is known as:
    a. Hashimoto's thyroiditis.
    b. Graves' disease.
    c. thyroid cancer.
    d. cretinism.

80. A lobectomy is a surgical procedure performed on the:
    a. ovary.
    b. pineal gland.
    c. thyroid gland.
    d. pancreas.

81. Hemoglobin A1C is:
    a. the hemoglobin that causes sickle cell anemia.
    b. associated with small red blood cells.
    c. a test used to monitor blood glucose over 3 to 4 months.
    d. decreased when there is increased urine output.

82. Which type of diabetes occurs only during pregnancy?
    a. insipidus
    b. type 1
    c. type 2
    d. gestational

83. Exophthalmos is associated with:
    a. diabetes mellitus.
    b. diabetes insipidus.
    c. Graves' disease.
    d. gigantism.

84. Which of these abbreviations is associated with diabetes?
    a. SIADH
    b. IDDM
    c. SAD
    d. TSH

85. Which of the following is true of antidiuretic hormone (ADH)?
    a. It is produced by the hypothalamus.
    b. It is stored and released by the posterior pituitary gland.
    c. It keeps excessive amounts of water from being lost in the urine.
    d. all of the above

86. Which hormone is associated with the wake-sleep cycle?
    a. epinephrine
    b. melatonin
    c. thyroid hormone
    d. testosterone

87. Which is the abbreviation for the hormone released by the anterior pituitary gland that stimulates the thyroid gland?
    a. FSH
    b. ACTH
    c. ADH
    d. TSH

88. The purpose of the parathyroid glands is to regulate the:
    a. amount of calcium in the blood.
    b. amount of glucose in the blood.
    c. amount of sodium in the blood.
    d. function of the thyroid gland.

89. Which of the following is true when glucose levels are low in the blood?
    a. Beta cells of the pancreas produce insulin.
    b. Alpha cells of the pancreas produce glucagon.
    c. Delta cells of the pancreas produce somatostatin.
    d. all of the above

90. Hormones from various endocrine glands affect:
    a. body metabolism.
    b. blood glucose.
    c. blood calcium and sodium.
    d. all of the above.

91. The hormone testosterone is produced by the:
    a. ovaries.
    b. testes.
    c. pituitary gland.
    d. thymus.

92. The chemical messengers of the endocrine system are known as:
    a. neurotransmitters.
    b. electrolytes.
    c. hormones.
    d. receptors.

93. Which of the following is true of hormones?
    a. Hormones are released through ducts.
    b. Hormones can stimulate a gland or organ.
    c. Hormones can inhibit a gland or organ.
    d. all of the above

94. Calcium levels in the blood are regulated by:
    a. parathyroid hormone from the parathyroid gland.
    b. calcitonin from the thyroid gland.
    c. both parathyroid hormone and calcitonin.
    d. neither parathyroid hormone nor calcitonin.

95. Which word is misspelled?
    a. adenohypophysis
    b. diabetes mellitis
    c. synergism
    d. hyperthyroidism

96. The suffix -ism means:
    a. condition of the blood.
    b. pertaining to.
    c. enlargement.
    d. disease from a specific cause.

Short Answer

Write the word or phrase that best completes each statement or answers the question.

97. It is important to write the abbreviation for drops, (gtt), in lower case because the upper case abbreviation, GTT, means _____ _____ _____.

98. Thyromegaly is also known as _____.

99. Hyposecretion of the growth hormone during childhood and puberty results in _____.

100. Severe hypothyroidism in adults is called _____.

101. Excessive growth of dark hair in the forearms and face of the female from hypersecretion of the male sex hormone is called _____.

102. Gigantism results from hypersecretion of the growth hormone in childhood, whereas _____ results from hypersecretion of the growth hormone in the adulthood.

103. The patient with diabetes insipidus exhibited the symptom _____, a medical need for excessive excretion of urine.

104. _____ syndrome is associated with a weight gain along with deposition of fat in the face (moon face) and the upper back (buffalo hump).

105. A pheochromocytoma is a benign tumor of the _____ of the adrenal gland.

106. Galact/o- and lact/o- are both combining forms that mean _____.

107. The nervous system uses neurotransmitters as chemical messengers. The endocrine system uses _____ as chemical messengers.

108. The endocrine system helps the body maintain a balance known as _____ through the use of hormones.

109. The outermost part of the adrenal gland is the adrenal _____.

110. The _____ system includes organs and glands that secrete hormones directly into the blood.

111. _____ is a condition caused by increased levels of growth hormone in adulthood.

112. A goiter is a chronic and progressive enlargement of the _____ gland.

113. _____ _____ is the most common form of hyperthyroidism.

114. _____ diabetes mellitus occurs only during pregnancy.

115. Enlargement of the male breasts because of an imbalance in androgens and estradiol is also known as _____.

116. All endocrine glands secrete _____.

117. The function of the endocrine system is to keep the body in a steady state of balance known as _____.

118. The _____ is located in the brain just below the thalamus.

119. The _____ gland is known as the master gland of the body.

120. The most abundant and biologically active of the mineralocorticoid hormones is _____.

121. The corpus luteum (ruptured ovarian follicle) produces and secretes estradiol and _____ when stimulated by LH from the anterior pituitary gland.

122. _____ is the most abundant and biologically active of all the androgens (male hormones).

123. The action of hormones can involve stimulation or the opposite action which is _____.

124. When hormones work in conjunction with one another is it called _____.

125. When too much of a hormone is secreted, this is known as _____.

126. _____ is a condition in which there is hyposecretion of all of the hormones of the anterior pituitary gland.

127. _____ is hypersecretion of prolactin. This causes secretion of milk from the breasts, even though the patient is not pregnant.

128. _____ is hypersecretion of growth hormone during adulthood.

129. _____ hemorrhage occurs after or following childbirth if there is not enough oxytocin.

130. _____ is chronic and progressive enlargement of the thyroid gland.

131. Excessive amounts of _____ hormone during puberty cause gigantism.

132. _____ is the male hormone that stimulates the development of the male sexual characteristics.

133. The symptoms of diabetes insipidus include excessive urine production, known as _____ and excessive thirst, known as _____.

134. The medical name for the sudden onset of severe hyperthyroidism is _____ _____.

135. Some endocrinologists specialize their practice and only treat patients with diabetes mellitus. These specialists are known as _____.

True/False

Write 'T' if the statement is true and 'F' if the statement is false.

_____ 136. During puberty testosterone from the testes produces primary and secondary sex characteristics in the male to include growth of internal and external genitalia, deepening of the voice, and appearance of body hair.

_____ 137. Exophthalmos is a symptom found in some patients with hypothyroidism.

_____ 138. Patients with gestational diabetes mellitus are at risk for developing type 2 diabetes mellitus later in life.

_____ 139. Gynecomastia can be a sign of hypersecretion of estrogen in the young female

_____ 140. Myxedema is the medical word for congenital hypothyroidism.

_____ 141. Diabetes mellitis is the correct spelling for the disease involving hyposecretion of insulin.

_____ 142. Galactorrhea, a secretion of breast milk, can occur even though the patient has not been pregnant.

_____ 143. Uterine inertia is associated with hypersecretion of oxytocin.

_____ 144. Diabetic nephropathy is a chronic complication of diabetes involving the nervous system.

_____ 145. The word endocrinology derives from the word parts meaning innermost, secrete, and specialty.

_____ 146. Organs and glands of the endocrine system all release substances called hormones.

_____ 147. All of the organs and glands of the endocrine system are influenced by the secretions of the pituitary gland.

_____ 148. Both the hypothalamus and the pituitary gland are located in the brain.

_____ 149. The thyroid gland has three lobes connected by a bridge of tissue called a peninsula.

_____ 150. The pancreas is both an endocrine gland and part of the digestive system.

_____ 151. Each adrenal gland functions as two separate glands that secrete different hormones.

_____ 152. The ovaries are part of both the female reproductive system and the endocrine system, and are in turn affected by the pituitary gland located in the brain.

_____ 153. Some hormones can inhibit actions in the body, other hormones can stimulate actions in the body.

_____ 154. The hormones released from some glands act to stimulate other glands.

_____ 155. Antidiabetic drugs like DiaBeta, Diabinese, and Glucotrol are given by subcutaneous injection to treat diabetes mellitus.

_____156. The thymus gland decreases in size and function with age.

_____157. Diabetic patients who need insulin inject it subcutaneously.

_____158. The glands of the endocrine system are all located within the abdominopelvic cavity.

_____159. The pituitary gland in females produces FSH to stimulate the follicles of the ovary, but the pituitary gland in males does not produce FSH.

_____160. Gynecomastia occurs only in females.

Essay

Write your answer in the space provided or on a separate sheet of paper.

161. The patient had a thyroidectomy for cancer. Postoperatively he complained of severe muscle cramping. Lab tests showed that he had depressed levels of calcium in his blood. What could account for his postoperative complication?

162. Why is it recommended that diabetes mellitus patients pay special attention to foot care?

163. Why is the pituitary gland known as the master gland of the body?

164. Briefly discuss the thyroid function test (TFT).

165. Briefly explain the purpose and function of the radioactive iodine uptake and thyroid scan.

166. Define the word endocrinology.

167. Explain the difference between stimulation and inhibition with respect to hormones.

CHAPTER 15

Multiple Choice

Choose the one alternative that best completes the statement or answers the question.

1. The physician noted in the physical examination that the patient had aniscoria. This means that the patient had:
   a. blood in the anterior chamber of his eye.
   b. a swelling of the optic nerve in the back of the eye.
   c. crossed eyes.
   d. pupils that were unequal in size.

2. Mydriatic eye drops are given to a patient before an eye examination in order to:
   a. dilate the pupils.
   b. anesthetize the conjunctiva.
   c. cleanse the eye of mucus.
   d. decrease the flow of tears.

3. The combining form irid/o- refers to the:
   a. white of the eye.
   b. eyelid.
   c. tear ducts.
   d. colored portion of the eye.

4. All of the following are true about the sclera except which sentence?
   a. It is known as the white of the eye.
   b. It bends or refracts light rays entering the eyes.
   c. It is the site of attachment for the extraocular muscles.
   d. It helps to maintain the shape of the eye.

5. In bright light the muscles of the iris contract, reducing the size of the pupil in order to keep too much light from entering the eye. This process is called:
   a. mydriasis.
   b. myopia.
   c. miosis.
   d. macula.

6. A slit lamp examination includes viewing the:
   a. retina and optic disk.
   b. optic nerve and macula.
   c. rods and cones.
   d. lens and anterior chamber.

7. A patient has a bacterial infection of the eye. What would be the antibiotic used for this condition?
   a. Mydriacyl
   b. Genoptic
   c. Viroptic
   d. Ocupress

8. The patient's prescription is for –4.25 diopters. This means that the patient is:
   a. nearsighted.
   b. farsighted.
   c. presbyopic.
   d. legally blind.

9. Which is the abbreviation for the left eye?
   a. OD
   b. OU
   c. OS
   d. IOL

10. The blind spot of the eye is found at the:
    a. macula.
    b. fundus.
    c. fovea.
    d. optic disk.

11. The border between the transparent edge of the cornea and the white of the fibrous sclera is the:
    a. pupil.
    b. anterior chamber.
    c. limbus.
    d. optic disk.

12. The ability of both eyes to turn medially toward the nose and maintain focus as an object approaches the face is called:
    a. accommodation.
    b. convergence.
    c. stereoscopic vision.
    d. conjugate gaze.
13. The patient complained of a recent painful swelling of the eyelid. The physician told the patient that he had a stye. The medical word for this condition is:
    a. keratitis.
    b. hyperopia.
    c. photophobia.
    d. hordeolum.
14. Robert Kovaleski needs to have a cataract removed from his eye. In order to have this surgery performed, this patient must see an:
    a. ophthalmologist.
    b. optician.
    c. optometrist.
    d. occultist.
15. Which is the condition in which the lower eyelid turns inward causing the eyelashes to come into contact with the conjunctiva?
    a. blepharoptosis
    b. chalazion
    c. entropion
    d. extropion
16. The patient has a herpes simplex infection of his eye. The medication prescribed for this condition is:
    a. Genoptic.
    b. Ocuflax.
    c. Viroptic.
    d. Flarex.
17. Which abbreviation would be found in a physical assessment relating to an examination of the eyes?
    a. HEENT
    b. PERRL
    c. EOM
    d. all of the above
18. The muscle that turns the eye downward is the:
    a. medial rectus.
    b. lateral rectus.
    c. superior rectus.
    d. inferior rectus.
19. All of the following words pertain to the eye except:
    a. uvea.
    b. macule.
    c. fovea.
    d. pupil.
20. Which is the medical word for pinkeye?
    a. dacryocystitis
    b. conjunctivitis
    c. chalazion
    d. blepharitis
21. Hyperthyroidism is known to cause the eyes to bulge out resulting in:
    a. diplopia.
    b. conjunctivitis.
    c. hyperopia.
    d. exophthalmos.
22. Which is an age-related disease with loss of central vision?
    a. macular degeneration
    b. papilledema
    c. retinitis pigmentosa
    d. presbyopia
23. Which is a specific medical word for lateral deviation of the eye or "wall eye"?
    a. astigmatism
    b. aphakia
    c. amblyopia
    d. exotropia
24. Which is a surgery done to correct myopia?
    a. photorefractive keratectomy
    b. capsulotomy
    c. angiography
    d. retinopexy
25. Glaucoma is a threat to vision because it involves a/an:
    a. build-up of protein molecules in the lens that gradually block light rays.
    b. deterioration of the macula as abnormal blood vessels grow under it.
    c. increase in intraocular pressure that gradually destroys structures in the eye.
    d. inflammation of the optic nerve due to increased intracranial pressure.
26. Red, painful swelling or pimple containing pus near the edge of the eyelid from a bacterial infection in a sebaceous gland is known as:
    a. hordeolum.
    b. blepharoptosis.
    c. entropion.
    d. nystagmus.
27. The eye disorder characterized by clouding of the lens, causing decreased vision is known as:
    a. cataract.
    b. chalazion.
    c. glaucoma.
    d. conjunctivitis.

28. The loss of flexibility of the lens of the eye with blurring vision and loss of accommodation caused by aging is known as:
    a. presbyopia.
    b. night blindness.
    c. cataract.
    d. xerophthalmia.

29. Medial deviation of one or both eyes is known as:
    a. retinoblastoma.
    b. glaucoma.
    c. esotropia.
    d. astigmatism.

30. In which of the following is the surface of the cornea curved more steeply on one side of the eye than on the other, so there is no single point of focus?
    a. hyperopia
    b. myopia
    c. astigmatism
    d. amblyopia

31. Which is a diagnostic procedure used to detect increased intraocular pressure and glaucoma?
    a. tonometry
    b. visual acuity test
    c. ophthalmoscopy
    d. visual field test

32. The abbreviation OD means:
    a. left eye.
    b. prism diopter.
    c. right eye.
    d. doctor of optometry.

33. The combining form lacrim/o- means:
    a. eyelid.
    b. tears.
    c. gland.
    d. retina.

34. The combining form aque/o- means:
    a. darkness.
    b. watery substance.
    c. light.
    d. old age.

35. Which surgical procedure is performed to seal leaking or hemorrhaging retinal blood vessels or to reattach a detached retina?
    a. capsulotomy
    b. laser photocoagulation
    c. enucleation
    d. keratoplasty

36. Which medical procedure is performed to test the ability of the ciliary muscles and ligaments to contract and flex the lens as demonstrated on near and distance visual acuity tests?
    a. retinopexy
    b. tonometry

    c. convergence
    d. accommodation

37. Insufficient production of tears with eye irritation is known as:
    a. dacryocystitis.
    b. scleral icterus.
    c. conjunctivitis.
    d. xerophthalmia.

38. The abbreviation OS means:
    a. left eye.
    b. both eyes.
    c. right eye.
    d. each eye.

39. The round opening in the iris that allows light rays to enter the internal eye is the:
    a. retina.
    b. iris.
    c. pupil.
    d. sclera.

40. Acute contagious bacterial conjunctivitis with mucus discharge is commonly known as:
    a. papilledema.
    b. scleral icterus.
    c. nystagmus.
    d. pinkeye.

41. The medical word for nearsightedness is:
    a. hyperopia.
    b. myopia.
    c. presbyopia.
    d. aphakia.

42. What is the medical word for the lateral deviation of the eye known as wall-eyed?
    a. exotropia
    b. esotropia
    c. blindness
    d. myopia

43. Which oil glands are located at the edges of the eyelids?
    a. sebaceous glands
    b. sweat glands
    c. lacrimal glands
    d. nasolacrimal glands

44. The combining form orbit/o- means:
    a. vision.
    b. eye socket.
    c. eyeball.
    d. visual cortex.

45. The combining form scot/o- in the medical word scotoma means:
    a. color.
    b. gray.
    c. light.
    d. old age.

46. Which medical procedure is used to test the extraocular muscles?
    a. visual acuity test
    b. visual field test
    c. papillary nespone test
    d. gaze test
47. The abbreviation IOL means:
    a. inner ocular lens.
    b. intracapsular optic lens.
    c. intraocular lens.
    d. interior ophthalmic lens.
48. Which is the medical word that includes the retina?
    a. optic nerve
    b. fundus
    c. anterior chamber
    d. choroid
49. Which condition occurs in patients with uncontrolled diabetes mellitus?
    a. color blindness
    b. aphakia
    c. retinopathy
    d. macular degeneration
50. The medical specialty that studies the anatomy and physiology of the eye, and uses diagnostic tests, medical and surgical procedures, and drugs to treat eye diseases is
    a. opthalmology.
    b. ophthalmology.
    c. optometry.
    d. opticianry.
51. The small area between the cornea and the surface of the iris through which the aqueous humor circulates is called the:
    a. posterior chamber.
    b. caruncle.
    c. fovea.
    d. anterior chamber.
52. The _____ gland produces and releases tears.
    a. endocrine
    b. ocular
    c. fundus
    d. lacrimal
53. The organ of the eye responsible for the color of the eye is the:
    a. lens.
    b. iris.
    c. optic chiasm.
    d. orbit.

54. A patient is admitted to the emergency room after being involved in a car accident. The patient hit his head on the steering wheel causing extensive damage. The surgeon diagnosed a fractured orbit, among other injuries. What is the orbit?
    a. a sensory nerve in the cranium
    b. a round opening in the iris
    c. a dark, yellow-orange area in the retina
    d. a bony socket in the skull
55. Inflammation or infection of the eyelid with redness, crusts, and scales at the bases of the eyelashes is called:
    a. blepharoptosis.
    b. conjunctivitis.
    c. blepharitis.
    d. dacryocystitis.
56. What is Xerophthalmia?
    a. insufficient production of tears
    b. inflammation of the lacrimal sac
    c. "crossed" eyes
    d. foreign object in the eyes
57. A condition which causes pronounced outward bulging of the anterior surface of the eye is called:
    a. scleral icterus.
    b. aniscoria.
    c. exophthalmos.
    d. hyphema.
58. Retinopathy often occurs in patients with what uncontrolled disease?
    a. diabetes
    b. atherosclerosis
    c. stroke
    d. cardiac insufficiency
59. The medical word for farsightedness is:
    a. myopia.
    b. hyperopia.
    c. strabismus.
    d. nystagmus.
60. Yellow coloration of the conjunctivae which makes the sclerae also appear yellow is called:
    a. scleral icterus.
    b. color blindness.
    c. glaucoma.
    d. photophobia.
61. Clouding of the lens is called:
    a. presbyopia.
    b. papilledema.
    c. cataract.
    d. retinopathy.

62. What class of drugs is used to dilate the pupil and prepare the eye for an exam?
    a. corticosteroid
    b. antiviral
    c. antibiotic
    d. mydriatic

63. What is the abbreviation for the right eye?
    a. OS
    b. OO
    c. RE
    d. OD

64. Which is the professional who cuts, grinds, and finishes corrective lenses?
    a. optician
    b. ophthalmologist
    c. optometrists
    d. optometry

65. Which is part of the anterior eye?
    a. sclera
    b. eyelashes
    c. limbus
    d. all of the above

66. Which is the oil-secreting part of the eye found at the edge of the eyelid?
    a. sebaceous (meibomian) glands
    b. optic nerve
    c. limbus
    d. lacrimal glands

67. The lens is enclosed in a clear membrane called the:
    a. lens.
    b. foveal.
    c. fundal.
    d. rectus.

68. The eye can move in all directions because of the many different extraocular muscles attached to the sclera. How many different muscles control the eye?
    a. 2
    b. 3
    c. 4
    d. 6

69. The white of the eye is called the:
    a. retina.
    b. iris.
    c. sclera.
    d. optic disk.

70. Which of the following is used to measure distance vision?
    a. Snellen chart
    b. tonometry
    c. visual field test
    d. fluorescein angiography

71. The cones of the eye are located in the retina and function in:
    a. distance vision.
    b. color vision.
    c. focusing the light rays.
    d. light and dark vision.

72. The point where the optic nerve enters the retina is known as the:
    a. optic disk.
    b. cornea.
    c. macula.
    d. lens.

73. Which test is used to diagnose glaucoma?
    a. LASIK procedure
    b. tonometry or air puff test
    c. Snellen chart or tumbling E test
    d. ophthalmoscope

74. The area of greatest visual acuity is the:
    a. lens.
    b. conjunctiva.
    c. retina.
    d. macula.

75. The operation phakoemulsification is performed on the:
    a. retina.
    b. iris.
    c. lens.
    d. vitreous humor.

76. An eye doctor who has an M.D. is known as a/an:
    a. optician.
    b. optometrist.
    c. ophthalmologist.
    d. primary care physician.

77. Presbyopia is characterized by:
    a. retinal detachment.
    b. legal blindness.
    c. blepharoptosis.
    d. decreased flexibility of the lens.

78. All of the following are true about vitreous humor EXCEPT:
    a. It is a clear, jelly-like substance.
    b. Light rays pass through it to reach the retina.
    c. It fills the anterior chamber between the cornea and the iris.
    d. There is much more vitreous humor in the eye than aqueous humor.

79. Reattaching and fixing the membrane that lines the back of the eyeball when it has become detached is a surgical procedure known as:
    a. pseudophakia.
    b. corneal transplant.
    c. otoplasty.
    d. retinopexy.

80. Repetitive, rhythmic movements of the eye when the patient looks to the one side or the other are known as:
    a. presbyopia.
    b. stye.
    c. nystagmus.
    d. conjunctivitis.
81. Which of the following is treated with a blepharoplasty?
    a. infection of the eyelid
    b. corneal abrasion or ulcer
    c. xerophthalmia
    d. sagging skin on the eyelids
82. Fluorescein is a dye used to diagnose:
    a. dilated pupil.
    b. corneal abrasion.
    c. myopia.
    d. glaucoma.
83. The meibomian glands secrete:
    a. oil.
    b. tears.
    c. sweat.
    d. all of the above.
84. Which of the following is NOT true about the sclera?
    a. It is the white of the eye.
    b. The extraocular muscles are attached to it.
    c. It produces aqueous humor.
    d. Its anterior portion is the clear cornea.
85. Which of these is the function of the ciliary body?
    a. to change the shape of the lens, make aqueous humor
    b. to produce tears and aqueous humor
    c. to change the shape of the lens and produce vitreous humor
    d. all of the above
86. Which two structures of the eye are involved in bending light rays to focus them on the retina?
    a. lens and posterior cavity
    b. cornea and retina
    c. pupil and retina
    d. cornea and lens
87. Which portion of the brain interprets visual impulses from the optic nerve?
    a. thalamus
    b. retina
    c. occipital lobe
    d. frontal lobe
88. To look for bleeding from the blood vessels in the retina, the physician would order:
    a. fluorescein angiography.
    b. Snellen chart testing.
    c. accommodation testing.
    d. phorometry.
89. Eye patching is used to treat patients with:
    a. blindness.
    b. amblyopia.
    c. nystagmus.
    d. myopia.
90. Which word is misspelled?
    a. ophthalmology
    b. conjunctivitis
    c. nystagmus
    d. acommodation

Short Answer

Write the word or phrase that best completes each statement or answers the question.

91. Chronic inflammation of the eyelid is termed _____.
92. The condition in which old age causes the lens to become less flexible resulting in blurry near vision is called _____.
93. The _____ gland releases tears continually to lubricate the eye.
94. An _____ is the surgical removal of the eyeball from its orbit.
95. Xerophthalmia is also known as _____ _____ .
96. Involuntary rhythmic motion of the eye that can point to an underlying disease such as multiple sclerosis is called _____.
97. Distance visual acuity can be initially assessed using the _____ eye chart.
98. The surgical process of _____ is associated with an extracapsular cataract extraction involving breaking up the lens with an ultrasonic probe.
99. Persons may arrange to donate their _____ upon their death to be transplanted into the eyes of persons with diseased _____.
100. When you define the prefix, hemi-, you can complete this sentence: Hemianopsia is a condition in which the patient cannot see _____ of the visual field, either right or left or up or down.
101. A diagnostic procedure to detect increased intraocular pressure and glaucoma is called _____.
102. _____ is a radiologic procedure that uses high-frequency sound waves to create an image of the eye.
103. A/an _____ is a handheld instrument with a light and changeable lenses of different strengths used to examine the retina from all angles.

104. Corneal _____ is a surgical procedure to replace a damaged or diseased cornea.

105. A surgical procedure to remove the eye from the orbit because of trauma or tumor is called _____.

106. A drug class called _____ drugs are used to dilate the pupil.

107. A doctor who diagnoses and treats patients with vision problems, but who does not perform surgery and is not a physician, is called a/an _____.

108. The _____ is a tough, fibrous connective tissue that forms a continuous outer layer around the eyeball.

109. A red, triangular tissue at the medial corner of the eye is called the _____.

110. The _____ is a delicate, transparent mucous membrane that covers the insides of the eyelids and continues across the anterior surface of the eye.

111. Across the anterior part of the eye, the sclera changes into a transparent layer known as the _____.

112. At the center of the iris is the _____, a round opening that allows light rays to enter the eye.

113. The process known as _____ keeps too much light from entering the eye.

114. The _____ duct carries tears to the inside of the nose.

115. The _____ chamber is a small area between the cornea and the iris.

116. The _____ disk is a bright, yellow-white circle with sharp edges on the side of the retina closest to the nose.

117. The _____ is a spongy membrane of blood vessels that is part of the internal structure of the eye.

118. The _____ is a clear, hard disk made of transparent protein molecules arranged in a crystalline fashion.

119. _____ _____ is a clear, watery fluid that is continuously produced by the ciliary body.

120. The _____ cavity is the largest area in the eye.

121. _____ in the retina are sensitive to all levels of light but not to color.

122. The _____ is a relay station that sends sensory nerve impulses to the right or left visual cortex.

123. _____ is a weakening of connective tissue in the lower eyelid in older patients.

124. Another name for pink eye is _____.

125. The optic nerve is cranial nerve _____.

126. The patient should stand _____ feet from the vision chart to accurately check distance vision.

127. The two types of strabismus are cross-eye or esotropia and wall-eye or _____.

128. In English words, the abbreviation OS means _____ _____ and OU means _____ _____.

129. A person with a best-corrected visual acuity (even with corrective lenses) of _____ is legally blind.

True/False

Write 'T' if the statement is true and 'F' if the statement is false.

_____130. Tonometry and gonioscopy are tests done to detect glaucoma.

_____131. The combining form, pupil/o- means pertaining to the round opening at the center of the iris.

_____132. The vitreous humor is the clear gel-like substance that fills the anterior chamber of the eye.

_____133. The combining forms phac/o- and lenticul/o- both refer to the lens of the eye.

_____134. Lasix surgery is used to reshape the cornea to correct nearsightedness.

_____135. The light sensitive cells in the retina that only respond to color are the rods.

_____136. At birth an infant is treated with antibiotics to the eyes prophylactically to prevent gonorrhea passed on by the birth canal of the mother.

_____137. An extracapsular cataract extraction will result in aphakia unless an artificial intraocular lens is inserted.

_____138. A retinoblastoma occurs most often in the elderly.

_____139. If the lacrimal ducts are obstructed, the patient will have difficulty with the flow of tears.

_____140. Aqueous humor is a clear, watery fluid produced by the caruncle of the eye.

_____141. The extraocular muscles are six muscles that control the movements of the eye in all directions.

_____142. A clear, hard disk in the internal eye is called the lacrimal sac.

_____143. Sebaceous glands at the edges of the eyelids are also called meibomian glands.

_____144. The clear, gel-like substance that fills the posterior cavity of the eye is called aqueous humor.

_____145. A combining form that means pertaining to the lens is lenticul/o.

_____146. Inflammation or infection of the eyelid is called blepharoptosis.

_____147. The lower eyelid turns outward with ectropion.

_____148. A red, painful swelling or pimple containing pus located near the edge of the eyelid and also known as a stye is called a hordeolum.

_____149. Hyphema is an abnormal sensitivity to bright light.

_____150. The anterior and posterior chambers are filled with vitreous humor.

_____151. The combining form blephar/o- means eyelash.

_____152. Loss of transparency of the lens is known as glaucoma.

_____153. Babies who inherit blue/blue or blue/green genes for eye color do not have melanocytes in their irises.

_____154. Tears contain an antibacterial enzyme to prevent bacterial infections in the eyes.

Essay

Write your answer in the space provided or on a separate sheet of paper.

155. Laser photocoagulation was performed on a patient with a detached retina. Explain what this procedure was intended to do.

156. Describe the abnormality in the eye that would signal to the physician that the patient has a liver disease.

157. How does the chart that is used to test vision in very young children differ from the chart used for adults?

158. Why are most babies' irises slate blue at birth?

159. Briefly explain the function of the lacrimal gland.

160. Explain the difference between the function of the rods and the cones in the retina.

161. Describe the conjunctiva and its function.

162. Describe blepharoptosis and its surgical treatment.

163. Describe fluorescein staining and what it is used for.

CHAPTER 16

Multiple Choice

Choose the one alternative that best completes the statement or answers the question.

1. The word buccal means pertaining to the:
   a. palate.
   b. jaw.
   c. cheek.
   d. tongue.

2. The infection of the mouth and tongue called oral candidiasis is also known as:
   a. thrush.
   b. leukoplakia.
   c. pharyngitis.
   d. glossitis.

3. Epistaxis is the medical word for:
   a. earache.
   b. nosebleed.
   c. dizziness.
   d. sore throat.

4. Rinne and Weber are eponyms for:
   a. instruments used in ear surgery.
   b. surgical procedures done to correct hearing difficulty.
   c. diseases of the ear.
   d. tests to assess hearing capability.

5. Which is the fleshy tissue in the back of the oral cavity that hangs from the soft palate?
   a. tragus
   b. uvula
   c. eustacian tube
   d. auricle

6. Hearing loss associated with old age is known as:
   a. tinnitus.
   b. otalgia.
   c. otosclerosis.
   d. presbycusis.

7. The eponym for the condition with edema in the semicircular canals causing hearing loss, ringing in the ears, and vertigo is:
   a. Hertz.
   b. Romberg.
   c. Ménière.
   d. Weber.

8. Kate was unhappy about her protruding ear so she elected to have an otoplasty performed on her:
   a. pinna.
   b. tragus.
   c. vestibule.
   d. external auditory canal.

9. A stapedectomy would be performed for which condition?
   a. cerumen impaction
   b. labyrinthitis
   c. otosclerosis
   d. sinusitis

10. Which medication is used to suppress the cough center in the brain?
    a. dextromethorphan (Robitussin)
    b. beclomethasone (Beconase)
    c. fexofenadine (Allegra)
    d. nystatin (Mycostatin)

11. The patient had removal of the bony prominence just behind his ear. This procedure is a:
    a. turbinectomy.
    b. stapedectomy.
    c. mastoidectomy.
    d. ethmoidectomy.

12. Which is a structure in the middle ear that can be partially visualized during otoscopy?
    a. cochlea
    b. malleus
    c. stapes
    d. vestibule

13. Rhinophyma is:
    a. polyp formation in the nasal mucosa.
    b. frequent nosebleeds.
    c. lateral displacement of the nasal septum.
    d. redness and hypertrophy of the nose.

14. An example of a URI is:
    a. nosebleed.
    b. hay fever.
    c. postnasal drip.
    d. common cold.

15. TMJ syndrome includes pain, clicking, and muscle spasm in the area of the:
    a. tongue.
    b. back of the throat.
    c. jaw.
    d. outer ear.

16. John is a six year old with chronic serous otitis media. Treatment for his condition would be:
    a. tympanostomy tube insertion.
    b. otoplasty.
    c. mastoidectomy.
    d. cheiloplasty.

17. Patients with allergic rhinitis can find relief by using:
    a. nystatin (Mycostatin).
    b. meclizine (Antivert).
    c. hydrocodone (Hycodan).
    d. fexofenadine (Allegra).

18. Which condition would produce an abnormal brainstem auditory evoked response (BAER)?
    a. otosclerosis
    b. acoustic neuroma
    c. cleft lip
    d. vertigo

19. Anacusis is:
    a. lack of the sense of smell.
    b. having no voice.
    c. deafness.
    d. inability to swallow.

20. Glue ear, a thick accumulation of middle ear secretions, is associated with:
    a. cerumen impaction.
    b. labyrinthitis.
    c. otitis externa.
    d. otitis media.

21. The patient has acute pharyngitis. What test would be done to identify the cause of the infection and identify the appropriate treatment?
    a. PND
    b. C&S
    c. ABR
    d. URI

22. The infant with a thrush infection was treated with:
    a. penicillin.
    b. flunisolide (Nasalide).
    c. nystatin (Mycostatin).
    d. Cerumenex.

23. A radical neck dissection for cancer would include partial removal of the:
    a. pharynx.
    b. mandible.
    c. epiglottis.
    d. maxillary sinus.

24. The frontal sinuses are located:
    a. above each eyebrow.
    b. behind the eye, deep within the skull.
    c. on either side of the nose.
    d. beneath the cheek bones.

25. Sounds (ringing, buzzing, hissing, roaring) that are heard constantly or intermittently in one or both ears, even in a quiet environment are a symptom of the condition known as:
    a. acoustic.
    b. vertigo.
    c. tinnitus.
    d. rales.

26. Which is the medical word that refers to the chin?
    a. helix
    b. ala
    c. mentum
    d. tragus

27. Which is an oral infection caused by the yeast-like fungus *Candida albicans*?
    a. gingivitis
    b. tonsillitis
    c. thrush
    d. pharyngitis

28. Otorrhea is the drainage of serous fluid or pus from the:
    a. throat.
    b. ear.
    c. nose.
    d. eye.
29. Acute or chronic bacterial infection of the middle ear with purulent (pus) material is known as:
    a. acoustic neuroma.
    b. suppurative otitis media.
    c. serous otitis media.
    d. otosclerosis.
30. The sudden, sometimes severe, bleeding from the nose is known as:
    a. epistaxis.
    b. hemotympanum.
    c. anosmia.
    d. rhinorrhea.
31. Which is the sensation of being off balance when the body is not moving?
    a. vertigo.
    b. tinnitus.
    c. syncope.
    d. transient.
32. The cause of cold sores is:
    a. herpes simplex virus type 1.
    b. herpes simplex virus type 2.
    c. thrush.
    d. leukoplakia.
33. The second bone of the middle ear is the:
    a. incus.
    b. stapes.
    c. malleus.
    d. ossicle.
34. The auricle is also called the:
    a. hammer.
    b. incus.
    c. anvil.
    d. pinna.
35. All of the following structures are found in the ear EXCEPT:
    a. vestibule.
    b. turbinates.
    c. oval window.
    d. ossicle.
36. Loss of the sense of smell is known as:
    a. anosmia.
    b. tinnitus.
    c. nasal decongestant.
    d. auditory.
37. The abbreviation AS means:
    a. both ears.
    b. right ear.

c. left ear.
d. each ear.
38. Which is a surgical procedure to repair the lip?
    a. polypectomy
    b. gingivoplasty
    c. cheiloplasty
    d. buccoplasty
39. Which is a benign, slow-growing mass in the middle ear composed of cholesterol deposits and epithelial cells?
    a. cholesteatoma
    b. serous otitis media
    c. suppurative otitis media
    d. cochlear implant
40. Which drugs are used to suppress the cough center in the brain?
    a. antihistamine drugs
    b. corticosteroid drugs
    c. decongestant drugs
    d. antitussive drugs
41. Which drugs constrict blood vessels and decrease swelling of the mucous membranes of the nose and sinuses due to colds and allergies?
    a. corticosteroid drugs
    b. antihistamine drugs
    c. antitussive drugs
    d. decongestant drugs
42. The abbreviation T & A means:
    a. tonsils and adenoids.
    b. teeth and adenoids.
    c. throat and adenoids.
    d. tonsillectomy and adenoidectomy.
43. Which diagnostic procedure analyzes the brain's response to sounds?
    a. audiometry
    b. tympanometry
    c. BAER
    d. Rinne and Weber hearing test
44. Bacterial or viral infection of the throat is known as:
    a. tonsillitis.
    b. laryngitis.
    c. pharyngitis.
    d. thrush.
45. The combining form ossicul/o- means:
    a. middle ear.
    b. little bone.
    c. eustachian tube.
    d. eardrum.

46. Which is a surgical procedure to reconstruct a ruptured eardrum?
    a. myringotomy
    b. otoplasty
    c. cheiloplasty
    d. tympanoplasty

47. Which medical procedure is performed to assess equilibrium?
    a. tonometry
    b. audiometry
    c. Romberg's sign
    d. rapid strep test

48. All of the following abbreviations relate to the ear or hearing EXCEPT:
    a. PND.
    b. BAER.
    c. HZ.
    d. BOM.

49. The medical specialty that studies the anatomy and physiology of the ears, nose, mouth, and throat and uses diagnostic tests and medical and surgical procedures is called:
    a. otolaryngology.
    b. otology.
    c. laryngology.
    d. laryngoscopy.

50. Which of the following words contains a combining form that means hammer?
    a. ossicular
    b. incudal
    c. mallear
    d. meatus

51. Which part of the ear do these structures belong to: vestibule, semicircular canals and cochlea?
    a. inner ear
    b. middle ear
    c. outer or external ear
    d. none of the above

52. Which of the following sinuses is actually a group of four pairs of sinuses?
    a. frontal sinuses
    b. maxillary sinuses
    c. ethmoid sinuses
    d. paranasal sinuses

53. Which of the following phrases contains a word part that means cheek?
    a. oral mucosa
    b. submandibular nodes
    c. buccal mucosa
    d. temporomandibular joint

54. The semicircular canals are oriented in all of the following planes EXCEPT:
    a. horizontal.
    b. vertical.
    c. midsagittal.
    d. oblique.

55. Hearing loss may be caused by all of the following EXCEPT:
    a. foreign body or infection in the external auditory canal.
    b. dysequilibrium.
    c. damage to the inner ear by exposure to loud music, especially on a long-term basis.
    d. degeneration of the ossicles of the middle ear.

56. Which of the following is NOT a benign tumor of some portion of the ENT system?
    a. acoustic neuroma
    b. cholesteatoma
    c. polyp
    d. cervical lymphadenopathy

57. Which of the following surgical procedures is done to correct hearing loss by surgically placing a small device behind the ear?
    a. cochlear implant
    b. cheiloplasty
    c. sinus endoscopy
    d. myringotomy

58. Which best describes the path sound travels?
    a. external ear, tympanic membrane, external auditory canal, middle ear, inner ear
    b. tympanic membrane, external ear, external auditory canal, middle ear, inner ear
    c. external auditory canal, external ear, tympanic membrane, middle ear, inner ear
    d. external ear, external auditory canal, tympanic membrane, middle ear, inner ear

59. Which is bilateral hearing loss due to aging?
    a. conductive
    b. presbyacusis
    c. anacusis
    d. sensorineural

60. Blood in the middle ear space is called:
    a. labyrinthitis.
    b. hemotympanum.
    c. Ménière's disease.
    d. presbyacusis.

61. Acute or chronic infection of the middle ear is known as:
    a. myringitis.
    b. otis media.
    c. mastoiditis.
    d. otalgia.

62. A collection of fluid behind the tympanic membrane that creates an air-fluid level is:
    a. effusion.
    b. serous.
    c. suppurative.
    d. otorrhea.

63. Infection of the air cells of the bone of the mastoid process is called:
    a. mastoiditis.
    b. mastitis.
    c. myringitis.
    d. tinnitus.

64. Abnormal formation of bone in the inner ear, particularly between the stapes and the oval window is called:
    a. otorrhea.
    b. tinnitus.
    c. otosclerosis.
    d. anosmia.

65. Vertigo is:
    a. ringing in the ears.
    b. inflammation of the nose.
    c. ruptured eardrum.
    d. dizziness.

66. Redness and hypertrophy of the nose with small to large, irregular lumps in the skin is known as:
    a. rhinophyma.
    b. URI.
    c. sinusitis.
    d. epistaxis.

67. A surgical procedure that uses plastic surgery to correct deformities of the external ear is called:
    a. otoplasty.
    b. glossectomy.
    c. laryngectomy.
    d. rhinoplasty.

68. The combining forms that mean eardrum are myring/o- and:
    a. ot/o-.
    b. lingu/o-.
    c. tympan/o-.
    d. gloss/o-.

69. The medical word otolaryngologist can be separated into the following component word parts:
    a. prefix, prefix, combining form, suffix.
    b. prefix, combining form, combining form, suffix.
    c. combining form, combining form, suffix, suffix.
    d. combining form, combining form, combining form, suffix.

70. The suffix -tome means:
    a. surgical excision.
    b. disease condition.
    c. process of measuring.
    d. instrument used to cut.

71. The combining form cheil/o- means:
    a. ear.
    b. lip.
    c. chin.
    d. neck.

72. The suffix -metry in the medical word audiometry means:
    a. instrument used to examine.
    b. pertaining to.
    c. process of measuring.
    d. state or condition.

73. The physician looks into the ear with a lighted instrument known as a/an:
    a. tuning fork.
    b. ophthalmoscope.
    c. otoscope.
    d. endoscope.

74. Otitis media is a bacterial infection of the:
    a. middle ear.
    b. cochlea.
    c. external ear.
    d. pharynx.

75. The _____ chain is the name given to the collection of the three small bones in the middle ear.
    a. ossicular
    b. eustachian
    c. tympanic
    d. auricular

76. Alligator forceps are used to remove:
    a. tonsils.
    b. turbinates.
    c. ossicles.
    d. cerumen.

77. All of the following abbreviations refer to the ear EXCEPT:
    a. TMJ.
    b. EAC.
    c. TM.
    d. AD.

78. Ear pinning, the surgery done for protruding ears, is known as:
    a. tonsillectomy.
    b. otoplasty.
    c. tympanoplasty.
    d. radical neck dissection.

79. Surgery to insert PE ventilating tubes to drain the middle ear is known as:
    a. audiometry.
    b. presbycusis.
    c. myringitis.
    d. tympanoplasty.
80. By pressing on the cheekbones, the physician is evaluating the patient for signs of:
    a. tonsillitis.
    b. sinusitis.
    c. allergic rhinitis.
    d. deviated septum.
81. What is the purpose of the vestibular branch of cranial nerve VIII?
    a. hearing
    b. balance
    c. swallowing
    d. smell
82. Air is warmed and moisturized in the nasal cavity by which structure?
    a. cochlea
    b. sinuses
    c. conchae
    d. tragus
83. A patient with epistaxis has:
    a. an earache.
    b. a nosebleed.
    c. poor hearing
    d. a sinus infection.
84. Another name for the chin is the:
    a. philtrum.
    b. nasolabial fold.
    c. vermilion border.
    d. mentum.
85. The vermilion border can be found:
    a. on the lips.
    b. around the tongue.
    c. at the end of the tympanic membrane.
    d. in the inner ear.
86. The adenoids are found in the:
    a. nasopharynx
    b. oropharynx
    c. hypopharynx
    d. larynx.
87. The opening to the larynx is covered by the _____ during swallowing.
    a. glottis
    b. vocal cords
    c. epiglottis
    d. Adam's apple

88. The bone that divides the nasal cavity from the oral cavity and forms the roof of the mouth is known as the:
    a. soft palate.
    b. maxillary sinus.
    c. hard palate.
    d. buccal mucosa.
89. A benign tumor of the auditory nerve is a/an:
    a. acoustic neuroma.
    b. cholesteatoma.
    c. hemotympanum.
    d. otosclerosis.
90. Edema of the semicircular canals with destruction of the cochlea, causing hearing loss, tinnitus, and vertigo, is caused by:
    a. otitis externa.
    b. otitis media.
    c. myringitis.
    d. Ménière's disease.
91. Which word is misspelled?
    a. otolaryngology
    b. myringitis
    c. tonsilectomy
    d. tinnitus
92. Which hearing test uses a tuning fork?
    a. tympanometry
    b. culture and sensitivity
    c. Rinne
    d. hertz
93. A rapid strep test would be done for a patient with:
    a. a ruptured tympanic membrane.
    b. sinusitis.
    c. serous otitis media.
    d. sore throat.
94. The inner ear consists off all of these structures EXCEPT:
    a. helix.
    b. cochlea.
    c. organs of Corti.
    d. semicircular canals.
95. Jimmie Jencks stuck a jellybean in his right ear. In that ear, he would have:
    a. presbyacusis.
    b. otitis media.
    c. conductive hearing loss.
    d. mastoiditis.
96. To examine the nose, the physician uses a nasal _____ and shines a penlight to light up into the area.
    a. otoscope
    b. endoscope
    c. speculum
    d. myringotome

97. A/an _____ is a flexible, fiberoptic scope with a magnifying lens and a light source that can be inserted into the nose, sinuses, or throat to examine the tissues and take a biopsy.
    a. speculum
    b. endoscope
    c. otoscope
    d. tuning fork

98. During a radical neck dissection, all of the following may be performed EXCEPT:
    a. myringotomy.
    b. glossectomy.
    c. removal of the jaw bone.
    d. laryngectomy.

99. Irene Stansbury suffered a sudden blow to the head that caused her tympanic membrane to rupture. This injury would be repaired by performing a/an:
    a. myringotomy.
    b. otoplasty.
    c. Weber test.
    d. tympanoplasty.

Short Answer

Write the word or phrase that best completes each statement or answers the question.

100. The common name for a condition with painful, recurring clusters of blisters erupting on the lips or nose caused by the herpes simplex virus is _____ _____.

101. The medical word for drainage of fluid or pus from the ear is _____ .

102. The precancerous lesion associated with tobacco use _____ looks like a thickened, flat white patch on the mucous membrane of the mouth.

103. The combining forms gloss/o- and lingu/o- refer to the _____.

104. An _____ is a test done to assess hearing acuity and hearing loss.

105. Elisa Marks elected to have a/an _____ to correct her oversized nose.

106. The abbreviation for the right ear is _____.

107. There are four pairs of _____ or hollow cavities within the skull.

108. When cerumen becomes thick and a large amount of it is wedged in the external auditory canal, this is known as a/an _____.

109. The external ear is also known as the _____.

110. The middle ear contains three tiny bones called the: _____, _____, and _____.

111. The _____ are three long projections of the ethmoid bone that jut into the nasal cavity

and function to break up the stream of air as it enters the nose. They are also known as the nasal conchae.

112. A/an _____ _____ is a benign tumor of the nerve cells of the auditory nerve.

113. _____ is the sound of buzzing, ringing, hissing, or roaring heard constantly or intermittently in one or both ears, even in a quiet environment.

114. _____ is a drug toxic effect in which certain drugs damage the cochlea.

115. _____ is sinusitis that involves all of the sinuses on one side of the face.

116. _____ is a medical procedure that uses a lighted scope to examine the external auditory canal and tympanic membrane.

117. _____ is the study of the ears, nose, and larynx.

118. The ear canal has glands that secrete _____, a waxy, sticky substance that traps dirt and has an antibiotic action against microorganisms that enter the canal.

119. The eardrum is also called the _____ membrane.

120. The middle ear is connected to the upper throat by the _____ tube.

121. The first structure of the inner ear is called the _____.

122. The end of the vestibule coils on itself to form a snail shell-shaped structure known as the _____.

123. The nasal _____ is a vertical wall of bone that divides the nose into right and left sides.

124. Along the walls of the nasal cavity are a series of three long, bony projections, known collectively as the nasal _____.

125. A _____ is a hollow cavity within a cranial or facial bone.

126. The _____ fold is the oblique skin crease in the cheek, going from the edge of the nose to the corner of the mouth.

127. The _____ border is the pink-red border around the lips.

128. Each end of the mandible is attached to the temporal bone of the cranium at the moveable _____ joint.

129. The oropharynx contains the _____ tonsils, areas of lymphoid tissue on either side of the throat where the soft palate arches downward.

130. The _____ or voice box is a short, triangular structure.

131. At the superior end of the larynx just below the base of the tongue is the _____, a lid-like structure.

132. Surgical excision of a polyp from the vocal cord is called a _____.

133. _____ is the medical name for clear but excessive discharge from the nose.

134. The medical word for earwax is _____.

135. The medical word for a sore throat is _____.

136. In audiometry, the frequency of a pure tone is measured in _____, while the intensity of a pure tone is measured in _____.

137. A feeling of dizziness and nausea from riding in a car, boat, or plane is known as motion sickness. The medical word for this condition is _____.

138. Prior to inserting PE tubes into the middle ear to drain fluid, the surgeon must first perform a/an _____, making an incision in the tympanic membrane. For this procedure, the physician uses an instrument known as a/an _____.

True/False

Write 'T' if the statement is true and 'F' if the statement is false.

_____139. The mentum refers to the vertical ridges on the upper lip.

_____140. A cholesteatoma is a benign, slow growing mass commonly found on the cochlea.

_____141. Removal of lymphoid tissue from the pharynx is abbreviated T&A.

_____142. When a physician tells the patient, "open your mouth wide and say ah," the physician wants to look at the patient's pharynx.

_____143. Audit/o- and aur/i- are combining forms that both mean the sense of hearing.

_____144. The plural spelling for both nostrils is naris.

_____145. An audiologist is a physician who specializes in the diseases of the ear.

_____146. If the patient is experiencing constant ringing in the ears, he has tinnitus.

_____147. Anosmia occurs when a person loses the sense of smell.

_____148. Tonsilitis is the correct spelling for the inflammation of the tonsils.

_____149. Otosclerosis means the external ear becomes hardened.

_____150. The ENT system shares some structures with the gastrointestinal system and the respiratory system.

_____151. Rhinoplasty is the treatment for a ruptured tympanic membrane.

_____152. Otosclerosis is hardening of the arteries of the ear, similar to arteriosclerosis of the cardiovascular system.

_____153. The suffix in the word otorrhea means the same thing as the suffix in the word diarrhea.

_____154. A 79-year-old patient presents to the emergency department complaining of feeling dizzy or off balance. It could be said that she has vertigo.

_____155. Glossitis is an inflammation of the tongue.

_____156. Audiometry is a diagnostic test that analyzes the brain's response to sounds.

_____157. Romberg's sign is a medical finding that helps a healthcare worker assess a patient's equilibrium.

_____158. A mastoidectomy is a surgical procedure to remove part of the tympanic membrane as a result of chronic middle ear infection.

_____159. Decongestant drugs dilate the blood vessels in order to decrease swelling of the mucous membranes of the nose and sinuses due to colds and allergies.

_____160. The nasal cavity is formed by the ethmoid bone and the mandible.

_____161. The tonsils and adenoids play a role in the immune response.

_____162. Inhaled air causes the vocal cords to vibrate.

_____163. A laryngectomy is a surgery that would be done for patients with rhinorrhea.

_____164. To test a patient's hearing, audiometry uses pure tones while speech audiometry uses spoken words.

_____165. The eustachian tube allows pressure in the inner ear to equalize with pressure in the throat and mouth and outside of the body.

Essay

Write your answer in the space provided or on a separate sheet of paper.

166. Why is otitis media common in young children?

167. Describe vocal polyps and describe the type of employment that would predispose a person to develop vocal cord polyps.

168. Name the three areas of the throat.

169. The three bones of the middle ear are the hammer, anvil, and stirrup. What are their correct medical names?

170. Explain the relationship between the function of the vocal cords and speech.

171. Briefly explain how hearing occurs.

172. Briefly discuss the three major types of hearing loss, and what may cause each.

173. Briefly discuss thrush and the type of patients in which it is seen.

174. What is brainstem auditory evoked response (BAER) and what is it used for?

CHAPTER 17

Multiple Choice

Choose the one alternative that best completes the statement or answers the question.

1. Which psychiatric disorder consists of behaviors such as repetitive handwashing, checking if doors are locked, and repeating words?
   a. anxiety disorder
   b. attention-deficit hyperactivity disorder
   c. obsessive-compulsive disorder
   d. panic disorder

2. The area of the brain involved in amnesia due trauma or disease is the:
   a. hippocampus.
   b. cingulated gyrus.
   c. hypothalamus.
   d. fornix.

3. Echolalia means:
   a. involuntary movements such as eye tics or arm thrusting.
   b. soiling clothing with feces in a person over the age of five.
   c. vocalizing vulgar or inappropriate words.
   d. repeating words that someone else has said.

4. Feigning medical or psychiatric symptoms to get attention is known by the eponym of _____ disorder.
   a. Tourette
   b. Munchausen
   c. Beck
   d. Rorschach

5. Valium and Tranxene belong to which classification of drugs?
   a. antianxiety
   b. antipsychotic
   c. antidepressant
   d. none of the above

6. ETOH is an abbreviation used to indicate a/an _____ odor of the breath associated with substance abuse.
   a. fruity
   b. alcohol
   c. foul
   d. metalliclike

7. Which mental health professional can prescribe drugs or medications?
   a. psychiatrist
   b. psychologist
   c. social worker
   d. all of the above

8. In which disorder might a patient demand to be the center of attention with an exaggerated sense of self worth and importance but not have a psychosis or mania?
   a. narcissistic personality
   b. person with a delusional disorder
   c. bipolar disorder
   d. avoidant personality

9. Which is a therapy for a severely depressed patient that involves inducing a seizure?
   a. SSRI
   b. TAT
   c. CBT
   d. ECT

10. Which condition would fall under the Axis II method used to classify psychiatric conditions?
    a. bulimia
    b. panic disorder
    c. schizophrenia
    d. mental retardation

11. Which neurotransmitter prepares the body for "fight or flight" and is seen in increased levels in patients with anxiety-related disorders?
    a. dopamine
    b. serotonin
    c. epinephrine
    d. norepinephrine

12. Treatment for anorexia nervosa would not include:
    a. antipsychotic drugs.
    b. antidepressant drugs.
    c. family therapy.
    d. psychotherapy.

13. A fear of heights is termed:
    a. claustrophobia.
    b. acrophobia.
    c. thanatophobia.
    d. agoraphobia.

14. *The Three Faces of Eve* is a movie made in 1957 about a woman who was described as having multiple personalities. The current name for this condition is:
    a. depersonalization.
    b. conversion disorder.
    c. identity disorder.
    d. anxiety disorder.

15. Without therapy the person with impulse control disorder and trichotillomania will eventually become:
    a. obese.
    b. blind.
    c. deaf.
    d. bald.

16. Chronic, mild bipolar disorder with mood swings is known as:

    a. attention deficit disorder.

    b. borderline personality.

    c. cyclothymia.

    d. delusional disorder.

17. Which drug will make a person physically ill when combined with alcohol?

    a. cocaine

    b. Litholoid

    c. Antabuse

    d. nicotine

18. The psychological "inkblot test" consists of a series of abstract shapes from which a patient is to describe what he sees. This is referred to as the:

    a. Rorschach test.

    b. Thematic Apperception Test.

    c. Beck Depression Inventory.

    d. psychiatric interview.

19. Decreased levels of the neurotransmitters norepinephrine and serotonin are associated with:

    a. anxiety.

    b. phobic behavior.

    c. euphoria and excitement.

    d. depression.

20. A patient whose fear of flying in an airplane is due to claustrophobia would most likely be treated with which psychotherapeutic technique?

    a. aversion therapy

    b. systematic desensitization

    c. psychoanalysis

    d. art therapy

21. Which is a drug used for the mood disorder mania?

    a. Antabuse

    b. Haldol

    c. Lithium (Lithobid)

    d. Prozac

22. The man was arrested after secretly peeping into his neighbor's bedroom windows so that he could attain sexual arousal. His condition is called:

    a. exhibitionism.

    b. sadism.

    c. voyeurism.

    d. transvestism.

23. Tardive dyskinesia, involuntary repetitive movements of the face and extremities, is a severe side effect of Thorazine, which is a/an:

    a. antidepressant drug.

    b. antipsychotic medication.

    c. antianxiety drug.

    d. abused substance.

24. What does it mean if a psychiatrist documented that the patient had a flat affect?

    a. There is no outward display on the face of any of the patient's emotions or thoughts.

    b. The patient is not able to feel guilt or shame.

    c. The patient does not receive any sexual arousal from images of the opposite sex.

    d. The patient is in a stuporous, fixed position like a statue.

25. A person with pyromania might break the law by:

    a. stealing to cover a gambling debt.

    b. shoplifting.

    c. setting fires for pleasure.

    d. assaulting someone.

26. Which is an example of a psychiatric test used to assess personality, emotions, attitudes, motivation, and conflicts? The patient is shown pictures of social or interpersonal situations and describes what is happening in the picture.

    a. Rorschach Test

    b. Axis II test

    c. Thematic Apperception Test

    d. psychiatric interview

27. The abbreviation DT means:

    a. delusion with toxicity.

    b. delirium tremors.

    c. delirium tremens.

    d. drug therapy.

28. Which word means pertaining to the mood or state of mind?

    a. emotion

    b. obsession

    c. affective

    d. therapy

29. Which disorder is characterized by constant, persistent, uncontrollable thoughts that occupy the mind, cause anxiety, and compel the patient to perform excessive, repetitive activities for fear of what might happen if these are not done?

    a. phobia

    b. dementia

    c. panic disorder

    d. obsessive-compulsive disorder

30. Microphobia is a fear of:

    a. germs.

    b. science.

    c. crowds.

    d. small things.

31. Which psychiatric test assesses the degree of depression?

    a. TAT

    b. BDI

    c. OCD

    d. ECT

32. False sensory impressions involving vision, smell, sound, taste, or touch are known as:
    a. hallucinations.
    b. delusions.
    c. paranoia.
    d. obsessions.

33. The combining form hebe/o- in hebephrenic schizophrenia means:
    a. dramatic.
    b. youth.
    c. pleasure.
    d. human being.

34. The word anhedonia means:
    a. lack of mature behavior.
    b. without suffering.
    c. lack of pleasure in any activity.
    d. antisocial behavior.

35. Which test is also known as the inkblot test?
    a. Holmes Rating Scale
    b. Beck's Inventory
    c. Rorschach test
    d. Thematic Apperception Test

36. Which drugs are used to inhibit the action of excessive norepinephrine while increasing the sensitivity of serotonin receptors?
    a. antianxiety drugs
    b. antidepressant drugs
    c. antipsychotic drugs
    d. drugs for mania

37. The abbreviation SAD means:
    a. stress anxiety disorder.
    b. standard anxiety disease.
    c. selective attention disorder.
    d. seasonal affective disorder.

38. Which type of psychiatric therapy uses toys and other objects to help young children express emotions and re-enact traumatic or abusive events?
    a. art therapy
    b. play therapy
    c. group therapy
    d. family therapy

39. Which psychiatric therapy involves the patient thinking about a destructive behavior, coupled with a mild electric shock or noxious smell like ammonia?
    a. aversion therapy
    b. systemic desensitization
    c. electroconvulsive therapy
    d. cognitive-behavioral therapy

40. Anxiolytic drugs and minor tranquilizers are also known as:
    a. antipsychotic drugs.
    b. drugs for mania.
    c. antidepressant drugs.
    d. antianxiety drugs.

41. Which condition is also known as manic-depressive disorder?
    a. catalepsy
    b. bipolar disorder
    c. schizophrenia
    d. delusional disorder

42. Which disorder involves repetitive pulling out of hair from the head?
    a. pedophilia
    b. pyromania
    c. trichotillomania
    d. kleptomania

43. Knowingly exhibiting factitious medical or psychiatric symptoms and lying in order to get a tangible reward, like narcotic drugs or disability payments is known as:
    a. malingering.
    b. hypochondriasis.
    c. Munchausen by proxy.
    d. Munchausen syndrome.

44. Thanatophobia is a fear of:
    a. spiders.
    b. snakes.
    c. strangers.
    d. death.

45. Which structure sends nerve impulses to the sympathetic nervous system during fear or anger to increase the heart rate and respiratory rate as part of the "fight or flight" response to danger?
    a. hypothalmus
    b. thalmus
    c. hippocampus
    d. fornix

46. The combing form limb/o- means:
    a. almond shape.
    b. edge, border.
    c. flexible.
    d. lower back.

47. An extreme, chronic fear of being fat, an obsession with becoming thinner and decreased food intake is characteristic of:
    a. bulimia.
    b. binge-purge disorder.
    c. appetite disorder.
    d. anorexia nervosa.

48. Obtaining sexual arousal by deliberately causing abuse, pain, humiliation, or bondage to another person is known as:
    a. voyeurism.
    b. sadism.
    c. rape.
    d. transvestism.

49. The abbreviation ETOH means:
    a. poisoning.
    b. alcohol.
    c. overdose.
    d. electrotherapy of the head.

50. Which of the following words means a fear of death?
    a. agoraphobia
    b. xenophobia
    c. ophidiophobia
    d. thanatophobia

51. The limbic system contains all of the following structures EXCEPT:
    a. cingulate gyrus.
    b. thalamus.
    c. hypothalamus.
    d. fornix.

52. Which of the following is caused by injury to or degeneration of the hippocampi?
    a. overeating and obesity
    b. disinterest in eating
    c. loss of all long-term memory
    d. insomnia

53. Decreased levels of which neurotransmitter may result in schizophrenia?
    a. dopamine
    b. epinephrine
    c. norepinephrine
    d. serotonin

54. An intense, unreasonable fear of a specific thing or situation is known as a/an:
    a. obsessive-compulsive disorder.
    b. seasonal affective disorder.
    c. generalized anxiety disorder.
    d. phobia.

55. Which type of psychiatric therapy is characterized by a patient thinking about a desired, but destructive behavior, coupled with a mild electrical shock or noxious smell?
    a. art therapy
    b. cognitive-behavioral therapy
    c. aversion therapy
    d. electroconvulsive therapy

56. Which of the following phobias is NOT associated with a fear or mental disorder?
    a. photophobia
    b. arachnophobia
    c. triskaidekaphobia
    d. claustrophobia

57. Which types of disorders are characterized by a temporary or permanent impairment of thinking and memory?
    a. post-traumatic stress disorder
    b. generalized anxiety disorder
    c. panic disorder
    d. cognitive disorders

58. Which type of drugs is also known as anxiolytic drugs?
    a. antidepressant drugs
    b. antipsychotic drugs
    c. antianxiety drugs
    d. Antabuse

59. Emotions are normal forms of expression. Which of the following is a sign of mental illness?
    a. extremely intense emotion
    b. long-lasting emotion
    c. inappropriate or absent emotion
    d. all of the above

60. Increased levels of this chemical in the brain caused by cocaine, narcotics, and alcohol produce the euphoria and excitement ("high") experienced by addicts.
    a. serotonin
    b. dopamine
    c. GABA
    d. epinephrine

61. Which type of disorder dwells on scenarios asking "What if . . .?"
    a. obsessive-compulsive disorder
    b. panic disorder
    c. phobia disorder
    d. generalized anxiety disorder

62. Which word means repeated passage of stool into the clothing in a child older than age five who does not have gastrointestinal illness or disability?
    a. autism
    b. reactive attachment disorder
    c. encopresis
    d. Tourette's syndrome

63. Which disorder is characterized by frequent, spontaneous, involuntary movement tics (eye blinking, throat clearing, arm thrusting) and vocal tics (grunts, barks), or comments that are socially inappropriate, vulgar, obscene, or racist?
    a. autism
    b. Tourette's syndrome
    c. ADHD
    d. echolalia

64. Which disorder is characterized by patients gorging themselves on excessive amounts of food (binge eating) and then, for fear of gaining weight, ridding (purging) themselves of food?
    a. anorexia nervosa
    b. bulimia
    c. depersonalization
    d. fad dieting

65. A loss of connection between personal thoughts and a sense of self and the environment is known as:
   a. depersonalization.
   b. fugue.
   c. malingering.
   d. Munchausen syndrome.

66. Which is a radiologic procedure that shows areas of abnormal metabolism in the brain related to dementia and Alzheimer's disease?
   a. x-ray
   b. CT scan
   c. MRI
   d. PET scan

67. Which psychological test uses cards with abstract shapes on them?
   a. TAT
   b. psychiatric interview
   c. Rorschach test
   d. aversion therapy

68. Which psychiatric therapy places the patient in a dream-like trance?
   a. hypnosis
   b. group therapy
   c. psychoanalysis
   d. play therapy

69. A _____ is a persistent, but irrational fear of a specific thing or situation.
   a. hallucination
   b. seizure
   c. phobia
   d. all of the above

70. _____ is a mental disorder characterized by a loss of contact with reality with hallucinations and delusions.
   a. Psychosis
   b. Neurosis
   c. Mental retardation
   d. Panic attack

71. Control of long-term memory and comparison between present and past emotions and events is the responsibility of the:
   a. amygdaloid bodies.
   b. thalamus.
   c. hypothalamus.
   d. hippocampus.

72. The extreme happiness that accompanies mania is known as:
   a. euphoria.
   b. hallucination.
   c. fugue.
   d. delirium.

73. The interpretation of facial expressions and new social situations is the responsibility of the:
   a. thalamus.
   b. amygdaloid bodies.
   c. hippocampus.
   d. hypothalamus.

74. Which types of emotions can be signs of mental illness?
   a. absent emotions
   b. extremely intense emotions
   c. inappropriate emotions
   d. all of the above

75. James Meade is unable to recognize his own face in the mirror because of advanced Alzheimer's disease. This is because of degeneration in the area of his:
   a. affect.
   b. neurotransmitter.
   c. hippocampus.
   d. fornix.

76. Which area of the brain is responsible for reasoning, judgment, planning, organization, and personality?
   a. frontal lobe
   b. serotonin
   c. thalamus
   d. hippocampus

77. Hyperstimulation of the amygdaloid bodies can produce:
   a. flat affect and disinterest.
   b. violent, aggressive behavior.
   c. inability to analyze.
   d. "fight or flight."

78. Decreased levels of which neurotransmitter are related to the development of schizophrenia and depression?
   a. serotonin
   b. dopamine
   c. norepinephrine
   d. GABA

79. Continued, disabling reaction to an excessively traumatic event is known as:
   a. OCD.
   b. SAD.
   c. ADHD.
   d. PTSD.

80. Acute confusion, disorientation, and agitation due to the effect of toxic levels of drugs or alcohol is known as:
   a. delirium.
   b. amnesia.
   c. dementia.
   d. dysthmia.

81. An exaggerated sense of self-worth and importance is characteristic of a _____ personality.
   a. delusional
   b. antisocial
   c. narcissistic
   d. schizophrenic

82. Which type of activity is NOT part of a psychiatric interview?
   a. noting the patient's general appearance
   b. asking patient's to interpret inkblots
   c. asking the patient why he came for care
   d. reviewing stressors in the patient's life

83. The process of helping a patient get through the symptoms of alcohol withdrawal is known as:
   a. substance abuse.
   b. alcohol intoxication.
   c. family therapy
   d. detoxication.

84. When a schizophrenia patient uses a new, made-up word that has no meaning, this is known as a/an
   a. delusion.
   b. hallucination.
   c. neologism.
   d. addiction.

85. Which of the following is true of global amnesia?
   a. Events before the onset of amnesia cannot be remembered.
   b. All present and past events cannot be remembered.
   c. Events after the onset of amnesia cannot be remembered.
   d. Selected events can be remembered.

86. When a pyromaniac sets a fire, he/she is:
   a. trying to conceal a crime.
   b. taking revenge.
   c. trying to collect insurance money.
   d. none of the above.

Short Answer

Write the word or phrase that best completes each statement or answers the question.

87. Bipolar disorder is also known as _____ disorder.

88. Alzheimer's disease is the most common cause of _____, the gradual deterioration of mental function.

89. A person who wears clothing that belongs to the opposite sex or poses as someone of the opposite sex is called a _____

90. The patient underwent _____ in order to stop smoking. He was put into a sleep-like trance during which time the therapist made suggestions to his unconscious mind to later act on consciously.

91. These three combining forms ment/o-, phren/o-, and psych/o- mean _____.

92. The patient admitted to binging on food, and purging with laxatives because she was driven by the fear of getting fat. This eating disorder is known as _____.

93. A person who attains sexual arousal with preadolescent children is called a _____.

94. Severe alcohol withdrawal symptoms are termed _____ tremens.

95. Hebephrenia, inappropriate, childish, and silly behavior, is a subtype of the psychosis known as _____.

96. The abbreviation _____ refers to the publication published by the American Psychiatric Association that includes psychological conditions arranged according to five axes.

97. _____ is the outward display on the face of the inward emotions and thoughts.

98. _____ is a sympathetic nervous system neurotransmitter that prepares the body for "fight or flight."

99. Related structures in the brain that control emotion, mood, memory, motivation, and behavior are called the _____ system.

100. _____ is prevailing, predominant emotion affecting a person's state of mind.

101. The _____ bodies are almond-shaped areas within each temporal lobe that interpret facial expression and new social situations to identify danger.

102. The tract of nerves that joins all the parts of the limbic is called the _____.

103. _____-_____ disorder is a mental disorder characterized by constant, persistent, uncontrollable thoughts that occupy the mind, cause anxiety, and compel the patient to perform excessive, repetitive, meaningless activities.

104. A _____ disorder is a sudden attack of severe, overwhelming anxiety without an identifiable cause.

105. Acute confusion, disorientation and agitation due to toxic levels of drugs or alcohol in the brain is known as _____.

106. The _____ test uses cards with abstract shapes on them to help determine a patient's mental state.

107. The _____ acts as a relay station, receiving nerve impulses from the five senses (sight, hearing, touch, taste, and smell) and relaying them to the sensory and motor areas of the cerebral cortex.

108. The _____ controls long-term memory and facilitates comparison between present and past emotions and experiences.

109. A/an _____ is an intense state of feelings.

110. The presence of an emotion in the thoughts produces an outward display on the face or the person's _____.

111. A person's emotional state of mind may reflect many emotions at the same time (fear, guilt, and anger), but the prevailing, predominant emotion is known as the person's _____.

112. _____ are chemicals that play an important role in emotions by relaying messages from one neuron to the next.

113. _____ is released when a person experiences fear or anger in order to prepare the body for "fight or flight."

114. _____ is the chemical that controls the day-to-day function of the involuntary processes in the body through the parasympathetic nervous system.

115. _____ is the fear of heights.

116. _____ is the fear of closed-in spaces.

117. _____ is the gradual but progressive deterioration of cognitive function due to old age or a neurological disease process.

118. _____ means exhibiting factitious medical or psychiatric symptoms and lying about them in order to get a tangible reward, like narcotic drugs or disability payments.

119. _____ is the disorder that is demonstrated by a preoccupation with and misinterpretation of minor bodily sensations with the fear that these indicate disease.

120. A person with a/an _____ personality has a disregard for written and unwritten rules and standards of conduct of society and shows lying, stealing, and a disregard for others.

121. If you feel a strong infatuation for someone of the opposite sex, you are experiencing high levels of the neurotransmitter _____ in your brain.

122. The feeling that someone is trying to hurt or kill you when this is not true is known as a _____ of persecution.

True/False

Write 'T' if the statement is true and 'F' if the statement is false.

_____123. PMDD is a continued, disabling reaction to a very traumatic event in which a patient has problems such as chronic anxiety, insomnia, and irritability.

_____124. When a patient represses overwhelming anxiety, a psychotic disorder can occur in which the patient shows physical disability such as blindness with no physical reason.

_____125. Fetishism is an overwhelming impulse to steal things.

_____126. Xenophobia is a fear of strangers.

_____127. With regard to substance-related disorders, the words dependence and tolerance mean the same thing.

_____128. Psychoanalysis is a therapeutic process developed by Sigmund Freud that includes dream analysis and hypnosis.

_____129. Seasonal affective disorder (SAD) is caused by hypersecretion of melatonin and shows itself as depression.

_____130. The limbic system in the brain consists of structures that control emotion, behavior, and memory.

_____131. ADHD is more common in boys than in girls, but most children outgrow the symptoms by later childhood.

_____132. Autism is an impulsive flight from one's life and familiar surroundings after a traumatic event.

_____133. Attention deficit hyperactivity disorder is characterized by memory loss.

_____134. Autistic children may be of normal intelligence or mentally retarded.

_____135. Oppositional defiant disorder is the inability to bond emotionally and form intimate relationships with others because of severe abuse or neglect of the patient's basic needs before age two.

_____136. Bulimia is an extreme eating disorder characterized by a decrease in food intake to the point of starvation.

_____137. Depersonalization is the loss of connection between personal thoughts and sense of self and the environment.

_____138. A malingerer is a patient who exhibits factitious medical or psychiatric symptoms and knowingly lies in order to get a tangible reward such as a narcotic drug or disability payment.

_____139. Somatoform disorders are characterized by excessive, dramatic physical complaints that do not fit any medical disease.

_____140. Bipolar disorder is characterized by chronic mood swings between mania and euphoria.

_____141. Delusional disorder is characterized by continued false beliefs concerning events of everyday life that are fixed and unchanging despite the efforts of others to persuade or evidence showing otherwise.

_____142. The PET scan is a radiologic procedure characterized by the use of ultrasound waves to diagnose mental disorders.

_____143. An overwhelming impulse to steal things that have little or no value is known as pyromania.

_____144. A cocaine addict is not aware of the serious medical conditions related to the use of that substance.

_____145. During hypnosis, the patient is able to remember who they are and what is happening.

_____146. Triskaidekaphobia is also known as a fear of snakes.

Essay

Write your answer in the space provided or on a separate sheet of paper.

147. Hypochondriasis refers to a patient's preoccupation with the fear that minor body sensations are indicative of a serious disease. Analysis of the word is as follows: Hypo- = beneath + chondr/o- = cartilage + -iasis = abnormal condition. How does the analysis of this word relate to the condition?

148. What are the two "poles" of bipolar disorder?

149. Which area of the brain is responsible for interpreting facial expressions and new social situations?

150. Which area of the brain regulates sexual behavior?

151. Name two substances that are classified as hallucinogens.

152. Describe the characteristics of posttraumatic stress disorder.

153. List the different types of amnesia and their characteristics.

154. Discuss the concept of dementia.

155. Describe hypochondriasis.

156. Describe the "Beck Depression Inventory."

CHAPTER 18

Multiple Choice

Choose the one alternative that best completes the statement or answers the question.

1. The process of single cell destruction or programmed cellular death is known as:
   a. apoptosis.
   b. mitosis.
   c. necrosis.
   d. oncosis.

2. The Philadelphia chromosome appears in:
   a. fibrosarcoma.
   b. chronic myelogenous leukemia.
   c. adenocarcinoma.
   d. small cell carcinoma.

3. An example of brachytherapy would be:
   a. insertion of radioactive substances intravenously for thyroid cancer.
   b. insertion of radioactive substances into the lymphatic system for leukemia.
   c. external beam radiation directed at the chest for lung cancer.
   d. positioning of a radioactive implant directly into the bladder for bladder cancer.

4. In addition to the lumpectomy performed for her breast carcinoma, Joan Bentley also had a/an _____ biopsy done to remove the first site that receives drainage from the primary breast tumor.
   a. punch
   b. incisional
   c. sentinel node
   d. stereotactic

5. The Hickman, Broviac, and Groshong are:
   a. implantable ports.
   b. intraperitonal catheters.
   c. central venous catheters.
   d. implantable wafers.

6. Debulking is a surgical procedure for cancer that has the intent of:
   a. reducing the size of the tumor.
   b. removing the tumor and surrounding tissues.
   c. taking a small portion of the tumor for biopsy purposes.
   d. removing organs that secrete hormones that encourage growth of certain cancers.

7. Following her surgery for breast cancer Mrs. Jaseene was put on _____ to create a hormone environment that attempts to prevent future cancer growth.
   a. Compazene
   b. Adriamycin
   c. Methotrexate
   d. Tamoxifen

8. A retinoblastoma is an embryonal cancerous tumor of the _____ that occurs in young children.
   a. brain
   b. liver
   c. eye
   d. testis

9. The Reed Sternberg cell appears on biopsy from which cancer?
   a. adenocarcinoma
   b. Hodgkin's lymphoma
   c. multiple myeloma
   d. chronic myelogenous leukemia

10. Which organ could develop an adenocarcinoma?
   a. pancreas
   b. skeletal muscle
   c. bone
   d. cartilage

11. Intravesical chemotherapy is a medical procedure using a catheter to instill cancer chemotherapy into the:
   a. stomach.
   b. bladder.
   c. uterus.
   d. colon.

12. Which of the following is a cancer of the skin?
   a. hepatocellular carcinoma
   b. malignant melanoma
   c. small cell carcinoma
   d. leukemia

13. An example of exfoliative cytology would be a:
   a. Pap smear of bronchial washings for suspected lung cancer.
   b. bone marrow aspiration for suspected leukemia.
   c. chromosomal abnormality examination for Ewing's sarcoma.
   d. frozen section of a breast tumor for possible cancer.

14. Which blood test can point to cancer of the prostate when the results are elevated?
   a. CA 15-3
   b. HCG
   c. CEA
   d. PSA

15. Mary McLaughlin's breast cancer is staged as: T3 N1 M0. This means that:
   a. she has a small localized tumor with no spread to other organs.
   b. she has a large tumor that has spread to lymph node tissue but not to other organs.
   c. she has a large tumor that has spread to lymph node tissue and spread to surrounding muscle tissue.
   d. she has three separate tumors with lymph node spread but no metastases.

16. Cryosurgery uses liquid nitrogen to _____ and destroy abnormal tissue.
   a. burn
   b. identify
   c. coagulate
   d. freeze

17. An intrathecal catheter will deliver the chemotherapy needed to treat cancer of the:
   a. bladder.
   b. bone marrow.

   c. spinal cord.
   d. peritoneum.

18. Which is a drug used to treat the nausea and vomiting that can accompany cancer chemotherapy?
   a. Adriamyan
   b. Compazine
   c. Protocol
   d. hormonal drug

19. Which is the abbreviation for a catheter used to deliver cancer chemotherapy to the entire body?
   a. PICC
   b. PR
   c. DNA
   d. BRCA

20. Cancer cells that are described as undifferentiated may also be referred to as:
   a. metastatic.
   b. hormonal.
   c. oncogenic.
   d. anaplastic.

21. Basal cell carcinoma is a type of _____ cancer.
   a. cervical
   b. skin
   c. breast
   d. bladder

22. Receptor assays are cytology tests done for which type of cancer?
   a. skin
   b. bone
   c. breast
   d. chronic lymphocytic leukemia

23. Elevated levels of _____ in the blood can point to liver cancer.
   a. alpha fetoprotein (AFP)
   b. karyotype
   c. progesterone receptors
   d. BRCA 1

24. Which procedure is done in conjunction with extensive cancer surgery to remove possible metastatic sites?
   a. exploratory laparotomy
   b. tumor ablation
   c. debulking
   d. lymph node dissection

25. Which word would not be used to describe a cancerous tumor?
   a. anaplastic
   b. metastatic
   c. encapsulated
   d. undifferentiated

26. The period of time during which there are no signs and symptoms of cancer is known as:
   a. prophylaxis.
   b. remedy.
   c. relapse.
   d. remission.

27. Which type of cancer affects the connective tissues?
   a. lymphoma
   b. myeloma
   c. carcinoma
   d. sarcoma

28. The medical and surgical procedures that classify cancer by how far it has spread in the body are known as:
   a. staging.
   b. layering.
   c. grading.
   d. sizing.

29. Which treatment involves radioactive implants (needles, wires, capsules, pellets/seeds) inserted into the tumor or the tissue around the tumor?
   a. intravenous radiotherapy
   b. external beam radiotherapy
   c. intracavitary radiotherapy
   d. interstitial radiotherapy

30. Which procedure uses a CT scan to pinpoint the location of the mass and guide the biopsy needle?
   a. incisional biopsy
   b. stereotactic biopsy
   c. punch biopsy
   d. sentinel node biopsy

31. CA 15-3 is a tumor marker to detect the presence of:
   a. breast cancer.
   b. ovarian cancer.
   c. pancreatic cancer.
   d. colon cancer.

32. Excision of the tumor as well as the nearby organs because of widely spread cancer is known as:
   a. brachytherapy.
   b. debulking.
   c. endoscopy.
   d. exenteration.

33. Which medical procedure involves liquid nitrogen being sprayed or painted onto a small malignant lesion to freeze and destroy the tissue?
   a. cryosurgery
   b. fractionation
   c. brachytherapy
   d. electrosurgery

34. Which is a cancer of a plasma cell?
   a. osteosarcoma
   b. adenocarcinoma
   c. leukemia
   d. multiple myeloma

35. Which is a nuclear medicine procedure that uses a radioactive tracer that collects in particular organs or tissues?
   a. scintigraphy
   b. ultrasound
   c. CT scan
   d. MRI

36. Which is an environmental substance that can contribute to the development of cancer?
   a. carcinogen
   b. oncogene
   c. genetic mutation
   d. heredity

37. Ewing's tumor is a cancer of the:
   a. liver.
   b. spinal cord.
   c. bone.
   d. lung.

38. Which is a medical procedure in which an intravenous catheter is inserted into the arm and threaded into the superior vena cava whereby chemotherapy drugs can be administered?
   a. Bx
   b. TNM
   c. BMT
   d. PICC

39. The process by which cells that were once mature and differentiated become undifferentiated and immature in appearance and behavior is known as:
   a. angiogenesis.
   b. encapsulated.
   c. apoptosis.
   d. anaplasia.

40. Which is a medical procedure that uses electrical current to remove small cancerous tumors on the skin?
   a. electrosurgery
   b. biopsy
   c. cryosurgery
   d. resection

41. Which is a medical procedure that classifies cancer by how well differentiated the cells appear under the microscope?
   a. staging
   b. layering
   c. grading
   d. sizing

42. Which is a process by which cancerous cells break off from a tumor and move through the blood vessels or lymphatic vessels to other sites in the body?
    a. metastasis
    b. mitosis
    c. mutation
    d. angiogenesis

43. Basal cell carcinoma is a type of:
    a. breast cancer.
    b. brain cancer.
    c. lung cancer.
    d. skin cancer.

44. Osteosarcoma is cancer of the:
    a. brain.
    b. lung.
    c. bone.
    d. muscle.

45. Which is a blood test that detects a protein present in an embryo but not in adults? Elevated levels are seen with several different cancers?
    a. HCG
    b. CEA
    c. AFP
    d. UA

46. Which classification system is used to detect cervical cancer?
    a. Bethesda system
    b. FIGO staging
    c. Dukes classification
    d. Gleason score

47. Which medical procedure involves the insertion of a catheter into the bladder for administration of chemotherapy drugs?
    a. intracavitary chemotherapy
    b. intravesical chemotherapy
    c. intrathecal catheter
    d. peripherally inserted catheter

48. Which cancerous tumors are not adversely affected by radiation therapy?
    a. radiodefiant
    b. radiosusceptible
    c. radiosensitive
    d. radioresistant

49. Programmed cell death rate is known as:
    a. cancer.
    b. mitosis.
    c. apoptosis.
    d. endoplasmic reticulum.

50. Which of the following is NOT a carcinogen?
    a. heredity
    b. radiation
    c. industrial chemicals
    d. some chemotherapy drugs

51. Cancerous tumors release a substance that causes blood vessels in the surrounding tissues to grow into the tumor to provide it with nutrients. This process is known as:
    a. encapsulation.
    b. angiogenesis.
    c. oncogenesis.
    d. carcinogenesis.

52. During the process of _____ , cancer cells break off and move to other sites within the body.
    a. invasion
    b. anaplasia
    c. genetic mutation
    d. metastasis

53. The process by which embryonic cells assume different shapes and functions in different parts of the body is called:
    a. metastasis.
    b. differentiation.
    c. oncogenesis.
    d. angiogenesis.

54. A condition of atypical cells that are abnormal in size, shape, or organization but have not yet become cancerous is called:
    a. carcinomatosis.
    b. dysplasia.
    c. neoplasia.
    d. adenocarcinoma.

55. Which of the following describes a cancer of the epithelial cells lining the duct of the gallbladder?
    a. cholangiocarcinoma
    b. lymphadenopathy
    c. hepatocellular carcinoma
    d. angiosarcoma

56. A patient with ovarian cancer has a series of blood tests done. The alpha fetoprotein level is high. Which of the following statements is true regarding this level?
    a. The high alpha fetoprotein level indicates that the cancer is responding well to treatment.
    b. The high alpha fetoprotein level is normal and has no relationship to the cancer.
    c. Alpha fetoprotein levels are not usually done in ovarian cancer patients.
    d. The high alpha fetoprotein level indicates that the cancer may be advanced.

57. What type of biopsy is done with a large-gauge needle inserted into the tumor to obtain several long pieces of tissue?
    a. core needle
    b. excisional
    c. fine-needle aspiration
    d. punch

58. Which cell organelles are small sacs that contain powerful digestive enzymes to destroy a bacterium or virus that invades the cell?
   a. mitochondria
   b. golgi
   c. lysosomes
   d. endoplasmic reticulum

59. Which is NOT a cell organelle?
   a. Golgi apparatus
   b. mitochondria
   c. endoplasmic reticulum
   d. cytoplasm

60. Through the action of DNA, which of the following controls all of the activities that take place within the cell, such as the production of cellular proteins and the production of enzymes to control metabolism in the cell?
   a. mitochondria
   b. nucleus
   c. ribosomes
   d. RNA

61. Which gene is the most important suppressor gene? It is located on chromosome 17 in every cell. It is inactive until DNA in the cell's nucleus is damaged?
   a. p53
   b. Herz/neu
   c. BRCA
   d. CEA

62. Which is NOT a factor contributing to the development of cancer?
   a. heredity
   b. a blow to the body
   c. pathogens
   d. carcinogens

63. The word metastasis means:
   a. encapsulated.
   b. moving to other parts of the body.
   c. caused by heredity.
   d. out of control.

64. The abbreviation Ca means:
   a. a tumor registry.
   b. a grading of a tumor.
   c. cancer.
   d. an estrogen receptor.

65. What is a PICC?
   a. a type of tumor
   b. a type of IV catheter
   c. a type of biopsy
   d. none of the above

66. Which statement is TRUE?
   a. Chemotherapy protocols use a combination of several different chemotherapy drugs that are administered together.
   b. Chemotherapy drugs never contain platinum.
   c. Chemotherapy drugs never include hormonal drugs because hormones will make a tumor grow.
   d. Antibiotics are never used in cancer treatment, because they are designed for infections and cancer is not an infection.

67. How does radiation therapy work to treat cancer?
   a. It disrupts the atoms in the DNA, which keeps them from dividing.
   b. It disrupts the atoms in the RNA, which keeps them from dividing.
   c. It causes the cells to kill themselves.
   d. It destroys only cancerous cells and not normal cells.

68. Loss of normal differentiated cell structure is known as:
   a. angiogensis.
   b. metastasis.
   c. anaplasia.
   d. encapsulation.

69. Carcinomatosis means:
   a. a state of cancer.
   b. abnormal cells that look like cancer.
   c. a condition of carcinoma in a specific site.
   d. cancerous tumors in multiple sites.

70. A benign dermoid cyst in the ovary that contains hair and sometimes teeth is known as a:
   a. Wilms' tumor.
   b. neuroblastoma.
   c. seminoma.
   d. teratoma.

71. All of the following are true about bone marrow aspiration EXCEPT:
   a. it is done in the posterior iliac crest.
   b. it is used to treat leukemia or lyphoma.
   c. it shows all stages of cell development.
   d. it is examined under the microscope.

72. Which of the following is NOT a blood test to detect early signs of cancer?
   a. Pap
   b. PSA
   c. HCG
   d. CEA

73. Fractionation refers to the treatment of cancer with:
    a. divided doses of radiation.
    b. implantable wafers of chemotherapy drugs.
    c. surgically implanted catheters.
    d. dividing a large tumor by doing debulking.

74. The use of chemotherapy drugs after another type of treatment like surgery has already been done as the primary treatment is known as _____ therapy.
    a. protocol
    b. biopsy
    c. oncology
    d. adjuvant

75. Which of the following is a career that deals with the field of oncology and cancer?
    a. DNA
    b. FIGO
    c. CTR
    d. PSA

76. Within each cell, there are small sacs that contain powerful digestive enzymes. These are known as:
    a. chromosomes.
    b. lysosomes.
    c. genes.
    d. mitochondria.

77. A cell has all of the following structures EXCEPT:
    a. cytoplasm.
    b. nucleus.
    c. cell wall.
    d. mitochondria.

Short Answer

Write the word or phrase that best completes each statement or answers the question.

78. _____ is the study of anatomy and physiology of cancer cells, including diagnostic tests, various treatments, and drugs.

79. The process of cancer cells spreading from the original site to other sites in the body is known as _____ .

80. _____ is a general word for the presence of cancer in multiple sites of the body.

81. A _____ is a malignant tumor of fatty tissue.

82. _____ is a radiological procedure used to screen for breast cancer.

83. To remove the basal cell carcinoma from Diane Jorgenson's face, the physician performed a wide _____: removal of the tumor plus a large margin of normal tissue surrounding it.

84. The abbreviation Bx means _____.

85. An astrocytoma is a type of cancer, found in the _____ .

86. _____ is a radiological procedure that uses dye to outline the lymphatic vessels.

87. Excision of a cancerous tumor as well as excision of all nearby lymph nodes, soft tissue, and muscle is a _____ resection.

88. The human papillomavirus causes genital warts and chronic inflammation that can lead to _____ cancer in women.

89. Lymph nodes release a substance called _____ _____ factor which causes cancer cells to become necrotic and die.

90. _____ is a process by which cells that were once mature and differentiated become undifferentiated and immature in appearance and behavior.

91. A _____ is the return of symptoms or signs of cancer after a period of improvement or even remission.

92. _____ carcinoma is cancer of the mucous membranes lining the bronchi of the lungs.

93. Hepatocellular carcinoma is cancer of the liver and is also known as a _____.

94. Hodgkin's disease is a type of _____.

95. _____ cytology is a cytology test that examines cells from secretions or from cells scraped or washed from a body surface.

96. A tumor with increased numbers of estrogen receptors or progesterone receptors is considered to be _____ dependent.

97. A _____ is the smallest independently functioning structure in the body that can reproduce itself by division.

98. The _____ is a gel-like substance that fills the cell.

99. Messenger _____ duplicates the information contained in a gene and carries that information to the ribosome where it is used to assemble amino acids to produce a protein molecule.

100. _____ is the process by which a cell divides.

101. _____ is a process by which a cancerous tumor causes blood vessels in the surrounding tissues to grow into the tumor and provide it with nutrients.

102. _____ is the condition of atypical cells that are abnormal in size, shape, or organization but have not yet become cancerous.

103. _____ is the general word for any growing tissue or tumor, benign or malignant, that is not part of normal body structure or function.

104. _____ cell carcinoma is a cancer of the deepest layer (base layer) of the epidermis of the skin.

105. _____ is cancer of a blood vessel or lymphatic vessel.

106. _____ sarcoma is a rare cancer of the skin and subcutaneous tissue usually seen in AIDS patients.

107. _____ is cancer of the bone.

108. Cancer of the white blood cells is known as _____.

109. Cancer of an embryonal cell of the kidney that occurs in young children is called Wilm's tumor or _____.

110. _____ is a radiologic procedure that uses ultra high-frequency sound waves to produce an image.

111. The acronym CAUTION can help you remember the ways in which early cancer can present itself; the C stands for _____ _____ _____ _____ _____ _____.

112. Dimpling of the surface of the skin caused by advanced breast cancer is known by the medical name of peau d' _____.

113. A procedure that uses radiopaque contrast dye to outline the structures of the lymphatic system is known as a _____ .

114. The FIGO Staging System is a classification system for cancer of the _____.

115. The Gleason Score is a classification system for cancer of the _____ _____.

116. A _____ is a written plan of how to treat a particular type of cancerous tumor.

117. The study of cancerous tumors, their diagnosis, and their treatment, is the medical specialty known as _____.

True/False

Write 'T' if the statement is true and 'F' if the statement is false.

_____118. The human papillomavirus that causes genital warts can lead to cervical cancer in women.

_____119. The process by which a cancerous tumor causes blood vessels to grow into the tumor and provide it with nutrients is called oncogenesis.

_____120. Dysplasia describes a cancer that is localized and still contained in the area of origin.

_____121. Remission is the return of the symptoms and signs of a cancer previously treated.

_____122. A malignancy of cartilage is known as chondrocarcinoma.

_____123. A rhabdomyosarcoma is a malignancy found, for example, in the biceps muscle of the upper arm.

_____124. Choriocarcinoma is an embryonal cell cancerous tumor of the ovary.

_____125. The patient's biopsy revealed a cervical cancer in situ. This means that the cervical cancer has metastasized to a secondary site.

_____126. Ewing's sarcoma of the subcutaneous tissues can appear as a complication of AIDS.

_____127. An incisional biopsy is a procedure to expose the suspected cancer and remove the entire tumor along with a surrounding margin or normal tissue.

_____128. When a CT scan is used to pinpoint the location of a mass and guide the biopsy needle, the procedure is called a stereotactic biopsy.

_____129. An implantable wafer containing a chemotherapy drug is implanted in a tumor before it has been removed.

_____130. Debulking is a surgical procedure where a surgeon removes only part of a large tumor, to reduce the size of the tumor.

_____131. A surgical procedure which excises the tumor as well as all of the nearby organs is called an exenteration.

_____132. Alkylating drugs are used to break DNA strands in the cancerous cells, and are considered a type of chemotherapy drug.

_____133. Antiemetic drugs are chemotherapy drugs that treat nausea and vomiting.

_____134. A cell is the smallest, independently functioning structure in the body that can reproduce itself by division.

_____135. Suppressor genes stimulate mitosis and keep each cell from dividing excessively.

_____136. Cancer in situ exists when a tumor is still contained to the primary site.

_____137. Suppressor genes promote the mitosis of cells.

_____138. A neoplasm is always a malignant tumor.

_____139. CAUTION is the acronym for the warning signs for some common cancers.

_____140. The skin or mucous membrane is the site where an adenocarcinoma will form.

_____141. Chemotherapy antibiotic drugs can be used to treat both cancer and bacterial infections due to cancer.

Essay

Write your answer in the space provided or on a separate sheet of paper.

142. If a cancerous cell is not destroyed by the p53 gene, describe at least one of the three ways that the body can destroy a cancer cell to prevent it from developing into a cancerous tumor.

143. Describe the significance of the Her2/neu cytology test.

144. What is the difference between adenocarcinoma and carcinoma?

145. What is a sarcoma?

146. What is a blood smear and why is it done?

147. What is tumor grading?

148. What is the TNM system and what is it used for?

CHAPTER 19

Multiple Choice

Choose the one alternative that best completes the statement or answers the question.

1. The metallic element in contrast dye that is instilled into the rectum to outline the colon and rectum for radiological examination is:
   a. iodine.
   b. thallium.
   c. gadolinium.
   d. barium.

2. How does a xeromammogram differ from a mammogram?
   a. The xeromammogram shows a three-dimensional image of the breast rather than a one-dimensional image.
   b. The xeromammogram is produced by nuclear medicine technology rather than by x-ray technology.
   c. The xeromammogram image is printed on paper rather than on x-ray film.
   d. The xeromammogram uses a magnetic field to scan the breast rather than x-ray beams.

3. X-rays are used in all of the following tests EXCEPT:
   a. arteriography.
   b. magnetic resonance imaging.
   c. roentgenography.
   d. fluoroscopy.

4. Radioactive substances that emit positrons are used in _____ scans.
   a. US
   b. KUB
   c. RAIU
   d. PET

5. If a chest x-ray is taken so that the x-rays penetrate the chest and exit through the back on an x-ray plate, this is a/an _____ chest x-ray.
   a. AP
   b. lateral
   c. IVP
   d. TEE

6. An open MRI is more comfortable to a person who suffers from a fear of:
   a. heights.
   b. water.
   c. being in closed spaces.
   d. needles.

7. The most common type of chest x-ray is done with the patient standing with the chest next to the x-ray plate. This is a/an _____ chest x-ray.
   a. posteroanterior
   b. anteroposterior
   c. lateral
   d. oblique

8. A person with which object in their body will be told that having an MRI is contraindicated for them because the metal in the object will be subjected to the magnetic field and become dislodged?
   a. hip prosthesis
   b. cochlear implant
   c. permanent dental crowns
   d. all of the above

9. Radiopharmaceuticals are also known as _____ because they can be located in a particular part of the body by the gamma rays they produce.
   a. dosimeters
   b. positrons
   c. tracers
   d. emissions

10. Technetium-99m, xenon-133, and gallium-67 are radiopharmaceuticals that:
    a. emit positrons.
    b. are combined with monoclonal antibodies.
    c. contain iodine.
    d. emit gamma rays.

11. Which test is considered to be screening and not diagnostic?
    a. angiography
    b. bone densitometry
    c. electron beam tomography
    d. intravenous cholangiography

12. Which is an abbreviation for an x-ray of urinary organs?
    a. KUB
    b. IVC
    c. US
    d. DSA

13. A grayscale ultrasonography or B scan is _____ dimensional.
    a. one
    b. two
    c. three
    d. four

14. A dosimeter is found in a:
    a. lead apron.
    b. transducer.
    c. film badge.
    d. flat plate.

15. Which is the eponym for the technology used to produce audible sounds from the body such as blood flowing though an artery or the heartbeat of a fetus?
    a. Curie
    b. Rem
    c. Becquerel
    d. Doppler

16. Xenon-133 and krypton-81m are radiopharmaceuticals used to diagnose cancer of the:
    a. lung.
    b. heart.
    c. colon.
    d. ovary.

17. A preliminary radiograph taken before contrast medium is introduced is referred to as a/an:
    a. enhanced film.
    b. bucky film.
    c. scout film.
    d. portable film.

18. An intravenous cholangiography will diagnose:
    a. pancreatic cancer.
    b. gastric ulcers.
    c. gallstones.
    d. diverticulitis.

19. The MUGA scan assesses _____ function.
    a. liver
    b. lung
    c. colon
    d. heart

20. Which is the correct position for a lateral decubitus x-ray?
    a. sitting
    b. lying on the side
    c. lying on the abdomen
    d. standing

21. Which is a diagnostic test of urinary organs in which contrast dye is injected into the ureters using a catheter through the bladder?
    a. kidneys, ureters, bladder film
    b. retrograde pyelography
    c. lymphangiography
    d. intravenous pyelography

22. Mrs. Jeanne Smith had a DEXA scan to determine if she had:
    a. breast cancer.
    b. kidney stones.
    c. gallstones.
    d. osteoporosis.

23. Mr. Isaiah Ritter had an abdominal aneurysm that showed up on a/an:
    a. coronary angiogram.
    b. venogram.
    c. aortogram.
    d. arthrogram.

24. In roentgenography, areas of low density are said to be:
    a. radiolucent.
    b. radiopaque.
    c. translucent.
    d. transopaque.

25. In which type of x-ray does the beam enter the patient's anterior chest, penetrate the upper body, exit the upper back, and enter the x-ray plate?
    a. PA chest x-ray
    b. AP chest x-ray
    c. lateral chest x-ray
    d. oblique x-ray

26. Which is a preliminary radiograph taken to provide an initial view of an area before contrast medium is administered?
    a. portable film
    b. scout film
    c. plain film
    d. lead film

27. A xeromammogram is printed on _____, rather than x-ray film.
    a. paper
    b. magnetic tape
    c. electronically
    d. microfilm

28. Which type of procedure uses an x-ray beam that is controlled by a computer?
    a. scan
    b. ultrasound
    c. CT scan
    d. x-ray

29. Which type of procedure uses a strong magnetic field inside a scanner to align protons in the atoms of the patient's body?
    a. MRI
    b. ultrasound
    c. CT scan
    d. x-ray

30. Which procedure is referred to as a full body scan and uses a beam of electrons?
    a. MRI
    b. PET
    c. EBT
    d. DSA

31. Which type of procedure uses pulses of inaudible, ultra high-frequency sound waves to create images of the internal structures of the body?
    a. sonography
    b. x-ray
    c. CT scan
    d. MRI

32. Which procedure involves the patient swallowing an endoscopic tube that contains a tiny sound wave-emitting transducer at its tip? The tip is positioned in the esophagus so that it is directly behind the heart.
    a. PET
    b. SPEC
    c. TEE
    d. Doppler

33. All of the following radiologic tests expose the patient to radiation EXCEPT:
    a. x-rays.
    b. ultrasonography.
    c. CT scan.
    d. fluoroscopy.

34. The length of time it takes for half of the atoms in an amount of a radioactive substance to decay and become stable is known as the:
    a. half-life.
    b. echo.
    c. dual energy.
    d. Roentgen.

35. Which is another name for radiopharmaceuticals?
    a. markers
    b. Roentgens
    c. tracers
    d. guiders

36. Which is given intravenously for nuclear medicine imaging of the thyroid gland?
    a. indium-111
    b. iodine-123
    c. gallium-67
    d. krypton-81m

37. Which is a gas that is inhaled for nuclear imaging of the lung?
    a. indium-111
    b. iodine-123
    c. gallium-67
    d. krypton-81m

38. In nuclear medicine, areas of increased uptake are called:
    a. hot spots.
    b. dark spots.
    c. cold spots.
    d. light spots.

39. Which contrast medium is used in MRI scans?
    a. iodine
    b. gold bond
    c. gadolinium
    d. barium

40. A shielding apron worn by radiologic personnel to protect themselves from radiation exposure is known as a:
    a. magnetic apron.
    b. lead apron.
    c. protective apron.
    d. metallic apron.

41. Which procedure uses an x-ray beam and iodinated contrast medium instilled into the subarachnoid space to create an image of the spinal cavity, spine, and spinal nerves?
    a. PET scan
    b. neurography
    c. myelography
    d. OncoScint scan

42. Which is the unit of measurement for radiation exposure?
    a. rem
    b. grams
    c. electrons
    d. positrons

43. A ventilation-perfusion (V/Q) scan uses an inhaled radiopharmaceutical and scintigraphy to create an image of the:
    a. lungs.
    b. heart.
    c. bones.
    d. thyroid gland.

44. The abbreviation KUB means:
    a. kidneys, ureters, bladder.
    b. kidneys and urinary bladder.
    c. kidneys, urethra, bladder.
    d. krypton, uranium, barium.

45. Which of the following is NOT a type of radiologic test using x-rays?
    a. fluoroscopy
    b. computerized axial tomography
    c. sonography
    d. mammography

46. Which of the following radiologic studies uses contrast dye to examine a joint?
    a. arthrography
    b. cholecystography
    c. cholangiography
    d. pyelography

47. Which of the following tests uses a magnetic field to examine the body?
   a. EBT
   b. CAT scan
   c. DEXA scan
   d. MRI

48. Which of the following things are NOT contraindicated in a magnetic resonance imaging study?
   a. hearing aids
   b. cloth hospital gowns
   c. insulin pumps
   d. pierced earrings

49. Which of the following types of ultrasonography produce images in shades of brown?
   a. two-dimensional
   b. three-dimensional
   c. echocardiography
   d. real-time ultrasonography

50. What substance is given intravenously in order to image the thyroid gland?
   a. Gallium-67
   b. Indium-111
   c. Krypton-81m
   d. Iodine-123

51. Which of the following words contains a word part that means point of light?
   a. emission
   b. scintigraphy
   c. cholecystography
   d. fluoroscopy

52. Which statement is NOT true regarding CAT scans?
   a. The computer creates a two-dimensional image or slice of the part of the body being examined.
   b. Bony structures are seen very clearly on CAT scan.
   c. CAT scans may be enhanced with iodinated radiopaque contrast dye injected intravenously.
   d. The x-ray emitter moves in a triangle around the patient.

53. In this test, liquid barium contrast medium is swallowed. It outlines the esophagus and stomach to show ulcers or areas of blockage.
   a. oral cholecystography
   b. upper gastrointestinal series
   c. pyelography
   d. lymphangiography

54. What type of procedure uses a computer to take many two-dimensional images or "slices" of the body?
   a. PET scan
   b. CAT scan

   c. X-ray
   d. mammography

55. What type of scan uses a strong magnetic field inside a scanner?
   a. PET scan
   b. CAT scan
   c. x-ray
   d. MRI

56. A liquid suspension of which solution creates a white and chalky contrast medium that is radiopaque?
   a. iodine
   b. barium
   c. krypton-81m
   d. all of the above

57. Which is NOT a contraindication for having an MRI?
   a. dental work
   b. body piercing
   c. transdermal patches
   d. hearing aid

58. Every radioactive substance is in a constant state of decay (changing from being unstable to being stable). What is the word used for the length of time it takes for half of the atoms in an amount of a radioactive substance to decay and become stable?
   a. half life
   b. term life
   c. stable time
   d. unstable time

59. What is EBT?
   a. electron beam tomography
   b. a sonogram
   c. an x-ray of the cranium
   d. a transducer

60. The terms spiral and helical refer to a/an:
   a. CT scan.
   b. x-ray.
   c. PET scan.
   d. radiopharmaceutical drug.

61. Which procedure uses contrast dye injected into the subarachnoid space at the level of the L3 and L4 vertebrae?
   a. pyelography
   b. lymphangiography
   c. CT scan
   d. myelography

62. In this type of x-ray, an x-ray beam enters the patient's chest from the side, penetrates the upper body, and exits through the other side.
   a. oblique x-ray
   b. AP chest x-ray
   c. lateral chest x-ray
   d. KUB

63. When you hear the word protons, you think of what type of radiologic procedure?
    a. MRI
    b. CT
    c. sonography
    d. roentgenography

64. When you hear the word positrons, you think of what type of radiologic procedure?
    a. MRI
    b. x-ray
    c. PET
    d. scintigraphy

65. All of the following are true about a virtual colonoscopy procedure EXCEPT which statement?
    a. It produces a three-dimensional image.
    b. It is done with electron beam tomography.
    c. It costs less than a standard colonoscopy.
    d. It is a screening test ordered by a physician.

66. When an entire fluoroscopy procedure is captured on videotape, this procedure is known as a:
    a. densitometry.
    b. arteriography.
    c. tomography.
    d. cineradiography.

67. An ultrasound transducer is placed on the _____, and an ultrasound probe is placed in a _____.
    a. organ; bone
    b. skin; duct
    c. head; chamber
    d. skin; cavity

68. The radiopharmaceutical indium-111 combined with monoclonal antibodies is used during scintigraphy to:
    a. detect cancerous cells.
    b. measure organ metabolism.
    c. create an image of bones
    d. estimate the gestational age of the fetus.

69. Which of these abbreviations stands for the most common radiologic procedure performed?
    a. PET
    b. V/Q scan
    c. KUB
    d. CXR

70. On an IVP report, which structure is certain to be mentioned?
    a. brain
    b. heart
    c. stomach
    d. kidneys

71. On an UGI series report, all of these structures would be mentioned EXCEPT
    a. stomach.
    b. heart.
    c. esophagus.
    d. small intestine.

72. The use of radioactive substances to create images of body structures is known as
    a. radiology.
    b. nuclear medicine.
    c. roentgenography.
    d. radiography.

73. The use of a continuous x-ray beam to capture motion of the internal organs is known as:
    a. mammography.
    b. xeromammography.
    c. fluoroscopy.
    d. DEXA.

74. An area of increased uptake of radiopharmaceutical on a scan is known as a/an:
    a. scintigram.
    b. cold spot.
    c. HIDA.
    d. hot spot.

75. The discovery of radium as a radioactive element was done by:
    a. Roentgen.
    b. Becquerel.
    c. Curie.
    d. Joliot.

76. PET scans are helpful in showing areas of abnormal brain activity in:
    a. Alzheimer's.
    b. Parkinson's.
    c. epilepsy.
    d. all of the above.

Short Answer

Write the word or phrase that best completes each statement or answers the question.

77. Nuclear medicine uses _____ substances that emit rays or particles to create images of internal structures of the body.

78. The image produced by ultrasonography is known as a _____.

79. A _____ _____ is worn by the x-ray technician to protect the body from x-rays.

80. A ventilation-perfusion scan is also known as a _____ scan.

81. The abbreviation for chest x-ray is _____.

82. Radiation exposure is measured in _____.

83. A _____ uses continuous x-ray beams to capture the motion of internal organs as it occurs.

84. Gadolinium is a chemical element that responds to a magnetic field and therefore is injected intravenously or instilled into a body cavity to enhance the image obtained by _____.

85. An arthrography involves injecting a contrast dye into a _____ to produce an image.

86. _____ is a radiopaque contrast medium made of small, chalky particles suspended in a liquid and used for radiologic procedures of the digestive tract. It is normally swallowed or instilled in the rectum and colon.

87. The _____ position is a lying down or on the back position used for radiologic imaging.

88. In the phrase transesophageal echocardiography, the word part that means across is _____.

89. A _____ measures the cumulative exposure of a health care worker to radiation.

90. A _____ film is a radiograph taken at the patient's bedside or in the emergency department when the patient cannot be transported to the radiology department.

91. An imaging study that uses injected contrast dye to visualize the gallbladder is called a _____.

92. _____ uses a continuous x-ray beam to capture motion of the internal organs as it occurs.

93. In x-ray technology, areas of low density are said to be _____.

94. On x-ray, areas of high density are said to be _____.

95. In a _____ x-ray, the x-ray beam enters patient's upper back, penetrates the upper body, exits through the anterior chest, and enters the x-ray plate.

96. _____ is the process of measuring the amount of radiation exposure as detected by a film badge.

97. Contrast dye is injected to outline a blood vessel. In _____, it is injected into an artery to show blockage, narrowed areas, or aneurysms.

98. When contrast dye is injected into the bloodstream for an x-ray of the gallbladder it is known as _____.

99. _____ uses an x-ray beam to create an image of the breast.

100. A _____ uses an x-ray beam to measure bone mineral density (BMD) and determine if demineralization (from osteoporosis) has occurred.

101. _____ uses ultra high-frequency sound waves to show real-time, moving images of the heart during contraction and relaxation.

102. _____ medicine is the medical specialty that uses radioactive substances to create images of internal structures of the body.

103. _____ are manmade or naturally occurring radioactive substances that have been processed and measured so that they can be given as a drug dose.

104. A _____ is a positively charged particle that has the same mass as an electron, but the opposite charge.

105. X-rays are a type of invisible ionizing _____.

106. Another name for an x-ray is _____ or a _____.

107. Standardized positions of the angle of the patient in relation to the x-ray machine are known as _____ or views.

108. A subatomic particle accelerator that generates positrons for PET scans is known as a _____.

109. The medical specialty that uses various forms of radiation and sound waves to create images of the human body is known as _____.

110. The process of recording an image of a vein is known as _____.

111. The combining form son/o- means _____.

True/False

Write 'T' if the statement is true and 'F' if the statement is false.

____112. A roentgenogram is also known as a radiograph.

____113. An echocardiography uses high-frequency sound waves to show the heart during contraction and relaxation.

____114. During roentgenography, bone has a high density and therefore is radiolucent on x-ray images.

____115. Radiopharmaceuticals are manmade or naturally occurring radioactive substances called radionuclides that have been made into a drug.

____116. Indium-111 is given intravenously for nuclear medicine imaging of the heart.

____117. An example of interventional radiology is using ultrasonography to guide the insertion of the needle for an amniocentesis.

____118. An MRI scan exposes the patient to radiation and x-rays.

____119. An upper gastrointestinal series is also known as a barium enema.

_____120. Both CT scans and MRI scans are types of tomography that show many individual "slice" images.

_____121. During a PA chest x-ray, the x-ray beam enters a patient's anterior chest, penetrates the upper body, exits through the upper back, and then enters the x-ray plate.

_____122. Angiography is a general word for injecting contrast dye into a blood vessel and taking x-ray images.

_____123. In oral cholecystography, contrast dye is not injected but rather is taken orally in the form of a tablet.

_____124. In a mammogram, an x-ray is used to create an image of the uterus.

_____125. Although the heel or wrist bones can be tested for bone density, the hip and spine bones give the most accurate results.

_____126. Magnetic resonance imaging does not expose either the patient or the health care worker to radiation.

_____127. In nuclear medicine, radioactive substances are often injected directly into the patient's vein or given by inhalation.

_____128. A positron emission tomography (PET) scan uses magnetic fields to create diagnostic images.

_____129. A barium enema uses an x-ray beam and radiopaque barium contrast medium instilled into the rectum to create an image of the colon.

_____130. The electron beam tomography uses an electron beam and a spiral CT scan to create an image.

_____131. Electron beam tomography used in the virtual physical and virtual colonscopy does not expose the patient to any radiation.

_____132. Ultrasonography does not expose a patient to radiation, but Doppler ultrasonography does.

_____133. Magnetic resonance imaging uses a strong x-ray field inside a scanner to align the electrons in the atoms of the patient's body and create an image.

Essay

Write your answer in the space provided or on a separate sheet of paper.

134. Why are PET scans only available in large hospitals?

135. The radiologist views an x-ray film by placing it in front of a light box. How does the radiologist communicate the findings seen on x-ray to the patient's attending physician?

136. What is the difference between the suffixes -graphy and -gram?

137. Describe color flow duplex ultrasonography.

138. Briefly define and discuss echocardiography.

139. Explain what x-rays are.

140. Briefly discuss the concepts of radiolucency and radiopacity.

141. Briefly explain the purpose of a film badge.

Test Bank
Answer Key

CHAPTER 1

Multiple Choice

1. c. CPR stands for computerized patient record. All of the other abbreviations could be found as headings in the history and physical examination. Page Ref: 22, 24

2. c. An- means without and -esthesia means feeling or sensation. Page Ref: 15

3. d. Brady- means slow and -cardia means pertaining to the heart. Page Ref: 16

4. a. The suffix for the process of the exam is -scopy. Page Ref: 10

5. d. The combining form, with its root and attached vowel, has a hyphen to signify that a suffix should be combined with it to make a complete medical word. Page Ref: 7

6. b. Post- means after or behind. For example, postnatal means pertaining to after birth. Page Ref: 16

7. c. Pneumon/o- means lung and -itis means inflammation. Page Ref: 8, 9

8. b. Vertebrae is the plural form of vertebra. Page Ref: 21

9. b. For Latin singular nouns ending in -ex or -ix, change the ending to -ices to make the plural form. Page Ref: 21

10. d. Intra- means within and -hepatic means pertaining to the liver. Page Ref: 15

11. c. Laryng/o- means larynx or voicebox and -ectomy means surgical excision. Page Ref: 8, 10

12. a. Answers c and d are true of suffixes. Not every medical word has a prefix. Page Ref: 15

13. c. Peri- means around, tonsill/o- means tonsil, and -ar means pertaining to. Page Ref: 15

14. d. Dys- means difficult or painful and uria means condition of the urine. Page Ref: 16

15. a. The singular of bronchi is bronchus. Page Ref: 21

16. b. A suffix can be a single letter, a suffix is never used alone, and a suffix ends a word but never begins it. Page Ref: 9

17. a. Gastr/o- means stomach and -scopy means the process of using an instrument to examine. Page Ref: 8, 10

18. d. Tachy- means fast and -cardia means condition of the heart. Page Ref: 8, 16

19. d. The Health Insurance Portability and Accountability Act (HIPAA) is federal legislation passed in 1996 to safeguard medical information and to ensure that such information is released only to parties authorized to receive it. Page Ref: 23

20. c. The prefix sub- means underneath or below, such as in subcutaneous, which means underneath or below the skin. Page Ref: 15

21. c. Other words with similar abbreviations include treatment (Tx) and prescription (Rx). Page Ref: 24

22. d. The suffix -ectomy indicates a surgical removal or excision, such as tonsillectomy (removal of the tonsils). Page Ref: 10

23. a. Thinking and analyzing is done as you think about what you have seen or heard and then memorize, categorize, analyze, and understand the information. Page Ref: 6

24. c. Speaking is a method of relaying medical language; another method is writing. Page Ref: 6

25. a. Many words have been taken or derived from other languages. Many medical words come from the ancient Latin or Greek languages. Page Ref: 20

26. a. Not every medical word includes a prefix, but when present a prefix is always found at the beginning of the word. Page Ref: 15

27. d. The combining form gives the word its medical meaning. Page Ref: 7

28. c. Arthritis is inflammation of the joint. Page Ref: 8

29. d. Mastectomy means surgical excision of the breast. Page Ref: 8

30. b. Hepatitis is inflammation of the liver. Page Ref: 8

31. c. There are many other suffixes that mean pertaining to, such as -ac, -ar, and -ary. Page Ref: 9

32. a. The suffix -oma means tumor or mass. The medical word carcinoma means cancerous tumor. Page Ref: 9

33. d. To form the plural of a Latin feminine noun that ends in -a, change the -a to -ae. Page Ref: 21

34. a. To form the plural of a Latin noun that ends in -is, change -is to -es. Page Ref: 21

35. a. Many healthcare facilities are converting to a computerized patient record. Page Ref: 22

36. c. Battery is the act of touching another person without their consent. Page Ref: 23

37. c. HIPAA is a federal regulation requiring all healthcare settings to provide patients with a statement verifying that their health information is kept secure and that it is only released to authorized inquiries from other healthcare providers, insurance companies for payment purposes, or to healthcare quality monitoring organizations. Page Ref: 23

38. a. S (subjective) is for the patient's symptoms. O (objective) is for results of the physical exam. A (assessment) is for the diagnosis. P (plan) is for the plan for follow-up care. Page Ref: 23

39. c. A chief complaint is documented as the reason for the patient encounter. Page Ref: 24

40. b. The O (objective) section is for results of the physical exam. Page Ref: 23

41. d. The P (plan) section is for the plan for follow-up care. Page Ref: 23

42. c. To form the plural of a Greek noun that ends in -nx, change -nx to -nges. Page Ref: 21

43. a. The combining form for artery is arteri/o- and for blood vessel is angi/o-. Page Ref: 8

44. b. Keep the combining vowel on the first combining form to join two combining forms, but drop the combining vowel when a suffix begins with a vowel. Page Ref: 19

45. a. Electrocardiography is the process of recording the electrical activity of the heart. Page Ref: 10

46. d. The suffix -pathy means disease or suffering depending how it is used. Examples include retinopathy and sympathy. Page Ref: 9

47. d. Every medical word contains a combining form and a suffix, but not necessarily a prefix. Page Ref: 7

48. b. Pneum/o means lung or air. Page Ref: 8

49. d. Several suffixes (-ac, -ar, and -al) mean pertaining to. Page Ref: 9

50. a. Hepat/o- means liver and -megaly means enlargement of. Page Ref: 9

51. b. Endo- means innermost, within and tracheal means pertaining to the trachea. Page Ref: 15

52. d. Bradycardia means a slow heart rate. Page Ref: 16

53. c. Dysfunctional means pertaining to abnormal function. Page Ref: 16

54. d. These prefixes have opposite meanings. Page Ref: 15

55. a. A prefix goes before a combining form. Page Ref: 16

56. a. The primary emphasis is on the third syllable and the secondary emphasis is on the first syllable. Page Ref: 19

57. d. Medical words are derived from many languages, including Latin, Greek, English, Dutch, and French. Page Ref: 20

58. b. Combining forms may occur in the middle or beginning of a medical term, but never at the end. Page Ref: 7

59. d. The combining form always gives a medical word its meaning. The prefix and suffix modify the combining form. Page Ref: 7

60. a. A combining form always has a slash, combining vowel, and hyphen. Page Ref: 8

61. b. The combining form pneumon/o- means lung or air. Page Ref: 8

62. d. Healthcare professionals must read, hear, analyze, speak (pronounce), and write (spell) medical words correctly. Page Ref: 6

63. c. The combining form is made up of a root, slash, combining vowel, and hyphen. Page Ref: 7

64. c. Ven/o- is a combining form that means vein. Page Ref: 8

65. a. The suffix -ia means condition, state, or thing. Page Ref: 9

66. a. These suffixes indicate medical specialties or specialists, as in psychiatry, dietitian, or cardiology. Page Ref: 10

67. d. A medical word can include all of these word parts, although a medical word does not always have to have a prefix. Page Ref: 15

68. c. These prefixes indicate amount or size, such as below or deficient or many and much. Page Ref: 15

69. a. These prefixes describe a characteristic such as being against or being painful, difficult, or abnormal. Page Ref: 15

70. c. Alcoholism is a disease from the specific cause of consumption of alcoholic beverages. Page Ref: 9

71. b. The suffix -graphy means process of recording. Page Ref: 10

72. c. After dividing the word into medical parts and defining those word parts, begin with the definition of the suffix. Page Ref: 12

73. d. Medical words come mainly from Latin and Greek but also from other languages. Page Ref: 20

74. c. Latin feminine nouns end in -a and follow the rule of changing -a to -ae. Page Ref: 21

75. d. Latin masculine singular nouns end in -us. Page Ref: 21

76. a. Form the plural of Latin neuter nouns by changing -um to -a. Page Ref: 21

77. a. Some Greek singular nouns end in -ion. Page Ref: 21

78. a. Latin neuter nouns always form the plural by changing -um to -a. Page Ref: 21

79. d. All of these things are drawbacks of the paper medical record. Page Ref: 21

80. b. HIPAA is the Health Insurance Portability and Accountability Act, a federal regulation that was passed in 1996. Page Ref: 23

81. d. The Subjective (S) section contains the patient's account of the medical problem in his or her own (subjective) words. Page Ref: 25

Short Answer

82. study. The suffix -ology means the study of. Page Ref: 10

83. pertaining to. For example, nasal means pertaining to the nose. Page Ref: 9

84. much. The prefix poly- means many or much. Page Ref: 15

85. within. For example, intravenous means pertaining to within the vein. Page Ref: 15

86. enlargement. The suffix -megaly means enlargement. Page Ref: 9

87. disease. The suffix -pathy means disease or suffering. Page Ref: 9

88. tumor or mass. The suffix -oma means tumor. Page Ref: 9

89. brady-. Bradycardia means slow heart rate. Page Ref: 16

90. diagnoses. Make a Latin singular noun ending in -is plural by changing the ending to -es. Page Ref: 21

91. Etymology. Etym/o- means word origin, and -logy means the study of. Page Ref: 20

92. combining form. The prefix and suffix always modify the combining form. Page Ref: 7

93. Pneumon/o-. Pneumonia means a condition of the lungs. Page Ref: 9

94. Cardi/o-. Cardiac means pertaining to the heart. Page Ref: 8

95. Retin/o-. Retinal means pertaining to the retina. Page Ref: 8

96. suffix. The suffix can only appear at the end of a word, but there can be more than one suffix in a medical word. Page Ref: 9

97. -graphy. Electrocardiography is the process of recording the electrical activity of the heart. Page Ref: 10

98. prefix. Not every medical word has to contain a prefix. Page Ref: 15

99. slow. Bradycardia means slow heart rate. Page Ref: 16

100. prefix. A prefix attaches to the beginning of a combining form, and a suffix attaches to the end of a combining form. Page Ref: 15

101. Etymology. Etym/o- means word origin and -logy means the study of. Page Ref: 20

102. medical record. The medical record is a permanent, legal document. Page Ref: 22

103. informed consent. The patient is informed of the alternatives, risks, and possible complications before consenting (agreeing) to the surgery. Page Ref: 23

104. (S) Subjective; (O) Objective; (A) Assessment; (P) Plan. Subjective (S) is for the patient's symptoms, objective (O) is for the results of the physical examination by the physician, assessment (A) is for the diagnosis, and plan (P) is for the plan for follow-up care. Page Ref: 23

105. chief complaint. The chief complaint is the reason the patient is seeking treatment. Page Ref: 25

106. Health Insurance Portability and Accountability Act. This is the federal regulation passed in 1996 that protects a patient's right to privacy by ensuring that medical records are released only to authorized inquiries. Page Ref: 25

107. cardiology. Cardi/o- means heart, and -logy means study of. Page Ref: 8, 10

108. combining form. The root and combining vowel, along with a slash and a hyphen, make up a combining form. Page Ref: 7

109. suffix. The suffix is positioned at the end of a medical word, and the prefix is positioned at the beginning. Page Ref: 9

110. diagnosis. Diagnosis and treatment are often thought of together; their abbreviations are Dx and Tx. Page Ref: 25

111. physical examination. The physical exam heading in a medical report can be abbreviated PE. Page Ref: 24

112. post-. For example, postnatal means pertaining to after childbirth. Page Ref: 17

113. gastr/o-. For example, gastrointestinal means pertaining to the stomach and intestines. Page Ref: 8

114. psych/o-. For example, psychology means the study of the mind. Page Ref: 8

True/False

115. True. Most medical words are combinations of Latin and Greek words, and may include other languages such as Dutch, French, and parts of English words. Knowing the origin of a word may help to remember it. Page Ref: 20

116. True. It is important to understand that medical word parts are just like any language, they

mean the same regardless of their context. Page Ref: 7

117. False. It is the combining form which gives the word its meaning. Page Ref: 7

118. True. Just like in regular English, prefixes and suffixes in medical terms modify the meaning of the word. Page Ref: 9, 15

119. False. Medical words may contain one or more combining forms in order to create a word. In complex medical terms there may be two or even three combining forms. Page Ref: 7

120. True. Not all medical words contain a prefix, but all medical words contain a suffix. Page Ref: 9

121. False. Not every medical word contains a prefix; it is an optional word part. Page Ref: 7

122. True. A- is a one-letter prefix meaning without. Page Ref: 15

123. True. By putting the word parts in this order, you can easily discover the meaning of the medical word. Page Ref: 17

124. True. Not only does the patient's health or medical record contain medical information, it is also considered a legal document. Page Ref: 22

125. False. They are the upper chambers of the heart. Page Ref: 21

126. True. Many suffixes mean pertaining to. They are all used to create adjective forms. Page Ref: 9

127. True. The assessment is another name for the diagnosis. Page Ref: 23

128. False. Some medical words originated in English, Dutch, French, and other languages. Page Ref: 20

129. False. It means an abnormal condition of a joint. Arthr/o- means joint and -osis means abnormal condition. Page Ref: 8, 9

130. False. The suffix -graphy means the process of recording. Page Ref: 10

131. True. Neur/o- means nerve and -oma means tumor. Page Ref: 9

132. False. Hypothyroidism is an underactive thyroid. The prefix hypo- means below or deficient. Page Ref: 15

133. False. Informed consent is the document that is signed to permit a surgical operation. Page Ref: 23

134. False. There is no substitute for a thorough, working knowledge of medical language obtained through formal study. Page Ref: 5

135. True. Success in the healthcare field comes from knowing medical language. Page Ref: 5

136. False. Healthcare professionals use medical language to communicate both with patients and with other healthcare professionals such as doctors, technicians, and nurses. Page Ref: 6

137. False. The combining form is the foundation of the medical word and gives meaning to the medical word. The combining vowel helps the

combining form connect to another combining form or a suffix. Page Ref: 7

138. True. Medical record is the older name for the health record. Page Ref: 22

139. False. A medical word must have a combining form and a suffix, but a prefix is an optional word part. Page Ref: 15

Essay

140. First, define each word part. Then put the definitions of the word parts in order beginning with the suffix, followed by the prefix, and then the combining form. Lastly, add small connecting words to make a correct and complete definition. Page Ref: 17

141. The great ancient Greek and Roman civilizations advanced the study and the practice of medicine. Their knowledge of anatomy, diseases, and treatments served as a foundation for modern medical knowledge and medical language is representative of this. Page Ref: 20

142. Reading, listening, thinking/analyzing, speaking, and writing. Page Ref: 6

143. Many medical words are derived from ancient Latin and Greek words. Sometimes the words are very similar to the original Latin and Greek words. Some medical words are also derived from other languages such as English, Dutch, and French. Page Ref: 20

144. These are some (but not all) of the characteristics of combining forms:
    - Every medical word contains a combining form.
    - Sometimes a medical word contains two or more combining forms, one right after the other.
    - A combining form is the foundation of a medical word and gives the word its medical meaning.
    - Prefixes and suffixes modify the meaning of the combining form. Page Ref: 7

145. These are some (but not all) of the characteristics of prefixes:
    - Not every medical word contains a prefix. It is an optional word part.
    - A prefix cannot be the foundation of a medical word.
    - A prefix always modifies the meaning of the combining form.
    - When present, a prefix always comes at the beginning of a medical word.
    - A prefix can only attach to the beginning of a combining form.
    - A prefix always ends with a hyphen to show that it is a word part, not a complete word. Page Ref: 15

146. These are some (but not all) of the characteristics of suffixes:

- Every medical word contains a suffix.
- Some medical words contain two suffixes, one right after the other.
- A suffix cannot be the foundation of a medical word.
- A suffix always modifies the meaning of the combining form.
- A suffix is always positioned at the end of a medical word.
- A suffix always begins with a hyphen to show that it is a word part, not a complete word. Page Ref: 9

CHAPTER 2

Multiple Choice

1. b. The transverse plane may also be described as having superior (top) and inferior (bottom) sections. Page Ref: 39

2. d. Onc/o- means tumor or mass and -logy means the study of. Page Ref: 51

3. c. Integument refers to a covering or the skin. Page Ref: 47

4. a. Pro- means before, gnos/o- means knowledge, and -osis means condition Page Ref: 65

5. d. Ventr/o- means front or abdomen. Page Ref: 36

6. b. Later/o- means side. Page Ref: 38

7. d. The diaphragm is a muscle that is superior to the abdominal cavity and inferior to the thoracic cavity. Page Ref: 42

8. b. Hypo- means below, gastr/o- means stomach, and -ic means pertaining to. Page Ref: 43

9. c. This may help you remember: "Lying on the spine is supine." Page Ref: 36

10. b. Etiology refers to the cause of a disease. Idiopathic means the cause of a disease is unknown. Page Ref: 62

11. c. Congenital means being born with a condition but this example is not inherited or related to genetic processes. Page Ref: 62

12. d. A stethoscope is an instrument used to listen to body sounds. Auscultation is listening to body sounds to determine abnormalities. Page Ref: 64

13. c. The physician assistant can perform some of the duties of a physician, such as ordering treatment, and prescribing medications. Page Ref: 66

14. a. A symptom is a deviation from health that can only be perceived by the patient. Choices B, C, and D are signs—conditions that can be detected by observation and examination. Page Ref: 63

15. c. Caud/o- means tailbone or lower part of the body. Page Ref: 40

16. d. Proximal is near the point of attachment and distal is the furthest part from the attachment. Page Ref: 41

17. d. Ot/o- means ear, rhin/o- means nose, laryng/o- means throat, and -logy means the study of. Page Ref: 55

18. b. Hospice cares for patients who are suffering from terminal diseases. Palliative care aims to help the patient to be comfortable but is not intended to cure the disease. Page Ref: 68

19. c. Viscera are soft internal organs. Page Ref: 43

20. a. The combining form inguin/o- means groin. Page Ref: 43

21. b. Remiss/o- means send back and -ion means action or condition. Page Ref: 65

22. a. D.P.M. stands for Doctor of Podiatric Medicine, also known as a podiatrist. Page Ref: 66

23. c. Many other suffixes, such as -ac, -ar, and -eal, also mean pertaining to. Page Ref: 60

24. a. A cavity is a hollow space surrounded by bone and containing organs. The thoracic cavity is the chest cavity. Page Ref: 42

25. a. A chronic condition is one that lasts three months or more. Choices B, C, and D do not describe this woman's disease course at this time. Page Ref: 65

26. b. The three body planes are coronal, midsagittal, and transverse. Page Ref: 35

27. c. The midsagittal plane is an imaginary vertical plane that divides the entire body into right and left sections. Page Ref: 38

28. a. The coronal plane is an imaginary vertical plane that divides the entire body into front and back sections, following the coronal suture. Page Ref: 35

29. d. The transverse plane is an imaginary plane that divides the entire body into top and bottom sections. Page Ref: 39

30. a. Cephalad and caudad are directional opposites. Moving in a cephalad direction is moving toward the head. Moving in a caudad direction is moving toward the tailbone or lower parts of the body. Page Ref: 40

31. c. Distal and proximal are directional opposites. Moving in a distal direction is moving from where the limb is attached to the body toward the fingers or toes (end of the limb). Moving in a proximal direction is moving from the fingers or toes toward where the limb is attached to the body. Page Ref: 41

32. a. The spinal cavity, a continuation of the cranial cavity, lies within and is protected by the bones (vertebrae) of the spinal column. Page Ref: 42

33. c. The mediastinum contains the trachea, esophagus, heart, and other central structures of the thoracic cavity. Page Ref: 42

34. a. There are four abdominopelvic quadrants and nine abdominopelvic regions. Page Ref: 43

35. b. The function of the respiratory system is inhalation and exhalation of air. Page Ref: 46

36. a. The cardiovascular system contains the heart, arteries, veins, and capillaries that circulate the blood. Page Ref: 46

37. c. Neonatology involves the study of newborn infants, whereas pediatrics refers to medical care for infants and children. Page Ref: 51

38. c. The hypogastric region is centered on and inferior to the umbilical region. Page Ref: 44

39. c. A woman with problems of the female genital system would see a gynecologist. A woman with urinary problems would see a urologist. Page Ref: 49

40. b. Examples of iatrogenic conditions are when the wrong drug is given to a patient or when surgery is performed on the wrong leg. Page Ref: 62

41. c. A nosocomial infection is caused by exposure to infection while the patient is in the hospital. Page Ref: 63

42. a. Patients who are asymptomatic can still have a disease, but it can only be detected by medical tests. Page Ref: 63

43. c. A stethoscope is used to listen to the sounds of the heart. Page Ref: 64

44. b. If a patient was burned two years ago and this burn has healed but has left a contracture, this contracture is an example of a sequela. Page Ref: 65

45. a. A cardiac catheterization is an example of a diagnostic procedure. A therapeutic procedure causes improvement in the symptoms or signs. Page Ref: 65

46. b. The attending physician is responsible for the care of the patient while in the hospital. Page Ref: 66

47. c. The prefix re- means again, backward or unable to. The combining form fract/o- means break up. The suffix -ory means having the function of. Page Ref: 65

48. a. The abbreviations for diagnosis (Dx), treatment (Tx), and symptoms (Sx) are all similar in form. Page Ref: 74

49. b. Primary care physicians specialize in family practice or pediatrics. Page Ref: 74

50. a. The Latin word hospice is related to the words hospitable, hospitality, and hospital. Page Ref: 68

51. a. When studying the body, disease is not an approach. The study of the body is approached from a point of wellness. Page Ref: 35

52. d. Inside-to-outside is not one of the body planes. The midsagittal plane divides the body into right and left sections, the transverse plane divides the body into top and bottom sections, and the coronal plane divides the body into front and back sections. Page Ref: 35

53. b. Coronal plane. It is named for the coronal suture where the anterior and posterior skull bones meet. Page Ref: 35

54. a. Gastroenterology. While several specialties study the pharynx, only gastroenterology studies the esophagus as well. Page Ref: 46

55. c. Degenerative. Examples of degenerative disease are multiple sclerosis and hearing loss. Page Ref: 62

56. c. Exacerbation is the sudden worsening of the severity of a patient's signs or symptoms. Page Ref: 65

57. a. Refractory. Certain diseases that cannot be treated with drugs or therapy may require surgery. Page Ref: 65

58. c. The most frequently used healthcare setting is a doctor's or physician's office. Seriously ill patients who cannot be quickly diagnosed or adequately treated in the office are sent to a hospital. Page Ref: 67

59. a. Perform an H & P. This is a history and physical, and is the hallmark of diagnosis. Page Ref: 63

60. b. Allied health professionals. These include technologists, technicians, and therapists. Page Ref: 67

61. b. Pulmonology (PUL-moh-NAWL-oh-jee). Pulmon/o- means lung and -logy means the study of. Page Ref: 46

62. a. Lumbar means pertaining to the lower back. Page Ref: 54

63. d. Thorax means chest. Page Ref: 42

64. a. Pharmacology (FAR-mah-KAWL-oh-jee), pharmac/o- means medicines, drugs and -logy means the study of. Page Ref: 51

65. d. Radiology (RAY-dee-AWL-oh-jee), radi/o- means x-rays; radiation and -logy means the study of. Page Ref: 51

66. c. Otolaryngology (OH-toh-LAIR-ing-GAWL-oh-jee), ot/o- means ear, laryng/o- means larynx (voicebox), and -logy means the study of. Page Ref: 50

67. b. Endocrinology (EN-doh-krih-NAWL-oh-jee), endo- means internal, within; crin/o- means secrete, and -logy means the study of. Page Ref: 53

68. b. Dermatology (DER-mah-TAWL-oh-jee), dermat/o- means skin, and -logy means the study of. Integumentary (in-TEG-yoo-MEN-tair-ee), integument/o- means skin, and -ary means pertaining to. Page Ref: 47

69. a. Gastrointestinal (GAS-troh-in-TES-tih-nal), gastr/o- means stomach, intestin/o- means in-

testines, and -al means pertaining to. Page Ref: 46

70. c. Oncology (ong-KAWL-oh-jee), onc/o- means tumor, mass, and -logy means the study of. Page Ref: 51

71. c. The coronal plane is named for the coronal suture in the cranium. Page Ref: 35

72. d. It might help to remember that the dorsal fin is on the back of a shark. Page Ref: 36

73. b. The coronal plane and the midsagittal plane derive their names from the coronal and sagittal sutures in the cranium. Page Ref: 36

74. d. The coronal plane is also known as the frontal plane. Page Ref: 36

75. b. The correct spelling is posteroanterior. Page Ref: 37

76. c. Later/o- means side. Page Ref: 38

77. c. The midsagittal plane follows the sagittal suture that divides the posterior of the cranium into right and left sides. Page Ref: 38

78. d. The proximal end of the humerus is at the shoulder and the distal end of the humerus is at the wrist. Page Ref: 41

79. a. Distal is moving from the body toward a limb. Page Ref: 41

80. b. The thoracic cavity holds all of these organs. Page Ref: 42

81. b. The abdominal cavity is inferior to or below the thoracic cavity. Page Ref: 42

82. d. The cranial cavity is continuous with the spinal cavity. Page Ref: 42

83. c. Microscopic structures cannot be seen with the unaided eye. Page Ref: 45

84. d. Viscera is a Latin word that means soft internal organs. Page Ref: 43

85. b. A cell is a microscopic structure that cannot be seen with the unaided eye. Page Ref: 45

86. d. Cardi/o- means heart. Page Ref: 46

87. b. Pulmonology is the study of the lungs. Page Ref: 46

88. c. The endocrine system contains glands that produce hormones. Page Ref: 50

89. b. Ophthalm/o- means eye. Page Ref: 50

90. d. Ger/o- means old age. Page Ref: 51

91. c. Onc/o- means tumor or mass. Page Ref: 51

92. a. Onc/o- means tumor or mass. Page Ref: 51

93. c. Disease is a change in the body's structure or function, whether slight or life threatening. Page Ref: 62

94. a. Eti/o- means cause of disease. Page Ref: 62

95. c. Congenit/o- means present at birth. Page Ref: 62

96. d. Health is wellness of all aspects of a person: physical, mental, social. Page Ref: 62

97. a. Asymptomatic means pertaining to without symptoms. Page Ref: 63

98. c. Acute is sudden and severe, while chronic may be less intense but continues over time. Page Ref: 64

99. a. Remission is a temporary improvement in symptoms and signs. Page Ref: 65

100. b. A terminal illness is one that eventually and always results in death. Page Ref: 65

101. a. Chiropractors are doctors who specialize in the alignment of the bones, muscles, and nerves. Page Ref: 66

102. c. The physician is the leader of the healthcare team. All others listed assist the physician in treating the patient. Page Ref: 66

103. a. An audiologist cannot prescribe medications like a physician extender can. Page Ref: 66

104. c. A technician is a skilled professional with technical skills. Page Ref: 67

105. b. Only physicians and physician extenders can prescribe medications. Page Ref: 67

106. a. Acutely ill patients need the facilities of a hospital in order to recover. Page Ref: 67

107. d. The hospice provides all of these services to dying patients and their families. Page Ref: 68

108. d. Ambulatory patients are able to leave the treatment facility on their own shortly after being treated. Page Ref: 68

109. d. Outpatients are not admitted to the facility where they receive care. Page Ref: 68

Short Answer

110. quadrants. The word quadrant means four parts. Page Ref: 43

111. cranial. The cranium is made of several bones in the head that surround and protect the brain. Page Ref: 42

112. microscopic. The special instrument is a microscope. Page Ref: 45

113. below. The prefix hypo- means below or deficient. Page Ref: 43

114. nosocomial. Nosocomial is derived from a Greek word that means hospital. Page Ref: 63

115. medical treatment. Psychiatry means study and treatment of the mind. Page Ref: 51

116. intestine. Both intestin/o- and enter/o- mean intestine. Page Ref: 46

117. hematology. Hemat/o- means blood and -logy means the study of. Blood is the carrier of oxygen and nutrients to the tissues and cells. Page Ref: 47

118. posterior. Posterior means pertaining to the back. Page Ref: 36

119. transverse. The transverse plane is also known as the horizontal plane. Page Ref: 39

120. proximal. Distal means moving away from the center or point of origin. Proximal means moving toward the center or point of origin. Page Ref: 41

121. cranial. The cranial cavity contains the brain and cranial nerves. Page Ref: 42

122. pulmonary. Pulmonary means pertaining to the lungs. Page Ref: 46

123. orthopedics. Orth/o- means straight. Page Ref: 47

124. Cephalad. Cephal/o- means head. Page Ref: 40

125. hematology. Hemat/o- means blood. Page Ref: 47

126. oncology. Onc/o- means tumor or mass. Page Ref: 51

127. Physiology. Physi/o- means physical function. Page Ref: 44

128. anterior; ventral. Anterior (an-TEER-ee-or), anter/o- means before, front part and -ior means pertaining to. Ventral (VEN-tral), ventr/o- means front, abdomen and -al means pertaining to. Page Ref: 36

129. posterior; dorsal. Posterior (pohs-TEER-ee-or), poster/o- means back part, and -ior means pertaining to. Dorsal (DOR-sal), dors/o- means back, dorsum and -al means pertaining to. Page Ref: 36

130. midsagittal. The midsagittal plane follows the sagittal suture that divides the posterior cranium into right and left sections. Page Ref: 38

131. transverse (or horizontal). Transverse (trans-VERS), trans- means across, through and -verse means to turn; to travel. Every medical word must contain a combining form. The medical word transverse looks like it only contains a prefix and a suffix, but the suffix actually contains the combining form (vers/o-) plus a one-letter suffix (-e). Horizontal (HOR-ih-ZAWN-tal), horizont/o- means boundary between the earth and sky and -al means pertaining to. Page Ref: 39

132. superior; inferior. Superior (soo-PEER-ee-or), super/o- means above and -ior means pertaining to. Inferior (in-FEER-ee-or), infer/o- means below and -ior means pertaining to. Page Ref: 39

133. cephalad. Cephalad (SEF-ah-lad), cephal/o- means head and -ad means toward, in the direction of. Page Ref: 40

134. caudad. Caudad (KAW-dad), caud/o- means tailbone, lower part of the body and -ad means toward, in the direction of. Page Ref: 40

135. distal; distally. Distal (DIS-tal), distally (DIS-tal-lee), dist/o- means away from the center or point of origin, -al means pertaining to, and -ly means going toward. Page Ref: 41

136. proximal; proximally. Proximal (PRAWK-sih-mal), proximally (PRAWK-sih-mah-lee), proxim/o- means near the center or point of origin, -al means pertaining to, and -ly means going toward. Page Ref: 41

137. superficial; external. Superficial (soo-per-FISH-al), superfici/o- means on or near the surface and -al means pertaining to. External (eks-TER-nal), extern/o- means outside and -al means pertaining to. Page Ref: 41

138. internal. Internal (in-TER-nal), intern/o- means inside and -al means pertaining to. Page Ref: 41

139. cavity. Cavity (KAV-ih-tee), cav/o- means hollow space and -ity means state or condition. Page Ref: 42

140. hypochondriac. Hypochondriac (HY-poh-KAWN-dree-ak), hypo- means below or deficient, chondr/o- means cartilage, and -iac means pertaining to. Hypochondrium is a Greek word for the area below the cartilage of the ribs on either side of the abdomen. Page Ref: 43

141. macroscopic. Macroscopic (MAK-roh-SKAWP-ik), macro- means large, scop/o- means to examine with an instrument, and -ic means pertaining to. There is no such instrument as a macroscope; a macroscopic examination uses the eye itself as the examining "instrument." Page Ref: 45

142. Anatomy; Physiology. Anatomy (ah-NAT-oh-mee), ana- means apart from, through, or up, and -tomy means process of cutting or making an incision. Every medical word must contain a combining form. The suffix of anatomy contains the combining form tom/o-. Physiology (FIZ-ee-AWL-oh-jee), physi/o- means physical function and -logy means the study of. Page Ref: 44

True/False

143. True. These terms are often used when positioning a patient to take chest x-rays. Page Ref: 37

144. False. SNF is a skilled nursing facility, also known as a nursing home. Page Ref: 68

145. True. The combining form ger/o- means old age. Page Ref: 51

146. True. An iatrogenic condition is one caused by medical treatment. Page Ref: 62

147. False. This describes the attending physician. Page Ref: 66

148. False. These patients are called outpatients. Page Ref: 68

149. True. Medial is moving toward the midline and lateral is moving away from the midline. Page Ref: 38

150. True. The lymphatic system is a source of the immune response. Page Ref: 47

151. False. The mediastinum is located in the thoracic or chest cavity. Page Ref: 42

152. True. Refractory refers to something that is unable to be broken up. Page Ref: 65

153. True. Diseases are detected in asymptomatic patients only through medical testing. Page Ref: 63

154. True. A neoplasm is a new growth or formation. It may be either benign or malignant. Page Ref: 63

155. False. Palliative care is supportive medical and nursing care given to keep the patient comfortable, but that does not cure the disease. Page Ref: 68

156. False. Organs are considered macroscopic, because they can be seen with the unaided eye. Page Ref: 45

157. True. There are a number of body systems that can be studied in this way. Page Ref: 45

158. True. In the medical specialty approach, the human body can be studied according to the medical specialties that make up the practice of medicine. Page Ref: 46

159. True. Both of these specialties study the female genital and reproductive system, although obstetrics concentrates more on pregnancy and childbirth. Page Ref: 49

160. False. The epigastric region is one of the nine regions of the abdominopelvic area, located *above* the stomach. Page Ref: 43-44

161. False. The body system that includes the skin, hair, nails, sweat glands, and oil glands is the integumentary system. Page Ref: 47

162. False. Neurology is the medical specialty; the nervous system is the body system. In medical terminology it is important to examine the suffixes and combining forms before deciding on the meaning of a word. Page Ref: 48

163. False. The diaphragm separates the thoracic and abdominal cavities. Page Ref: 42

164. True. Viscera is a Latin word that means soft internal organs. Page Ref: 43

165. True. Internal means deep inside the body and superficial means on or near the surface. Page Ref: 41

166. False. A cavity is a hollow space surrounded by bones or muscles. Page Ref: 43

167. True. The immune system contains cells from the blood and the lymphatic system. Page Ref: 47

168. False. The abbreviation for dentist is D.D.S., for Doctor of Dental Surgery. D.P.M. is the abbreviation for Doctor of Podiatric Medicine. Page Ref: 74

Essay

169. Inspection (viewing), auscultation (listening), palpation (feeling), and percussion (tapping). Page Ref: 64

170. Any two of the following are correct.
    Body planes and body directions approach
    Body cavities approach
    Quadrants and regions approach
    Anatomy and physiology approach
    Microscopic-to-macroscopic approach
    Body systems approach
    Medical specialties approach Page Ref: 35

171. The pancreas is posterior to the stomach. The opposite of anterior is posterior. Page Ref: 36

172. Both conditions are caused by pathogens such as bacteria, viruses, and fungi. However, the word communicable describes an infectious disease that is passed on by direct contact with people, animals, or insects. Page Ref: 63

173. Health is a state of optimum wellness. It includes not only the health of the body but also includes wellness of all aspects of life: physical, mental, emotional, spiritual, and social. Page Ref: 35

174. The anatomical position is the standard position of the body for the purpose of studying it. The body is erect, with the head up, hands by the side with palms facing forward, and legs straight with toes pointing forward. Page Ref: 34

175. An ancillary department provides services that support the medical and surgical care given in a hospital. Examples of ancillary departments are radiology, physical therapy, dietary, pharmacy, and emergency. Page Ref: 67

176. A hospice is a facility for patients who have a terminal illness and require palliative supportive care and counseling. Hospices also provide emotional support for the patients and their families. Hospice services may also be provided in the patient's home. Page Ref: 68

CHAPTER 3

Multiple Choice

1. b. The antrum immediately precedes the pylorus. Page Ref: 91

2. b. The correct spelling is ileus. Page Ref: 110

3. b. Degluti/o means swallowing. Page Ref: 90

4. d. The cystic duct from the gallbladder empties into the common bile duct. Page Ref: 95

5. c. Emesis is a Greek word meaning ejected contents. Page Ref: 109

6. c. Steatorrhea is improperly digested fat in the feces from certain pancreatic diseases. Page Ref: 116

7. a. Diverticulum is the singular form of this Latin neuter noun; the plural is diverticula. Page Ref: 112

8. d. Hepat/o- means liver and -megaly means enlargement. Page Ref: 119

9. a. The esophagogastroduodenoscopy (EGD) views the upper intestinal tract ending at the duodenum. Page Ref: 134

10. a. Albumin is manufactured in the liver. Page Ref: 123

11. b. Hepatomas are malignant and could metastasize or spread the cancer. Page Ref: 120

12. d. Ingui/o- means groin. Page Ref: 116

13. a. Nexium is a proton pump inhibitor that blocks production of hydrochloric acid in patients with gastroesophageal reflux disease (GERD). Page Ref: 133

14. b. Percutaneous endoscopic gastrostomy (PEG) is a permanent feeding tube in the stomach. Page Ref: 131

15. b. Although the symptoms may be similar in all of these conditions, only irritable bowel syndrome would show a normal colon. Page Ref: 113

16. c. Colonic polyps have a high tendency to become malignant. Page Ref: 114

17. c. The appendix is the only organ of those listed above which is located in the right lower quadrant of the abdomen. Page Ref: 111

18. b. This is also called an irreducible hernia. Page Ref: 116

19. d. Choledocholithiasis is defined as stones in the common bile duct. Page Ref: 121

20. b. Intussuscep/o- means to receive within. Page Ref: 111

21. a. Bright red blood per rectum (BRBPR) and hematochezia, blood in the stool, could be describing the same condition in a patient. Page Ref: 134

22. a. Volvulus is a Latin word that means to roll. Page Ref: 111

23. c. Anastom/o- means to unite two tubular structures. Page Ref: 128

24. d. The haustra allow large amounts of undigested food fibers and water to be held in the intestine. Page Ref: 93

25. c. The symptoms of intussusception include vomiting and abdominal pain. The cause is unknown. Page Ref: 111

26. a. Symptoms of volvulus include vomiting and abdominal pain. Blood vessels to the intestines can also be twisted, decreasing the blood supply and causing the tissues to die. This is also known as malrotation. Page Ref: 111

27. d. A diverticulum can be in the shape of a pouch or a tube. Diverticula are not hereditary. They are thought to be caused by eating a low-fiber diet that forms small, compact stools. Page Ref: 112

28. a. The symptoms of IBD (inflammatory bowel disease) are diarrhea, bloody stools, abdominal cramps, and fever. Inflammation of the mucosa is seen. Page Ref: 113

29. a. Polyp is derived from a Latin word that means many footed. The base or stalk (foot) of a polyp comes in different shapes and sizes. Page Ref: 114

30. c. The source of hematochezia can be an ulcer, cancer, Crohn's disease, polyps, diverticula, or hemorrhoids. Bright red blood indicates active bleeding in the lower gastrointestinal system. Page Ref: 115

31. b. During an ERCP, an endoscope is passed through the mouth and into the duodenum. A catheter is passed through the endoscope, and the contrast material is injected. Page Ref: 125

32. b. Barium enema is a radiologic procedure that uses a liquid opaque contrast dye (barium) introduced through the rectum. Page Ref: 124

33. a. The combining form mastic/o- means chewing. Page Ref: 90

34. b. Hepat/o- means liver, splen/o- means spleen, and -megaly means enlargement. Page Ref: 119

35. a. Examples of antiemetic drugs are Antivert, Compazine, and Phenergan. Page Ref: 133

36. b. Gastr/o- means stomach and -ectomy means surgical excision. Page Ref: 131

37. c. Stomat/o- means mouth and -itis means inflammation. Page Ref: 107

38. d. PTC stands for percutaneous transhepatic cholangiography. Per- means through or throughout, cutane/o- means skin, and -ous means pertaining to. Trans- means across or through, hepat/o- means liver, and -ic means pertaining to. Chol/o- means gall or bile, angi/o- means vessels, and -graphy means process of recording. Page Ref: 118-119

39. b. Hepatitis B is caused by exposure to the blood (or serum) of a person who is already infected with the hepatitis B virus (HBV). Page Ref: 118-119

40. c. The symptoms of cirrhosis include nausea, vomiting, weakness, and jaundice. Cirrhosis can be caused by alcoholism, viral hepatitis, or chronic obstruction of the bile ducts. Severe cirrhosis can progress to liver failure. Page Ref: 118

41. a. Hemorrhoids are caused by increased intra-abdominal pressure from straining to pass hard stools. This repeatedly dilates the veins until they permanently protrude. Page Ref: 114

42. c. Patients with paralysis of the lower extremities lack sensation and motor control of the external anal sphincter and are said to be incontinent. Page Ref: 115

43. c. Patent is derived from a Latin word that means to lie open. Page Ref: 114

44. a. A peduculated polyp has a thin stalk; whereas a sessile polyp is shaped like a mound with a broad, rounded base. Page Ref: 114

45. c. The symptoms of dysentery include watery diarrhea mixed with blood and mucus. Page Ref: 113

46. d. Peptic ulcer disease (PUD) involves chronic irritation, burning pain, and erosion of the mucosa to the point of forming an ulcer. Page Ref: 110

47. b. The source of hematemesis is the stomach or esophagus. The cause can be an esophageal ulcer, esophageal varies, or a gastric ulcer. Coffee-grounds emesis contains old, dark blood that has been partially digested in the stomach. Page Ref: 108

48. d. Uvula is derived from a Latin word that means little grape. The uvula looks like a little grape hanging in the posterior oral cavity. Page Ref: 89

49. b. The oral cavity is where food or drink enters the gastrointestinal system. Page Ref: 89

50. d. Salivary glands is a general phrase for the specific pairs of parotid, submandibular, and sublingual glands. Page Ref: 90

51. c. The pharynx is the medical word for throat. Page Ref: 90

52. a. The uvula is in the oral cavity, not in the stomach. The cardia is one of the five areas of the stomach, even though it sounds like it is related to the heart. Page Ref: 91

53. d. The stomach is a primary organ of digestion, not an accessory organ. Page Ref: 94-96

54. a. Hydrochloric acid is a strong acid, which kills microorganisms on ingested food. It also breaks down food fibers and converts pepsinogen into pepsin. Page Ref: 97

55. c. This process is known as emulsification. Page Ref: 97

56. d. Lactase breaks down the sugar in milk. The combining form lact/o- means milk. Page Ref: 97

57. c. Dysphagia. Dys- means painful or difficult, phag/o- means swallowing. Page Ref: 107

58. b. Percutaneous transhepatic cholangiography. The key to this answer is the word percutaneous, which means through the skin. Page Ref: 125

59. a. Oncologist (ong-KAWL-oh-jist), onc/o- means tumor or mass, log/o- means the study of, and -ist means one who specializes in. Page Ref: 135

60. a. Omphalocele (OM-fal-oh-ceel), omphal/o- means umbilicus, navel, and -cele means hernia. Page Ref: 116

61. *c.* Adhesion (ad-HEE-zhun), adhes/o- means to stick and -ion means action or condition. *Page Ref:* 116

62. d. Malrotation (MAL-roh-TAY-shun), mal- means bad or inadequate, rotat/o- means to rotate, and -ion means action or condition. Page Ref: 111

63. c. Colic (KAWL-ik), col/o- means colon and -ic means pertaining to. A symptom of colic is crampy abdominal pain that occurs shortly after eating. Page Ref: 111

64. d. Ulcer (UL-ser) means a sore. A gastric ulcer is found in the stomach. Page Ref: 110

65. b. Gravidarum (GRAV-ih-DAIR-rum) is a Latin word meaning of pregnancy. Hyperemesis gravidarum only occurs during pregnancy. Page Ref: 109

66. b. Polyphagia (PAWL-ee-FAY-jee-ah), poly- means many or much, phag/o- means eating or swallowing, and -ia means condition, state, or thing. Page Ref: 107

67. *c.* Gloss/o- and lingu/o- both mean tongue. Page Ref: 102

68. *d.* Peritone/o- means peritoneum. Page Ref: 102

69. d. The gastrointestinal system begins at the oral cavity and ends at the anus. Page Ref: 89, 93

70. c. The uvula is the fleshy part of the soft palate that hangs in the back of the throat. Page Ref: 89

71. a. The combining form gloss/o- means tongue. Page Ref: 89

72. c. Taste receptors on the tongue send nerve impulses about tastes to the gustatory cortex in the brain. Page Ref: 89

73. a. The pharynx is the medical word for the throat. Page Ref: 90

74. b. The combining form degluti/o- means swallowing. Page Ref: 90

75. d. There are no wavelike contractions in the oral cavity to propel the food. Food in the oral cavity moves as it is pushed by the tongue and then swallowed. Page Ref: 90, 91

76. c. Rugae are mucosal folds in the stomach that open out to accommodate large amounts of food. Haustra are outpouchings in the intestinal wall that allow the intestine to hold large amounts of undigested food fibers and water. Page Ref: 91

77. d. The cardia, the superior aspect of the stomach, is near the heart but is not part of it. Page Ref: 91

78. c. The villi project outwardly as thin structures to increase the surface area available to absorb nutrients. Page Ref: 92

79. d. The large intestine includes the cecum, the ascending colon, transverse colon, descending colon, sigmoid colon, rectum, and anus. Page Ref: 93

80. a. Peyer's patches are part of the immune system and contain white blood cells to destroy disease-causing bacteria in the intestines. Page Ref: 93

81. c. Vermiform means wormlike. This word is used to describe the appendix. Page Ref: 93

82. a. Bile produced by the liver is stored in the gallbladder. Gall is an Old English word meaning bitter or bile. Page Ref: 95

83. b. Food is broken down chemically by the chemical action of enzymes and hydrochloric acid. Page Ref: 97

84. c. Bile breaks up large globules of fat in the process of emulsification. Page Ref: 97

85. d. Emulsification uses bile to break down large globules of fat. Then the enzyme lipase from the

pancreas chemically breaks fat globules into fatty acids. Page Ref: 97

86. c. Lactase. The combining form lact/o- means milk. Page Ref: 97

87. a. Food nutrients in the blood are taken via the portal vein to the liver. Page Ref: 97

88. b. All of these answers have to do with stool, but defecation is the actual process of passing stool (elimination). Page Ref: 98

89. b. A sphincter is a muscular ring in the gastrointestinal tract. The cardiac sphincter prevents food in the stomach from going back into the esophagus. Page Ref: 91

90. a. Saliv/o- and sial/o- both mean saliva. Page Ref: 135

91. d. Gastr/o- means stomach, enter/o- means intestines, and -itis means inflammation of. Page Ref: 108

92. c. The appendix is the pouch that hangs from the cecum. Page Ref: 111

93. d. A surgical suture line is an incision and a hernia there is known as an incisional hernia. Page Ref: 116

94. c. Ascitic fluid accumulates in the abdominopelvic cavity because liver disease causes backup of blood in the portal vein. Page Ref: 117

95. a. A hepatocyte is a liver cell. Page Ref: 94

96. d. Chol/e- means bile, gall (gallbladder). Page Ref: 121

97. a. An enema is administered through the rectum and the dye outlines the rectum and colon. Page Ref: 124

98. c. Lapar/o- means abdomen. Page Ref: 131

99. a. Enter/o- means intestine. Page Ref: 135

100. c. Cholecystitis is inflammation of the gallbladder. Page Ref: 121

101. b. Gastr/o- means stomach and -ostomy means surgically created opening. Page Ref: 131

102. d. The gallbladder stores bile produced by the liver and releases bile when you eat a fatty meal. The gallbladder can develop stones in it. Page Ref: 95, 121

103. d. The combining form colon/o- and the suffix -scopy make up the word colonoscopy. Page Ref: 130

104. d. Emesis is vomiting, but vomiting blood is hematemesis. Page Ref: 108

105. c. Melena is derived from a Greek word that means black. Page Ref: 116

106. d. Barium is an opaque contrast dye that is swallowed and outlines the upper GI tract. Page Ref: 126

107. a. Gastric ulcers are most commonly caused by *H. pylori*. Page Ref: 110

108. b. Hepat/o- means liver and -itis means inflammation of. Page Ref: 118

109. b. Volvulus is a Latin word meaning to roll. Page Ref: 111

110. d. The suffix -ase (as in the enzyme lipase) means enzyme. Page Ref: 97

111. c. The small intestine contains the C-shaped duodenum, then the jejunum, and then the ileum. Page Ref: 92

112. a. Lumen is a Latin word that means window. Page Ref: 92

113. c. In countries with diets high in fiber and low in processed foods, diverticulosis is uncommon. Page Ref: 112

114. a. Obstip/o- means severe constipation. Page Ref: 115

115. c. The correct spelling is cirrhosis. Page Ref: 118

116. d. A stone blocking the bile ducts increases levels of unconjugated bilirubin in the blood, giving the tissues a yellow color known as jaundice. Page Ref: 120

117. b. Gallstones have no effect on the pancreas. Bacterial or viral infections or chronic alcoholism can cause inflammation or infection of the pancreas. Page Ref: 122

118. d. Guaiac is a resin from a tropical plant that turns blue in the presence of blood. Page Ref: 123

119. d. A gallbladder ultrasound does not use any contrast dye. Page Ref: 126

120. a. O&P stands for ova and parasites. Page Ref: 124

121. c. Bi/o- means living tissue and -opsy means process of viewing. Page Ref: 127

122. d. Stoma is a Greek word that means a mouth. Page Ref: 129

123. c. The abdomen is explored through a wide incision. Lapar/o- means abdomen and -tomy means process of cutting or making an incision. Page Ref: 131

124. a. Emet/o- means to vomit. Page Ref: 133

Short Answer

125. Appendix. Append/o- means small structure hanging from a larger structure. Page Ref: 93

126. Meconium. Meconium is a Latin word meaning waste from a newborn child. Page Ref: 98

127. Cholelithiasis. Chol/e- means bile or gall (gallbladder in this word) and lith/o- means stone. Page Ref: 121

128. colic. Colic means pertaining to the colon. Page Ref: 111

129. or/o-. Oral means pertaining to the mouth. Page Ref: 89

130. inguinal; inguinal. The combining form inguin/o- means groin. Page Ref: 116

131. liver. ALT and AST are enzymes found mainly in the liver. Page Ref: 123

132. Intravenous cholangiography. Intravenous means pertaining to within a vein. Cholangi/o- means bile duct. Page Ref: 125

133. dyspepsia. Dys- means painful, difficult, or abnormal and peps/o- means digestion. Page Ref: 108

134. peristalsis. Peritalsis means the process of contraction around. Page Ref: 91

135. oral cavity. Oral (OR-al), or/o- means mouth and -al means pertaining to. Oral is the adjective form for mouth. Page Ref: 89

136. saliva. Saliv/o- means saliva and -ary means pertaining to. Page Ref: 90

137. mastication. Mastication (MAS-tih-KAY-shun), mastic/o- means chewing and -ation means a process; being or having. Page Ref: 90

138. cardia, fundus, body, antrum, pylorus. Cardia (KAR-dee-ah) is derived from a Greek word meaning heart. The cardia of the stomach and the cardiac sphincter of the esophagus are near, but not part of, the heart. Fundus (FUN-dus) is a Latin word meaning the part of a hollow organ that is the farthest from the opening. The body is the largest, curved part of the stomach. Antrum (AN-trum) is a Latin word meaning cave. Pylorus (py-LOR-us) is derived from a Greek word meaning gatekeeper. The pyloric sphincter acts as a gatekeeper, keeping food in the stomach and then opening to let food into the duodenum. Page Ref: 91

139. Chyme. Chyme (KIME) is derived from a Greek word meaning juice. Page Ref: 92

140. small intestine; small bowel. Bowel (BAH-ool) is derived from a Latin word meaning sausage. The loops and sections of intestine can look like a string of sausages. Page Ref: 92

141. duodenum. Duodenum (DOO-oh-DEE-num), (doo-AWD-ah-num) is derived from a Latin word meaning twelve. Ancient Roman physicians measured the duodenum as being 12 fingerbreadths in length. Page Ref: 92

142. appendix. Appendix (ah-PEN-diks), append/o- means small structure hanging from a larger structure and -ix means a structure. Page Ref: 93

143. mesentery. Mesenteric (mez-en-TAIR-ik), meso- means middle, enter/o- means intestine, and -ic means pertaining to. The mesentery is attached to the jejunum and ileum, the middle parts of the small intestine. Page Ref: 94

144. bilirubin. Bilirubin (BIL-ih-ROO-bin), bil/i- means bile, gall, rub/o- means red, and -in means substance. Bilirubin is not a red pigment. The combining form rub/o- indicates that bilirubin comes from the breakdown of old red blood cells. Page Ref: 94-95

145. gallbladder. Gallbladder (GAWL-blad-er), gall is an Old English word meaning bitter (the taste of bile) and bladder is an Old English word meaning a fluid-filled sac. Page Ref: 95

146. enzymes. Enzyme (EN-zime) is a Greek word meaning leaven. Enzymes speed up chemical reactions just as leaven (yeast) speeds up the rising of bread. Page Ref: 97

147. meconium. Meconium (meh-KOH-nee-um) is a Latin word meaning waste from a newborn child. Page Ref: 98

148. Antiemetic. Antiemetic (AN-tee-eh-MET-ik), anti- means against, emet/o- means to vomit, and -ic means pertaining to. Page Ref: 133

149. gastroesophageal reflux disease. GERD is a chronic inflammation and irritation of the esophagus due to reflux (a backward flow) of stomach acid into the esophagus. Page Ref: 134

150. Chyme. Chyme is derived from a Greek word meaning juice. Page Ref: 92

151. inflammation. Gastritis is inflammation of the stomach. Page Ref: 108

152. Peritoneal. The abdominopelvic cavity is lined with a membrane called the peritoneum, which secretes peritoneal fluid. Page Ref: 94

153. flatus. Excessive flatus can be caused by certain types of food. Page Ref: 98

154. epiglottis. It protects the lungs from aspirated food. Page Ref: 100

155. hyperemesis gravidarum. Gravidarum is a Latin word meaning pregnancy. Page Ref: 109

156. Ileus. Ileus is a Latin word meaning rolled up tightly or obstructed. Page Ref: 110

157. hematochezia. The source of bleeding can be an ulcer, cancer, Crohn's disease, polyp, diverticulum, or hemorrhoid. Page Ref: 115

158. infectious. Hepatitis A is an acute, short-lived infection from which most people completely recover. There is no vaccination to prevent hepatitis A. Page Ref: 118

159. appendectomy. The suffix -ectomy means surgical excision. Page Ref: 127

160. gallbladder. Chol/e- means bile or gall, cyst/o- means bladder or fluid-filled sac. Page Ref: 95

161. Possible answers include digestive tract, alimentary canal, or gastrointestinal (GI) system.. The different names highlight the different functions of the digestive system. Page Ref: 94

162. Gastroenterology. Gastr/o- means stomach, enter/lo- means intestine, and -logy means the study of. Page Ref: 87

163. wormlike. The appendix is a thin, pink, fleshy appendage that can be as long as eight inches. Page Ref: 93

True/False

164. False. They are produced by the pancreas. Page Ref: 97

165. True. This test measures the presence of blood in the stool. Page Ref: 116, 123-124

166. True. Compazine is used to treat nausea and vomiting. Page Ref: 133

167. True. The suffix -ase means enzyme. Page Ref: 97

168. False. This condition is known as anorexia. Page Ref: 107, 117

169. True. Aliment/o- means food, nourishment. Food enters the body and is processed by the GI tract. Page Ref: 99

170. False. They are combining forms for tongue. Page Ref: 89

171. True. Bile breaks apart large globules of fat. Page Ref: 95

172. True. This is also referred to as gastric stapling. Page Ref: 132

173. False. The patient with ascites will show a distended abdomen from fluid accumulation in the abdominopelvic cavity. Yellow-orange discoloration is known as jaundice. Page Ref: 117, 120

174. False. The sublingual glands are located under the tongue. The combining form lingu/o- means tongue. Page Ref: 90

175. True. Although the liver participates in the digestive process, it is not directly involved in digestion. Page Ref: 94

176. False. Polyphagia means excessive overeating. Page Ref: 107

177. False. A cholecystectomy is the surgical removal of the gallbladder. The suffix -ectomy means surgical excision. Page Ref: 128

178. False. Serum hepatitis is another name for Hepatitis B. Page Ref: 118

179. True. The word part hemat/o- means blood. Hematemesis means vomiting of blood. Page Ref: 108

180. False. High-fiber diets and laxatives are often used to treat irritable bowel syndrome. Page Ref: 113

181. False. Although all polyps are benign, they can become cancerous and are usually removed in order to prevent this. Polyps are considered risk factors for cancer of the colon. Page Ref: 114

182. False. A chronic, progressive inflammation and eventual irreversible degeneration of liver tissue characterized by nodules and scarring is called cirrhosis. Page Ref: 117

183. True. Polypectomy does not need to be an invasive surgery. Page Ref: 132

184. True. Dys- means painful, difficult, or abnormal, phag/o- means eating, and -ia means condition, state, thing. Page Ref: 107

185. False. The first part of the small intestine is the duodenum. Page Ref: 92

186. True. Hepat/o- means liver and -cyte means cell. Page Ref: 94

187. True. Anorexia nervosa is a psychiatric disorder in which patients have an obsessive desire to be thin and decrease food intake to the point of starvation. Page Ref: 107

188. True. The pancreas releases digestive enzymes, but does not directly digest food itself. Page Ref: 96

189. False. Cholecystokinin stimulates the gallbladder to release bile. Page Ref: 97

190. True. After manipulation of the intestines during surgery, peristalsis is often slow to resume. Postoperative means after surgery. Ileus is a Latin word that means rolled up and tightly obstructed. Page Ref: 110

191. False. Dys- means painful, difficult, abnormal; phag/o- means eating, swallowing, and -ia means condition, state, thing. Page Ref: 107

192. True. Hemorrhoids are distended veins just like varicose veins in the leg, but they are in the rectum and are caused by straining to pass stool. Page Ref: 114

193. True. Benign familial polyposis is the condition of multiple family members all with benign polyps. Page Ref: 114

194. True. Emesis is a Greek word that means vomiting; vomitus is a Latin word that means the same thing. Page Ref: 109

195. False. Hematochezia is the presence of blood in the stool. Hematemesis is the presence of blood in vomited stomach contents. Page Ref: 115

196. False. Both gloss/o- and lingu/o- mean tongue. Page Ref: 135

Essay

197. CLO is a laboratory test done to detect the presence of *Helicobacter pylori,* a bacterium that is a major cause of gastric ulcers. Page Ref: 123

198. Hepatitis A is carried by contaminated food or water, which would account for several people contracting the virus at the same time. Hepatitis B, C, and D are caused by exposure to contaminated body fluids such as blood. Page Ref: 118-119

199. Varices are swollen, protruding veins in the mucosa of the lower esophagus or stomach. Liver disease causes the blood to back up in the portal vein. The blood then goes through the gastroesophageal veins as another route to return to the heart. However, these vessels cannot handle the load and eventually become engorged from the blood flow and pressure. Esophageal and gastric varices are easily irritated by passing food. They can hemorrhage suddenly, causing death. Page Ref: 108

200. Mechanical digestion consists of mastication, deglutition, and peristalsis. Chemical digestion consists of the action of enzymes and acid, which break down foods into molecules of nutrients that can be absorbed and used by the body. Page Ref: 96-97

201. C & S is a diagnostic test that determines which bacterium is causing an intestinal infection and which antibiotics it is sensitive to. A stool specimen is swabbed on a culture dish that contains a nutrient medium for growing bacteria. As the colonies grow, they are examined both by physical appearance of the colonies and under a microscope. Disks containing various antibiotics are placed in the colonies to determine which ones inhibit the growth of the bacteria. Page Ref: 124

202. An endoscopy is a surgical procedure that uses an endoscope (a flexible, fiberoptic scope with a magnifying lens and a light source) to internally examine the gastrointestinal tract. Endoscopy can be coupled with another procedure such as a biopsy or removal of a polyp. Page Ref: 130

203. A gastroplasty is a surgical procedure to treat severely obese patients. Staples are placed down one side of the stomach, making the stomach much smaller. It is also known as gastric stapling. Page Ref: 132

204. A surgical incision (-otomy) into the common bile duct (choledoch/o-) to remove a stone (lith/o-). Page Ref: 129

CHAPTER 4

Multiple Choice

1. d. The correct spelling is expiration. Page Ref: 160

2. b. Pulmonology is the study of the lungs. Page Ref: 158

3. c. Antibiotics are effective only against bacterial infections. Page Ref: 187

4. c. Orth/o- means straight and -pnea means breathing. Page Ref: 178

5. b. Pneumoconiosis is a chronic lung disease caused by particle inhalation. Anthracosis, or black lung disease, is a type of pneumoconiosis caused by inhaling coal dust. Page Ref: 174

6. a. Alveolus is a Latin word meaning small hollow cell or cavity; alveoli is the plural form. Page Ref: 158

7. b. Carboxyhemoglobin is a blood test that measures the amount of carbon monoxide in the blood. A car left running in a closed area would produce considerable carbon monoxide. Page Ref: 100

8. c. Anti- means against, tuss/o- means cough, and -ive means pertaining to. Page Ref: 187

9. a. The sternum is the breast bone. Page Ref: 159

10. c. A stethoscope is an instrument used to listen to body sounds. Page Ref: 182

11. b. COPD is chronic obstructive pulmonary disease, any condition involving long-standing air flow problems. Chronic bronchitis is the only example of COPD of those listed. Page Ref: 171

12. a. Failure of the heart to adequately pump blood causes fluid to accumulate in the alveoli. Page Ref: 175

13. c. PPD means packs per day or purified protein derivative. Page Ref: 189

14. a. URI is an upper respiratory infection. The nose and throat are part of the upper respiratory tract but the bronchi, lungs, and pleura are not. Page Ref: 189

15. c. Arterial blood gases measure oxygen and carbon dioxide in the blood. Hypercapnia is above-normal levels of carbon dioxide in the blood. Page Ref: 179, 180

16. b. Rales are crackling sounds heard when air is passing through fluid or mucus filled air passages. Page Ref: 170

17. d. The Mantoux test is done to screen for tuberculosis. Page Ref: 182

18. a. Asthma is called reactive airway disease because it occurs as a hypersensitivity reaction to a triggering agent. Page Ref: 169

19. c. The pulse oximeter is attached to a patient's finger or ear lobe to monitor oxygen levels in the blood. Page Ref: 180

20. a. A tracheostomy is an incision into the trachea to make a permanent opening for respiration either with or without mechanical ventilation. Page Ref: 186

21. b. INH is a drug for tuberculosis. Page Ref: 187

22. c. Larynx is a Greek word meaning voice box. Page Ref: 156

23. d. The turbinates jut out into the nasal cavity to slow down inhaled air so it can pick up warmth and moisture. Page Ref: 155

24. a. Carried by a recessive gene, cystic fibrosis affects all glands that secrete mucus, digestive enzymes, and sweat. Page Ref: 171-172

25. a. Pulmon/o- means lung and -logy means the study of. Page Ref: 154

26. d. The mucous membranes of the pharynx also warm and moisten the inhaled air and trap inhaled particles. Page Ref: 155

27. c. During swallowing, muscles in the neck pull the larynx up to meet the epiglottis so that food moves across the top of the epiglottis and into the esophagus, not into the larynx. Page Ref: 156

28. a. Each bronchus enters the lung and then further divides into many smaller passageways known as bronchioles. They carry inhaled and exhaled air to and from the alveoli. Page Ref: 157

29. d. The mediastinum is the smaller cavity within the thoracic cavity that contains the trachea and other structures not related to the respiratory system. Page Ref: 159

30. b. The respiratory system exchanges oxygen for carbon dioxide. It also traps and expels foreign particles, bacteria, and other pathogens in the incoming air. Page Ref: 160

31. b. Status is the Latin word for standing still. A person with status asthmaticus stays in a state of continuous, severe asthma. Page Ref: 169

32. a. COPD, chronic obstructive pulmonary disease, is the combination of chronic bronchitis and emphysema caused by chronic exposure to pollution or smoking. Page Ref: 171

33. c. Normal inspiration sounds like a soft wind rushing through a tunnel. Page Ref: 170

34. c. Em- means in, py/o- means pus, and -ema means condition. This condition is also known as pyothorax. Page Ref: 172

35. d. Legionnaire's disease was first identified in 1976 when many people at an American Legion convention in Philadelphia became sick from breathing air from an air conditioning system that was contaminated by a bacterium attracted to the environment of the lungs. The bacterium was subsequently named *Legionella pneumophilia*. Page Ref: 173

36. b. Anthracosis is also known as coal miner's lung or black lung disease and is caused by inhaling coal dust. Page Ref: 174

37. b. Pan- means all, lob/o- means lobe of an organ, and -ar means pertaining to. Page Ref: 175

38. c. Hem/o- means blood and -ptysis means abnormal condition of coughing up. Hemoptysis is coughing up blood. Page Ref: 176

39. d. The bacterium that causes tuberculosis has a unique waxy coating. It can be identified because it only holds an acid stain, so it is known as an acid-fast bacillus. Page Ref: 189

40. c. Paroxysmal nocturnal dyspnea (PND) is an attack of shortness of breath that occurs at night and awakens the patient. Page Ref: 189

41. a. Asphyxia can occur at any age if the patient chokes, drowns, or is suffocated. Page Ref: 179

42. d. Hypo- means below or deficient, ox/o- means oxygen, and -ia means condition, state, or thing. Page Ref: 180

43. b. Carbox/y- means carbon monoxide. Page Ref: 180

44. c. A pulmonary function test is a diagnostic procedure in which a spirometry is used to graph the measurements of the lung capacity. Page Ref: 180

45. b. An Ambu bag is attached to a face mask or an endotracheal tube and squeezed to force air into the lungs. Page Ref: 185

46. a. A pneumonectomy is usually performed to treat lung cancer. Page Ref: 186

47. a. Antitussive drugs are used to treat chronic bronchitis and nonproductive coughs. Some of these drugs are narcotic. Page Ref: 187

48. d. Ox/y- means oxygen and hem/o- means blood. Page Ref: 161

49. b. Alveoli is plural; the singular form is alveolus. Page Ref: 158

50. a. Carbon dioxide molecules contain one carbon atom and two oxygen atoms. Page Ref: 161

51. d. Inter- means between and cost/o- means rib. Page Ref: 164

52. b. It is not considered chronic bronchitis because it has only been present for two days. Page Ref: 169

53. a. Atel/o- means incomplete and -ectasis means dilation. Page Ref: 170

54. d. Although cystic fibrosis (CF) affects many body parts, the most debilitating effects are on the lungs. Page Ref: 171-172

55. c. Em- means in and py/o- means pus. Page Ref: 172

56. a. Lobar means pertaining to one lobe of an organ. Page Ref: 175

57. c. Hyper- means above or more than normal, capn/o- means carbon dioxide, and -ia, means condition or state. Page Ref: 179

58. c. Mucous membrane lines the respiratory tract and warms and humidifies incoming air. It produces mucus to trap foreign particles. Page Ref: 164

59. b. Parenchyma refers to the functional part of the lung (i.e., the alveoli) as opposed to the connective tissue framework. Page Ref: 164

60. b. Thorac/o- means thorax (chest) and cav/o- means hollow. Page Ref: 165

61. d. Rales (RAWLZ) are irregular crackling or bubbling sounds during inspiration. Wet rales are caused by obstruction of the alveoli by fluid or infection. Dry rales are caused by chronic irritation or fibrosis. Page Ref: 170

62. b. Atelectasis (AT-eh-LEK-tah-sis), atel/o- means incomplete and -ectasis means dilation. Page Ref: 170

63. a. Emphysema (EM-fih-SEE-mah), em- means in, phys/o- means inflate or distend; grow, and -ema means condition. Page Ref: 171

64. b. Empyema (EM-py-EE-mah), em- means in, py/o- means pus, and -ema means condition. Also known as pyothorax. Page Ref: 172

65. a. Opportunistic (AWP-or-too-NIS-tik), opportun/o- means well-timed, -istic means pertaining to. Page Ref: 175

66. c. Dyspnea (DISP-nee-ah), dys- means painful, difficult, -pnea means breathing. Page Ref: 178

67. c. Chronic obstructive pulmonary disease (COPD) is a combination of chronic bronchitis and emphysema. Page Ref: 171, 189

68. a. *Pneumocystis carinii* pneumonia is an opportunistic infection that attacks the weakened immune system of patients with AIDS. Page Ref: 175

69. c. Blood not pumped out by the left ventricle backs up into the pulmonary circulation. Then fluid comes out of the blood and fills the lungs. Page Ref: 175

70. d. Another name for empyema is pyothorax. Page Ref: 172

71. b. Hem/o- means blood and -thorax means chest cavity. Page Ref: 177

72. d. All of these healthcare workers can perform endotracheal intubation if the patient needs it. Page Ref: 183

73. c. Atel/o- means incomplete and -ectasis means dilation. Page Ref: 170

74. b. A laryngoscope is an instrument that is used to view the larynx prior to endotracheal intubation. Page Ref: 183

75. b. Dyspnea on exertion (DOE) means shortness of breath or difficulty breathing when exercising. Page Ref: 178, 189

76. d. A metered-dose inhaler (MDI) delivers a puff of medication when the patient inhales. Page Ref: 187, 189

77. d. Lob/o- means lobe of an organ (the lobe is part of the lung) and -ectomy means surgical excision. Page Ref: 186

78. a. Lobar pneumonia affects a lobe of the lung. Page Ref: 175

79. c. Inter- means between and cos/to- means ribs. Page Ref: 176

80. c. The Heimlich maneuver creates a burst of air in the chest that pushes the obstruction into the mouth where it can be expelled. Page Ref: 183

81. d. Respiration consists of breathing in (inspiration or inhalation) and breathing out (expiration or exhalation). Page Ref: 160

82. b. Eu- means normal or good, -pnea means breathing. Page Ref: 161

83. d. Orth/o- means straight and -pnea means breathing. Page Ref: 178

84. c. A pulse oximeter is a device clipped onto the finger that measures the oxygen saturation in the blood. An arterial blood gas is a laboratory test that measures all the gases in the blood, including oxygen. Page Ref: 180, 181

85. d. Steth/o- means chest. A stethoscope is used to listen to the chest. Page Ref: 190

86. c. The correct spelling is pneumonia. Page Ref: 175

Short Answer

87. eupnea. Eu- means normal and -pnea means breathing. Page Ref: 161

88. oncologist. Onc/o- means cancer. Page Ref: 190

89. hemoptysis. Hem/o- means blood and -ptysis means abnormal condition of coughing up. Page Ref: 176

90. cyanosis. Cyan/o- means blue. Page Ref: 179

91. thoracotomy. Thorac/o- means thorax (chest) and -tomy means process of cutting or making an incision. Page Ref: 186

92. atelectasis.. Atel/o- means incomplete and -ectasis means dilation. Page Ref: 170

93. metered-dose inhaler or MDI. Bronchodilator drugs dilate constricted airways by relaxing the smooth muscles that surround the bronchioles and bronchi. Corticosteroid drugs block the immune system from causing inflammation in the lung. Page Ref: 187, 188

94. AIDS. *Pneumocystis carinii* pneumonia is an opportunistic infection. Page Ref: 175

95. embolus or embolism. Embolus is a Greek word meaning a plug or wedged stopper. Page Ref: 176

96. Reye. Using aspirin for a viral infection such as influenza carries the risk for Reye syndrome. Acetaminophen (Tylenol) should be used instead. Page Ref: 172

97. trachea. The trachea, a muscular tube about 1 inch in diameter and 4 inches in length, is a passageway for inhaled and exhaled air. Page Ref: 157

98. phrenic. Phrenic means pertaining to the diaphragm. Page Ref: 161

99. surfactant. Surfactant is secreted by the alveoli. Page Ref: 158

100. turbinates. The turbinates are also known as the nasal conchae. Page Ref: 155

101. Eupneic. Eu- means good and -pneic means breathing. Page Ref: 161

102. deoxygenated. Deoxygenated blood travels back to the heart and then the lungs where carbon dioxide enters the alveoli and is exhaled. Page Ref: 162

103. Stridor. Other abnormal breath sounds include rales, rhonchi, and wheezes. Page Ref: 170

104. Anthracosis. Anthracosis is caused by inhaling coal dust. Page Ref: 174

105. Pneumoconiosis. Anthracosis and asbestosis are two types of pneumoconiosis. Page Ref: 174

106. pneumonia. Pneumon/o- means lung or air and -ia means condition, state, or thing. Page Ref: 174

107. embolus. Embolus is a Greek word meaning a plug or wedged stopper. Page Ref: 176

108. septum. Septum (SEP-tum) is derived from a Latin word meaning a partition. Page Ref: 155

109. pharynx. Pharynx (FAIR-ingks) is a Greek word meaning throat. Page Ref: 156

110. epiglottis. Epiglottis (EP-ih-GLAWT-is), epi- means upon or above, glottis is a Greek word meaning opening of the larynx. Page Ref: 156

111. Bronchopulmonary. Bronchopulmonary (BRONG-koh-PUL-moh-nair-ee), bronch/o- means bronchus, pulmon/o- means lung, and -ary means pertaining to. Page Ref: 157

112. alveolus. Alveolus (al-VEE-oh-lus) is a Latin word meaning small hollow cell or cavity. Page Ref: 158

113. parenchyma. The parenchyma contains the functional cells of any organ. Page Ref: 158

114. thorax; sternum. Thorac/o- means chest. The sternum is the breast bone. Page Ref: 159

115. mediastinum. Mediastinum (MEE-dee-as-TY-num) is derived from a Latin word meaning a lower servant who performs routine duties. Perhaps the mediastinum seemed like a smaller, less important area compared to the larger, active thorax. Page Ref: 159

116. diaphragm. Nerve impulses from the phrenic nerve cause the diaphragm to contract during inspiration. Page Ref: 159

117. phrenic. Phrenic (FREN-ik), phren/o- means diaphragm; mind, -ic means pertaining to. Page Ref: 161

118. Respiration. Respiration (RES-pi-RAY-shun), re- means again and again; backward; unable to, spir/o- means breathe, and -ation means a process; being or having. Page Ref: 160

119. inhalation; inspiration. Inhalation (IN-hah-LAY-shun), in- means in, within; not, hal/o- means breathe, -ation means a process; being or having. Inspiration (IN-spih-RAY-shun), in- means in, within; not, spir/o- means breathe, -ation means a process; being or having. Page Ref: 160

120. exhalation; expiration. Exhalation (EKS-hah-LAY-shun), ex- means out, away from, hal/o- means breathe, -ation means a process; being or having. Expiration (EKS-pih-RAY-shun), ex- means out, away from, spir/o- means breathe, -ation means a process; being or having. The s is deleted from spir/o- because the prefix ex- already provides an s sound. Expire also means to die or to take a last breath. Page Ref: 160

121. Asthma. Asthma (AZ-mah) is a sudden onset of hyperreactivity of the bronchi and bronchioles with bronchospasm. Asthma is a Greek word meaning bronchospasm (contraction of the smooth muscle), inflammation, and panting. Page Ref: 169

122. Trachea. The trachea is the passageway that allows air to flow from the mouth and nose to the lungs. Page Ref: 157

123. Pharynx. The pharynx is the throat and the larynx is the voice box. Page Ref: 156

124. Pack-years. Pack-years equals the number of packs smoked per day multiplied by the number of years the person has been smoking. Page Ref: 169

125. cockroaches. Contact with cockroaches as well as cockroach droppings and carcasses behind walls are asthma triggers. Page Ref: 169

126. oxygen. The two prongs in the nose are connected to tubing that goes to an oxygen source. Page Ref: 184

127. bronchioles. Bronchi divide into smaller branches known as bronchioles. Page Ref: 157

128. cilia. Cilia are small hairs that move to push inhaled particles away from the lungs. Page Ref: 157

129. diaphragm. The respiratory control center directs the phrenic nerve to cause the diaphragm to contract and initiate inhalation. Page Ref: 161

130. apnea. A- means without and -pnea means breathing. Page Ref: 177

True/False

131. True. To expire is to take the last breath. Page Ref: 160

132. True. A tube is inserted into the trachea to manually or mechanically assist the patient in breathing. Page Ref: 183

133. False. It is called an Ambu bag. Page Ref: 185

134. False. Mucus is misspelled. In the sentence, the word is used as an adjective, and it should be spelled mucous. Page Ref: 162

135. False. Pne/o- means breathing; pneumon/o- and pulmon/o- mean lung. Page Ref: 158, 161

136. True. Hypo- means below, ox/o- means oxygen, and -emia means substance in the blood. Page Ref: 180

137. False. PA (posteroanterior) or AP (anteroposterior) are the abbreviations used to describe the entry and exit direction of the x-rays. Page Ref: 189

138. True. It can help to prevent postoperative atelectasis or collapsed lung. Page Ref: 184

139. True. Acid-fast bacillus is used to describe a microorganism that could turn out to be *Mycobacterium tuberculosis*. Page Ref: 176

140. False. Walking pneumonia is caused by *Mycoplasma pneumoniae*. Page Ref: 175

141. False. Abnormally low level of oxygen in the arterial blood is called hypoxemia. Oxyhemoglobin carries oxygen in the blood. Page Ref: 180

142. True. Asthma attacks recur intermittently and can be triggered by a number of things. Page Ref: 169

143. False. The small tubular branches of airway that carry air into and out of the alveoli are called bronchioles. Page Ref: 157

144. False. Carbon dioxide is a waste product of metabolism. Page Ref: 161

145. True. The left lung is slightly smaller than the right. Page Ref: 158

146. True. Carboxyhemoglobin competes with oxygen for receptor sites on the hemoglobin molecule. If there is too much carboxyhemoglobin, the patient may die. Page Ref: 180

147. True. The device emits light waves that penetrate the skin and are absorbed or reflected depending on how saturated the hemoglobin is. Page Ref: 181

148. True. The supplemental oxygen can help raise blood oxygen levels and relieve symptoms related to hypoxemia. Page Ref: 184-185

149. False. The bronchoscope is the name of the lighted instrument. The procedure is called a bronchoscopy. Page Ref: 185

150. True. Often in medicine there are two names for the same thing. In this case, the two words are very similar. Page Ref: 186

151. True. Endotracheal intubation inserts an endotracheal tube to establish an airway. Page Ref: 183

152. True. The prefix epi- means upon or above, and the glottis is the opening into the larynx. Page Ref: 156

153. False. Pneumonectomy is surgical removal of the entire lung because of lung cancer. Page Ref: 186

154. False. The right lung has three lobes and the left lung has two lobes. Page Ref: 157

155. True. COPD has components of both chronic bronchitis and emphysema. Page Ref: 171

156. False. Double pneumonia involves both lungs. Page Ref: 175

157. False. Tuberculosis is caused by a bacterium, *Mycobacterium tuberculosis*. *Page Ref:* 176

158. True. Eupnea means normal breathing. Page Ref: 161

Essay

159. Surfactant is present in the alveoli of the lungs to keep these air sacs open. The alveoli of premature infants often do not produce enough surfactant. Without surfactant the alveoli cannot inflate sufficiently and the infant develops respiratory distress syndrome. Page Ref: 165

160. The barrel chest is an enlargement of the diameter of the chest. In the disease process of emphysema the elasticity of the alveoli is lost. This creates an inability to exhale adequate amounts of air and leaves air trapped in the lungs. As the disease progresses, the overinflated lungs create an expansion of the chest. Page Ref: 172

161. A tracheotomy is an incision into the trachea. A tracheostomy is a permanent opening created by a tracheotomy. A tube is inserted to keep the opening patent (open) and to help facilitate removal of secretions. A tracheostomy helps provide access to the lungs in a patient who needs long-term respiratory support or mechanical ventilation. Page Ref: 186

162. Bronchodilator drugs dilate constricted airways by relaxing the smooth muscles that surround the bronchi and bronchioles. These drugs are used in asthma and any condition that causes bronchoconstriction. Page Ref: 187

163. Mast cell stabilizer drugs help stabilize mast cells in the respiratory tract. When a mast cell is stabilized, it will not break down and release histamine and other chemicals that cause bronchoconstriction. These drugs are used primarily to help prevent asthma attacks. Page Ref: 187

164. The respiratory system begins in the nose and mouth and continues to the pharynx (throat), larynx (voice box), and trachea (windpipe). The trachea divides into the right and left mainstem bronchi and right and left lungs. The bronchi further divide into smaller and smaller bronchi branches, and eventually into the smallest airway branches—bronchioles. The bronchioles eventually lead to the alveoli, tiny air sacs that comprise the actual functional tissue of the lungs. Page Ref: 155

165. The pleura is a membrane that lines the outer surface of the lungs, and doubles back on itself to line the thoracic cavity. There is fluid between the layers of the pleura, which makes it easy for the pleura to slide against itself during breathing. Page Ref: 159

CHAPTER 5

Multiple Choice

1. c. The radial artery carries blood to the lower arm along the side by the thumb. Page Ref: 213, 249

2. b. Choices A, C, and D involve blockage of coronary arteries, whereas endocarditis involves the inner lining and valves of the heart. Page Ref: 229

3. a. The tricuspid valve is named for its three triangular leaflets, or cusps. Page Ref: 208

4. c. Although an elevated level of low density lipoprotein (LDL) is a risk factor for development of a myocardial infarction, it is not a diagnostic indicator as the others are. Page Ref: 241-242

5. c. Coronary artery bypass graft is a surgical procedure that transplants a vein harvested from the leg into the coronary artery that is blocked, creating a new avenue for blood supply to a part of the myocardium. Rerouting of the internal mammary artery can also be done to provide a new source of blood supply to the myocardium. Page Ref: 251

6. d. Demands put on the heart from other conditions cause the heart to enlarge and eventually it is unable to contract sufficiently to send an adequate amount of blood to the body. Page Ref: 229-230

7. a. A sphygmomanometer measures blood pressure. The pressure is measured in millimeters (mm) of mercury (Hg). Page Ref: 250

8. c. Regurgitat/o- means flow backward and -ion means action or condition. Page Ref: 233

9. c. The left atrium receives the blood from the lungs. Page Ref: 215-216

10. b. Blocked coronary arteries with a decreased blood flow and oxygen to the myocardium will cause chest pain referred to as angina pectoris. Page Ref: 229

11. a. Sclerotherapy is done by injecting a substance into the varicose vein to harden and occlude it. Page Ref: 249

12. d. Ventricular fibrillation is a very dangerous arrhythmia. The defibrillator is applied to the chest of the patient to deliver a strong electrical shock to the heart to restore normal sinus rhythm. Page Ref: 248

13. d. Tampon/o- means stop up, and -ade means action or process. Page Ref: 231

14. d. The impulses from the SA node in the right atrium are not relayed to the ventricles due to a complete block at the AV node. Page Ref: 235

15. b. The heart valves in rheumatic heart disease are vulnerable to pathology such as scarring and narrowing. Page Ref: 233

16. c. Digitalis decreases the heart rate and strengthens its contraction. Page Ref: 255

17. b. An aneurysm is an area of arterial wall weakness that must be removed because it bulges outward and can rupture without warning. Page Ref: 251

18. d. Narrowing of the arteries of the legs with decreased circulation causes pain on walking. Page Ref: 239

19. c. The bundle of His is the next part of the conduction system after the AV node. Page Ref: 217

20. c. Sick sinus syndrome is a condition in which rapid and then slow heart rates occur. Patients with this condition benefit from anti-arrhythmia drugs and pacemaker insertion to control the abnormal heart rhythms. Page Ref: 235, 252

21. d. In right-sided heart failure, the right ventricle is unable to adequately pump blood. Page Ref: 229

22. c. A thrombolyic medication is used to break apart formed blood clots. Page Ref: 256

23. a. A narrowed pulmonary valve along with a ventricular septal defect, enlarged right ventricle, and malposition of the aorta are the anomalies of the tetralogy of Fallot. Page Ref: 233

24. a. X-ray studies performed during a cardiac catheterization show how much coronary artery blockage is present. Page Ref: 242

25. d. Telemetry is a monitoring of a patient's heart rate and rhythm with transmission of the information to a central monitoring system. Cardiac arrest is the stopping of effective heart action. Page Ref: 244

26. c. The cardiovascular system is a continuous, circular body system that includes the heart and all of the vascular structures or blood vessels (arteries, capillaries, and veins). Page Ref: 207

27. d. There are four hollow chambers inside the heart—the right atrium and left atrium on top and the right ventricle and left ventricle on the bottom. Page Ref: 207

28. a. The mitral valve with its two leaflets opens as blood flows into the left ventricle and then closes to prevent blood from flowing back into the left atrium. This valve is also known as the bicuspid valve. Page Ref: 208

29. a. My/o- means muscle, cardi/o- means heart, and -um means structure or tissue. Page Ref: 209

30. b. The aorta receives oxygenated blood from the heart and distributes it to the body. Page Ref: 212

31. d. Perone/o- means fibula (lower leg bone), -al means pertaining to. Page Ref: 213

32. c. All veins have one-way, cup-shaped valves that keep the blood flowing in one direction, toward the heart. These valves prevent the blood from flowing backwards toward the capillaries. Page Ref: 214

33. b. The sinoatrial node or pacemaker of the heart is a small area of tissue in the posterior wall of the right atrium. Page Ref: 217

34. c. Epinephrine overrides the normal sinus rhythm and causes the heart to beat faster to support increased activity during exercise or periods of physical stress. Page Ref: 218

35. d. In dilated cardiomyopathy, the left ventricle is dilated and the myocardium is so stretched that it can no longer contract to pump blood. Idiopathic cardiomyopathy has an unknown cause. Page Ref: 229

36. a. Myocardial infarction is death of myocardial cells due to severe ischemia. Page Ref: 230

37. b. Endocarditis occurs in patients who already have a structural defect of the valves of the heart. Page Ref: 231

38. a. The foramen ovale is a normal opening in the septum that closes at birth. It is not a congenital abnormality. ASD, VSD, and tetralogy of Fallot are congenital abnormalities of the heart. Page Ref: 233

39. c. An aneurysm is an area of dilation and weakness in the wall of the artery. Page Ref: 235

40. c. Hyper- means above or more than normal, and tens/o- means pressure. Page Ref: 238

41. a. Raynaud's phenomenon was discovered by Maurice Raynaud, a French physician. Page Ref: 240

42. b. CRP is a blood test to measure the level of inflammation in the body. Page Ref: 241

43. a. The suffix -metry means the process of measuring. Telemetry is a diagnostic procedure to monitor a patient's heart rate and rhythm on a

monitor at the nurses' station in the CCU or ICU. Page Ref: 244

44. d. Radiopaque contrast dye is injected. It flows into the coronary arteries and shows stenosis or blockage. The x-ray image is known as a coronary angiogram. Page Ref: 245

45. c. A SPECT scan is a nuclear medicine procedure that uses the radioactive tracer technetium-99m. Page Ref: 246

46. a. A Doppler image can also show blockages or clots in the vessel. Doppler technology is also used in automatic blood pressure machines and in fetal monitors. Page Ref: 247

47. b. A vital sign is a medical procedure during a physical examination to measure the temperature, pulse, and respirations (TPR), as well as the blood pressure. Page Ref: 249

48. d. Heart transplantation is a surgical procedure to remove a severely damaged heart from a patient with end-stage heart failure and insert a new heart from a donor (a patient that has recently died). Page Ref: 251

49. c. Septum is a Latin word meaning a partition. Page Ref: 208

50. b. Chordae tendinae is a Latin phrase meaning cords like tendons. Page Ref: 208

51. a. The myocardium is the muscular layer of the heart. Page Ref: 209

52. d. The coronary arteries are the first arteries to branch off from the aorta. Page Ref: 213

53. d. Capillaries connect the arteries and veins. Page Ref: 214

54. b. The sinoatrial node is an area of specialized nervous tissue in the heart that is also called the pacemaker of the heart. Page Ref: 217

55. a. The refractory period is normal and helps the heart rest between beats. Page Ref: 218

56. c. The ductus arteriosus allows oxygenated blood from the mother to go directly from the pulmonary artery to the aorta and to the whole body. Page Ref: 220

57. d. Angina pectoris is caused by coronary artery disease that blocks the flow of oxygenated blood to the myocardium. Page Ref: 229

58. c. Endocarditis occurs in patients who already have a structural defect of the valves or heart. Page Ref: 231

59. c. Intra- means within. Intraventricular blood is found within the right and left ventricles. Page Ref: 208

60. c. Bicuspid (by-KUS-pid), bi- means two, cusp/o- means projection, point, and -id means resembling; source or origin. Page Ref: 208

61. a. Septum (SEP-tum) is derived from a Latin word meaning a partition. Page Ref: 208

62. b. Epicardium (EP-ih-KAR-dee-um), epi- means upon, above, cardi/o- means heart, and -um means a structure. Page Ref: 209

63. a. Pericardial (PAIR-ih-KAR-dee-al), peri- means around, cardi/o- means heart, and -al means pertaining to. Page Ref: 209

64. b. Cardiothoracic (KAR-dee-oh-thoh-RAS-ik), cardi/o- means heart, thorac/o- means thorax, (chest), and -ic means pertaining to. Page Ref: 210

65. b. Lumen (LOO-men) is a Latin word meaning window. Page Ref: 210

66. a. Vasoconstriction (VAY-soh-con-STRIK-shun), vas/o- means blood vessel; vas deferens, constrict/o- means drawn together, narrowed, and -ion means action; condition. Page Ref: 211

67. d. Femoral (FEM-oh-ral), femor/o- means femur (thigh bone), -al means pertaining to (see Figure 5-9). Page Ref: 212

68. d. Popliteal (pop-LIT-ee-al) (pop-lih-TEE-al), poplite/o- means back of the knee, -al means pertaining to. Page Ref: 213

69. c. High-density lipoproteins (HDLs) are carriers for cholesterol in the blood. Page Ref: 242

70. a. Lumen is a Latin word meaning window. Page Ref: 210

71. d. Angina pectoris is a condition that precedes a myocardial infarction. Ischemia is a condition that precedes cell death. Page Ref: 229

72. b. Peri- means around, card/i- means heart, and -itis means inflammation of. Page Ref: 231

73. d. The septum is the dividing wall between the chambers of the heart. Page Ref: 208

74. c. An electrocardiogram creates a record of the electrical activity of the heart, which includes P waves and QRS complexes. Page Ref: 243

75. a. Essential hypertension is the most common type of hypertension. Page Ref: 238

76. b. Aneurysm means a dilation. Page Ref: 236

77. d. Blood backs up in the inferior vena cava because the right side of the heart cannot pump it out quickly enough. Fluid in the blood goes out into the tissues of the legs and feet and causes edema. Page Ref: 230

78. b. Intra- means within, ventricul/o- means ventricle, and -al means pertaining to. Page Ref: 208

79. a. The apex of the heart is the tip of the heart that surrounds the ventricles where the point of maximum impulse (PMI) of the heart sounds is heard most distinctly for auscultation. Page Ref: 249, 257

80. b. The coronary arteries supply oxygenated blood to the myocardium of the heart. Page Ref: 213

81. c. The common carotid artery brings oxygenated blood to the brain, head, and face. Page Ref: 213

82. a. The popliteal artery carries blood behind the knee to the lower leg. Page Ref: 213

83. d. The common iliac arteries are the two artery branches that arise where the abdominal aorta ends. Page Ref: 212

84. a. The systemic circulation goes to the body and is separate from the pulmonary circulation that goes to the lungs. The coronary arteries provide blood to the heart but are not a separate type of circulation. Page Ref: 212

85. c. The foramen ovale is a temporary opening in the septum of the fetal heart that allows oxygenated blood from the umbilical cord to circulate throughout the body. Page Ref: 216

86. b. Cardi/o- means heart and -megaly means enlargement. Page Ref: 229

87. b. Ather/o- means soft, fatty substance [plaque], scler/o- means hard, and -osis means abnormal condition. Page Ref: 237

88. a. High-density lipoproteins (HDL) carry cholesterol in the blood and take it to the liver where it is made into bile and excreted from the body. Page Ref: 217

89. d. The echo of sound waves bounced off the heart create the image. Page Ref: 247

90. a. Phleb/o- is the Greek combining form meaning vein. Page Ref: 258

91. c. Arteriosclerosis is hardening of the arteries due to plaque and the formation of collagen fibers under the plaque that make the artery wall hard and non-elastic. Page Ref: 217

92. d. Defibrillation uses an electrical shock to the patient's chest to restore the heart to a regular rhythm. Page Ref: 248

93. d. Ather/o- means fatty substance. Atherosclerosis is a disease of the blood vessels, but ather/o- refers to the disease process, not the blood vessel itself. Page Ref: 217

94. b. The correct spelling is arrhythmia. Page Ref: 233

95. d. High-density lipoproteins (HDL) carry cholesterol in the blood and are known as "good cholesterol." Page Ref: 257

96. a. Coronary artery bypass graft (CABG) is pronounced as "cabbage" or as "C-A-B-G." Page Ref: 251

Short Answer

97. cardiomegaly. Cardi/o- means heart and -megaly means enlargement. Page Ref: 229

98. coronary. Coronary means pertaining to an encircling structure because these arteries encircle the heart. Page Ref: 213

99. asystole (or cardiac arrest). A- means without and systole means contracting. Page Ref: 234

100. aorta; venae cavae. The aorta takes blood from the heart to the body, and the superior and inferior vena cavae bring blood from the body to the heart. Page Ref: 212, 214

101. electrocardiography or EKG. Occasional arrhythmias are difficult to detect except with a 24-hour monitor. Page Ref: 244

102. bradycardia. Brady- means sow, card/i- means heart, -ia means condition. Page Ref: 234

103. saphenous. The saphenous vein from the leg is used as a graft vessel. Page Ref: 251

104. Raynaud's. Vasoconstriction and arterial spasm are characteristic of this disease. In Raynaud's phenomenon, blood vessels become smaller in diameter and blood flow is decreased. Page Ref: 240

105. arteriosclerotic heart disease. This is the presence of plaque and collagen fibers that narrow and harden the arteries. Page Ref: 236

106. carotid. The common carotid artery branches into the external carotid artery to the neck, mouth, and face, and the internal carotid artery to the brain. Page Ref: 213

107. valves. There are four valves in the heart: the tricuspid valve, pulmonary valve, mitral valve, and aortic valve. Page Ref: 208

108. Auscultation. Ascult/o- means listening. Page Ref: 248

109. mediastinum. Mediastinum is derived from a Latin word meaning a lower servant who performs duties. Perhaps the mediastinum seemed like a smaller, less important area compared to the larger, active thoracic cavity. Page Ref: 210

110. pacemaker. The SA node is a small area of tissue in the posterior wall of the right atrium. Page Ref: 217

111. epinephrine. Epinephrine is released during exercise and periods of physical stress. Page Ref: 218

112. Cardiomegaly. Cardi/o- means heart and -megaly means enlargement. Page Ref: 229

113. septum. Septum is a Latin word meaning a partition. Page Ref: 233

114. Bradycardia. Brady- means slow, -cardia means pertaining to the heart. Page Ref: 234

115. premature. Premature contraction is also known as extrasystole Page Ref: 235

116. aneurysm. An aneurysm is a bulging, weak area in the arterial wall. Page Ref: 236

117. Cardiology. Cardi/o- means heart, -logy means the study of. Page Ref: 206

118. tricuspid. Tricuspid (try-KUS-pid), tri- means three, cusp/o- means projection, point, and -id means resembling; source or origin. Page Ref: 208

119. mitral. Mitral (MY-tral), mitr/o- means structure like a miter (tall hat with two points), -al means pertaining to. Page Ref: 208

120. myocardium. Myocardium (MY-oh-KAR-dee-um), my/o- means muscle, cardi/o- means heart, and -um means a structure. Page Ref: 209

121. endocardium. Endocardium (EN-doh-KAR-dee-um), endo- means innermost, within, cardi/o- means heart, and -um means a structure. Page Ref: 209

122. mediastinum. Mediastinum (MEE-dee-as-TY-num) is derived from a Latin word meaning a lower servant who performs duties. Perhaps the mediastinum seemed like a smaller, less important area compared to the larger, active thoracic cavity. Page Ref: 210

123. Vasculature. Vasculature (VAS-kyoo-lah-chur), vascul/o- means blood vessel, -ature means system. Page Ref: 210

124. endothelium. Endothelium (EN-doh-THEE-lee-um), endo- means innermost, within, theli/o- means tissue layer, and -um means a chemical element; a structure. Page Ref: 210

125. arterioles. Arteriole (ar-TEER-ee-ohl), arteri/o- means artery, -ole means small thing. Page Ref: 211

126. vasoconstriction. Vasoconstriction (VAY-soh-con-STRIK-shun), vas/o- means blood vessel; vas deferens, constrict/o- means drawn together, narrowed, and -ion means action; condition. Page Ref: 211

127. coronary. Coronary (KOR-oh-nair-ee), coron/o- means encircling structure and -ary means pertaining to. Coronary is derived from a Latin word meaning crown. The coronary arteries sit on the surface of the heart and encircle it like a crown. Page Ref: 212

128. systole; diastole. Systole is the contraction of the heart muscle, and diastole is the resting of the heart muscle while the chambers fill with blood. Page Ref: 217

129. cardiologist. Cardi/o- means heart, log/o- means the study of, and -ist means one who specializes in. Page Ref: 258

130. Myocardial infarction. Myocardial means pertaining to the heart muscle. Infarct/o- means area of dead tissue, and -ion means condition. Page Ref: 230

131. Cardiology. Cardi/o- means heart, and -logy means the study of. Page Ref: 206

132. process of reshaping by surgery. Valvoplasty is a surgical procedure to reconstruct a heart valve to correct stenosis or prolapse. Page Ref: 253

133. digitalis. Digitalis dosages were not regulated in the late 1800s, and the drug can easily reach toxic levels in the blood. Page Ref: 255

134. bradycardia. Tachy- means fast, and brady- means slow. Page Ref: 234, 236

135. aneurysmectomy. -Ectomy means surgical excision. Page Ref: 251

True/False

136. True. Secondary hypertension has a known cause, such as kidney disease. Page Ref: 239

137. False. It is the sinoartrial node or SA node. Page Ref: 217

138. True. Systole means a contracting, and diastole means an expansion (resting and filling). Page Ref: 217

139. False. This is called a pharmacologic stress test using Persantine, a drug injected into the patient to dilate the coronary arteries. Doppler is a type of ultrasound to test blood flow. Page Ref: 244, 247

140. False. These are palpitations. Palpation is using the fingers to feel or palpate the body. Page Ref: 235

141. True. Paroxysmal tachycardia is an episode of rapid heart rate that occurs suddenly. Page Ref: 236

142. False. It is the endocardium. Page Ref: 209

143. True. These drugs can also be used to treat other heart problems as well. Page Ref: 255, 256

144. False. It stands for acute myocardial infarction. Page Ref: 257

145. True. The gamma camera records multiple images that are coordinated (gated) with the EKG during a multiple-gated acquisition (MUGA) scan. Page Ref: 246

146. False. A heart murmur is an abnormal sound that the heart makes as blood leaks past a defective heart valve. Page Ref: 231

147. True. This is a structural abnormality in which the leaflets of the mitral valve do not close tightly, letting blood in the left ventricle come back into the left atrium. Page Ref: 233

148. True. These are all disturbances to the heart rhythm and are known as arrhythmias. Page Ref: 234-235

149. False. Because the blood pressure is higher than normal, it can be said that the patient is hypertensive, not hypotensive. Page Ref: 238-239

150. True. Hyperlipidemia is a general word for any condition with elevated levels of fats (including cholesterol) in the blood. Page Ref: 241

151. True. Several cardiac enzymes appear within specific time frames after a heart attack. Page Ref: 241

152. False. A cardiac catheterization can be done to diagnose a problem with either the left side or the right side of the heart. Page Ref: 242

153. True. The resulting x-ray image is known as an angiogram. Page Ref: 245

154. True. The drug causes irritation and inflammation that later becomes hardened fibrosis that occludes the vein. Page Ref: 249

155. False. Antihypertensive drugs are used to treat high blood pressure. Page Ref: 254

156. False. The pericardium creates the pericardial sac. The bundle of His is part of the electrical conduction system of the heart. Page Ref: 209

157. False. The endocardium is the inner lining of the heart chambers. The endothelium is the smooth inner lining of the blood vessels. Page Ref: 209, 210

158. False. The pulmonary arteries carry deoxygenated blood away from the heart to the lungs. Page Ref: 216

159. False. The largest artery in the body is the aorta. Page Ref: 212

160. True. Men experience angina pectoris as crushing chest pain, while women are more likely to experience angina pectoris as indigestion, fatigue, or nausea. Page Ref: 229

161. True. A Holter monitor is worn for 24 hours to record arrhythmias that only happen occasionally. Page Ref: 244

162. False. The heart can only get oxygenated blood through the coronary arteries. Page Ref: 213

163. False. Triglycerides are a fatty substance that is formed from excessive amounts of sugar in the diet. Triglycerides are not related to cholesterol. Page Ref: 237

164. False. A prolapse occurs when the valve leaflets do not close tightly because they are drooping down. Page Ref: 233

165. False. During angina pectoris, the heart muscle cells are in need of oxygen, but they do not die. Page Ref: 229

166. True. Auscult/o- means listening, and -ation means a process. Page Ref: 248

Essay

167. Ventricular fibrillation is a very fast, irregular heart rate. Because the heart is beating so quickly, the chambers do not have time to fill with blood. Cardiac output is severely decreased and blood is not distributed to the body including to the myocardium. If this arrhythmia continues, the heart will stop. Page Ref: 234

168. In the percutaneous transluminal coronary angioplasty (PTCA), a catheter with a balloon attached is inserted into a coronary artery that is blocked with plaque. The balloon is inflated and the plaque is compressed against the arterial walls. This then allows for a larger area for the blood to flow. A stent may be inserted with the balloon. The stent is left in place after the balloon and catheter are withdrawn, leaving improved coronary artery blood flow. Page Ref: 253

169. High-density lipoprotein (HDL) is a lipoprotein that carries cholesterol in the blood. It is ordered as part of a lipid profile. Lactic dehydrogenase (LDH) is an enzyme present in the heart muscle. Its levels rise after a myocardial infarction. It is one of the tests done to help diagnose a myocardial infarction. Page Ref: 241, 242

170. Aspirin helps prevent heart attacks in patients with known risk. It helps prevent blood clots from forming by keeping platelets from aggregating and sticking together. Page Ref: 254

171. Calcium channel blockers are drugs that block the movement of calcium ions into myocardial cells and smooth muscle cells of the artery walls, causing the heart rate and blood pressure to decrease. They are used to treat angina pectoris, congestive heart failure, and hypertension. Page Ref: 255

172. The pulmonary arteries carry blood that is low in oxygen and high in carbon dioxide. This blood is passed through capillaries in the lungs, where the carbon dioxide is released and oxygen is picked up. The capillaries then join into the pulmonary veins where the oxygen-rich blood is carried to the heart to be distributed to the body through the systemic circulation. Page Ref: 216

173. The conduction system of the heart starts with the sinoatrial node (SA), which initiates the electrical rhythm. From the SA node, the electrical impulse travels to the atrioventricular node (AV), to the bundle of His, and then down the right and left bundle branches in the interventricular septum. At the apex of the heart, the right and left bundles separate, and the electrical impulse spreads across the ventricles in a network of nerves called the Purkinje fibers, causing both ventricles to contract simultaneously. Page Ref: 217-218

174. Angina pectoris is mild-to-severe chest pain, jaw pain, pain radiating down the arm, or indigestion-like pain caused by ischemia of the myocardium. It is caused by coronary artery disease in which atherosclerosis blocks the flow of oxygenated blood through the coronary arteries to the myocardium. Page Ref: 229

CHAPTER 6

Multiple Choice

1. c. Aplastic anemia is a decrease of all types of blood cells due to a failure of bone marrow production. Pancytopenia: pan means all, cyto means cell, and penia means decrease. Page Ref: 300

2. b. Multiple myeloma is a malignancy of plasma cells. These cells produce the abnormal immunoglobin Bence Jones protein. Page Ref: 314

3. a. Red bone marrow cells are collected from a matched donor and inserted into the patient intravenously. Page Ref: 317

4. b. Procrit stimulates the bone marrow to produce erythrocytes. Page Ref: 319

5. c. Coagul/o- means clotting and -ation means a process. Page Ref: 307

6. a. Also called the MonoSpot, this test detects antibodies formed against the virus that causes infectious mononucleosis. Page Ref: 313

7. d. Folic acid and vitamin B_{12} are among the necessary nutrients to form healthy erythrocytes. Page Ref: 302

8. b. RBC indices include testing for the mean (or average) cell volume as well as the mean cell hemoglobin and mean cell hemoglobin concentration. Page Ref: 311

9. d. These are examples of drugs used for HIV infections and AIDS. None of the other abbreviations are diseases that require drug therapy. Page Ref: 320

10. a. Albumin is a large protein molecule that stays in the blood and holds water in the blood by osmotic pressure. Page Ref: 284

11. c. Factor VIII is the antihemophilic factor that is missing due to a genetic abnormality in hemophilia A. Page Ref: 308

12. b. As a storage area for whole blood, the spleen can release extra blood into circulation upon need. Page Ref: 289

13. d. The red blood cells in iron deficiency anemia are small in size, or microcytic, and pale in color, or hypochromic. Page Ref: 302

14. a. Antibodies made in the recipient's blood attack the donor's blood cells and cause them to break apart. Hem/o- means blood and -lysis means break apart. Page Ref: 304

15. a. Maternal IgA antibodies passed on through breast milk are absorbed into the infant's bloodstream. This provides a borrowed source of immunity until the infant produces his own antibodies. Page Ref: 291

16. d. These are various names used to refer to the specialized lymphocyte that is invaded by the AIDS virus. Page Ref: 290

17. b. The laboratory test for partial thromboplastin measures the time it takes for a sample of blood to clot. Heparin is an anticoagulant so the clotting time is lengthened. Page Ref: 312

18. c. Neutrophils specifically act as destroyers of bacteria by phagocytosis. Phag/o- means swallowing, cyt/o- means cell, and -osis means condition. Page Ref: 280

19. a. The hematocrit reports the percentage of red blood cells. Page Ref: 311

20. d. Lack of exercise causes blood to pool in the veins and predisposes the patient to development of a blood clot. Heparin is an anticoagulant used to prevent clotting. Page Ref: 307

21. b. This is a test using radioactive vitamin B_{12}. The patient's inability to absorb B_{12} is measured, confirming the diagnosis. Page Ref: 314

22. c. During circulation these red blood cells become misshapen like crescents. Page Ref: 303

23. b. Apheresis is a Greek word meaning removal. Page Ref: 316

24. c. Testing for ferritin indirectly measures the amount of iron stored in the patient's body. Page Ref: 313

25. d. This category would include any abnormally shaped RBC, such as the crescent-shaped erythrocyte found in sickle cell anemia. Page Ref: 301

26. a. Hematopoiesis occurs in the sternum, ribs, hip bones, bones of the spinal column, and the long bones of the legs. Page Ref: 279

27. b. Serum is a Latin word that means whey. When milk curdles, it separates into the curds (solids) and whey (liquid). Page Ref: 277

28. a. Neutrophils are the most common leukocyte. Page Ref: 280

29. c. Thrombocytes are also called platelets. Within seconds of an injury, they form clumps that help to block the flow of blood. Thrombocytes also contain some clotting factors that may be released to begin the formation of a blood clot. Page Ref: 284

30. d. A antigens are present on the erythrocytes of a person with type A blood. Anti-B antibodies are present in the plasma of a person with type A blood. Page Ref: 285

31. d. Blood type O is the universal donor because its erythrocytes do not have antigens against either the type A or type B blood. In an emergency situation, blood type O negative can be given to patients with any other blood type without causing a transfusion reaction. Page Ref: 285

32. c. The combining form aggreg/o- means crowding together. When thrombocytes stick to the damaged area of the blood vessel and form clumps to block the blood flow, this process is called aggregation. Page Ref: 286

33. b. The immune response detects pathogens that arise in the body. Page Ref: 289

34. a. In active immunity, B cells become plasma cells and produce the antibody IgG specific to that pathogen. When the pathogen again invades the body, the antibodies coat it and target it for destruction. Page Ref: 291

35. b. Immunoglobulin D is present in B cells. It stimulates the B cell to become a plasma cell. Page Ref: 291

36. d. There are five classes of immunoglobin: IgA, IgD, IgE, IgG, and IgM. Page Ref: 291

37. c. Mega- means large, kary/o- means nucleus, and -cyte means cell. A megakaryocyte contains a large nucleus and a large amount of cytoplasm. Page Ref: 284

38. d. Anemia can have many causes. An- means without and -emia means substance in the blood. Page Ref: 301

39. b. A- means without, plast/o- means being formed, and -ic means pertaining to. In aplastic

anemia, the total number of erythrocytes is decreased, even though individual erythrocytes are normocytic (normal size) and normochromic (normal in color). Page Ref: 301

40. a. Polycythemia vera is due to uncontrolled production by the red marrow. The cause is unknown. Page Ref: 303

41. a. Leukemia is named according to the type of immature or mature leukocyte that is most prevalent and whether the onset of symptoms is acute or chronic. Page Ref: 305

42. c. The symptoms of mononucleosis include lymphadenopathy, fever, and fatigue. It is often referred to as the kissing disease because it commonly affects young adults and is transmitted through contact with saliva that contains the virus. Page Ref: 306

43. d. Activated clotting time (ACT) is more accurate than partial thromboplastin time (PTT) when the patient is on high-dose heparin. A prolonged (rather than normal) clotting time is desirable to prevent blood clots. Page Ref: 312

44. b. During plasmapheresis, a donor gives a unit of blood which is rapidly spun in a centrifuge. Centrifrugal force pulls the blood cells to the bottom of the bag. The plasma portion at the top is siphoned off, and the blood cells are given back to the donor. Page Ref: 317

45. d. Corticosteroid drugs are anti-inflammatory drugs that are also given to organ transplant patients to prevent rejection of the donor organ. Page Ref: 319

46. d. Hemat/o- means blood and -poiesis means condition of formation. Page Ref: 279

47. a. Plasma is the clear, straw-colored liquid portion of the blood. Page Ref: 277

48. a. The erythrocyte is the most numerous type of blood cell. Page Ref: 280-282

49. a. Leukocytes are also known as white blood cells. Erythrocytes are also known as red blood cells. Page Ref: 280-282

50. d. Thrombocytes or platelets are active in the blood clotting process. Page Ref: 284

51. c. Albumin is the plasma protein that exerts an osmotic pressure that keeps water in the plasma. Page Ref: 288

52. d. Aggregation is the crowding together of thrombocytes as they stick in damaged tissue. Page Ref: 286

53. d. The immune response can detect and destroy all of these things. Page Ref: 289

54. c. Blood dyscrasia includes any disease of the blood cells. Page Ref: 300

55. b. The red blood cells are the keys to diagnosing anemia. Page Ref: 312

56. a. DVT stands for deep vein thrombus, a blood clot in one of the deep veins of the lower leg. Page Ref: 307

57. b. Thrombocytopenia (THRAWM-boh-SY-toh-PEE-nee-ah), thromb/o- means thrombus (blood clot), cyt/o- means cell, and -penia meanscondition of deficiency. Page Ref: 308

58. c. Lymphedema (LIM-fah-DEE-mah), lymph/o- means lymph, lymphatic, and -edema means swelling. Page Ref: 309

59. c. Agglutination (ah-GLOO-tih-NAY-shun), agglutin/o- means clumping, sticking, and -ation means a process. Agglutination is derived from a Latin word meaning glue. Page Ref: 310

60. a. Lymph is derived from a Latin word meaning clear spring water. Node is derived from a Latin word meaning a knob or mass of tissue. Page Ref: 287

61. a. Prothrombin (pro-THRAWM-bin), pro- means before, thromb/o- means thrombus (blood clot), and -in means a substance. Page Ref: 286

62. a. Platelet (PLAYT-let) is a combination of the English word plate and the suffix -let (little). Aggregation (AG-reh-GAY-shun), aggreg/o- means crowding together, and -ation means a process; being or having. Page Ref: 286

63. b. Lymphocyte (LIM-foh-site), lymph/o- means lymph, lymphatic system, and -cyte means cell. Page Ref: 282

64. a. The spleen does not produce red blood cells. That is done in the red marrow of the long or flat bones. Page Ref: 287

65. c. The lymphatic vessels or ducts empty into large veins in the neck. Page Ref: 287

66. d. The thymus is in the mediastinum, posterior to the sternum. Page Ref: 288

67. c. Interleukin is a chemical released by macrophages that have engulfed a virus. Page Ref: 290.

68. b. Micr/o- means small and -cyte means cell. Page Ref: 300, 302

69. c. During a transfusion reaction, antibodies in the patient's serum attack the red blood cells of the donor blood, causing hemolysis. Page Ref: 304

70. c. Leukemia is always classified as either acute or chronic. Page Ref: 307

71. c. Women are carriers of hemophilia, but only males contract the disease. Page Ref: 308

72. d. Auto- means self. Autologous blood is collected from the patient and given back to him or her. Page Ref: 317

73. b. The correct spelling is splenectomy. Page Ref: 318

74. c. Viscos/o- means thickness. Page Ref: 303

75. d. The correct spelling is hematocrit. Page Ref: 311

76. b. Rh factor is an antigen in the blood. Page Ref: 285

77. a. The white blood cell (WBC) differential measures the numbers of the five types of white blood cells. Page Ref: 313

78. b. Packed red blood cells (PRBCs) are a blood product given during a blood transfusion. Page Ref: 320

79. c. A red blood cell or erythrocyte contains hemoglobin that binds to oxygen. Page Ref: 278

80. c. Leukocytes are white blood cells that function in the immune response, not in blood clotting. Page Ref: 280

81. b. Eryth/o- means red. Page Ref: 278

82. c. Leukemia is a malignancy in which the white blood cells multiply uncontrollably. Page Ref: 305

83. a. Path/o- means disease and -gen means that which produces. Page Ref: 289

84. c. Anemia is a decreased number of red blood cells or poorly formed red blood cells that do not function properly. Page Ref: 301

85. a. Sickle cell anemia is an inherited genetic defect in an amino acid in the hemoglobin. Page Ref: 303

86. d. A bad sore throat would cause pathogens to be collected by the lymphatic capillaries, causing lymphadenopathy in that area. Page Ref: 309

87. a. The axillary lymph nodes filter lymphatic fluid from the breast tissues. Page Ref: 288, 309

88. a. A lymphoma is a cancerous tumor of lymphocytes or of lymph nodes. Page Ref: 309

89. d. T lymphocytes mature in the thymus, and B lymphocytes mature in the red marrow. Page Ref: 290

90. c. Meg/a- means large. Page Ref: 284

91. c. Albumin is the major protein molecule in the blood. Page Ref: 285

92. d. Erythrocytes contain the antigen for blood groups. Page Ref: 285

93. d. Too few red blood cells cause anemia. Page Ref: 301

94. d. Both sickle cell anemia and hemophilia are inherited disorders that are present at birth. Page Ref: 303, 308

95. b. Mononucleosis is caused by the Epstein-Barr virus and can be transmitted by contact with infected saliva. Page Ref: 306

96. c. The CD4 count is used to monitor the progress of AIDS. Page Ref: 313

97. d. Phlebotomy and venipuncture are the same procedure. Page Ref: 315

Short Answer

98. splenomegaly. Splen/o- means spleen, and -megaly means enlargement. Page Ref: 310

99. phlebotomy. Phleb/o- means vein and -otomy means incision. Page Ref: 315

100. plasma. This is the straw-colored liquid that is about 55% of the total volume of blood. Page Ref: 277

101. stem. Stem cells in the bone marrow give rise to every different type of blood cell. Page Ref: 279

102. Epstein-Barr. The Epstein-Barr virus is transmitted through contact with infected saliva. Page Ref: 307

103. hemorrhages. Petechiae are pinpoint hemorrhages caused by thrombocytopenia. Page Ref: 308

104. leukemia; leukemia. Leuk/o- means white, and -emia means substance in the blood. Page Ref: 305

105. hemoglobin. This forms the compound oxyhemoglobin. Page Ref: 278

106. autoimmune. Auto- means self and -immune means immune response. Page Ref: 310

107. Hematology. Hemat/o- means blood, and -logy means study of. Page Ref: 276

108. hematopoiesis. Hemat/o- means blood, and -poiesis, means condition of formation. Page Ref: 279

109. erythroblast. Erythr/o- means red, and -blast means immature cell. Page Ref: 279

110. neutrophil. The neutrophil is one of five different types of white blood cells. Page Ref: 280

111. macrocytes. The prefix in the term, macr/o-, gives a hint to the fact that this cell can handle large amounts of cellular debris. Page Ref: 282

112. fibrin. This is the last step in the activation of the clotting factors. Page Ref: 286

113. complement. They coat the pathogen and kill it by making holes in it. Page Ref: 291

114. Passive. The maternal antibodies, which are present as passive immunity, provide protection from all of the diseases that the mother has had. Page Ref: 291

115. Hematology. Hemat/o- means blood, and -logy means the study of. Page Ref: 276

116. Immunology. Immun/o- means immune response, and -logy means the study of. Page Ref: 276

117. plasma. Plasma is left when the cells are removed from the blood. Page Ref: 277

118. serum. Serum (SEER-um) is a Latin word meaning whey. When milk curdles, it separates into the curds (solids) and whey (liquid). Page Ref: 277

119. Erythrocytes. Erythrocyte (eh-RITH-roh-site), erythr/o- means red, and -cyte means cell. Page Ref: 278

120. Hemoglobin. Hemoglobin (HEE-moh-GLOH-bin), hem/o- means blood, glob/o- means shaped like a globe; comprehensive, and -in means a substance. Page Ref: 278

121. Hematopoiesis. Hematopoiesis (HEE-mah-toh-poy-EE-sis), hemat/o- means blood, and -poiesis means condition of formation. Page Ref: 279

122. erythropoietin. Erythropoietin (eh-RITH-roh-POY-eh-tin), erythr/o- means red, and -poietin means a substance that forms. Add words to make a correct definition of erythropoietin: a substance that forms red [blood cells]. Page Ref: 279

123. Phagocytes. Phagocyte (FAG-oh-site), phag/o-means eating, swallowing, and -cyte means cell. Page Ref: 280

124. Basophils. Basophil (BAY-soh-fil), bas/o- means basic (alkaline), and -phil means attraction to, fondness for. Page Ref: 281

125. Monocytes. Monocyte (MAWN-oh-site), mon/o- means one, single, and -cyte means cell. Add words to make a correct and complete definition of monocyte: Cell [that has a] single [lobe in its nucleus]. Page Ref: 282

126. electrolytes. Electrolyte (ee-LEK-troh-lite), electr/o- means electricity, and -lyte means dissolved substance. An electrolyte is so named because it will conduct electricity when it is in a solution. Page Ref: 293

127. hemorrhage. Hemorrhage (HEM-oh-rij), hem/o- means blood, and -rrhage means excessive flow or discharge. Loss of a large amount of blood, externally or internally. Injury to an artery causes a forceful spurting of a large amount of bright red blood. Treatment: Tourniquet, pressure, or suturing to stop the bleeding. Page Ref: 300

128. neutrophil. Neutrophils are granulocytes because their cytoplasm shows large granules, which do not stain either red or blue (i.e., they are neutral), and there are more than three lobes in the nucleus. Page Ref: 283

129. lymphocyte. The lymphocyte has a round nucleus, nearly invisible granules in the cytoplasm, and there is little cytoplasm. Page Ref: 283

130. Lymphocytes; macrophages. Lymphocytes are present in both the blood and the lymph nodes. Macrophages are blood cells that play a role in the immune response by engulfing cells and cellular debris. Page Ref: 282

131. spleen. The spleen is a lymphoid organ located behind the stomach. Page Ref: 287, 289

True/False

132. True. Hemat/o- means blood and -poiesis means condition of forming. Page Ref: 279

133. False. They are called segmented neutrophils or segs. Bands or stabs are the immature neutrophils. Page Ref: 280

134. True. Antigens are proteins on the cell membrane of an erythrocyte. Page Ref: 285

135. False. These are abnormal lymphocytes found in the lymph nodes of patients with Hodgkins' disease. Page Ref: 309

136. True. Reticulocytes have a nucleus because they are not yet mature red blood cells. Page Ref: 279

137. False. Aspirin does not dissolve clots; it is used to prevent blood clot formation. Page Ref: 319

138. True. Hem/o- means blood, and -stasis means condition of standing still. Page Ref: 286

139. True. Removal of axillary lymph nodes is often part of breast cancer surgery. Absence of these lymph nodes leaves inadequate drainage for lymph in the arm on the side where the surgery was performed. Page Ref: 309

140. False. While it is true that donated blood is tested for HIV, the lab will perform a p24 antigen test. MonoSpot is a test to detect mononucleosis. Page Ref: 313

141. False. Immunology is the medical specialty that studies the anatomy and physiology of the lymphatic system. Page Ref: 276

142. True. These bones may include the sternum, ribs, hip bones, bones of the spinal column, and long bones of the legs. Page Ref: 279

143. False. The amount of plasma in the blood is related both to how much water is taken into the body and how much water is excreted from the body. Page Ref: 277

144. True. The center of a red blood cell is depressed, is not as thick, and is paler in color. Unlike most other cells, there is no nucleus. Page Ref: 278

145. True. These are the most active leukocytes in allergic reactions. Page Ref: 281

146. False. Monocytes are the largest of the leukocytes, and they are able to engulf large numbers of cells and cellular debris. They are also known as macrophages. Page Ref: 282

147. True. The prefix in the term anticoagulant is anti-, which means against. In this case it means against coagulation. Page Ref: 318

148. False. Thrombolytic enzymes dissolve blood clots by breaking the fibrin strands. Page Ref: 319

149. True. These drugs are given to prevent rejection of a transplanted organ. Page Ref: 319

150. True. Both of these drugs inhibit substances which the virus needs to reproduce itself. Page Ref: 319

151. True. Microorganisms or cancerous cells are carried by the lymphatic fluid in the lymphatic capillaries to a lymph node where they are destroyed. Page Ref: 287

152. False. The lymphatic system is not continuous. It begins at lymphatic capillaries and ends as large lymphatic ducts empty into large veins in the neck. Page Ref: 287

153. True. The tonsils and adenoids are lymphatic tissue, but their function is discussed in Otolaryngology (Chapter 16). Page Ref: 288

154. True. Cytokines are part of the immune response. Page Ref: 289

155. True. Tumor necrosis factor (TNF) is one of the substances produced by monocytes as part of the immune response. Page Ref: 290

156. False. The hematocrit measures the percentage of red blood cells compared to the entire sample. Page Ref: 311

157. False. Immunization and vaccination produce active immunity by stimulating the body's own immune system to identify a pathogen and make antibodies against it. Page Ref: 291

158. False. Red blood cells are the most numerous cells in the blood. Page Ref: 278

159. True. Thromb/o- means thrombus (blood clot) and -cyte means cell. Page Ref: 284

160. False. Hem/o- means blood, and -rrhage means excessive flow or discharge. Page Ref: 300

161. False. Leukemia is a cancer of the lymphocytes. Page Ref: 305

162. False. BA is not a blood type. Page Ref: 285

Essay

163. The red blood cells in these patients change into a crescent shape after releasing oxygen. These misshaped cells do not easily move through the capillaries. They tend to jam up in microcirculation, interfering with blood flow and causing pain. Page Ref: 303

164. For unknown reasons people with this disease produce too many erythrocytes. The patient's blood becomes thick and the increased blood volume causes a strain on the heart. Using phlebotomy and draining some blood reduces the blood volume. Page Ref: 303

165. A phlebotomist draws blood from a patient's vein. Phleb/o- means vein, tom/o- means a cut, and -ist means one who specializes in. Page Ref: 321

166. When the body is injured, the injured blood vessel constricts to decrease the amount of blood flow. Then circulating thrombocytes stick to the damaged area of the blood vessel wall and form clumps to block the blood flow, known as platelet aggregation. Next, clotting factors in the blood are activated and begin to produce strands of fibrin that trap erythrocytes and form a thrombus or blood clot. This process, known as coagulation, stops the bleeding. Page Ref: 286

167. Lymphangiography is a radiologic procedure in which a radiopaque contrast medium is injected into a lymphatic vessel. X-rays are taken of the lymph node chains as the dye travels through the lymphatic vessels. Page Ref: 314

168. This is an invasive procedure done to remove a specimen of bone marrow from the hip bone. It is done to help diagnose patients with known or suspected leukemia, lymphoma, and anemia to examine the stages of development of the blood cells. This procedure is also done to harvest bone marrow from a healthy donor to give to a patient as a bone marrow transplant. Page Ref: 315

169. A vaccination is a medical procedure that injects a vaccine into the body. A vaccine is a solution of killed or attenuated bacteria or viral cells or cell fragments. The body produces antibodies and memory B lymphocytes specific to that pathogen. If the vaccinated patient encounters that pathogen again, the patient will have mild or no symptoms of the disease. Vaccinations are routinely used to prevent diseases that could be fatal or cause serious disability if contracted. Page Ref: 316

170. A blood donation is a medical procedure by which a unit of whole blood is collected from a volunteer donor. After the blood has been donated, it can be given as a blood transfusion to a patient to correct or treat a number of medical problems. Page Ref: 316, 317

CHAPTER 7

Multiple Choice

1. c. Eschar is derived from a word meaning burn scab. Page Ref: 355

2. d. This is a slow-growing cancer that arises from the deepest layer of the epidermis of the skin. Page Ref: 363

3. a. Alopecia means hair falling out. Page Ref: 367

4. b. Electr/o- means electricity, sect/o- means to cut, and -ion means action. Page Ref: 371

5. c. PUVA stands for psoralen drug and ultraviolet A light therapy, which is used to treat psoriasis. Page Ref: 377

6. b. Cold sores are also known as fever blisters and have recurrent outbreaks. Page Ref: 358

7. c. Scleroderma is an autoimmune disorder with an unknown cause. Page Ref: 365

8. d. A furuncle is a boil. An incision and drainage (I & D) is done by making a cut into the abscess allowing the contents to come out. Page Ref: 357

9. a. Excori/o- means to take out skin and -ation means process. Page Ref: 357

10. d. Sudoriferous glands, or sweat glands, are a type of exocrine gland. Page Ref: 342

11. a. A verruca is a wart, and is a type of viral disease. Page Ref: 359

12. c. Tinea cruris is a fungal disease in the skin of the groin. Page Ref: 358

13. d. Xer/o- means dry. Although the other conditions may exhibit dryness of the skin, the med-

ical word for dry skin is xeroderma. Page Ref: 352

14. a. Comedos are blackheads, a characteristic of acne vulgaris. Page Ref: 365

15. b. Ecchymosis is also a type of contusion. Page Ref: 350

16. b. The Tzanck test is a laboratory test performed on fluid from viral lesions. Shingles is herpes varicella-zoster, a viral disease causing blister lesions on the skin. Page Ref: 370

17. d. Collagen is a firm, white protein in tissue fibers through the skin. Some people have the tendency to deposit excess collagen in the formation of scar tissue, creating keloids rather than normal scars. Page Ref: 356

18. b. Body hair becomes erect when the body gets cold. Pil/o- means hair and erect/o- means to stand up. Page Ref: 342

19. b. Skin turgor is an assessment of the skin's ability to snap back when pinched. A dehydrated patient's skin will stay elevated when pinched. Page Ref: 352

20. c. A macule is a flat, pigmented skin lesion. Page Ref: 351

21. a. Debridement is a surgical or medical procedure done in various ways to remove dead tissue or foreign bodies from wounds. Page Ref: 371

22. b. Rhytidectomy is commonly known as a face lift. Page Ref: 374

23. d. Vitiligo is patches of white skin without pigment caused by an autoimmune response. The albino person has depigmented skin from a condition acquired genetically. Page Ref: 354

24. d. Nix is a drug used to treat the infestation of lice or pediculosis. Page Ref: 359

25. b. Dermat/o- means skin, and -logy means the study of. Page Ref: 338

26. a. The purpose of the integumentary system is to protect the body. It is the body's first line of defense against invading microorganisms. Page Ref: 339

27. b. Melanin is a dark brown or black pigment. Page Ref: 340

28. d. The dermis contains arteries, veins, and nerves, as well as hair follicles, sebaceous glands, and sweat glands. Page Ref: 340

29. c. The subcutaneous tissue is composed of adipose tissue or fat that is the layer beneath the dermis. Page Ref: 341

30. a. Sebaceous glands secrete oil, and sudoriferous glands secrete sweat. Page Ref: 342

31. d. The combining form pil/o- means hair. Piloerection is when the hair follicles contract causing the hair to stand up and form a goosebump. Page Ref: 342

32. c. This severe systemic allergic reaction can cause a hypersensitive individual to go into anaphylactic shock. Page Ref: 344

33. c. A macule is a little spot or blemish in the skin. Page Ref: 351

34. b. Certain systemic diseases have distinctive characteristic rashes. Page Ref: 352

35. a. Albinism is a genetic mutation that causes nonfunctioning melanocytes that do not produce melanin. There is a lack of pigment in the skin, hair, and iris of the eyes. The patient is said to be an albino. Page Ref: 352

36. d. Striae or stretch marks in the skin of the abdomen and buttocks are the result of small tears in the dermis as the skin stretches to accommodate the pregnant uterus. Page Ref: 354

37. a. A first degree burn involves only the epidermis. A second degree burn involves the epidermis and the upper layer of the dermis. A third degree burn involves the epidermis and the entire dermis. There is no such thing as a fourth degree burn. Page Ref: 355

38. d. Keloid means resembling a tumor, because of its excessive size. Page Ref: 355

39. c. Herpes simplex virus type 2 is a sexually transmitted disease that causes vesicles in the genital area. These lesions tend to recur during illness and stress. Page Ref: 358

40. c. Tinea cruris is also known as jock itch. Page Ref: 358

41. a. Freckles contain groups of melanocytes that absorb sunlight and then produce more melanin, causing the skin to tan. Page Ref: 351

42. b. Poly- means many, much and -dactyly means condition of finger or toes. Page Ref: 362

43. b. Color varies from black to brown to red within the *same* lesion. Page Ref: 363

44. a. SLE is an autoimmune disorder characterized by deterioration of the collagen in the skin and connective tissues. Page Ref: 364

45. d. Schiz/o- means split, trich/o- means hair, and -ia means condition. Page Ref: 368

46. c. Arnault Tzanck was a Russian dermatologist; the Tzanck test was named after him. Page Ref: 370

47. c. Alphahydroxy acid (glycolic acid) provides the mildest chemical peel. Stronger chemical peels using trichloroacetic acid and phenol are usually done in surgery. Page Ref: 372

48. a. The combining form excis/o- means to cut out. The suffix -ion means action or condition and -al means pertaining to. An excisional biopsy involves cutting out the entire lesion. Page Ref: 373

49. b. Benadryl is an antipruritic drug, which is used to decrease itching. Page Ref: 376

50. d. Dermatology uses diagnostic tests, medical procedures, surgical procedures, and drugs to treat diseases of the skin. Page Ref: 338

51. d. The muscles are part of the musculoskeletal system. The skin, hair, and nails are all part of the integumentary system. Page Ref: 339-343

52. a. Only the epidermis and dermis are layers of the skin, and the epidermis is the thin, outermost layer of the skin. Page Ref: 339

53. c. The sebaceous glands are exocrine glands. The endocrine glands secrete substances directly into the blood. Adipose is a tissue, not a gland. Keratin is a fibrous protein, not a gland. Page Ref: 342

54. d. While the other choices could progress into life-threatening reactions, only anaphylaxis is considered life-threatening. Page Ref: 344

55. a. Lesions can result from any number of causes including disease or injury. Benign is a specific word meaning a tumor that is not cancerous. Malignant is a specific word meaning a tumor that is cancerous. Dermatitis is a specific word meaning inflammation of the skin. Page Ref: 351

56. b. The medical word for itching is pruritus. While poison ivy may be accompanied by rash, rash is not another name for itching. Xeroderma is excessive dryness of the skin. Dermatitis is the general category for any inflammation of the skin. Page Ref: 352

57. a. Only intradermal injections injected antigens into the skin to try to elicit a local allergic reaction. Page Ref: 369

58. d. Only curettage uses a curette to scrape off the superficial part of a skin lesion. Page Ref: 371

59. d. Only dermabrasion uses a wire brush or diamond to scrape the epidermis. Micro-dermabrasion uses aluminum oxide crystals to abrade and remove the epidermis. Chemical peel uses chemicals. Laser skin resurfacing uses a computer-controlled laser to vaporize the epidermis and some of the dermis. Page Ref: 372

60. d. Only a punch biopsy uses a cutter to remove a plug-shaped core of skin. Page Ref: 373

61. a. Psoriasis has silvery scales and plaques of excessive epidermal cells. Page Ref: 364

62. c. Deposits of collagen harden the internal organs in scleroderma. Page Ref: 365

63. a. Seborrhea is overproduction of sebum, but seborrheic dermatitis includes that plus dry skin and dermatitis. Page Ref: 367

64. d. Schiz/o- means split, trich/o- means hair, and -ia means condition. Page Ref: 368

65. a. Onych/o- means nail, myc/o- means fungus, and -osis means abnormal condition. Page Ref: 368

66. c. Clubbing refers to the curved, clublike appearance of the nail. Page Ref: 369

67. a. None of the answers other than skin resurfacing use chemicals, abrasions, or lasers. Page Ref: 372

68. a. Biopsy is the only answer that is performed for the purpose of diagnosis. Page Ref: 373

69. d. Ringworm is caused by a fungus that is treated with an antifungal drug. Page Ref: 376

70. c. Intra- means within, and derm/o- means dermis. The dermis is just beneath the epidermis. Page Ref: 377

71. a. First-degree burns involve the epidermis and cause redness but not blisters. Page Ref: 355

72. c. Normal flora are bacterial that grow on the skin but do not cause disease. Page Ref: 343

73. d. As we age, melanocytes die and the hair contains no melanin and so is white. Page Ref: 342

74. a. Follicles are cells in the dermis that produce hairs. Page Ref: 342

75. b. Adipocere is the waxy decomposition of adipose tissue in a dead body. Page Ref: 342

76. d. Dermat/o- means skin and -itis means inflammation of. Page Ref: 350

77. c. A cyst is an elevated circular mound that is semisolid or partly fluid filled. Page Ref: 351

78. b. A scale is a flat, thin flake and is characteristic of psoriasis and dandruff. Page Ref: 351

79. a. An abrasion is also known as a brush burn. Page Ref: 354

80. c. Bullae means bubble because it is a large, raised blister filled with fluid. Page Ref: 355

81. d. Decubitus is derived from a Latin word meaning lying down. Page Ref: 356

82. a. A caruncle is composed of several furuncles or abscesses. Page Ref: 357

83. b. Herpes varicella-zoster virus causes chickenpox and shingles. Page Ref: 358

84. c. Herpes varicella-zoster virus causes chickenpox and shingles. Page Ref: 358

85. b. Contact with these allergens can produce contact dermatitis in sensitive people. Page Ref: 360

86. c. Hem/o- means blood, angi/o- means blood vessel, and -oma means tumor or mass. Page Ref: 361

87. d. Nevus is a Latin word meaning mole or birthmark. Page Ref: 361

88. b. Kaposi's sarcoma is a rare cancer that attacks the skin and other parts of the body in patients with poor immune system function. Page Ref: 364

89. c. Sebum trapped in pores becomes black and forms a blackhead or comedo. Page Ref: 365

90. a. Rhin/o- means nose and -phyma means tumor or growth. Page Ref: 366

91. c. Eczema is a type of seborrheic dermatitis with crusty, yellow exudates in infants and adults. Page Ref: 367

92. b. Diaphor/o- means sweating. Page Ref: 367

93. a. Lip/o- means fat and -oma means tumor. Page Ref: 361

94. d. Alopecia is derived from a Greek word meaning hair falling out. Page Ref: 367

95. a. Cry/o- means cold. Page Ref: 370

96. d. Sutures are used to close the deep layers and then the skin itself. Page Ref: 373

97. d. Dermatome is a homonym that has different meanings. Page Ref: 375

98. b. The correct spelling is eschar. Page Ref: 355

99. a. The correct spelling is rhytidectomy. Page Ref: 374

100. a. Ungu/o- is Latin for nail and onych/o- is Greek for nail. Page Ref: 379

101. c. Adip/o- means fat. Page Ref: 379

102. d. Epi- means above. Page Ref: 339

103. b. Exfoliation is similar to the falling of dead leaves (foliage) from trees. Page Ref: 340

104. c. Alopecia is baldness while hirsutism is excessive hairness. Page Ref: 367, 368

105. b. A comedo is another name for a blackhead in acne vulgaris. Page Ref: 365

106. d. Acne rosacea has all these characteristics. Rosacea means rose-colored or reddened. Page Ref: 366

107. b. Necr/o- means dead. Page Ref: 353

108. a. Pedicul/o- means lice. Page Ref: 359

109. c. Vitiligo is the progressive loss of skin pigment in patches until the entire skin is white. Page Ref: 354

110. a. Cicatrix is a Latin word for scar, while kel/o- means tumor and -oid means resembling. Page Ref: 356

111. a. Lip/o- means fat. Page Ref: 374

112. d. Epithelium or epithelial tissues is the large category that includes the skin and mucous membranes. Page Ref: 339

113. b. Kerat/o- means hard, fibrous protein. Page Ref: 339

114. b. The epidermis is very thin and the subcutaneous tissue is not part of the skin. Page Ref: 339, 341

115. d. The dermis contains arteries, veins, and nerves. Page Ref: 340

116. d. Cut/i- means skin and -cle means small thing. Page Ref: 343

117. a. All/o- means other or strange and refers to something outside the body. Page Ref: 344

118. a. Phylact/o- means guarding or protecting and, when used in the medical word anaphylaxis, it means excessive guarding or protecting. Page Ref: 344

119. d. Ungu/o- and onych/o- are both combining forms that mean nail. Page Ref: 343

120. d. Macule is derived from a Latin word meaning a spot. Page Ref: 351

121. c. Lacer/o- means a tearing. Page Ref: 357

Short Answer

122. yellow. Xanth/o- is the combining form for yellow. Page Ref: 362

123. cutane/o-. Cutane/o- is the Latin combining form for skin. Page Ref: 379

124. reddish. Erythemat/o- means redness. Page Ref: 353

125. nails. Onych/o- means nail, myc/o- means fungus, and -osis means condition. Page Ref: 368

126. lesion. Lesion means to injure. Page Ref: 351

127. hives. Urticaria is sudden edema and wheals from an allergic reaction. Page Ref: 360

128. color. Cyanosis refers to blue; icterus refers to yellow-orange; port wine refers to purple-red. Page Ref: 353, 361

129. Cellulitis. Cellul/o- means cell and -itis means inflammation. Page Ref: 356

130. cicatrix. Cicatrix is a Latin word meaning scar. Page Ref: 356

131. malignant melanoma. ABCD stands for asymmetry, border, color, and diameter. Page Ref: 363

132. incisional. Incis/o- means to cut into. Page Ref: 373

133. Dermatoplasty. Dermat/o- means skin and -plasty means process of reshaping by surgery. Page Ref: 374

134. autograft. Auto- means self. Page Ref: 374

135. psoriasis. Coal tar drugs cause the epidermal cells to multiply more slowing and decrease itching. Page Ref: 376

136. epidermis. Epi- means upon, above and dermis refers to the skin. Page Ref: 339

137. Melanocytes. Melan/o- means black. Page Ref: 340

138. dermis. Collagen is a firm, white protein and elastin is an elastic, yellow protein. Page Ref: 340

139. exocrine. Exocrine glands secrete to the outside of the body. Page Ref: 342

140. skin. The skin is the largest organ of the body. Page Ref: 339

141. Anaphylaxis. It can be caused by food allergies, bee stings, latex, or certain drugs in hypersensitive individuals. Page Ref: 344

142. integumentary system. Integumentary (in-TEG-yoo-MEN-tair-ee), integument/o- means skin, and -ary means pertaining to. Integumentary is derived from a Latin word meaning a covering. Page Ref: 339

143. epithelium. Epithelium (EP-ih-THEE-lee-um), epi- means upon, above, theli/o- means tissue layer, and -um means a structure. Page Ref: 339

144. dermis. Dermis (DER-mis) is derived from a Greek word meaning skin. Page Ref: 340

145. subcutaneous. Subcutaneous (SUB-kyoo-TAY-nee-us), sub- means below; underneath; less than, cutane/o- means skin, and -ous means pertaining to. Page Ref: 341

146. sudoriferous. Sudoriferous (soo-doh-RIF-er-us), sudor/i- means sweat, fer/o- means to bear, and -ous means pertaining to. Sudor is a Latin word meaning sweat. Page Ref: 342

147. follicle. A follicle is a small sac that contains a hair. Page Ref: 342

148. lunula. Lunula (LOO-nyoo-lah), lun/o- means moon, and -ula means little. Lunula is a Latin word meaning little moon. Page Ref: 343

149. allergy. Allergy (AL-er-jee), all/o- means other; strange, and -ergy means activity; process of working. Page Ref: 344

150. anaphylaxis. Anaphylaxis (AN-ah-fih-LAK-sis), ana- means apart from; excessive, and -phylaxis means condition of guarding or protecting. Page Ref: 344

151. contusion. Contusion (con-TOO-zhun), con-tus/o- means bruising, and -ion means action; condition. Page Ref: 350

152. turgor. Turgor (TER-gor) is derived from a Latin word meaning fullness. Page Ref: 352

153. cyanosis. Cyanosis (SY-ah-NOH-sis), cyan/o- means blue, and -osis means condition; condition; process. Page Ref: 353

154. Polydactyly. Polydactyly (PAWL-ee-DAK-tih-lee), poly- means many, much, and -dactyly means condition of fingers or toes. Page Ref: 362

155. Basal cell carcinoma. Carcinoma (KAR-sih-NOH-mah), carcin/o- means cancer, and -oma means tumor, mass. Basal refers to the deepest layer of the epidermis. Page Ref: 363

156. Dermatology. Dermat/o- means skin and -logy means the study of. Page Ref: 338.

157. rhytidectomy. Rhytid/o- means wrinkes and -ectomy means surgical excision. Page Ref: 374

158. melanin. Melan/o- means black and -in means a substance. Page Ref: 340

159. dermatome. Derm/a- means skin and -tome means area with distinct edges. Page Ref: 341

160. Athlete's foot. Pedis is a Latin word referring to the foot. Page Ref: 358

161. Shingles. The same virus causes both chicken-pox rash and shingles. Page Ref: 358

162. Decubitus ulcer. Decubitus means lying on the back, which is the cause of most bedsores. Page Ref: 356

True/False

163. False. The subcutaneous tissue is directly beneath the skin but is not anatomically considered part of the skin as the dermis and epidermis are. Page Ref: 341

164. True. Skin pigmentation or coloration is related to the melanin production but not to the number of melanocytes in the skin. Page Ref: 340

165. True. Sunlight converts cholesterol in the epidermis to vitamin D. Page Ref: 340

166. False. Pil/o- refers to the hair. Page Ref: 342

167. False. The correct spelling is pruritus. Page Ref: 352

168. True. A bedsore is also called a decubitus ulcer or pressure ulcer. Page Ref: 356

169. True. A pilondial sinus is located toward the end of the spine and is an abnormal passageway that contains hair that is never shed. Page Ref: 368

170. False. A mole is a nevus; a wart is a verruca. Page Ref: 361

171. False. This describes acne rosacea. Page Ref: 366

172. True. Par- means beside, onych/o- means nail, and -ia means condition. Page Ref: 369

173. True. The integumentary system is the most extensive system of the body. Page Ref: 339-343

174. False. The process of dead skin cells being sloughed of is called exfoliation. Page Ref: 340

175. False. The subcutaneous tissue is a connective tissue beneath the dermis. It is not a type of nervous tissue. Page Ref: 341

176. True. When the sweat evaporates from the skin, the body cools. Page Ref: 342

177. False. Hair cells are filled with keratin, which make the hair shaft strong. Page Ref: 342

178. False. It is the melanin in the epidermis that absorbs ultraviolet light. Page Ref: 340

179. True. There are several types of allergic or hypersensitivity reactions. Page Ref: 344

180. True. Besides the elastin, the fat layer conserves body heat and protects the internal organs as the infant learns to walk. Page Ref: 344

181. False. A neoplasm may be either malignant or benign. Page Ref: 352

182. True. Debridement removes dead tissue and creates a clean surface that can heal. Page Ref: 371

183. True. Lip/o- means fat. Suction removes the fat and reshapes the body. Page Ref: 374

184. False. The skin presents a dry and slightly acidic environment that discourages the growth of microorganisms. Page Ref: 344

185. True. Arsenic poisoning produces characteristic white bands on the nails. Page Ref: 342

186. True. Acne vulgaris occurs in adolescence, but acne rosacea occurs in middle age. Page Ref: 366.

187. True. Chronic sun exposure causes these roughened areas on the skin. Page Ref: 360

188. False. Anhidrosis is congenital absence of the sweat glands. Diaphoresis is excessive sweating. Page Ref: 367

189. False. Hirsutism is the presence of excessive dark hair on the upper lip and forearms in women. Page Ref: 368

190. False. This describes paronychia, not onychomycosis. The combining form myc/o- shows that onychomycosis is caused by a fungus. Page Ref: 369

191. False. Transdermal drugs are in the form of patches and the drugs are absorbed through the skin. Page Ref: 377

192. True. Coal tar causes epithelial cells to multiply more slowly so that plaques do not form in patients with psoriasis. Page Ref: 376

193. True. Botox is a drug that keeps muscles from contracting and forming wrinkles in the skin. Page Ref: 370

194. True. Intact skin forms a barrier against disease. Page Ref: 339

195. True. Bas/o- means base of a structure. Page Ref: 340

196. True. Neoplasm means a new growth, which can be either benign or malignant. Page Ref: 352

197. False. The outermost layer is the epidermis, which is above (epi- means above) the dermis. Page Ref: 339

198. False. Sunburn occurs when melanin cannot absorb any more ultraviolet light from the sun. Page Ref: 340

199. True. The subcutaneous tissue contains fatty tissue that acts as insulation to conserve body heat. Page Ref: 341

200. False. Petechiae are pinpoint hemorrhages, while a hematoma is an elevated collection of blood under the skin. Page Ref: 350

Essay

201. Anaphylaxis is a severe systemic allergic reaction with respiratory distress (difficulty breathing), hypotension (abnormally low blood pressure), and shock (compromised circulation). Page Ref: 344

202. Moh's surgery is done for skin cancer in some patients. The surgery uses a microscope to view excised pieces of tissue to try to make certain that all of the cancer is removed. Page Ref: 374

203. The integumentary system covers the entire surface of the body and consists of the skin, hair, and the nails. It is an extremely large, flat, flexible body system that covers the entire surface of the body. The purpose is to protect the body from invading microorganisms. The sense of touch is also part of the integumentary system. Page Ref: 339-343

204. A local allergic reaction occurs when an allergen touches the skin or mucous membranes of a hypersensitive individual. Histamine and other substances are released and cause redness, swelling, irritation, and itching in the area. A systemic allergic reaction occurs when allergens are inhaled, ingested, or injected into a hypersensitive person, causing symptoms in one or more body systems. Some effects include bronchoconstriction, dilation of blood vessels throughout the body, hives, and in very rare cases anaphylaxis. Page Ref: 344

205. Anaphylaxis is a severe systemic allergic reaction in hypersensitive individuals that can be life threatening. It is a medical emergency. Symptoms include bronchoconstriction with respiratory distress, hypotension, and shock. Page Ref: 344

206. Necrosis is a gray-to-black discoloration of the skin in areas where the tissue has died. Necrosis can be a result of a burn, decubitus ulcer, wound, or tissue with a poor blood supply. Gangrene follows necrosis and is the subsequent bacterial invasion and decay of necrotic tissue. Page Ref: 353

207. Second-degree burns involve the epidermis and the upper layer of the dermis. They cause erythema, pain, and swelling. Frequently there are small blisters or larger ones called bullae, as the dermis detaches from the dermis. Second-degree burns are known as partial-thickness burns. Third-degree burns involve the epidermis and the entire dermis. Further, third-degree burns may involve the subcutaneous tissue and muscle. The area is black where the skin is burned. Third-degree burns are also known as full thickness burns. Page Ref: 355

CHAPTER 8

Multiple Choice

1. d. Talus means ankle bone, pes means foot; equin/o- means horse (as a horse walks on hooves), -varus means bent toward the midline. Page Ref: 434

2. b. The correct spelling is humerus. Page Ref: 406

3. a. Comminut/o- means break into minute pieces. Page Ref: 426

4. c. The meniscus is the crescent-shaped cartilage located in some synovial joints, such as the knee. Page Ref: 411

5. a. Rheumatoid arthritis is a disease of connective tissue, particularly the joints, involving autoimmunity. The patient's own antibodies attack its connective tissue. Page Ref: 432, 441

6. b. The abbreviations indicate above or below the knee amputation. Page Ref: 438

7. c. The zygomatic bones are the cheekbones. Page Ref: 400

8. d. In a greenstick fracture, one side of the bone is broken while the other side is bent. Page Ref: 426

9. c. An open reduction and internal fixation (ORIF) involves an incision, followed by application of devices applied to a compound fracture to keep the bone ends in alignment. Page Ref: 426, 440

10. c. THR means total hip replacement: removing the hip joint and replacing it with a prosthesis. Page Ref: 440

11. a. The acetabulum is a small, shallow cup. Page Ref: 408

12. b. Kyph/o- means bent; humpbacked. Page Ref: 429

13. b. Oste/o- means bone, por/o- means small openings, -osis means abnormal condition. Page Ref: 428

14. d. Lord/o- means swayback. Page Ref: 429

15. c. An inborn metabolic defect causes patients with gout to create a build-up of uric acid that forms crystal deposits in the soft tissues, particularly in the large toe. Page Ref: 431

16. a. Crepitus is a Latin word meaning a rattle. Page Ref: 432

17. b. Oste/o- means bone; -clast means break down. Page Ref: 414

18. d. ankyl/o- means fused and -osing means doing; spondyl/o- means vertebra and -itis means inflammation. Page Ref: 429

19. a. Scoliosis is a lateral curvature of the spine. A spinal fusion can stabilize the curvature. Page Ref: 430

20. c. Spondyl/o- means vertebra, olisthe/o- means slipping, and -osis means abnormal condition. Page Ref: 430

21. c. The epiphysis is the area of bone growth found at end of bones. Avascular necrosis involves death of cells at the end of a bone. The femur is the only bone described above. Page Ref: 424

22. a. Occipit/o- means back of the head. Page Ref: 398

23. d. Oste/o- means bone, and -tome means instrument used to cut. Rongeur is a French word that means to gnaw. Page Ref: 440

24. c. Degenerative joint disease (DJD) is a chronic inflammatory disease of joints, particularly weight-bearing joints. Page Ref: 432

25. a. The sphenoid bone is not a facial bone; it is a cranial bone. Page Ref: 399

26. b. Ribs 8 through 10 are attached to the spinal column, but are only indirectly attached to the sternum by long lengths of costal cartilage. Page Ref: 402

27. a. The lumbar vertebrae in the lower back are larger than the cervical or thoracic vertebrae because they bear the weight of the entire head, neck, and trunk of the body. Page Ref: 403

28. c. The clavicle is a rodlike bone on each side of the anterior neck. Page Ref: 405

29. c. The distal end of the radius connects to the bones of the wrist on the thumb side of the forearm. Page Ref: 406

30. b. The medial malleolus is a bony prominence on the distal end of the tibia. The lateral malleolus is a bony prominence on the distal end of the fibula. Page Ref: 409

31. c. Carp/o- means wrist and -al means pertaining to. Page Ref: 407

32. b. The coccyx is a group of several small, fused vertebrae below the sacrum. Page Ref: 403

33. a. The femur is the long bone of the upper leg. Page Ref: 409

34. c. Comminut/o- means break into minute pieces and -ed means pertaining to. Page Ref: 426

35. a. In osteomyelitis, bacteria enter the bone following an open fracture, crushing injury, or surgical procedure. Page Ref: 428

36. c. Kyphosis is an abnormal, excessive, posterior curvature of the thoracic spine, also called humpback or hunchback. Page Ref: 429

37. b. Genu valgum is also known as knock-knee because valgum is a Latin word that means bent away from the midline. Page Ref: 433

38. b. Goni/o- means angle and -metry means process of measuring. Page Ref: 437

39. a. Arthr/o- means joint and -desis means procedure to fuse together. Page Ref: 438

40. b. Bone resorption inhibitor drugs are used to treat osteoporosis. Page Ref: 441

41. d. The distal interphalangeal joint is in the phalanges (fingers or toes). Page Ref: 407

42. c. A bone density test is a radiologic procedure that measures the bone mineral density (BMD) to determine if demineralization from osteoporosis has occurred. Page Ref: 435

43. a. Arthralgia is pain in the joint caused by injury, inflammation, or infection from various causes. Page Ref: 431

44. a. An open fracture is any type of fracture in which the bone breaks through the overlying skin. It is also known as a compound fracture. Page Ref: 426

45. c. Chondr/o- means cartilage and -oma means tumor or mass. Page Ref: 424

46. b. The sternum is also known as the breast bone. Page Ref: 401

47. a. Synovial joints are fully moveable joints that have a joint capsule and a synovial membrane. Page Ref: 411

48. b. The calcaneous is also known as the heel bone. Page Ref: 410

49. a. The axial skeleton forms the central bony structure of the body around which other parts move. The combining form axi/o- means axis. Page Ref: 397

50. d. All of these are parts of the head except sacrum, which is part of the back. Page Ref: 398-400

51. c. The rib, clavicle, and thorax are parts of the chest; the sternum is the breast bone. Page Ref: 401

52. b. There are 12 pairs of ribs. Page Ref: 401

53. a. The scapula, acromion, and glenoid fossa are bones of the shoulders. Page Ref: 401

54. c. The carpal bones are the individual bones of the wrist. They connect other bones of the wrist and hand together. The other bones listed are in the hands and feet and fingers and toes, not the wrists. Page Ref: 407

55. b. Bone is a type of connective tissue also known as osseous tissue. Page Ref: 411

56. d. New bone is also formed along the epiphysial growth plates. Page Ref: 413

57. d. In a comminuted fracture, the bone is crushed or broken into several pieces. Page Ref: 426

58. a. There are two kinds of synovial joints: hinge-type joints (such as the elbow and knee) that only allow motion in two directions and ball-and-socket joints (such as the shoulder and hip) that allow motion in many directions. Page Ref: 411

59. b. Synovial (sih-NOH-vee-al), synov/o- means synovium (membrane) and -ial means pertaining to. Page Ref: 411

60. c. Osseous (AW-see-us), osse/o- means bone and -ous means pertaining to. Page Ref: 411

61. c. Diaphysis (dy-AF-ih-sis) is a Greek singular noun for the straight shaft of a long bone. Page Ref: 429

62. a. Ossification (AWS-ih-fih-KAY-shun), ossificat/o- means changing into bone and -ion means action; condition. Page Ref: 413

63. b. Humer/o- means upper arm bone, -al means pertaining to. Page Ref: 406

64. d. Menisc/o- means meniscus (crescent-shaped cartilage). Page Ref: 411

65. c. Uln/o- means ulna (forearm bone). Page Ref: 406

66. a. Zygomat/o- means zygoma (cheek bone). Each zygomatic bone is known as a zygoma. Page Ref: 400

67. d. Chondroma (kon-DROH-mah), chondr/o- means cartilage, -oma means tumor, mass. Page Ref: 424

68. c. Transverse means to travel across. Page Ref: 427

69. d. Diaphys/o- means shaft of a bone. Page Ref: 411

70. b. Chondr/o- is the Greek combining form for cartilage. Cartilag/o- is the Latin combining form. Page Ref: 443

71. d. Spondyl/o- is the Greek combining form for vertebra and vertebr/o- is the Latin form. Page Ref: 443

72. d. Symphysis means a state of growing together. The pubic bone is located in the pelvis. Page Ref: 408

73. c. Arthr/o- means joint, alg/o- means pain, and -ia means condition or state. Page Ref: 431

74. d. Arthr/o- means joint and -plasty means process of reshaping by surgery. A prosthesis is an artificial replacement part. Page Ref: 440

75. a. Overstretching or tearing of a ligament is a strain. Page Ref: 433

76. c. Spondyl/o- means vertebra and -olisthesis means abnormal condition and process of slipping. Page Ref: 430

77. a. Ligaments are strong bands of fibrous tissue that hold bone ends together in a synovial joint. Page Ref: 411

78. a. Coccyg/o- means tailbone. Page Ref: 403

79. b. Osteoarthritis shows degeneration of the joint. Page Ref: 432

80. c. Osse/o- means bone. Page Ref: 411

81. d. In degenerative joint disease, cartilage is gone and the bone ends rub together with movement and produce crepitus. Page Ref: 432

82. b. Rheumatoid arthritis is an autoimmune disease that responds to treatment with gold. Page Ref: 441

83. b. Perone/o- means fibula (lower leg). Page Ref: 409

84. a. The shin bone in the lower leg is the tibia. Page Ref: 409

85. c. Cost/o- is the combining form for rib. Page Ref: 402

86. d. Chondr/o- means cartilage, malac/o- means softening, and -ia means condition. Patellae refers to the kneecap (patella). Page Ref: 424

87. b. DIP stands for distal interphalanageal joint. Interphalangeal means between the bones of the phalanges or fingers. Page Ref: 442

88. d. The patient had degenerative joint disease (DJD) and had a total hip replacement (THR). Page Ref: 442

89. c. Pectus excavatum is the correct spelling. Page Ref: 433

90. b. Above-the-knee amputation (AKA) and below-the-knee amputation (BKA) are surgeries to remove a leg. Page Ref: 442

91. a. Hemarthrosis is an abnormal condition of blood in the joint. Page Ref: 431

92. a. The suffix -ics means knowledge or practice. Page Ref: 398

93. c. The patella is the medical word for the kneecap. Page Ref: 424

94. a. The sternum is the location of the bony deformity pectus excavatum. Page Ref: 433

95. d. Genu valgum is knock-knee. Page Ref: 433

96. c. The nucleus pulposis is the gelatinous substance inside each intervertebral disk. Page Ref: 404

97. c. The olecranon process or olecranon is the bony point of the elbow. Page Ref: 404, 406

98. b. Cancellous means pertaining to a lattice structure, rather than solid bone. Page Ref: 412

99. d. It tracks the actual height and weight as well as the percentile compared to other children. Page Ref: 413

100. d. Osteoclasts and osteoblasts are two types of osteocytes. Page Ref: 414

101. b. The fracture fragments might not be in alignment when they heal. Page Ref: 425

102. a. Gout has increased levels of uric acid in the blood. Page Ref: 434, 444

103. d. An intra-articular injection of cortisone is placed within the joint. Page Ref: 433, 436

104. b. Sound waves shock and break up the bone spurs. Page Ref: 437

105. b. Hallus valgus, a deformity of the toes, often creates a bunion at the base of the big toe. Page Ref: 433, 439

106. a. A fontanel closes as the infant matures. A foramen always stays open. Page Ref: 400

107. d. The sphenoid bone is located behind the nose and has a bony cup that holds the pituitary gland near the brain. Page Ref: 399

108. b. The hyoid bone in the neck anchors the muscles of the tongue but does not connect to any other bones. Page Ref: 401

109. d. All of these diseases can weaken the bone and cause a pathological fracture. Page Ref: 425

110. b. Scoliosis is a congenital S-shaped curvature of the spine in children. Page Ref: 430

111. d. While visual inspection may reveal some severe fractures and dislocations, an x-ray is able to reveal all fractures and dislocations and confirm the diagnosis. Page Ref: 435

Short Answer

112. chondroma. Chondr/o- means cartilage, -oma means tumor. Page Ref: 424

113. scoliosis. Scoli/o- means curved or crooked. Page Ref: 430

114. bunionectomy. A bunion is a swelling and inflammation of the base of the great toe. Page Ref: 439

115. arthralgia. Arthr/o- means joint, -algia means condition of pain. Page Ref: 431

116. hemarthrosis. Hem/o- means blood, arthr/o- means joint, -osis means abnormal condition. Page Ref: 431

117. Colles'. This fracture occurs by falling onto an outstretched hand. Page Ref: 426

118. articul/o-. Arthr/o- is Greek and articul/o- is Latin. Page Ref: 443

119. osteomalacia. Oste/o- means bone and -malacia means condition of softening. Page Ref: 428

120. straight. Orth/o- means straight. Page Ref: 398

121. tibia. The tibia is the anterior leg bone. Page Ref: 409

122. Ewing's. Ewing's sarcoma is named for James Ewing, and American pathologist. This is an example of an eponym: a person from whom something takes its name. Page Ref: 424

123. pathological. Path/o- means disease or suffering, log/o- means the study of, and -ic means pertaining to. Page Ref: 425

124. arthralgia. Arthr/o- means joint, alg/o- means pain, and -ia means condition, state, or thing. Page Ref: 431

125. dislocation. Dislocation is usually caused by injury or trauma. Page Ref: 431

126. scintigraphy. A gamma scintillation camera detects gamma rays from the radioactive tracer. Page Ref: 435

127. reduction. Reduct/o- means to bring back, decrease and -ion means action, condition. Page Ref: 436

128. Amputation. Amputat/o- means to cut off and -ion means action, condition. Page Ref: 438

129. Arthroscopy. Arthr/o- means joint and -scopy means process of using an instrument to examine. Page Ref: 438

130. analgesics. Examples include aspirin and Tylenol (acetaminophen). Page Ref: 441

131. appendicular. The skeleton can be divided into two areas of bones: the axial skeleton and the appendicular skeleton. Page Ref: 397

132. axial. Axial (AK-see-al), ax/o- means axis and -ial means pertaining to. An axis is a central structure around which something rotates. Page Ref: 397

133. frontal. Frontal (FRUN-tal), front/o- means from and -al means pertaining to. Page Ref: 398

134. foramen magnum. Foramen is a Latin word meaning an opening. Magnum is a Latin word meaning large. The foramen magnum is the largest foramen in the body. Page Ref: 399

135. ethmoid. Ethmoid (ETH-moyd), ethm/o- means sieve and -oid means resembling. The ethmoid bone is very porous with many small, hollow spaces that resemble a sieve. Page Ref: 399

136. fontanels. Fontanel (FAWN-tah-NEL) is a Latin word meaning fountain or spring, referring to the pulse that could be felt in the fontanel and was thought to be the fountain or spring of life. Page Ref: 400

137. vomer. Vomer (VOH-mer) is derived from a Latin word meaning plowshare, the cutting part of a plow. The vomer bone is shaped somewhat like the blade on a plow. Page Ref: 400

138. mandible. The mandible (MAN-dih-bl) is the lower jaw; the maxilla is the upper jaw. Page Ref: 400

139. manubrium. Manubrium (mah-NOO-bree-um) is a Latin word meaning handle. The manubrium is like the handle of the sternum with the xiphoid at the other end being its pointed tip. Page Ref: 401

140. costochondral. Costochondral (KAWS-toh-KAWN-dral), cost/o- means rib, chondr/o- means cartilage, and -al means pertaining to. Page Ref: 402

141. cervical. Cervical (SER-vih-kal), cervic/o- means neck; cervix and -al means pertaining to. Page Ref: 403

142. lumbar. Lumbar (LUM-bar), lumb/o- means lower back between the ribs and pelvis and -ar means pertaining to. Page Ref: 403

143. intervertebral disks. Intervertebral (IN-ter-VER-teh-bral), inter- means between, vertebr/o- means vertebra, and -al means pertaining to. Disk may also be spelled disc. Page Ref: 404

144. clavicle. The clavicle is a horizontal rodlike bone attached to either side of the manubrium. Page Ref: 405

145. scapula. Scapula is a Latin singular noun meaning shoulder blade. Form the plural by changing -a to -ae. Page Ref: 405

146. carpal. Carpal (KAR-pal), carp/o- means wrist and -al means pertaining to. Carpus is a Latin word meaning wrist. Page Ref: 407

147. shoulder; hip. Ball-and-socket joints are fully moveable and allow motion in many directions. Page Ref: 411

148. radius; ulna. The other bone in the arm is the upper arm bone or humerus. Page Ref: 406

149. tibia; fibula. The other bone in the leg is the upper leg bone or femur. Page Ref: 409

150. amputee. Amput/o- means to cut off and -ee means person who is the object of an action. Page Ref: 438

151. 206. Infants have more bones that later to fuse together. Page Ref: 397

True/False

152. False. The correct word is resorption. Page Ref: 441

153. False. The olecranon is the elbow; the calcaneus is the heel bone. Page Ref: 406, 410

154. False. A DEXA scan is done for osteoporosis to determine bone density. Page Ref: 435

155. False. This describes a prosthesis. An orthosis is a device such as a brace that is used to immobilize or correct an orthopedic problem. Page Ref: 437

156. False. Analgesics such as aspirin or Tylenol would be useful in this situation. Prednisone is not an over-the-counter medication and it is not used to treat minor injuries. Page Ref: 441

157. False. Hallux means great toe. Page Ref: 433

158. True. Because the cranium encases a cavity, the bones of the cranium can be depressed inwardly by a fracture. Page Ref: 426

159. True. Genu refers to knee. Valgum means bent away from the midline. It is the lower leg rather than the knee that is bent away. Page Ref: 433

160. False. The instruments used for arthrocentesis would be a needle or a trocar (a sharp, pointed instrument). The osteotome is used to cut into bone. Page Ref: 438

161. False. The skeletal system consists of 206 bones and other structures that are found throughout the body. Page Ref: 397

162. True. The axial skeleton is the part of the body around which other parts move. Page Ref: 397

163. True. All of these structures are protected by the facial bones. Page Ref: 398

164. True. The fontanels are open at birth, but gradually close as the cranial bones grow together. Page Ref: 400

165. True. The meaning of the word in English is the same as the meaning of the word in Latin. Page Ref: 408

166. True. The humerus is the upper arm bone; the radius and ulna are the lower arm bones. Page Ref: 406

167. False. Avascular necrosis is the death of cells in the epiphysis at the end of the femur. Gangrene can occur in the skin of the fingers and toes after exposure to cold. Page Ref: 424

168. False. Osteomyelitis is an infection in the bone and bone marrow. Page Ref: 428

169. True. After the dye is injected, an x-ray or CT scan is taken. Page Ref: 434

170. True. Red bone marrow produces these cells that function in the blood and the immune system. Page Ref: 412

171. False. A joint is also known as an articulation. The meniscus is a crescent-shaped cartilage. Page Ref: 410

172. True. Phalanx is a Greek word that means a line of soldiers, like the ten fingers and toes. Page Ref: 407

173. False. The kneecap is the patella; the point of the elbow is the olecranon. Page Ref: 406, 409

174. False. A physical therapist develops treatment and rehabilitation plans based on a physician's order. Page Ref: 443

175. True. The skull is the bony structure of the head that includes the cranium and facial bones. Page Ref: 398

176. False. The tarsal bones are the bones of the ankle. The carpal bones are in the wrist. Page Ref: 407

177. False. The glenoid fossa is in the shoulder joint. The acetabulum is the bony socket in the hip joint. Page Ref: 408

178. False. A hairline fracture can occur in any bone of the body. It has a very thin fracture line. Page Ref: 427

179. False. A prosthesis is an artificial limb or artificial joint. Page Ref: 437

180. True. A goniometer is a protractor-like device used to measure angle and range of motion. Page Ref: 437

Essay

181. Cervical, thoracic, lumbar, sacrum, coccyx. These correspond to vertebrae. The cervical vertebrae (C1-C7) are located in the neck. The thoracic vertebrae (T1-T12) arelocated in the chest. The lumbar vertebrae (L1-L5) are located in the lower back. The sacrum is a group of five fuesd vertebrae that are not individually numbered, except for the first sacral vertebra (S1). The coccyx (tailbone) is a group of several small, fused vertebrae that are not individually numbered. Page Ref: 403

182. The patient had a broken bone in the lower leg. The ends of the broken bone were not in alignment. The physician externally and manually moved the broken bone ends to place them into alignment. Then a wet plaster wrap was applied to the leg and allowed to dry and harden to keep the ends of the broken bones from moving. Page Ref: 436, 440

183. 1. Estrogen loss: estrogen stimulates bone formation so that if estrogen is decreased, new bone formation will be adversely affected. 2. Lack of dietary calcium. 3. Lack of exercise also contributes to the problem of bone breakdown. Page Ref: 428

184. Lordosis is an abnormal, excessive anterior curvature of the lumbar spine. Scoliosis is an abnormal, excessive, C- or S-shaped lateral curvature of the spine. Page Ref: 429, 430

185. Gout is a metabolic disorder that occurs most often in men. There are excessive levels of uric acid in the blood and severe pain as uric acid moves from the blood into the soft tissues and forms masses of crystals and soft tissue swelling known as tophi. Page Ref: 431

186. Bone density tests are radiologic procedures that measure the bone mineral density (BMD) to determine if demineralization from osteoporosis has occurred. The hip and spine bones give more accurate results. There are two types of bone densitometry, one using a CT scan and a DEXA scan using two x-ray beams. Page Ref: 435

187. A bone graft is a surgical procedure that uses whole bone or bone chips to repair fractures with extensive bone loss or defects due to bone cancer. Bone taken from the patient's own body is known as an autograft. Frozen or freeze-dried bone taken from a cadaver is known as an allograft. Page Ref: 439

188. Approximately 10% of the entire skeleton is broken down and rebuilt each year. This change takes place where bones have been damaged or are repeatedly subjected to mechanical stress. There are two types of osteocytes that are important in this process: osteoclasts, which break down areas of old or damaged bone, and osteoblasts, which deposit new bone tissue in those areas where bone has been broken down. Page Ref: 413, 414

CHAPTER 9

Multiple Choice

1. d. Oblique means slanted or on a diagonal. Page Ref: 469

2. b. A- means without, and tax/o- means coordination. Page Ref: 486

3. a. A contracture is permanently fixed in one position. Page Ref: 482

4. c. Torticollis is also known as wryneck, a contracted condition of the neck muscles on one side causing the neck to be in an abnormal position. Page Ref: 485

5. b. Striated or skeletal muscle tissue. Rhabd/o- means rod shaped, my/o- means muscle, sarc/o- means connective tissue, and -oma means tumor. Page Ref: 485

6. d. The glutus maximus forms the buttocks. Page Ref: 470

7. b. The physiatrist is a physician, either M.D. or D.O., who has training in physical medicine and rehabilitation or sports medicine. Page Ref: 496

8. d. The flexor hallucis brevis muscle is located in the big toe; hallux is the big toe. A podiatrist is limited to treating disorders of the feet. Page Ref: 496

9. c. A- means away from, vuls/o- means to tear away, and -ion means action or condition. Page Ref: 482

10. b. My/o- means muscle and -clonus means condition of rapid contracting and relaxing. Page Ref: 486

11. d. Tendin/o- means tendon and -itis means inflammation of. Page Ref: 488

12. a. Acetylcholine receptor antibodies are diagnostic of myasthenia gravis. Page Ref: 489

13. d. Fasci/o- means fascia and -otomy means process of cutting or making an incision. Page Ref: 492

14. c. Ab- means away from, and duct/o- means bring or move. Page Ref: 464

15. b. The palmar fascia of the hand becomes thickened and shortened, creating a contracture of the fingers. Page Ref: 487

16. d. The tibia is the shin bone of the lower leg. The condition described in the question is shin splints. Page Ref: 488

17. a. Fibr/o- means fibrous, my/o- means muscle, and -algia means pain. Page Ref: 482

18. d. Bradykinesia indicates slow movements or a decrease in the number of spontaneous movements. Brady- means slow. Page Ref: 486

19. c. This is a tear in the rotator muscles of the shoulder that surround the head of the humerus. Page Ref: 485

20. a. Electromyography is a test that records electrical activities as muscles contract and relax. Page Ref: 489

21. b. The thymus gland is the source of antibodies that are involved in the muscular weakness associated with myasthenia gravis. Page Ref: 493

22. c. A bruise or contusion causes bleeding in the muscle but does not break the skin. Page Ref: 483

23. c. This condition shows abnormal fatigue from the body's inability to produce sustained muscle contractions. Page Ref: 484

24. b. The three types of muscles are skeletal, smooth, and cardiac. Page Ref: 459

25. c. Smooth muscle forms a continuous thin layer in various organs and structures. Page Ref: 459

26. a. Muscle is attached to the bone at its origin or insertion by a tendon. Page Ref: 461

27. c. Gluteus means buttocks. Maximus means large. Page Ref: 470

28. a. Flexor means flexes. Hallucis means big toe (hallux). Brevis means short. Page Ref: 463

29. c. Flexion of the elbow causes the angle between the upper arm and lower arm to decrease. Page Ref: 464

30. b. The frontalis muscle lies on the forehead directly over the frontal bone of the cranium. Page Ref: 466

31. c. This is the upper arm muscle you show when you want people to see how strong you are. Page Ref: 468

32. a. The gastrocnemius muscle is on the posterior lower leg and is not related to the stomach. Page Ref: 471

33. c. Atrophy can be caused by malnutrition or it can occur in any part of the body that is paralyzed where the muscles receive no electrical impulse from the nerves. Page Ref: 482

34. c. Torticollis is also known as wryneck. Page Ref: 485

35. b. Ataxia is caused by diseases of the brain or spinal cord, cerebral palsy, or an adverse reaction to a drug. A- means without, and tax/o- means coordination. Page Ref: 486

36. b. The symptoms of restless leg syndrome occur mainly at night. The exact cause is unknown. Page Ref: 487

37. d. This condition is known by all three synonyms (golfer's elbow, pitcher's elbow, and medial epicondylitis). Page Ref: 487

38. c. A needle electrode is inserted into a muscle to record the electrical activity as the muscle contracts and relaxes. Page Ref: 489

39. a. For muscles in the hand, the physician asks the patient to grasp two of the physician's fingers and to squeeze them as tightly as possible. Page Ref: 491

40. c. Muscle or motor strength is measured on a scale of 0 to 5, with 0 being the inability to move the muscles being tested and 5 being normal strength. Page Ref: 491

41. a. Bursitis is an inflammation of the bursal sac because of repetitive muscular activity or pressure on the bone underneath the bursa. Page Ref: 487

42. b. Tremor is a Latin word that means a shaking. Page Ref: 486

43. c. Dyskinesia is associated with cerebral palsy. Dys- means difficult, and kines/o- means movement. Page Ref: 486

44. b. Rigor is a Latin word that means stiffness. Mortis is a Latin word that means of death. Page Ref: 485

45. a. CTD is a condition that affects the muscles, tendons, and sometimes the nerves. It occurs as a result of trauma due to repetitious movements over an extended period of time. Page Ref: 484

46. c. A muscle spasm is also known as a muscle cramp. Page Ref: 483

47. b. A- means without, and -trophy means process of development. Page Ref: 482

48. c. Delt/o- means triangle and -oid means resembling. Page Ref: 467

49. d. There are approximately 700 skeletal muscles in the body. Page Ref: 459

50. c. There are three types of muscles in the muscular system: skeletal, cardiac, and smooth muscle. Page Ref: 459

51. a. Plantar flexion of the foot causes the toe to point downward. Dorsiflexion of the foot causes the toe to point upward. Page Ref: 464

52. d. Rotation is moving a body part around on its axis. Page Ref: 465

53. c. These muscles work in pairs to either spread the ribs out or cause the ribs to move closer together during inspiration and expiration. Page Ref: 467

54. c. Maximus is a Latin word that means the largest one of a group. Page Ref: 470

55. a. Acetylcholine is the neurotransmitter involved in muscle contraction. Page Ref: 472

56. c. A fluid-filled sac that decreases friction where a tendon rubs against a bone near a synovial joint is a bursa. Page Ref: 461

57. d. A result of a crushing injury to the muscles of the leg causes compartment syndrome, which in turn causes all of the following except cardiac arrhythmias. Page Ref: 482

58. b. Muscle relaxant drugs have many uses, including being used to treat muscle spasms in patients with multiple sclerosis. Page Ref: 493

59. a. Anterior (an-TEER-ee-or), anter/o- means before, front part and -ior means pertaining to. Page Ref: 470

60. b. Contracture (con-TRAK-choor), contract/o- means pull together and -ure means system, result of. Page Ref: 482

61. a. Polymyalgia (PAWL-ee-my-AL-jah), poly- means many, much; alg/o- means pain; and -ia means condition, state, thing. Page Ref: 484

62. c. Bradykinesia (BRAD-ee-kin-EE-zee-ah), brady- means slow, kines/o- means movement, and -ia means condition, state, thing. Page Ref: 486

63. c. Bursitis (ber-SY-tis), burs/o- means bursa and -itis means inflammation of. Page Ref: 487

64. b. Electromyography uses electricity to diagnose muscle disease or nerve damage. Page Ref: 489

65. c. Biopsy (BY-awp-see), bi/o- means life; living organisms; living tissue and -opsy means the process of viewing. Page Ref: 492

66. a. Nonsteroidal (non-stair-OY-dal), non- means not, steroid/o- means steroid, -al means pertaining to. Anti-inflammatory (AN-tee-in-FLAM-ah-TOR-ee), anti- means against, inflammat/o- means inflammation, and -ory means having the function of. Page Ref: 494

67. a. Rehabilitation exercises include range of motion (ROM). Page Ref: 492

68. a. Abbreviations are commonly used and can have more than one meaning. Page Ref: 495

69. d. Rotation is movement around a central point or axis, such as the head turning on the vertebral column. Page Ref: 465

70. b. The suffix -or means person or thing that produces or does. Page Ref: 462

71. d. My/o- is the Greek combining form for muscle; muscul/o- is the Latin form. Page Ref: 495

72. b. Rhabdomyosarcoma is a cancerous tumor of the muscle. Page Ref: 485

73. a. The suffix -ics means knowledge or practice. Page Ref: 458

74. b. Stern/o- means sternum, cleid/o- means clavicle, and mastoid is the bony process behind the ear. Page Ref: 466

75. a. Tennis elbow occurs from the stress of repetitive hitting of tennis balls. Page Ref: 484, 488

76. c. OSHA is the Occupational Safety and Health Administration. Page Ref: 484

77. a. The latissimus dorsi muscle goes around the midback. Dorsal means pertaining to the back. Page Ref: 467

78. c. The outstretched arm is in extension; the palm down is known as pronation. Page Ref: 465

79. d. The skeletal muscles are voluntary muscles that move in response to conscious thought. Page Ref: 459

80. d. Brady- means slow, kines/o- means movement, and -ia means condition. Page Ref: 486

81. b. Flexion of the neck muscles produces "yes" and rotation produces "no." Page Ref: 464, 465

82. c. Plantar refers to the bottom of the foot. Page Ref: 464

83. b. Pector/o- means chest. Page Ref: 467

84. d. The lateral epicondyle is a bony projection on the side of the humerus where tendons of the extensor and supinator muscles originate. Page Ref: 488

85. c. Ten/o- means tendon and -rrhaphy means procedure of suturing. Page Ref: 493

86. b. A- means without and tax/o- means coordination. Page Ref: 486

87. a. Muscular dystrophy is a genetic inherited disorder of the gene that makes the muscle protein dystrophin. Page Ref: 483

88. b. Inter- means between and cost/o- means ribs. Page Ref: 467

89. d. The masseter muscle is in the jaw. Page Ref: 468

90. b. The correct spelling is ganglion. Page Ref: 487

91. d. Hyperkinesia means more than normal movement, while bradykinesia is slowed movement. Page Ref: 486

92. a. An assistive device increases mobility and independence in activities of daily living (ADLs). Page Ref: 490

93. b. A bursa acts as a cushion where a tendon rubs against a bone. Page Ref: 461

94. d. An aponeurosis is a flat, wide, white fibrous sheet of connective tissue that is sometimes composed of several tendons. Page Ref: 461

95. d. Muscle names are derived from their shape (deltoid), their size (gluteus maximus), their location (frontalis muscle), and other factors. Page Ref: 462

96. b. A contracture is a contraction that is now fixed and immobile. Page Ref: 482

97. d. The percussion hammer taps the tendon and tests the deep tendon reflexes as the muscle contracts. Page Ref: 491

Short Answer

98. myorrhaphy. My/o- means muscle and -rrhaphy means suture. Page Ref: 493

99. myalgia. My/o- means muscle and -algia means condition of pain. Page Ref: 484

100. bursitis. Burs/o- means bursa and -itis means inflammation of. Page Ref: 487

101. strain. A strain is an overstretching of the muscle. Page Ref: 483

102. atrophy. A- means without, and -trophy means process of development. Page Ref: 482

103. myopathy. My/o means muscle; -pathy means disease. Page Ref: 484

104. tremor. Tremor is a Latin word that means a shaking. Page Ref: 486

105. NSAID. NSAIDs are non-steroidal anti-inflammatory drugs. Page Ref: 494

106. whiplash. Whiplash is a common word for this type of injury. Page Ref: 483

107. myositis. Myos/o- means muscle and -itis means inflammation of. Page Ref: 484

108. musculature. Muscul/o- means muscle and -ature means system composed of. Page Ref: 459

109. origin. The insertion or ending point is where the muscle attaches to the bone that it moves when it contracts and relaxes. Page Ref: 460

110. tendon. A tendon is a cordlike, non-elastic, white fibrous band of connective tissue. Page Ref: 461

111. extension. Muscles that produce extension are known as extensors. Page Ref: 464

112. fascicle. These muscle fibers run parallel to each other so that, when they contract, they all pull in the same direction. Page Ref: 472

113. acetylcholine. Acetylcholine is a chemical messenger that moves across the neuromuscular junction and acts as a key to unlock receptors on the muscle fiber. Page Ref: 472

114. aponeurosis. An aponeurosis is sometimes composed of several tendons. Page Ref: 461

115. bursa. Bursa is a Latin noun meaning a purse. Page Ref: 461

116. gluteus maximus. Gluteus is a Latin word meaning buttocks and maximus is a Latin word meaning the largest one of a group. Page Ref: 470

117. spasm. A muscle spasm is also known as a muscle cramp. It is often brought on by overexercise. Page Ref: 483

118. voluntary. Voluntary (VAWL-un-tair-ee), volunt/o- means done by one's own free will and -ary means pertaining to. Page Ref: 479

119. striated. Striated (STRY-aa-ted) is derived from a Latin word meaning stripe. Page Ref: 459

120. origin. The origin is the point of beginning. Page Ref: 460

121. insertion. Insertion (in-SER-shun), insert/o- means to put in or introduce and -ion means action; condition. Page Ref: 480

122. tendon. A tendon attaches a muscle to a bone. A ligament attaches a bone to another bone. Page Ref: 461

123. abduction. Abduction (ab-DUK-shun), ab- means away from, duct/o- means bring or move; a duct, and -ion means action; condition. Page Ref: 464

124. supination. Supination (soo-pih-NAY-shun), supinat/o- means lying on the back and -ion means action; condition. Page Ref: 465

125. extension. Extension (eks-TEN-shun), extens/o- means straightening and -ion means action; condition. Page Ref: 464

126. deltoid. Deltoid (DEL-toyd), delt/o- means triangle and -oid means resembling. This muscle name is derived from the Greek capital alphabet letter delta, which is shaped like a triangle. Page Ref: 467

127. brachioradialis. Brachioradialis (BRAY-kee-oh-RAY-dee-AL-is), brachi/o- means arm, radi/o- means radius (forearm bone), and -alis means pertaining to. Page Ref: 468

128. fascicle. Each muscle is composed of several fascicles wrapped in fascia. Page Ref: 472

129. Acetylcholine. Acetylcholine (AS-ee-til-KOH-leen) is a neurotransmitter or chemical messenger. Page Ref: 472

130. hypertrophy. Hypertrophy (hy-PER-troh-fee), hyper- means above; more than normal and -trophy means process of development. Page Ref: 473

131. quadriceps femoris. Quadriceps (KWAD-rih-seps), quadri- means four and -ceps means head. Femoris (FEM-oh-ris) is a Latin word meaning of the femur. Page Ref: 471

132. flexion. Extension and flexion are opposite muscle movements. Page Ref: 464

133. inversion. Eversion and inversion are opposite muscle movements. Page Ref: 465

134. upward; downward. Try this mnemonic device to remember the difference: dorsiflexion means toes pointing upward, as a shark's dorsal fin points upward when it is swimming. Planar flexion means toes pointing downward toward the bottom of the foot, as plantar warts are on the bottom of the foot. Page Ref: 463

135. leg. The Achilles tendon attaches the gastrocnemius muscle to the calcaneous (heelbone). Page Ref: 470

136. biceps; triceps. The biceps brachii is the muscle of the anterior forearm that flexes the arm, and the triceps brachii is the muscle of the posterior forearm that extends the arm. Page Ref: 468

137. Orthopedics. Orth/o- means straight, ped/o- means child, and -ics means knowledge, practice. Add words to make a complete definition: The knowledge and practice of [producing] straight[ness] in a child [or an adult]. Page Ref: 458

138. Wryneck. Tort/i- means twisted position, and -collis means condition of the neck. Page Ref: 485

True/False

139. False. Pronation means to turn the palm down; supination means to turn the palm up. Page Ref: 465

140. True. Rhabd/o- means rod shaped; my/o- means muscle; -oma means tumor. Page Ref: 485

141. False. This is a change in the muscles of the dead body that creates contraction or stiffness. Page Ref: 485

142. False. The Tensilon test is confirmatory, although the EMG may be abnormal. Page Ref: 489

143. False. The ending point is known as the insertion. Page Ref: 460

144. False. The collective name is the quadriceps femoris. Hamstrings are on the posterior aspect of the upper leg. Page Ref: 471

145. False. The correct word is intramuscular. The prefix inter- means between; intra- means within. The drug is injected within the muscle. Page Ref: 494

146. True. The mutated gene cannot correctly make the muscle protein dystrophin. Page Ref: 483

147. True. It runs from the cheek to the jaw and moves the jaw upward. Page Ref: 466

148. True. If an incision is made to remove a portion of the muscle, it would be an open biopsy. Page Ref: 492

149. False. The combining form orth/o- means straight. Page Ref: 458

150. True.Voluntary muscles move in response to conscious thought. Page Ref: 459

151. False. The flexor hallucis brevis muscle is a muscle of the foot. Hallus means great toe. Page Ref: 462

152. True. Examples are the brachioradialis muscle, the biceps brachii, and the triceps brachii. Page Ref: 462, 468

153. False. The word pronation means turning the palm of the hand downward. Page Ref: 465

154. True. The key to this is the word oculi, which means eye. Page Ref: 466

155. False. The word hamstrings is a collective name for three muscles on the posterior aspect of the thigh. Page Ref: 471

156. True. Muscle fibers are called multinucleated because of their many nuclei. Page Ref: 472

157. False. Each muscle fiber is an individual cell, which may be as long as 12 inches. Page Ref: 472

158. True. Myalgia means pain in a muscle. Poly- means many. Page Ref: 484

159. False. The response to a deep tendon reflex test is an automatic, not conscious, reflex. Page Ref: 491

160. False. Rectus means straight; this muscle of the abdomen is oriented straight up and down. Page Ref: 469

161. False. Thenar refers to the thumb. Page Ref: 468

162. True. The biceps is a muscle that has two heads. Page Ref: 468

163. False. Rhabdomyosarcoma is a malignant tumor of the muscle. My/o- means muscle, sarc/o- means connective tissue, and -oma means tumor. Page Ref: 485

164. False. The Tensilon test is used to diagnose myasthenia gravis because Tensilon blocks the enzyme that breaks down acetylcholine. Page Ref: 489

165. True. Muscles decrease in size and strength with age. Page Ref: 471

166. False. The gastrocnemius muscle is located in the posterior lower leg. Page Ref: 470

167. False. Rigor mortis is a temporary muscle contraction after death. Page Ref: 485

168. True. Tremor is a Latin word meaning a shaking. Page Ref: 486

Essay

169. Surgical excision of a ganglion. A ganglion is a semisolid or fluid-containing cyst that develops on a tendon, often on the wrist, hand, or foot. It is clearly visible as a rounded lump under the skin that may or may not be painful. Page Ref: 492

170. CPK-MM is an isoenzyme found in skeletal muscle. It is released from muscle cells when injury or death occurs to these cells. High levels of serum CPK-MM point to diseases like muscular dystrophy in which skeletal muscle tissue is being destroyed. Page Ref: 489

171. The fascia around the muscle acts like a compartment. When significant amounts of blood build up, the tissues are compressed. If this pressure is not relieved, nerve and blood vessel necrosis will occur destroying these structures and resulting in the loss of function of the foot. Page Ref: 482

172. A contraction is a normal shortening of a muscle as actin filaments slide between myosin filaments in response to an electrical impulse from a nerve. A contracture is an abnormal, fixed position of a muscle in which it shortens due to inactivity or paralysis. Page Ref: 472, 482

173. The three types of muscle in the body are skeletal muscle, cardiac muscle, and smooth muscle. Skeletal muscles provides the means by which the body can move. They are voluntary, striated muscles that contract and relax in response to conscious thought. Cardiac muscle is an involuntary muscle that is not under conscious control. Smooth muscles are involuntary, nonstriated muscles. They are found in organs such as the stomach and intestines. Page Ref: 459

174. Muscles function in pairs to produce movement. When the first muscle contracts, the second muscle relaxes to allow movement in one direction. When the second muscle contracts, the first one relaxes to allow movement in the opposite direction. Page Ref: 463

175. Each muscle fiber is connected to a single nerve cell at the neuromuscular junction. When the electrical impulse reaches the end of the nerve cell, the nerve cell releases the neurotransmitter acetylcholine. Acetycholine is a chemical mes-

senger that moves across the neuromuscular junction and acts as a key to unlock receptors on the muscle fiber. This changes the permeability of the cell membrane and allows calcium ions to flow into the muscle fiber. Calcium ions cause the thin filaments to slide between the thick filaments, shortening the muscle and producing a muscle contraction. Page Ref: 472

176. Muscular dystrophy is a genetic inherited disease caused by a mutation of the gene that makes the muscle protein dystrophin. Without dystrophin, the muscles weaken and then atrophy. Symptoms appear in early childhood as weakness first in the lower extremities and then in the upper extremities. Weakness in the extremities is the most visible disability, but weakness of the diaphragm and inability to breathe is the most frequent cause of death. Page Ref: 483

177. An electromyography is a diagnostic procedure to diagnose muscle disease or nerve damage. A needle electrode inserted into a muscle records electrical activity as the muscle contracts and relaxes. The electrical activity is displayed as waveforms on an oscilloscope screen and permanently recorded on paper as an electromyogram. Page Ref: 489

CHAPTER 10

Multiple Choice

1. a. These drugs inhibit the enzyme that breaks down acetylcholine. Page Ref: 561

2. d. The combining form, radicul/o-, refers to spinal nerve root. The disk is displaced and presses on a spinal nerve root. Page Ref: 548

3. c. The patient who has this type of headache often has nausea, vomiting, and photophobia or sensitivity to light. Photo- means light; phob/o- means fear; -ia mean condition. Page Ref: 546

4. c. Gradual brain neuron destruction with plaques and tangles found on autopsy characterize Alzheimer's disease. Page Ref: 542

5. b. An aura can consist of a sign in the form of something seen, heard, or smelled that is not there. Page Ref: 543

6. b. The face loses animation and the walk appears as if the feet are dragging. Page Ref: 546

7. c. The visual cortex lies within the occipital lobe of the brain. Page Ref: 514

8. b. The suffix -cele refers to a protrusion or herniation of the spinal cord and meninges from a defect in the spinal column. Myel/o- is the combining form for spinal cord and mening/o- is the combining form for the lining of the spinal cord. Page Ref: 547

9. d. Endorphins is a combination of endo- meaning within and morphine, a drug that relieves pain. Page Ref: 525

10. b. During the seizure the body alternates between rigidity (tonic) and jerking movements (clonic). Page Ref: 543

11. d. A- means without and phas/o- means speech. Page Ref: 536

12. a. These cells regulate the amount of oxygen, nutrients, and other substances coming into the neurons. Page Ref: 522

13. b. TIA means transient ischemic attack. Transient means temporary. Page Ref: 539

14. a. Paraesthesias often result from chronic nerve damage. The prefix para- means abnormal and -esthesia means pertaining to feeling or sensation. Page Ref: 552

15. b. Tom/o- means a cut, slice, or layer and -graphy means process of recording. Page Ref: 554

16. c. Lou Gehrig suffered from amyotrophic lateral sclerosis. Page Ref: 549

17. b. The scores range from 3 to 15 and are the sum of individual scores for eye opening, motor response, and verbal response following a painful stimulus. Page Ref: 556

18. a. The causes of the lack of oxygen vary but can include compression of the umbilical cord. Page Ref: 537

19. d. Most often there is obstruction of the flow of cerebrospinal fluid that creates the build-up of the fluid. Hydr/o- means water; cephal/o- means head. Page Ref: 545

20. c. Nuchal rigidity is a stiff neck. This along with fever and headache are some of the signs of meningitis. Page Ref: 546

21. c. A severing of the spinal cord at this level of the spine would show a loss of sensation and movement below the waist, including paralysis of both legs as well as loss of bowel and bladder control. Page Ref: 549

22. d. This is a test known as a sleep study to determine why she falls asleep during the day while engaged in activity. Narc/o- means sleep; -lepsy means seizure. Page Ref: 555

23. a. Seizures are not considered one of the signs of a syncopal episode. Page Ref: 546

24. c. The arachnoid is located between the dura mater and the pia mater. Page Ref: 518

25. a. The hypothalamus is located inferior to the thalamus and regulates all of these body activities. Page Ref: 517

26. a. The glossopharyngeal is the ninth (IX) cranial nerve and it controls swallowing. Page Ref: 519

27. c. Efferent nerves carry impulses away from the spinal cord; whereas afferent nerves carry impulses toward the spinal cord. Page Ref: 521

28. c. The axon is covered by a fatty, white insulating layer of myelin that insulates the electrical impulse received from the nerve body. Page Ref: 524

29. c. The 12 pairs of cranial nerves carry sensory and motor impulses to and from the brain and

are numbered using Roman numerals. Page Ref: 518

30. b. A- means without or not, phas/o- means speech, and -ia means condition, state, or thing. Page Ref: 536

31. d. Arteriovenous malformation is an abnormality in which arteries in the brain connect directly to veins (rather than to capillaries), forming a twisted nest of blood vessels. Page Ref: 537

32. c. Cephal/o- means head and -algia means condition of pain. Page Ref: 537

33. b. Cerebral palsy (CP) can include spastic muscles; lack of coordination in walking, eating, and talking; muscle paralysis; seizures; and mental retardation because of lack of oxygen during birth. Page Ref: 537

34. b. Hemi- means one half, pleg/o- means paralysis, and -ia means condition. Page Ref: 540

35. a. TIA stands for transient ischemic attack, also known as a mini stroke. Its effects only last 24 hours. Page Ref: 539

36. c. Contusion is used to describe bruising of an internal organ. Page Ref: 540

37. d. This type of seizure results in unconsciousness with excessive motor activity. Page Ref: 543

38. b. Early symptoms of Parkinson's disease include muscle rigidity, tremors, and a slowing of voluntary movements due to an imbalance in the levels of dopamine and acetylcholine. Page Ref: 546

39. a. ALS is a chronic, progressive disease of the motor nerves of the spinal cord. Lou Gehrig, a professional baseball player, had this disease. Page Ref: 549

40. d. Trigeminal neuralgia is pain along the path of a nerve and its nerve branches caused by an injury to the nerve. Tic deuloreux is French for repeated muscle contractions that are painful. Page Ref: 551

41. d. PET stands for positron emission tomography. Page Ref: 554

42. a. Evoked potential is a diagnostic procedure in which an EEG is used to record changes in brain waves that occur following various stimuli. Page Ref: 555

43. c. A normal test or negative Babinski shows downward curling of the toes. Page Ref: 556

44. b. TENS stands for transcutaneous electrical nerve stimulation. Page Ref: 558

45. a. COMT inhibitor drugs inhibit the enzyme that metabolizes the drug levodopa. This allows more levadopa to reach the brain. Page Ref: 561

46. c. CVA is also known as stroke. Page Ref: 539

47. a. LP stands for lumbar puncture, which is another name for a spinal tap. Page Ref: 557

48. c. The cranial nerves are part of the peripheral nervous system. All of the other choices are part of the central nervous system. Page Ref: 513

49. a. The cranium is the bony structure that houses the brain. Page Ref: 513

50. d. The prefix hemi- means half and is a clue to the meaning. Page Ref: 516

51. b. The frontal lobe coordinates and analyzes information received by the other lobes and uses it to predict future events and the benefits or consequences of actions taken. Page Ref: 514

52. b. The olfactory nerve controls the sense of smell. Page Ref: 519

53. a. They are classified as afferent nerves, which carry nerve impulses toward the spinal cord and brain. Page Ref: 521

54. d. The astrocyte has radiating branches that support nearby neurons and connects them to capillaries. Page Ref: 522

55. d. Endorphins are the neurotransmitters which are located between neurons in the hypothalamus, thalamus, and brainstem and are the body's own natural pain relievers. Page Ref: 525

56. b. The inability to verbally express thoughts is called expressive aphasia. Page Ref: 536

57. a. Hemisphere (HEM-ih-sfeer), hemi- means one half, -sphere means sphere or ball. Page Ref: 516

58. b. Thalamus (THAL-ah-mus) is a Greek word meaning an inner chamber. Page Ref: 517

59. c. The midbrain is the most superior part of the brainstem. Page Ref: 517

60. d. Dendrites (DEN-dryt), dendr/o- means branching structure, -ite means thing that pertains to. Page Ref: 524

61. b. Petit mal (peh-TEE MAWL) is a French phrase meaning minor disorder. Page Ref: 544

62. c. Subdural (sub-DYOO-ral), sub- means below, underneath, or less than, dur/o- means dura mater, and -al means pertaining to. Hematoma (HEE-mah-TOH-mah), hemat/o- means blood, and -oma means tumor, mass. Page Ref: 545

63. b. Migraine (MY-grayn) is derived from a Greek phrase meaning half of the cranium because migraines often affect just one side of the head. Page Ref: 546

64. a. Neuropathy (nyoo-RAWP-ah-thee), neur/o- means nerve, and -pathy means disease, suffering. Page Ref: 552

65. b. Magnetic (mag-NET-ik), magnet/o- means magnet, and -ic means pertaining to. Page Ref: 554

66. a. Craniotomy (KRAY-nee-AWT-oh-mee), crani/o- means cranium (skull), and -tomy means process of cutting or making an incision. Page Ref: 559

67. b. Myel/o- means spinal cord. It should not be confused with the combining form my/o-, which means muscle. Page Ref: 547

68. a. Meningitis is the only one of these diseases that is an infection. Page Ref: 546

69. d. A hematoma develops in response to a trauma. Page Ref: 545

70. b. Quad- means four (all four extremities below the neck), pleg/o- means paralysis, and -ia means condition. Page Ref: 548

71. c. A neuron, an individual nerve cell, is the functional unit of the nervous system. Page Ref: 521

72. b. The arachnoid is one of the meninges. It has attached fibers that create a web-like structure. Arachn/o- means spider web and -oid means resembling. Page Ref: 518

73. d. The temporal lobe contains the auditory cortex for hearing and the olfactory cortex for smelling. Page Ref: 515

74. a. Syncope is a Greek word that means to faint. Page Ref: 546

75. a. Multiple sclerosis develops slowly over time, beginning in adolescence or early adulthood. Page Ref: 550

76. d. Electroencephalography (EEG) records brain wave patterns. Page Ref: 554

77. b. Radiculopathy is caused by a pinching of a spinal nerve root by an intervertebral disk in the spine. Page Ref: 548

78. b. The lamina or flat area of the arch of the vertebra is removed. Page Ref: 559

79. b. The carpal tunnel in the wrist becomes inflamed from repetitive movement, such as typing, and compresses the median nerve. Page Ref: 550

80. a. The vagus nerve travels through the chest and abdomen. Vagus is a Latin word that means wandering. Page Ref: 519

81. d. The epidural space is between the dura mater and the vertebra and contains fatty tissue and blood vessels. There is no epidural space in the brain. Page Ref: 520

82. c. The sympathetic nervous system constricts smooth muscles around arteries to raise the blood pressure in preparation for "fight or flight." Page Ref: 523

83. b. The cerebrospinal fluid (CSF) circulates around the brain and spinal cord. Page Ref: 562

84. d. A neurofibroma is a benign tumor of the peripheral nerve. Page Ref: 538, 552

85. b. Anesthesia is the absence of pain. Page Ref: 549, 551

86. b. A positron emission scan (PET) measures metabolism rather than anatomic structures. Page Ref: 554

87. d. Rhiz/o- is the Greek combining form for nerve root and radicul/o- is the Latin combining form. Page Ref: 563

88. a. Rhizotomy is a pain management technique that cuts the spinal nerve roots. Page Ref: 559

89. c. Proprioception is the sense of body position. Page Ref: 558

90. c. Meningitis is the correct spelling. Page Ref: 546

91. a. Stereotactic neurosurgery uses a three-dimensional apparatus to perform brain surgery to remove a brain tumor. Page Ref: 559

92. a. The cerebrum is the largest part of the brain. Page Ref: 514

93. a. Oligodendroglia are cells that form myelin to insulate neurons on the brain and spinal cord. Page Ref: 522

94. b. The parasympathetic nervous system controls functions like peristalsis in the GI tract and the release of saliva from the salivary glands. Page Ref: 523

95. d. A baby's head is heavy and the neck lacks muscle to control it. Shaking can cause any of these traumas. Page Ref: 540

96. c. Spin/o- refers to the spinal column or spinal cord. Page Ref: 543

97. a. Amnesia is a loss of memory. Page Ref: 536

98. c. Hydr/o- means water and -cephalus means head. Page Ref: 545

99. a. Photophobia is an aversion to light. Light often hurts the eyes of a patient having a migraine headache. Page Ref: 546

100. c. A lumbar puncture removes cerebrospinal fluid through a needle inserted between the vertebrae and into the spinal cavity. Page Ref: 557

Short Answer

101. lumbar puncture. A spinal tap is a medical procedure to obtain cerebrospinal fluid for testing. Page Ref: 557

102. Parkinson's disease. Early symptoms include muscle rigidity, tremors, and a slowing of voluntary movements. Later, the patient shows a mask-like facial expression, shuffling gait, or inability to ambulate. Page Ref: 546

103. electroencephalography. Electr/o- means electricity, encephal/o- means brain, and -graphy means process of recording. Page Ref: 554-555

104. reflex. Reflex is a Latin word meaning to bend back. Page Ref: 521

105. seizures. Seizure is derived from an Old French word meaning to grab. Page Ref: 543

106. dysphasia. Dys- means difficult; -phasia means condition of speech. Page Ref: 536

107. carpal tunnel syndrome. It is caused by repetitive motions of the hand and wrist, such as typing or data entry. Page Ref: 550

108. quadriplegic. Quadri- means four and indicates paralysis in all four extremities. Page Ref: 549

109. intervertebral. Inter- means between, and verteb/o- means vertebra. Page Ref: 548

110. Myelography. Myel/o- means spinal cord, and -graphy means process of recording. Page Ref: 554

111. Evoked potential. It is used to evaluate the potential ability of a particular nervous pathway to conduct nerve impulses. Page Ref: 555

112. Polysomnography. During sleep, the patient's EEG, eye movements, muscle activity, heartbeat, and respirations are monitored. Polysomnography is also known as a sleep study. Page Ref: 555

113. Babinski's. A normal (negative) test shows downward curling of the toes; an abnormal (positive) test shows upward extension of the great toe and lateral fanning of the other toes, and indicates injury to the parietal lobe or to the spinal nerves. Page Ref: 556

114. endarterectomy. This opens up the lumen of the artery, restores blood flow to the brain, and decreases the possibility of a stroke. Page Ref: 559

115. ventriculoperitoneal. This procedure is done to treat hydrocephalus. Page Ref: 560

116. anticonvulsant. Exampls are Depakene, Dilantin, Tegretol, and Zarontin. Page Ref: 560

117. cranial. The cranial cavity is surrounded by the cranium. Page Ref: 513

118. reflex. Reflex is derived from a Latin word meaning to bend back. Page Ref: 521

119. ventricles. Ventricle (VEN-trih-kl) is a Latin word meaning little belly. Page Ref: 517

120. central. Centr/o- means center; dominant part and -al means pertaining to. Page Ref: 513

121. cerebrum. Cerebrum (SER-eh-brum) (seh-REE-brum) is a Latin word meaning brain. Page Ref: 514

122. cortex. Cortex (KOR-teks) is a Latin word meaning the bark of a tree. Page Ref: 515

123. fissure. Fissure (FISH-ur), fiss/o- means splitting and -ure means system; result of. Page Ref: 516

124. corpus callosum. Corpus callosum (KOR-pus kah-LOH-sum) is a Latin phrase meaning body of tough fibers. Page Ref: 516

125. medulla. The medulla oblongata is part of the brainstem. Page Ref: 517

126. meninges. Meninges (meh-NIN-jeez) is the plural form. Meninx, the singular form, is seldom used. Page Ref: 518

127. reflex. Reflex (REE-fleks) is derived from a Latin word meaning to bend back. Page Ref: 521

128. neuron. Neuron (NYOOR-on) is a Greek word meaning a nerve. Page Ref: 521

129. somatic. Somatic (soh-MAT-ik), somat/o- means body and -ic means pertaining to. Page Ref: 521

130. sympathetic. Sympathetic (sɪM-pah-THET-ik), sym- means together, with; pathet/o- means suffering; and -ic means pertaining to. The sympathetic nervous system is active when the body is suffering from fear. Page Ref: 523

131. Narcolepsy. Narcolepsy (NAR-koh-lep-see), narc/o- means stupor, sleep and -lepsy means seizure. Page Ref: 546

132. spina bifida. Spina bifida (SPY-nah BIF-ih-dah) is a Latin phrase meaning backbone that is split into two parts. Page Ref: 547

133. multiple sclerosis. Sclerosis (skleh-ROH-sis), scler/o- means hard; sclera (white of the eye) and -osis means condition; abnormal condition; process. Page Ref: 550

134. Folic acid. Folic acid supplements taken by the mother during pregnancy reduce the incidence of neural tube defects. Page Ref: 547

135. TENS. A TENS unit transmits electrical impulses through the skin (transcutaneous) to block pain sensation. Page Ref: 558

136. neurology. Neur/o- means nerve and -logy means the study of. Page Ref: 512

137. gyri (singular: gyrus); sulci (singular: sulcus). The surface of the cerebrum is covered with these folds and grooves. Page Ref: 515

138. smell. Olfact/o- means the sense of smell. Page Ref: 515, 519

139. comatose. Comat/o- means deep unconsciousness and -ose means full of. Page Ref: 540

140. Down. Down syndrome was named by John Down, an English physician. Page Ref: 542

141. Shingles. Shingles is caused by the herpes zoster virus, the same virus that causes chicken pox in children. Page Ref: 551

142. Corpus callosum. The corpus callosum is a white band of nerves between the two hemispheres of the cerebrum. Page Ref: 516

143. 12; 31. The cranial nerves originate in the brain and carry nerve impulses to the face, head, neck, and upper back; the exception is cranial nerve X, which carries nerve impulses to the organs of the thoracic and abdominal cavities. The spinal nerves orginate from the spinal cord; each pair consists of a nerve to the right side of the body and anerve to the left side of the body. Page Ref: 519, 521

True/False

144. False. This condition is termed Bell's palsy. Page Ref: 550

145. False. This describes causalgia. Page Ref: 551

146. True. Endarterectomy opens the lumen of the artery, restoring blood flow to the brain. Page Ref: 559

147. False. This x-ray is termed a myelography. My/o- is the combining form for muscle, whereas myel/o- refers to spinal cord. Page Ref: 554

148. True. Sciatica is derived from a Greek word meaning related to the ischium (hip bone). The sciatic nerve passes through a large notch in the ischium. Page Ref: 548

149. True. Areas of demyelinization of the nerves of the brain and spinal cord cause scar tissue or plaques. Page Ref: 550

150. False. This is a Morton's neuroma. Page Ref: 552

151. True. Electrical impulses from this instrument travel through the skin to inhibit pain sensations to the brain. Page Ref: 558

152. True. The shunt runs from the ventricle of the brain to the peritoneal cavity in the abdomen. Page Ref: 560

153. False. This collection of blood would be located below the outermost layer of the meninges, the dura mater. Page Ref: 545

154. True. This is the inability to understand the spoken or written word and the inability to verbally express thoughts. Page Ref: 536

155. False. An arteriovenous malformation is an abnormality in which arteries in the brain connect to veins (not arteries or capillaries), forming a twisted nest of blood vessels. Page Ref: 537

156. True. Lymphoma may occur in any part of the body, including the brain. Page Ref: 538

157. False. A cerebrovascular accident is disruption or blockage of blood flow to the brain, which causes tissue death. Page Ref: 539

158. False. Coma is a deep state of unconsciousness and unresponsiveness caused by trauma or disease in the brain. Brain death is defined as an irreversible loss of all brain function as confirmed by an electroencephalogram. Page Ref: 540

159. True. The only way to unequivocally diagnose Alzheimer's is through autopsy of the brain. Page Ref: 541

160. False. The alpha fetoprotein test is actually conducted to diagnose a neural tube defect in a fetus before birth. Page Ref: 553

161. False. The Glasgow Coma Scale is a numerical scale that measures the depth of a coma. It has no relationship to aphasia. The scores range from 3-15. Page Ref: 556

162. True. If the patient's answers are all correct, the patient is said to be oriented to person, time, and place, or "oriented x 3." Page Ref: 557

163. False. A craniotomy is a surgical incision into the skull to expose the brain tissue, and is the first phase of any type of brain surgery, including diagnosing and/or excising a brain tumor. It may also be used for diagnosis and treatment of other brain-related problems. Page Ref: 559

164. False. Epilepsy is diagnosed based on the characteristics of the seizure and the results of the electroencephalography (EEG). Page Ref: 554

165. False. Tardive dyskinesia is a side effect of drugs used to treat Parkinson's disease. Page Ref: 561

166. False. White matter, not the gray matter, contains myelin. Myelin is a white, insulating coating on the neuron. Page Ref: 524

167. True. Cerebrospinal fluid is formed in the ventricles but circulates throughout the cranial cavity and spinal cavity. Page Ref: 517

168. False. A nerve impulse crosses the synapse in the form of a neurotransmitter, as a chemical signal. Page Ref: 524

169. False. It should be an intervertebral disk. Inter- means between; the disk is between two vertebrae. Page Ref: 548

170. True. A myelomeningocele is a protrusion (hernia) of the spinal cord and meninges. Page Ref: 547

171. True. A neurotransmitter transmits a message from one neuron to the next. Page Ref: 525

172. False. A reflex is an involuntary reaction controlled by the spinal cord. Page Ref: 521

173. True. The blood clot causes a CVA with lack of oxygenated blood to the left side of the brain, which affects the right side of the body. Page Ref: 539

174. True. The pons is a relay station where nerves cross. Page Ref: 517

175. True. Cauda equina is a Latin phrase that means horse's tail. These nerves resemble the many hairs of a horse's tail that originate from one area. Page Ref: 520

176. False. The spinal cord attaches to and is continuous with the medulla oblongata. Page Ref: 520

177. True. New variant Creutzfeldt-Jakob disease is caused by a prion (small, infectious protein particle) that also causes mad cow disease. Page Ref: 541

178. False. Down syndrome is a congenital defect in chromosome 21. Page Ref: 542

179. True. Psych/o- means mind and mot/o- means movement. These seizures cause some degree of impairment of consciousness and some muscle movements. Page Ref: 544

Essay

180. An interruption of blood flow from a problem in an artery providing blood to brain tissue in a particular site can create a lack of oxygen to that part of the brain and cause brain cells to die. This area of dead cells is called an infarct. Page Ref: 539

181. An electroencephalography (EEG) maps electrical currents that move along neurons of the brain. Epilepsy is characterized by nerve groupings in the brain that send abnormal, uncontrolled impulses. The EEG shows the distinct patterns of the abnormal electrical brain activity found in epilepsy. Electr/o- means electricity; encephal/o- means brain; -graphy means process of recording. Page Ref: 554-555

182. dura mater, arachnoid, pia mater. The dura mater is the outer, tougher layer, while the pia mater is delicate and lies next to the brain. The arachnoic is a spiderweb-like membrane between the dura mater and pia mater. Page Ref: 518

183. The dendrites are multiple branches at the beginning of a neuron that receive a neurotransmitter from the previous neuron, convert it to an electrical impulse, and send it to the cell body. The cell body contains the nucleus that di-

rects cellular activities, produces neurotransmitters, and provides energy for the cell. The cell body sends the electrical impulse to the axon, a single, elongated branch at the end of the neuron. There is a space called a synapse between the axon and the dendrites of the next neuron. A chemical neurotransmitter allows the electrical message to be transmitted across the synapse. Page Ref: 524

184. The parasympathetic nervous system is responsible for functions such as raising or lowering the heart rate, changing the diameter of the irises in response to changing levels of light, gastrointestinal peristalsis, salivary gland stimulation, and preparing the body for sexual activity. Norepinephrine is the neurotransmitter for the parasympathetic nervous system. Page Ref: 523

185. A cerebrovascular accident (CVA) is a disruption or blockage of blood flow to the brain, which causes tissue death and an area of necrosis known as in infarct. The blood flow can be disrupted by an embolus, thrombus, arteriosclerosis, or hemorrhage. CVAs affect the opposite side of the body from where they occur. The severity of the CVA depends on how much brain tissue was damaged. Results may range from hemiparesis (weakness on one side of the body) to death. Treatment may include thrombolytic drugs or surgery. Page Ref: 539

186. Dementia is disease of the brain in which many neurons in the cerebrum die, the cerebral cortex shrinks in size, and there is progressive deterioration in mental function. Symptoms include gradual decline in mental ability, forgetfulness, inability to learn new things, inability to perform daily activities, and difficulty making decisions. The symptoms progress over time and may eventually lead to psychiatric symptoms and complete memory loss. Page Ref: 541

187. Cerebral angiography is a radiologic procedure in which a radiopaque contrast dye is injected into the carotid arteries, and an x-ray is taken to visualize the arterial circulation in the brain. This test can show aneurysms, stenosis, tumors, or plaque in the arteries. A tumor can be seen as an interwoven collection of new blood vessels, or it can be seen indirectly when it distorts normal anatomy and forces arteries into abnormal positions. The x-ray image is known as an angiogram or arteriogram. Page Ref: 553

CHAPTER 11

Multiple Choice

1. c. The urethral meatus is the opening of the urethra to the outside of the body. The word meatus is derived from Latin meaning a passage. Page Ref: 586

2. a. In- means not; contine/o- means keep together; -ence means state. Page Ref: 604

3. a. The overactive bladder has urinary frequency and urgency due to involuntary contractions of the bladder. Page Ref: 619

4. c. The x-ray of the kidney, ureters, bladder is a preliminary or scout film without contrast material. Page Ref: 609

5. d. The nephropexy is a surgical suspension for a downwardly displaced kidney, nephroptosis. Nephr/o- means kidney; -pexy means process of surgically fixing in place. Page Ref: 616

6. b. Pyuria indicates the presence of pus, a product of a bacterial infection. Py/o- means pus; ur/o- means urine; -ia means condition. Page Ref: 605

7. a. Glomerulus is a Latin masculine noun. Form the plural by changing -us to -i. Page Ref: 588

8. c. K+ is the chemical symbol for potassium. Page Ref: 618

9. a. Hydr/o- means water. The ureter is the tube that carries urine from the kidney to the bladder. Page Ref: 597

10. c. Ketones are the byproduct of metabolism of fats and can be present in the urine of a diabetic. Page Ref: 605

11. c. I&O stands for intake and output. Monitoring body fluids can be important in patient care of diseases such as renal failure, dehydration, or diuretic use. Page Ref: 614

12. b. The trigone is the triangular area of the bladder between the two ureteral orifices and the opening to the urethra. Page Ref: 585

13. d. Incontinence is due to relaxation of the muscles in the pelvic wall. Page Ref: 604

14. c. Creatinine is a waste product from skeletal muscle activity that is normally removed from the body through urination. The presence of the other choices is an indication of some pathology. Page Ref: 588, 607

15. a. Voiding means expelling of urine. Cyst/o- means bladder; urethr/o- means urethra; -graphy means process of recording. Page Ref: 611

16. b. A Foley catheter contains an inflatable balloon that keeps it in the bladder. Page Ref: 612

17. c. The patient with end-stage renal disease (ESRD) requires dialysis to remove the wastes that the kidney is not capable of removing. Page Ref: 613

18. d. Macrobid and Gantrisin are antibiotics used for urinary tract infections. Page Ref: 618

19. a. Blood urea nitrogen is a laboratory test done to measure the amount of urea left in the blood that is not removed by the kidney. The patient with uremia is unable to adequately remove the urea, and this waste product accumulates in the blood. Ur/o- means urine; -emia means substance in the blood. Page Ref: 606

20. a. Wilms' tumor is also known as nephroblastoma. Page Ref: 600

21. d. Red blood cell production through secretion of erythropoietin; blood pressure through production of renin; pH through adjustments in bicarbonate retained or excreted. Page Ref: 590

22. d. Vesic/o- is a Latin combining form meaning bladder. Page Ref: 620

23. c. In response to the streptococci, the body produces antibodies that combine with the antigen of the bacterium to form complexes that clog the tiny pores of the glomerular basement membrane. This causes a kidney inflammation. Page Ref: 597

24. b. This is the measurement of the concentration of urine compared to water. Page Ref: 608

25. c. Both conditions are names for a congenital, incorrectly located urethral meatus. The urethroplasty would reposition the urethral meatus to the proper location. Page Ref: 617

26. c. A hilum is an indentation in an organ. There is a hilum in the kidney and a hilum in the lung. Page Ref: 583

27. c. The urethra carries urine between the bladder and the outside of the body. Page Ref: 586

28. a. The parenchyma contains the cortex and medulla. Page Ref: 592

29. b. Peristalsis also occurs in the digestive tract where muscles contract to move food. Page Ref: 584

30. d. The combining form vesic/o- means bladder. The combining form cyst/o- also means bladder. Page Ref: 585

31. a. Calculus is a Latin masculine singular noun meaning a pebble. Page Ref: 597

32. a. Albumin in the urine changes the osmotic pressure of the blood. Edema occurs in the extremities and fluid goes into the abdominal cavity. Page Ref: 599

33. c. Acute renal failure occurs suddenly and is usually due to trauma, severe blood loss, or overwhelming infection. Page Ref: 600

34. c. In renal failure, the kidneys are unable to remove the waste product urea. It reaches toxic levels in the blood. Page Ref: 600

35. c. Wilms' tumor is a cancerous tumor of the kidney (nephroblastoma) that occurs in children and arises from residual embryonic or fetal tissue. Page Ref: 600

36. c. Cystocele is also known as vesicocele. The suffix -cele means hernia. Page Ref: 601

37. c. Vesicovaginal fissure causes urine to flow from the bladder into the vagina and is excreted through the vagina. Page Ref: 602

38. a. Epi- means above or upon. Page Ref: 602

39. c. Enuresis is also called nocturnal enuresis or bedwetting. Page Ref: 603

40. a. The underlying cause of anuria is acute or chronic renal failure. Page Ref: 603

41. c. Dysuria can be due to many factors, such as kidney stones and cystitis. Page Ref: 603

42. d. This may be gross or frank blood (easily seen with the naked eye) or microscopic blood. Page Ref: 604

43. d. Glyc/o- means glucose. Page Ref: 603

44. a. Hyp/o- means below or deficient, kal/i- means potassium, and -emia means substance in the blood. Hypokalemia can be caused by diuretic drugs that cause the kidney to excrete excessive amounts of urine. Page Ref: 604

45. a. BUN stands for blood urea nitrogen. Page Ref: 606

46. c. Cyst/o- means bladder, urethr/o- means urethra, and -graphy means process of recording. Page Ref: 610

47. a. In continuous ambulatory peritoneal dialysis (CAPD), the patient is able to walk around between the three or four daily episodes of dialysis. Page Ref: 613

48. a. Diuretic drugs cause sodium to be excreted in the urine, and it brings water and potassium with it because of osmotic pressure. Page Ref: 618

49. c. UTI stands for urinary tract infection. Page Ref: 619

50. a. The pulmonary parenchyma is located in the lungs. The renal parenchyma is part of the urinary system. The kidneys, ureters, and bladder are part of the urinary system. Page Ref: 583-585

51. b. Only the word trigone cannot be paired with the word renal. Page Ref: 585

52. d. The nephron is a structural unit of the kidney, not a waste product. Page Ref: 588

53. a. Red blood cells are too large to pass through the pores and so they remain in the blood and are not filtered out. Page Ref: 589

54. d. Reabsorption is the process of moving water and non-waste substances out of the tubule and into the blood in a nearby capillary. Urination, micturition, and voiding are all words that mean eliminating urine from the body. Page Ref: 589

55. a. Enlargement of the kidney due to constant pressure from urine is called hydronephrosis. The urine is backed up in the ureter and kidney because of an obstructing stone or stricture. Page Ref: 597

56. d. Inflammation and infection of the pelves of the kidneys is pyelonephritis. This is caused by a bacterial infection of the bladder that ascends the ureters to the pelves of the kidneys. Page Ref: 600

57. d. Chronic renal failure always develops slowly. Page Ref: 600

58. a. Wilms' tumor, also known as nephroblastoma, is a type of cancer that occurs in children and arises from residual embryonic or fetal tissue. Page Ref: 600

59. a. A urinometer is used to measure specific gravity. Specific gravity is the measurement of the concentration of the urine as compared to that of water. Page Ref: 608

60. b. Micturition (MIK-choo-RISH-un), mictur/o- means making urine and -ition means a process; being or having. Page Ref: 589

61. a. The kidneys also help the body maintain a normal and constant internal environment by excreting less water and urine to increase the blood pressure if it falls. Page Ref: 590

62. b. Congenital (con-JEN-ih-tal), congenit/o- means present at birth, -al means pertaining to. Page Ref: 599

63. c. Ambulatory (AM-byoo-lah-TOR-ee), ambulat/o- means walking, -ory means having the function of. Page Ref: 613

64. b. Suprapubic (soo-prah-PYOO-bik), supra- means above, pub/o- means pubis (hip bone), -ic means pertaining to. Page Ref: 612

65. c. I&O is a nursing procedure that documents the total amount of fluid intake (oral, nasogastric tube, intravenous line, and so forth) and the total amount of fluid output (urine, wound drainage, and so forth). Page Ref: 614

66. a. Transplantation (TRANS-plan-TAY-shun), transplant/o- means move something to another place, -ation means a process; being or having. Page Ref: 616

67. b. The parenchyma (pah-RENG-kih-mah) is the functional or working area of any organ (as opposed to the organ's structural framework). The renal parenchyma is made up of the cortex and the medulla because these areas contain nephrons. Page Ref: 588

68. a. See Figure 11-8. Page Ref: 590

69. d. The collecting duct is the common passageway that collects fluid from many nephrons. The final step of reabsorption takes place there and the fluid is known as urine. Page Ref: 591

70. d. *E. coli* is present in the intestines and can enter the urethra. Page Ref: 605

71. c. The nephron is the functional unit of the kidneys. Page Ref: 588

72. b. The kidney stone blocks the flow of urine and the backed up urine dilates the ureter. Page Ref: 597

73. d. A catheter is a tube that drains urine. Page Ref: 612

74. a. Hemodialysis, peritoneal dialysis, or renal transplantation can take the place of nonfunctioning kidneys. Page Ref: 613, 615

75. a. A flat plate is a regular x-ray that is positioned over the kidneys, ureters, and bladder. Page Ref: 609

76. b. The stress of increased intra-abdominal pressure while sneezing, laughing, or coughing forces urine out. Page Ref: 604

77. d. Hemat/o- means blood, ur/o- means urine, and -ia means abnormal condition. Page Ref: 604

78. d. A culture and sensitivity identifies the bacterium and what antibiotic drugs its is sensitive to. Page Ref: 606

79. c. Retro- means behind. The retroperitoneal space is a small area that contains the kidneys and is located behind the peritoneum. Page Ref: 583

80. c. Rugae are folds in the mucosa that allow the bladder to expand when it is full of urine. Page Ref: 585

81. d. All are waste products of cellular metabolism. Page Ref: 588

82. d. The pH measures acidity and alkalinity. Page Ref: 607

83. a. Cyst/o- means bladder and -scopy means process of using an instrument to examine. Page Ref: 615

84. a. Ren/o- is the Latin combining form for kidney and nephr/o- is the Greek combining form. Page Ref: 620

85. d. The suffix -scope indicates the instrument used, while the suffix -scopy indicates the procedure itself. Page Ref: 615

86. c. Continuous ambulatory peritoneal dialysis (CAPD) is a treatment for renal failure. Page Ref: 613, 619

87. d. Pyel/o- is a combining form, nephr/o- is a combining form, and -itis is a suffix. Page Ref: 600

88. c. The suffix -meter means instrument used to measure. Page Ref: 608

89. a. End-stage renal disease (ESRD) affects the kidneys. The other abbreviations are not diseases. Page Ref: 619

Short Answer

90. stone. Calculus is a synonym for a stone. Page Ref: 617

91. nocturia. Noct/o- means night; ur/o- means urine; -ia means condition. Page Ref: 605

92. nephrolithiasis. Nephr/o- means kidney; lith/o- means stone; -iasis means state of. Page Ref: 597

93. cystoscopy. Cyst/o- means bladder; -scopy means process of using an instrument to examine. Page Ref: 615

94. anuria. An- means without; ur/o- means urine; -ia means condition. Page Ref: 603

95. pyelonephritis. Pyel/o- means renal pelvis; nephr/o- means kidney; Page Ref: 600

96. frost. This occurs during kidney failure when the kidneys cannot excrete urea from the blood. Page Ref: 600

97. urination. Urin/o- means urine and -ation means a process. Page Ref: 589

98. dysuria. Dys- means painful or difficult; ur/o- means urine; - ia means condition. Page Ref: 603

99. nephrectomy. Nephr/o- means kidney; -ectomy means surgical excision. Page Ref: 616

100. ureter. The ureter is a 12-inch tube that extends from the renal pelvis of the kidney to the bladder. There are two of them in every human. Page Ref: 584

101. peristalsis. The wall of the ureter contracts every 30 seconds to propel urine into the bladder in a process known as peristalsis. Page Ref: 584

102. rugae. When the bladder is empty, the mucosa collapses into folds called rugae. Page Ref: 585

103. prostate. In the male, as the urethra leaves the bladder, it travels through the prostate gland. Page Ref: 586

104. Filtration. Filtration is the process through which blood in the capillary pushes water, waste products, electrolytes, glucose and other substances through pores in the glomerulus and out into the Bowman's capsule. Page Ref: 589

105. distal. The loop of Henle widens to become the distal convoluted tubule. Page Ref: 589

106. bicarbonate. If the pH of the blood decreases, this causes bicarbonate to be reabsorbed, increasing the pH of the blood. Page Ref: 590

107. Glomerulonephritis. Glomerulonephritis is a complication that develops following an acute infection with streptococcus bacteria or viruses. Page Ref: 597

108. stone. In the word nephrolithiasis, the combining form lith/o- means stone. Page Ref: 597

109. Hematuria. Hematuria means blood in the urine. Page Ref: 604

110. ureter. Ureter (YOO-ree-ter) (yoo-REE-ter) is derived from a Greek noun meaning urinary canal. Page Ref: 584

111. hilum. Hilum (HY-lum) is a Latin singular neuter noun meaning an indentation in an organ. The plural form is hila (HY-lah). Form the plural by changing -um to -a. Page Ref: 583

112. cortex. Cortex (KOR-teks) is a Latin word meaning bark. Page Ref: 584

113. bladder. The bladder is a fluid-filled sac. Page Ref: 585, 587

114. urethra. Urethra (yoo-REE-thrah) is derived from a Greek word meaning passage for urine. Page Ref: 586

115. prostate. The prostate gland is part of the male reproductive system. Page Ref: 586

116. genitourinary. Genitourinary (JEN-ih-toh-YOO-rih-nair-ee), genit/o- means genitalia, urin/o- means urine; urinary system, and -ary means pertaining to. Page Ref: 587

117. nephron. The nephron is the microscopic functional unit of the kidney. Page Ref: 588

118. erythropoietin. Erythropoietin (eh-RITH-roh-POY-eh-tin), erythr/o- mens red, -poietin means a substance that forms. Page Ref: 590

119. Nephropathy. Nephropathy (neh-FRAWP-ah thee), nephr/o- means kidney; nephron, -pathy means disease, suffering. Page Ref: 598

120. nephroblastoma. Nephroblastoma (NEF-roh-blas-TOH-mah), nephr/o- means kidney; nephron, blast/o- means immature; embryonic, and -oma means tumor, mass. Page Ref: 600

121. hemodialysis. Hemodialysis (HEE-moh-dy-AL-ih-sis), hem/o- means blood, dia- means complete; completely through, and -lysis means process of breaking down or dissolving. Page Ref: 613

122. catheter. Catheter (KATH-eh-ter) is derived from a Greek word meaning to send down. Page Ref: 612

123. cystometrogram. Cystometrogram (SIS-toh-MET-roh-gram), cyst/o- means bladder; fluid-filled sac; semisolid cyst, metr/o- means measurement, and -gram means a record or picture. Page Ref: 611

124. Lithotripsy. Lithotripsy (LITH-oh-trip-see), lith/o- means stone, -tripsy means process of crushing. Page Ref: 616

125. kidneys, ureters, bladder. The KUB is an x-ray of these structures. Page Ref: 609

126. adrenal gland. The adrenal gland is directly above the kidney, but it is part of the endocrine system, not the urinary system. Page Ref: 583

127. many or much. There are many cysts in the kidney in polycystic kidney disease. Page Ref: 599

128. polyuria. A- means without and poly- means many, much. Page Ref: 603, 605

129. urology. Ur/o- means urine, urinary system and -logy means study of. Page Ref: 582

True/False

130. True. Enuresis is an involuntary passing of urine during sleep. Page Ref: 603

131. False. It is the presence of blood in the urine. Page Ref: 604

132. True. The renal cortex and medulla contain the nephrons, the structures involved in removing wastes from the body and creating urine. Parenchyma is a word used to describe the functional or working part of an organ. Page Ref: 588

133. False. This describes the ureter, of which there are two. Because both organs begin with the letter U they can be mistaken for each other. Page Ref: 584, 586

134. False. Polyuria means excessive urination. Pyuria is the condition that always means the presence of a urinary tract infection. Page Ref: 605

135. False. *Escherichia coli* (*E. coli*) is the most common cause of bacterial urinary tract infections. Page Ref: 605

136. True. Extracorporeal shock wave lithotripsy crushes a stone so that the patient can urinate the gravel or particles of the broken stone. Page Ref: 616

137. True. The ureters or bladder go into a spasm as the jagged edges of the passing stone scrape the mucosa. Page Ref: 598

138. False. The abnormal passageway is a vesicovaginal fistula. Vesic/o- means bladder; vagin/o- means vagina; fistula means tube. Page Ref: 602

139. False. The word is nephropathy. Nephr/o- means kidney; -pathy means disease. Page Ref: 598

140. True. The word is composed of three word parts: retr/o- meaning behind, peritone/o- meaning peritoneum, and -al meaning pertaining to. Page Ref: 583

141. False. Actually, electrolytes and glucose molecules are small enough to pass through the pores in the glomerulus, but they are reabsorbed back into the blood. Page Ref: 589

142. True. Non-waste substances are reabsorbed back into the blood in this arteriole. Page Ref: 589

143. False. The proximal convoluted tubule is the correct name of a normal renal structure. Page Ref: 589

144. True. How much water and non-waste substances (including glucose) are reabsorbed depends on the concentration of that substance in the blood. Page Ref: 589

145. True. As a person ages, some nephrons deteriorate and die, causing a decrease in kidney function. Page Ref: 589

146. True. If the blood pressure decreases, certain hormones are secreted, which in turn cause more sodium and water to be reabsorbed, concentrating the urine but raising the blood pressure back to normal. Page Ref: 590

147. True. The word calculus is Latin for pebble. Calculogenesis is also known as lithogenesis. Page Ref: 598

148. False. The medical word for any disease process involving the kidney is nephropathy. Nephroptosis means abnormally low position of a kidney. Page Ref: 598

149. False. A urinalysis is a test done to describe the characteristics of the urine while the leukocyte esterase is a urine test specifically to detect esterase. Page Ref: 606

150. True. Urea is a waste product of protein metabolism that is excreted in the urine. Page Ref: 588

151. False. A diuretic drug increases urine production. Page Ref: 618

152. True. Nephr/o- means kidney, lith/o- means stone, and -tomy means process of cutting or making an incision. Page Ref: 616

153. True. In hemodialysis, the shunt is placed between an artery and vein. In peritoneal dialysis, the shunt is placed in the abdomen. Page Ref: 613

154. True. A urine dipstick has several chemical pads to perform several different urine tests from one dip in a urine specimen. Page Ref: 607

155. False. The urethra travels through the prostate gland, but the prostate gland is part of the male reproductive system. Page Ref: 586

156. False. The male urethra is longer than the female urethra because it has to travel through the penis. Page Ref: 587

157. False. It tests the blood, not the urine, for the presence of urea. Page Ref: 606

158. True. Nephroptosis is a prolapsed or drooping kidney. Page Ref: 599

159. False. A biopsy is done to examine tissue for signs of cancer or kidney failure. Page Ref: 617

Essay

160. The location of the female urethra is close to the anus, a source of bacteria. The female urethra is shorter in length than the male urethra and that makes it easier for bacteria to travel upward toward the bladder. Page Ref: 605

161. When it is suspected that the patient has a urinary tract infection, the physician orders tests to find the cause of the infection and the best treatment for it. The culture involves using some of the patient's urine to grow organisms that are present in the urine. The organisms are identified and subjected to sensitivity testing with antibiotic disks to determine which antibiotic would be the most effective in killing the bacterium causing the patient's urinary tract infection. Page Ref: 606

162. Blood urea nitrogen (BUN) is a blood test that measures the amount of urea in the blood. It is used to monitor kidney function and the progression of kidney disease or to watch for signs of nephrotoxicity in patients taking aminoglycoside antibiotics. Page Ref: 606

163. A culture and sensitivity test is a urine test that puts urine onto culture medium in a Petri dish to grow and identify the microbial cause of a urinary tract infection. The specific disease-causing microorganism is identified and tested to determine its sensitivity to various antibiotic drugs. Page Ref: 606

164. Polycystic kidney disease is a congenital disease characterized by cysts in the kidney that eventually obliterate the nephrons, causing kidney failure. The early state of this progressive degenerative disease shows few symptoms and is not detected until hypertension and already-enlarged kidneys are palpated on physical examination. Page Ref: 599

165. Renal failure is a disease process in which the kidneys progressively decrease and then stop urine production. Symptoms do not appear until 80% of kidney function has been lost. The disease process can be divided into acute renal failure and chronic renal failure. Page Ref: 600

166. Erythropoietin is a hormone secreted by the kidneys when the number of red blood cells

decreases. It stimulates the bone marrow to produce more red blood cells. Page Ref: 590

CHAPTER 12

Multiple Choice

1. d. The origin of the word phimosis means a muzzling or a closure. Page Ref: 651

2. d. Balan/o- means glans penis; -itis means inflammation. Page Ref: 650

3. b. A transurethral resection of the prostate would be done for benign prostatic hypertrophy to reduce the size of the prostate. Page Ref: 656

4. d. Genital herpes is a viral disease and Zovirax is an antiviral drug. Page Ref: 657

5. b. The epididymis, located above and behind the testes, receives and stores spermatozoa from the seminiferous tubules. Page Ref: 639

6. c. Erectile dysfunction or impotence is the inability to achieve or sustain an erection. Page Ref: 650

7. b. Human papillomavirus causes genital warts. Page Ref: 652

8. c. The vas deferens are severed to prevent the passage of spermatozoa to the outside of the body and into a woman. Page Ref: 656

9. a. Crypt/o- means hidden; orch/o- means testis; -ism means process. Orchi/o- means testis; -pexy means surgically fixing in place. Page Ref: 656

10. a. The prostate produces some of the semen. The rest of the functions listed above relate to the testes and epididymis. Page Ref: 640

11. d. Prostate specific antigen. Increased levels can point to the presence of prostate cancer. Page Ref: 653

12. b. Chlamydia is the only choice that is caused by a bacterium. All the other choices are viral diseases. Page Ref: 651

13. b. A varicocele is the presence of a varicose vein in the spermatic cord to the testes and can cause a low sperm count. Page Ref: 649

14. d. Priapism is a continuing erection of the penis causing considerable discomfort. Page Ref: 651

15. a. The correct spelling is prostate. Prostrate means lying face down. Page Ref: 640

16. c. In a digital rectal exam, the examining physician inserts a gloved finger into the rectum to feel the prostate. Page Ref: 655

17. b. Gonorrhea is the only choice that is caused by a classification of bacteria called diplococci. Page Ref: 652

18. c. Located in the testes, these coiled tubules produce spermatozoa and the interstitial cells of these structures secrete testosterone. Page Ref: 638

19. d. The seminal vesicles produce most of the semen while the prostate and the bulbourethral glands produce some. Page Ref: 640

20. a. The corpora cavernosa consists of two columns of erectile tissue found on the upper side of the penis. Page Ref: 641

21. c. Elevated levels of acid phosphatase can point to prostate cancer that may have metastasized. Page Ref: 653

22. a. A routine semen analysis for infertility would not include examining the genetic structure (DNA) of the sperm. Page Ref: 654

23. b. The VDRL and RPR are blood tests to screen for syphilis antibodies. Page Ref: 652

24. c. The man with erectile dysfunction is unable to achieve or sustain an erection of the penis. An implant can help this condition. Page Ref: 656

25. c. The term flagellum is derived from a Latin word meaning little whip. The spermatozoon is the only cell in the body to have a flagellum. Page Ref: 643

26. c. The male genitourinary system is located in the pelvic cavity and outside the body in the area below the pelvic cavity. Page Ref: 642

27. d. The male genitourinary system is composed of the external and internal genitalia. Extern/o- means outside and intern/o- means inside. Page Ref: 637

28. a. The scrotum is a pouch that contains the testes. Page Ref: 637

29. a. During puberty, testosterone causes the development of the male sex characteristics: enlargement of the external genitalia, large body muscles, deepening of the voice, body hair, and sexual drive. Page Ref: 638

30. b. The Cowper's glands are small, bulblike glands about the size of peas that are located on either side of the urethra just below the prostate gland. Page Ref: 640

31. d. In uncircumcised males, the urethral meatus is covered by the prepuce or foreskin of the penis. Page Ref: 641

32. c. Mitosis is a process in which the 46 chromosomes in the nucleus duplicate and then split, creating two identical cells, each with 46 chromosomes. Page Ref: 643

33. a. Each spermatozoon is composed of a head that contains the 23 chromosomes and a tail or flagellum that propels it. Page Ref: 643

34. d. The combining form crypt/o- means hidden. The medical word cryptorchism means failure of one or both of the testicles to descent through the inguinal canal into the scrotum. Page Ref: 649

35. b. Orch/o- means testis. Orchitis is caused by a bacterium, the mumps virus, or trauma. Page Ref: 649

36. c. A cancerous tumor of one of the testes is known as testicular cancer or seminoma. Page Ref: 649

37. b. Chordee is caused by a constricting, cordlike band of tissue along the underside of the penis. Page Ref: 650

38. c. Erectile dysfunction (ED) is the inability to achieve or sustain an erection of the penis. It is also known as impotence. Page Ref: 650

39. a. Venereal disease is a contagious disease that is contracted during sexual intercourse with an infected individual. Venereal is derived from the Latin word Venus, meaning the goddess of love. Page Ref: 651

40. a. The *Neisseria gonorrhoeae* bacteria are present in the sexually transmitted disease gonorrhea. Page Ref: 652

41. d. Chancre is a lesion and sign of syphilis that is caused by the pathogen *Treponema pallidum,* a spirochete (spiral) bacterium. Page Ref: 652

42. b. Also known as genital warts, *Condylomata acuminats* is a sexually transmitted disease. Page Ref: 652

43. c. Gynecomastia, or enlargement of the male breast, is caused by an imbalance of androgens and estrogens. Page Ref: 653

44. a. Hormone testing is a blood test used to determine the levels of FSH and LH from the anterior pituitary gland and testosterone from the testes. Page Ref: 653

45. d. PSA is increased in men with prostate cancer. The higher the level, the more advanced the cancer. PSA levels fall after successful treatment of the cancer. Page Ref: 653

46. b. A semen analysis is done as part of the workup for infertility. The motility, or forward movement, and morphology, or shape, of the spermatozoa are evaluated. Page Ref: 654

47. d. ProstaScint is a combination of a radioactive tracer and a monoclonal antibody that binds to receptors on cancer cells from the prostate. Page Ref: 654

48. a. The combining form orchid/o- means testes. The suffix -pexy means process of surgically fixing in place. Page Ref: 656

49. c. Androgen drugs treat the lack of production of testosterone by the testes. Page Ref: 657

50. c. Proscar is a drug prescribed for benign prostatic hypertrophy. It inhibits the enzyme that causes the prostate to enlarge. Page Ref: 657

51. c. The vas deferens is an internal organ of the male genitourinary system. Page Ref: 637

52. a. The suffix -ary means pertaining to. Page Ref: 637

53. d. The scrotum contains the testes. Page Ref: 637

54. a. The suffix -cle means small. Page Ref: 638

55. c. Spermatozoon is a Greek noun. Form the plural by changing -on to -a. Page Ref: 638

56. a. The prefix inter- means within or between. Page Ref: 638

57. d. The suffix -ory means having the function of. Page Ref: 640

58. a. The bulbourethral glands are also known as Cowper's glands. Page Ref: 640

59. a. The male urethral meatus is covered by tissue known as the prepuce. Page Ref: 641

60. c. Failure of one or both of the testicles to descend through the inguinal canal into the scrotum is cryptorchism. Page Ref: 649

61. d. The prefix dys- means painful, difficult, or abnormal. Page Ref: 650

62. a. Flagellum (flah-JEL-um) is a Latin word meaning a little whip. A spermatozoon is the only cell in the human body that has a flagellum. Page Ref: 643

63. b. Luteinizing (LOO-tee-ih-ny-zing) hormone (LH) is so named because it stimulates interstitial cells of the testes as well as the corpus luteum of the ovary. Luteinizing hormone comes from the anterior pituitary gland. It causes the interstitial cells of the testes to secrete testosterone. Page Ref: 642

64. b. Meiosis (my-OH-sis) is a Greek word meaning lessening. Page Ref: 645

65. c. Prepuce (PREE-poos) is a combination of the prefix pre- (before, in front of) and the Latin word putos (penis). In uncircumcised men, the urethral meatus is covered by the prepuce or foreskin of the penis. Page Ref: 641

66. a. Spermatogenesis (SPER-mah-toh-JEN-eh-sis), spermat/o- means spermatozoon; sperm, gen/o- means arising from; produced by, and -esis means condition. Page Ref: 645

67. d. Androgen (AN-droh-jen), andr/o- means male, -gen means that which produces. Page Ref: 657

68. c. Vasectomy (vah-SEK-toh-mee), vas/o- means blood vessel; vas deferens, -ectomy means surgical excision. Page Ref: 656

69. b. Circumcision (SER-kum-SIZH-un), circum- means around, cis/o- means to cut, and -ion means action; condition. Page Ref: 656

70. c. Morphology (mor-FAWL-oh-jee), morph/o- means shape, -logy means the study of. Page Ref: 654

71. b. Crypt/o- means hidden, orch/o- means testis, and -ism means disease from a specific cause. Page Ref: 649

72. d. Dys- means difficult or painful, pareun/o- means sexual intercourse, and -ia means condition. Page Ref: 650

73. c. Human immunodeficiency virus (HIV) causes AIDS. Page Ref: 652

74. c. The prepuce or foreskin covers the glans penis in an uncircumcised male. Page Ref: 641

75. d. Circumcision does not cause male infertility. Page Ref: 656

76. b. A sexually transmitted disease (STD) is contracted through sexual contact with an infected partner. Page Ref: 651

77. a. Orchi/o- means testis and -ectomy means surgical excision. Page Ref: 656

78. d. None of the listed structures are in the external genitalia; all are internal. Page Ref: 640

79. c. The pituitary gland secretes follicle-stimulating hormone (FSH) to stimulate the testes to produce spermatozoa. Page Ref: 642

80. b. Balan/o- means penis, and -itis means inflammation of. Page Ref: 650

81. b. TURP stands for transurethral resection of the prostate gland. Page Ref: 656

82. c. Orchi/o- means testis. Page Ref: 659

83. c. The suffix -ile means pertaining to. Page Ref: 641

Short Answer

84. testes. Gon/o- means seed (spermatozoon or ovum). Page Ref: 638

85. syphilis. A chancre is a characteristic of syphilis infection. Page Ref: 652

86. testis. Semin/o- means spermatozoon and -oma means tumor or mass. Spermatozoa are produced in the testes. Page Ref: 649

87. breast. Gynec/o- means female; mast/o- means breast; -ia means condition. Page Ref: 653

88. scanty or too little. Oligospermia is defined as less than the normal amount of spermatozoa produced by the testes. Page Ref: 649

89. sexual intercourse. Dys- means painful; pareun/o- means sexual intercourse; -ia means condition. Page Ref: 650

90. spermatogenesis. Spermat/o- means spermatozoon, gen/o- means produced by; -esis means condition. Page Ref: 643

91. incisional. Incisi/o- means cut into; -ion means action; -al means pertaining to. Page Ref: 655

92. orchiectomy. Orchi/o- means testis; -ectomy means surgical excision. Page Ref: 656

93. ultrasonography. Ultra- means beyond; son/o- means sound; -graphy means process of recording. Page Ref: 654

94. urethra. The male genitourinary system shares the urethra with the urinary system. Page Ref: 637

95. epididymis. A long coiled tube that is attached to the wall of each testis is called the epididymis. Page Ref: 639

96. corpora cavernosa. The penis contains two columns of erectile tissue. The column of paired erectile tissue is called the corpora cavernosa. Page Ref: 641

97. spermatocytes. Immature sperm cells found in childhood are known as spermatocytes. Page Ref: 642

98. spermatogenesis. The process of forming mature spermatozoa is known as spermatogenesis. Page Ref: 643

99. inguinal. The passageway in the groin through which the testes travel as they descend from the abdomen to the scrotum is called the inguinal canal. Page Ref: 639

100. testosterone. The most abundant and most biologically active of the male sex hormones secreted by the testes is testosterone. Page Ref: 638

101. condition; abnormal condition. The suffix in the word phimosis means condition or abnormal condition. Page Ref: 651

102. 2. The pathogen that causes genital herpes is herpes simplex type 2. Page Ref: 651

103. human papillomavirus. The pathogenic organism that causes genital warts (condylomata acuminata) is human papillomavirus. Page Ref: 652

104. scrotum. Scrotum is a Latin word meaning a bag. Page Ref: 637

105. gonads. Gon/o- means seed (ovum or spermatozoon), -ad means toward, in the direction of. The gonads include the testes in men that produce spermatozoa and the ovaries in women that produce ova. Page Ref: 638

106. testosterone. Testosterone (tes-TAWS-teh-rohn) is a hormone secreted by the testes. Page Ref: 638

107. seminiferous. Seminiferous (SEM-ih-NIF-er-us), semin/i- means spermatozoon; sperm, fer/o- means to bear, -ous means pertaining to. Page Ref: 638

108. epididymis. Epididymis (EP-ih-DID-ih-mis), epi- means upon or above, and -didymis means twin structures. Page Ref: 638

109. spermatic. Spermatic (sper-MAT-ik), spermat/o- means spermatozoon; sperm, -ic means pertaining to. Page Ref: 639

110. prostate or prostate gland. Prostate is derived from a Greek word meaning one who stands before. Page Ref: 640

111. bulbourethral. Bulbourethral (BUL-boh-yoo-REE-thral), bulb/o- means like a bulb, urethr/o- means urethr, and -al means pertaining to. Page Ref: 640

112. erectile. Erectile (ee-REK-tile), erect/o- means to stand up, -ile means pertaining to. Page Ref: 641

113. Follicle. Follicle-stimulating hormone is so named because it stimulates both spermatocytes as well as follicles in the female ovaries that contain immature eggs. Page Ref: 642

114. puberty. Puberty (PYOO-ber-tee), puber/o- means growing up, -ty means quality or state. Puberty is derived from a Greek word meaning grown up. Puberty is a series of physical events of growth and the development of sexual maturity. Page Ref: 642

115. mitosis. Mitosis (my-TOH-sis), mit/o- means threadlike structure, -osis means condition; abnormal condition; process. When a cell is not dividing, the chromosomes appear as loosely arranged threads in the nucleus. Page Ref: 643

116. gametes. Gamete (GAM-eet) is derived from two closely related Greek words, one of which means husband and the other means wife. A gamete can be either the spermatozoon or the ovum (egg). Page Ref: 643

117. spermatocytes. Spermatocyte (SPER-mah-toh-site), spermat/o- means spermatozoon; sperm, -cyte means cell. Page Ref: 642

118. vas deferens. Vas is a Latin word meaning a vessel. Deferens is derived from a Latin word meaning to carry away. Page Ref: 640

True/False

119. True. A circumcision would remove the tight foreskin of the penis. Page Ref: 656

120. False. This condition is called chordee. Page Ref: 650

121. False. The prepuce is also known as the foreskin. Page Ref: 641

122. True. Genital warts are caused by viruses. Page Ref: 652

123. True. The muscles in the scrotum contract or relax to adjust for temperature changes in the environment. Page Ref: 637

124. True. Vas/o- means vas deferens; -stomy means surgically creating an opening. Page Ref: 656

125. True. Post- means after; coit/o- means sexual intercourse; -al means pertaining to. Page Ref: 650

126. False. These drugs along with Viagra are used to increase blood flow to the penis, therefore produce an erection. Page Ref: 657

127. True. Olig/o- means scanty; sperm/o- means sperm; -ia means condition. Page Ref: 649

128. True. The GU system is composed of parts that are both external (i.e., penis, testicles) and internal (i.e., vas deferens, prostate gland, etc.). Page Ref: 637

129. False. The scrotum is a few degrees cooler than the core body temperature. Page Ref: 637

130. True. In addition to storing and processing spermatozoa, it also destroys defective spermatozoa. Page Ref: 639

131. True. The urethra is a tube that allows both prostatic fluid and urine to flow to the outside of the body. Page Ref: 640-641

132. False. The word benign means not cancerous, indicating that BPH is a noncancerous condition. Page Ref: 649

133. True. The suffix -itis means inflammation of. Page Ref: 650

134. False. A- means without or lack of. Aspermia means without sperm. Page Ref: 654

135. False. The sound waves are transmitted across the rectum to create an image of the prostate gland. Page Ref: 654

136. True. Orchi/o- means testis, and -ectomy means surgical excision. Page Ref: 656

137. False. A prostatectomy is a surgical procedure to remove the entire prostate gland. It has nothing to do with the testicles. Page Ref: 656

138. False. A spermatocyte with 46 chromosomes is an immature cell that undergoes mitosis and meiosis until it becomes a spermatozoon with 23 chromosomes. Page Ref: 643

139. False. Treponema pallidum causes syphilis. Page Ref: 652

140. True. VDRL and RPR are two blood tests to detect syphilis. Page Ref: 652

141. False. The suffix -cle on testicle means small thing; however, both testes and testicle refer to the same structure and have the same meaning. Page Ref: 638

142. True. A vasovasostomy reconnects a previous vasectomy. Page Ref: 656

143. True. Self-examination of the testes can reveal an early cancer. Page Ref: 655

144. True. A gamete is a spermatozoon (or ova in the female) that has 23 chromosomes. Page Ref: 643

145. True. The urethral meatus is covered by the foreskin or prepuce. Page Ref: 641

146. False. Semen contains fluid from the bulbourethral glands. The penis does not contribute spermatozoa or fluid to the semen. Page Ref: 640

147. True. Testicular cancer arises from abnormal sperm, not the tissues of the testis. Page Ref: 649

Essay

148. The testes are developed before birth in the abdominal cavity. The inguinal canal serves as a passageway for the descent of the testes from the abdominal cavity. If this passageway fails to close after the descent, a loop of intestine can go through the inguinal canal and cause an inguinal hernia. Page Ref: 639

149. The vas deferens receives spermatozoa from the epididymis during ejaculation. Severing the vas deferens through an incision in the base of the scrotum prevents the spermatozoa from leaving the man's body. Therefore, without spermatozoa in the ejaculated fluid, the man cannot get the woman pregnant. Page Ref: 656

150. Proper development of spermatozoa depends on an environment in which the temperature is a few degrees cooler than body temperature, like the temperature of the scrotum because it is outside the body. Page Ref: 637

151. Testosterone is the most abundant and biologically active of all the male sex hormones. During puberty, testosterone causes the development of

the male sex characteristics that include enlargement of the external genitalia, large body muscles, deepening of the voice, body hair on the face and in the axillary and genital areas, and sexual drive. Testosterone also stimulates the maturation of spermatozoa. Page Ref: 638

152. The prostate gland is a round gland at the base of the bladder. It completely surrounds the first part of the urethra and produces prostatic fluid, which is a milky substance that makes up some of the volume of the semen. The prostatic fluid contains an antimicrobial that acts against bacteria in the woman's vagina, as well as a substance that activates enzymes in the head of the spermatozoa so that they penetrate the woman's ovum to fertilize it. Page Ref: 640

153. Cryptorchism is the failure of one or both of the testicles to descend through the inguinal canal into the scrotum. This causes a low sperm count and male infertility. Page Ref: 649

154. Gynecomastia is an enlargement of the male breast caused by an imbalance of androgens and estrogens because of puberty, aging, surgical removal of the testes or estrogen drug treatment for prostate cancer. Page Ref: 653

155. The digital rectal exam is a medical procedure to palpate the prostate gland. A gloved finger is inserted through the rectum and is used to feel for tenderness, nodules, hardness, or enlargement. This examination is a screening test for prostate cancer and should be done yearly for men over age 40. Page Ref: 655

CHAPTER 13

Multiple Choice

1. c. The term uterine prolapse means a falling downward of the uterus from loss of elasticity of the supporting structures. Descensus is a Latin word meaning falling from a higher position. Page Ref: 704

2. c. The gestation period for a term neonate is 38 to 42 weeks. Page Ref: 686

3. a. A colposcope is inserted into the vagina to view with magnification tissues of the cervix and vagina. Cryosurgery applies cold liquid nitrogen to the lesions. Page Ref: 720

4. a. episi/o- = vulva; -otomy = incision. Page Ref: 729

5. a. In placenta previa the placenta is abnormally implanted in the lower part of the uterus, obstructing the delivery of the fetus and requiring the removal of the fetus surgically. Page Ref: 729

6. d. Hysterosalpingography is a radiological examination done with contrast dye to see if the tubes are open to allow the egg and sperm to travel through for fertilization. Page Ref: 718

7. d. Os is the Latin word for an opening into a vessel. Page Ref: 680

8. d. Basal body temperature rises sharply on the day a woman is releasing an egg from an ovary. Page Ref: 684

9. d. Fibroid tumors or leiomyomata are benign smooth muscle tumors. They can be surgically excised from the uterus without removing the entire uterus. Page Ref: 725

10. c. Hormone replacement therapy, such as estrogen and progestin, is given to women during menopause. Page Ref: 731

11. a. The normal position of the uterus is to be tipped anteriorly. Page Ref: 679

12. b. Leukorrhea is a white, vaginal discharge. Of the choices above, only candidiasis is a yeast infection. Page Ref: 706

13. c. Pre- = before; -eclampsia = sudden development. This is a disorder of pregnancy involving the kidneys with fluid retention and protein in the urine. Page Ref: 711

14. b. Excessive glucose not metabolized by the mother is metabolized by the fetus and contributes to the large size of the fetus. Page Ref: 709

15. c. The Bartholin, urethral, and Skene glands are in the area of the vagina. Page Ref: 681

16. d. Peau d'orange describes dimpling of the skin as it resembles the peel of orange. Page Ref: 707

17. b. Pelvic inflammatory disease is an infection of the internal female reproductive organs often caused by a sexually transmitted disease. Page Ref: 703

18. a. Having the BRCA 1 or 2 gene increases the risk of developing these cancers. BRCA stands for breast cancer. Page Ref: 714

19. d. Pitocin stimulates the frequency and strength of uterine contractions. Page Ref: 730

20. b. Braxton Hicks contractions are irregular contractions of the uterus before the actual onset of labor. Page Ref: 687

21. d. Surfactant is found in the lungs to keep the air sacs open. The lack of surfactant results in respiratory distress syndrome in the infant. Page Ref: 713

22. c. Crowning occurs in the second stage of labor. Page Ref: 688

23. b. Meconium contains mucus, bile, and skin cells swallowed and excreted by the fetus in the amniotic fluid. Page Ref: 690

24. a. Dys- = difficult; toc/o- = labor; -ia = condition. Page Ref: 709

25. c. A fertilized ovum is known as an embryo until eight weeks, then it is called a fetus. Page Ref: 686

26. c. Normal cessation of menstrual periods occurs around age 40. Menopause is also known as climacteric and change of life. Page Ref: 704

27. c. Galact/o- means milk and -rrhea means flow. Galactorrhea is a discharge of milk from the

breasts when the patient is not pregnant or breastfeeding. It is caused by increased levels of prolactin from an adenoma (benign tumor) in the anterior pituitary gland in the brain. Page Ref: 707

28. a. Placenta previa is a Latin phrase that mean the placenta is before something else (the fetus). Page Ref: 710

29. b. The prefix multi- means many. The combining form -par means birth. The suffix -ous means pertaining to. Page Ref: 722

30. c. The abbreviation G means number of pregnancies. The abbreviation P means number of deliveries. The abbreviation Ab means number of abortions. Page Ref: 722

31. b. When a woman is pregnant, the last menstrual period is used as a guide to determine the estimated due date of the mother. Page Ref: 722

32. d. A dilation and curettage is a surgical procedure performed to remove abnormal tissue from inside the uterus. The other answers have misspelled words. Page Ref: 724

33. a. Premenstrual syndrome (PMS) occurs a few days before the onset of menses. The symptoms include breast tenderness, fluid retention, bloating, and mild mood changes (irritability, anger, sadness). It is caused by the high levels of estradiol and progesterone just prior to menstruation. Page Ref: 705

34. d. A cesarean section is a surgical procedure performed to deliver a fetus. The other answers have misspelled words. Page Ref: 729

35. a. The combining form men/o- means monthly menses. The suffix -arche means a beginning. Page Ref: 683

36. b. Salping/o- is a combining form for fallopian tube. Page Ref: 701

37. b. The prefix dys- means painful, difficult, or abnormal. The combining form toc/o- means childbirth or labor. The suffix -ia means condition, state, or thing. Page Ref: 709

38. a. The combining form colp/o- means vagina. Page Ref: 733

39. c. The prefix bi- means two. The combining form later/o- means side. The suffix -al means pertaining to. The combing form salping/o- means fallopian tube. The combining form oophor/o- means ovary. The suffix -ectomy means surgical excision. Page Ref: 725, 726

40. a. A total abdominal hysterectomy with bilateral salpingo-oophorectomy involves the removal of the entire uterus, both fallopian tubes, and both ovaries through an abdominal incision. Page Ref: 724, 725, 726

41. c. Pelvic inflammatory disease (PID) is an infection of the cervix that ascends to the uterus, fallopian tubes, and ovaries. It is often caused by a sexually transmitted disease. Page Ref: 703

42. c. HCG stands for human chorionic gonadotropin. A pregnancy test is a blood test performed to detect the presence of HCG that is secreted by the fertilized ovum. Page Ref: 717

43. d. The Apgar score was developed by Virginia Apgar, an anesthesiologist. Page Ref: 721

44. c. These drugs contain estrogen as a replacement for estradiol. Page Ref: 731

45. b. Cerclage reinforces the cervix and prevents it from dilating during pregnancy. The sutures are removed prior to delivery. Page Ref: 729

46. c. A radical mastectomy is performed infrequently. Page Ref: 728

47. b. The uterus is also referred to as the womb. Page Ref: 679

48. a. Hysterosalpinography is a radiologic procedure in which radiopaque contrast dye is injected through the cervix into the uterus. It coats and outlines the uterus and fallopian tubes and shows narrowing, scarring, and blockage. Page Ref: 718

49. a. A loose nuchal cord can be an incidental finding that causes no problems. A tight nuchal cord with one or more loops around the neck can impair blood flow to the brain, causing brain damage or fetal death. Page Ref: 713

50. a. Epinephrine is the hormone not secreted by the female reproductive system. This is the major fight or flight hormone secreted by the sympathetic nervous system. Page Ref: 676

51. d. The ovary is part of the internal genitalia of the female reproductive system. Page Ref: 675

52. d. A woman is most likely to lose a small amount of blood during the menstrual phase. Approximately 30 ml of blood, endometrial tissue, and mucus is shed from the uterus during this phase. Page Ref: 684

53. a. Adenocarcinoma of the breasts is a cancerous condition. Any word with the word part carcinoma is a type of cancer. Page Ref: 707

54. d. Cystocele is the most likely culprit, given the list of possibilities. The herniation of a cystocele occurs because of a weakness in the vaginal wall. Page Ref: 706

55. a. Galactorrhea is caused by increased levels of prolactin from an adenoma in the anterior pituitary gland. Page Ref: 707

56. b. Oligohydramnios is a decreased volume of amniotic fluid. The fetus swallows amniotic fluid but does not excrete a similar volume in its urine because of a congenital abnormality of the fetal kidneys. Page Ref: 710

57. a. An Apgar score of 0 reflects that there is a lack of breathing, heart rate, respiratory effort, muscle tone, and response to stimulation and skin color. Page Ref: 721

58. b. An infant that is not breathing is said to be apneic. Page Ref: 712

59. a. A medical procedure in which a hook is inserted into the cervix to catch and rupture the amniotic sac is called *amniotomy*. An amniotomy is used to induce labor. Page Ref: 721

60. a. Genitalia (JEN-ih-TAY-lee-ah), Genitalia is a Latin word meaning pertaining to generation and birth. Page Ref: 675

61. d. Estradiol (ES-trah-DY-awl), estr/a- female, di- two, -ol chemical substance. A molecule of estradiol contains two atoms of oxygen. Page Ref: 677

62. b. Acrocyanosis (AK-roh-SY-ah-NOH-sis), acr/o- extremity; highest point, cyan/o- blue, -osis condition; abnormal condition; process. Page Ref: 690

63. d. Fontanel (FAWN-tah-NEL), Also spelled fontanelle. Fontanel is derived from a Latin word meaning fountain because sometimes a pulse (thought to be the fountain or spring of life) can be felt there. Page Ref: 690

64. b. See Figure 13-14. Page Ref: 688

65. c. See Figure 13-9. Page Ref: 684

66. a. Pregnancy (PREG-nan-see), pregn/o- being with child, -ancy state of. Pregnancy is derived from a Latin word meaning before being born. Page Ref: 685

67. b. Fraternal (frah-TER-nal), fratern/o- close association or relationship, -al pertaining to. Although a fraternity usually is an association of all male members, fraternal twins can be two males, one male and one female, or two females. Page Ref: 685

68. a. Parturition (PAR-tyoo-RIH-shun), parturit/o- to be in labor, -ion action; condition. Page Ref: 687

69. c. Colostrum (koh-LAWS-trum). Colostrum contains maternal antibodies for the newborn. Page Ref: 689

70. b. The broad ligament is a sheet of peritoneum that attaches to the walls of the pelvic cavity. Page Ref: 676

71. b. Vertex or top of the head is a normal cephalic presentation. Page Ref: 687

72. a. Effacement and dilation occur normally to the cervix during labor. Page Ref: 687

73. b. Ne/o- is a combining form, nat/o- is a combining form, log/o- is a combining form, and -ist is a suffix. Page Ref: 733

74. a. A- is a prefix, men/o- is a combining form, and -rrhea is a suffix. Page Ref: 704

75. b. Lei/o- means smooth, my/o- means muscle, and -oma means tumor. Page Ref: 703

76. d. Men/o- means monthly and -arche means a beginning. Page Ref: 683

77. b. Colp/o- means vagina and -scopy means process of using an instrument to examine. Page Ref: 720

78. a. Dysplasia is a condition of an abnormal growth of cells on the cervix. Page Ref: 706

79. d. Augmentation means a process to increase in size. Page Ref: 727

80. d. The other choices are not related to the placenta. Page Ref: 708

81. d. It is possible to have a vaginal birth after cesarean section (VBAC). Page Ref: 729

82. d. Son/o- means sound. Page Ref: 719

83. c. The corpus luteum secretes these hormones after ovulation (release) of the ovum. Page Ref: 684

84. a. The chorion develops into the placenta. The amnion develops into the amniotic sac and fluid. Page Ref: 686

85. a. Oophor/o- means ovary. O/o- means ovum. Page Ref: 725

86. d. Lact/o- means milk. Page Ref: 733

87. b. Anovulation is the failure to ovulate and produce an ovum, which means that the woman is infertile and cannot get pregnant. Page Ref: 701

88. a. Salping/o- means fallopian tube and -itis means inflammation of. Page Ref: 701

89. d. Mast/o- means breast and -itis means inflammation of. Page Ref: 709

90. d. Nuchal means pertaining to the neck. Page Ref: 713

91. b. A Pap smear is performed on the cells of the cervix. Page Ref: 717

92. d. The biparietal diameter measures the distance between the two parietal bones of the head of the fetus to calculate gestational age. Page Ref: 719

93. b. The Apgar score rates a newborn for heart rate, respiratory rate, muscle tone, response to stimulation, and skin color. Page Ref: 721

94. c. Estimated gestational age (EGA) is the approximate age of the fetus in weeks. Page Ref: 723

95. b. Null/i- means none and -gravida means pregnancy. Page Ref: 722

Short Answer

96. bladder. Cyst/o- = bladder; -cele = hernia. Page Ref: 706

97. D & C or dilation and curettage. This procedure involves widening the cervix and scraping the uterine contents. Page Ref: 724

98. embryo. Embryo is a Greek word meaning that which swells and grows. Page Ref: 686

99. abortion. A spontaneous abortion is also known as a miscarriage. Page Ref: 711

100. neck. An umbilical cord that is too tight around the neck can impair blood flow to the brain. Page Ref: 713

101. amniocentesis. Amni/o- = amnion; -centesis = procedure to puncture. Page Ref: 717

102. oviducts. Ov/i = egg; duct = tube. Page Ref: 679

103. vagina. Colp/o- = vagina; -rrhaphy = suture. Page Ref: 724

104. endometriosis. Endometrial tissue is forced out of the uterine tubes and implants itself on organs in the pelvic cavity. Page Ref: 702

105. stereotactic. A stereotactic biopsy uses three different angles of mammography to precisely locate the mass in the breast. Page Ref: 714

106. exfoliative. A Pap smear is known as exfoliative cytology because it examines cells that have been scraped from the cervix. Page Ref: 715

107. Amniocentesis. Amniocentesis is a diagnostic test that examines the fluid in the amniotic sac. Page Ref: 717

108. anovulation. Failure of the ovaries to release a mature ovum at the time of ovulation is called anovulation. Page Ref: 701

109. endo-. endo- means internal or within. Page Ref: 702

110. oogenesis. The process of forming a mature ovum is known as oogenesis. Page Ref: 683

111. cephalic. A head-down presentation of a baby in the birth canal is called a cephalic presentation. Page Ref: 687

112. colostrum. A mother's first milk is known as colostrum. Page Ref: 689

113. vernix caseosa. The skin of a newborn is covered with a thick, white, cheesy substance called vernix caseosa. Page Ref: 690

114. gynecology. Gynecology, gynec/o- female, woman. Page Ref: 674

115. fallopian. Fallopian (fah-LOH-pee-an), fallopi/o- fallopian tube, -an pertaining to. The fallopian tubes were named by Gabriele Fallopius (1523-1562), an Italian anatomist. This is an example of an eponym: a person from whom something takes its name. Page Ref: 678

116. fundus. Fundus (FUN-dus). Fundus is a Latin word meaning part farthest from the opening. Page Ref: 679

117. corpus. Corpus (KOR-pus), Corpus is a Latin word meaning body. Page Ref: 679

118. genitalia. Genitalia (JEN-ih-TAY-lee-ah), Genitalia is a Latin word meaning pertaining to generation and birth. Page Ref: 675

119. mons pubis. Mons pubis (MAWNZ PYOO-bis), Mons is a Latin word meaning mountain. Pubis means of the pubic bone. Page Ref: 681

120. Luteinizing. Luteinizing (LOO-tee-ih-ny-zing), Luteinizing hormone is so named because it stimulates the corpus luteum of the ovary (as well as the interstitial cells of the testis). Page Ref: 683

121. prenatal. Prenatal (pree-NAY-tal), pre- before; in front of, nat/o- birth, -al pertaining to. Page Ref: 687

122. Braxton Hicks. Braxton Hicks (BRAK-ston HIKS), Braxton Hicks contractions were named by John Braxton Hicks (1823-1897), a British gynecologist. Page Ref: 687

123. oxytocin. Oxytocin (AWK-see-TOH-sin), ox/y- oxygen; quick, toc/o- labor and childbirth, -in a substance. Page Ref: 687

124. effacement. Effacement (eh-FAYS-ment), efface/o- do away with; obliterate, -ment action; state. Page Ref: 687

125. gestation. Gestation (jes-TAY-shun), gestat/o- from conception to birth, -ion action; condition. Page Ref: 686

126. embryo. Embryo (EM-bree-oh), Embryo is a Greek word meaning that which swells and grows within. Page Ref: 686

127. placenta. Placenta (plah-SEN-tah), Placenta is a Latin word meaning flat cake. Page Ref: 686

128. meconium. Meconium (meh-KOH-nee-um), Meconium is a Latin word meaning waste from a newborn child. Page Ref: 690

129. pica. Pica is a Latin word meaning magpie, because those birds look for all kinds of material to build their nests. Page Ref: 712

130. fimbriae; cilia. Fimbriae is a Latin word meaning fringe. The cilia are hairs. Page Ref: 678

131. oxytocin. Oxytocin released from the posterior pituitary gland begins labor by stimulating uterine contractions. Page Ref: 687

132. TAH-BSO. TAH-BSO stands for total abdominal hysterectomy and bilateral salpingo-oophorectomy. Page Ref: 732

True/False

133. False. This is called lochia. Colostrum is the first milk. Page Ref: 689

134. True. Tocolytics act by relaxing the smooth muscle contractions of the uterine wall. Toc/o- means labor and ly/o- means break down. Page Ref: 730

135. True. This is the age of the female's first menstrual period. Page Ref: 683

136. True. Detection of HCG in the female is used in pregnancy testing. Page Ref: 717

137. False. The placenta is expelled during the third stage of labor after the delivery of the child. Page Ref: 689

138. True. This thinning is a process that occurs in the first stage of labor. Page Ref: 687

139. True. Early separation of the placenta can cause hemorrhage in the mother and lack of oxygen in the fetus. Page Ref: 708

140. False. It predisposes to cervical cancer. Page Ref: 705

141. False. Obstetrics is the medical specialty that studies the anatomy and physiology of the female reproductive system during pregnancy and childbirth. Page Ref: 674

142. True. As part of the endocrine system they act as glands, and as part of the reproductive system they produce mature eggs. Page Ref: 676

143. False. The myometrium contains smooth muscle fibers. You can tell that it is muscular because the word part my/o- means muscle. Page Ref: 680

144. True. Certain hormones released at puberty help the eggs to mature. Page Ref: 683

145. False. The mature ovum is created by both mitosis and meiosis. Page Ref: 683

146. False. These events occur during the ischemic phase. Page Ref: 684

147. True. The moment that the spermatozoon penetrates the ovum, fertilization has occurred. After that, the surface of the ovum repels other spermatozoa. Page Ref: 685

148. True. If untreated, PID can cause scars in the fallopian tubes and infertility. Page Ref: 703

149. False. Fibrocystic disease of the breasts is a benign condition. Page Ref: 707

150. False. The perineum is present in both the female and male, but only the female has a vulva. Page Ref: 681

151. True. The ovaries are glands that secrete hormones and so are included in the endocrine system. Page Ref: 676

152. True. The breast structure contains mammary glands that secrete to the outside skin so they belong to the integumentary system, but because these glands secrete milk that is used to feed the newborn, the breasts are also part of the reproductive system. Page Ref: 682

153. False. Pregnancy begins at the moment of conception or fertilization of the ovum. Page Ref: 685

154. False. Braxton Hicks contractions are false labor contractions as the uterine muscle strengthens in preparation for future labor. Page Ref: 687

155. True. Climacteric is derived from a Greek word meaning the rungs of a ladder, a progression toward menopause. Page Ref: 705

156. False. An intrauterine pregnancy occurs in the uterus but an ectopic pregnancy occurs in the fallopian tube. Page Ref: 709

157. False. Uterine inertia is the abnormal condition of a lack of strong contractions during labor. Page Ref: 711

158. False. BRCA1 increases the risk of breast (BR) cancer (CA). Page Ref: 714

159. False. A TRAM flap is a reconstructive surgery performed after a mastectomy. Page Ref: 728

160. True. Leukorrhea is a white, cheesy discharge characteristic of candidiasis. Page Ref: 706

Essay

161. A tubal ligation is the surgery for removing of part of both fallopian tubes. The fallopian tube is the passageway for the egg to travel from the ovary to the uterus and also the passageway for the sperm to travel to the egg. The ligation blocks the possibility of the egg meeting with the spermatozoa and prevents conception. Page Ref: 726

162. The pelvimetry is a measurement of the maternal bony pelvis to ensure that she has enough room for the fetal head to pass through during labor and delivery. If there is not enough room, a cesarean section would be necessary. Page Ref: 722

163. The cervix has dilated from closed (0 cm) to completely open (10 cm) and the walls have thinned from 0% to 100% during labor. Page Ref: 687

164. Lecithin is a component of surfactant-a protein-fat substance that lowers surface tension to keep the alveoli from collapsing with each breath. Sphingomyelin levels are higher until the fetal lungs are mature, and then lecithin levels are higher than sphingomyelin. The L/S ratio (lecithin/sphingomyelin) helps predict the maturity of fetal lungs and thus the likelihood of fetal survival after birth. Page Ref: 717

165. A breast biopsy can be one of several types.
    1. A fine-needle aspiration, which uses a very small caliber needle to aspirate the mass.
    2. A vacuum-assisted biopsy, which uses a probe with a cutting device.
    3. A surgical incisional biopsy, which is an incision into the tumor with subsequent removal of some-but not all-of the tissue.
    4. A surgical excisional biopsy, where the entire mass is removed).
    5. A stereotactic biopsy, which uses three different angles of mammographyto precisely locate the mass. Page Ref: 714

166. A leiomyoma is a tumor of the myometrium, but it is benign. It is also called a uterine fibroid. Leiomyosarcoma is also a tumor of the myometrium, but it is cancerous. Page Ref: 703

167. During the first stage of labor, uterine contractions occur approximately every 30 minutes, becoming greater in intensity and duration. Cervical dilation progresses from 0 cm to 5 cm, and effacement progresses from 0% to 50%. Rupture of the membranes (ROM) also occurs during this stage and releases amniotic fluid. It takes 8 to 20 hours of labor for the cervix to completely dilate to 10 cm and 100% effacement. At this point, the second stage of labor begins. Page Ref: 687

CHAPTER 14

Multiple Choice

1. c. Hypocalcemia is the word for low levels of calcium in the blood. Hyp/o- = deficient; calc/o-

= calcium; -emia = blood. One of the functions of calcium in the body is to maintain normal functioning of the nerves and muscles. Nerve irritability and muscle spasms or tetany occur with low levels of blood calcium. Page Ref: 777

2. b. Alpha cells secrete glucagon, beta cells secrete insulin, and delta cells secrete somatostatin. Page Ref: 759

3. b. Addison's disease involves hyposecrection of cortisol, a hormone from the adrenal cortex that regulates glucose in the blood and that has an anti-inflammatory effect on the body. Page Ref: 782

4. a. Because the pituitary secretes hormones involved in many vital functions in the body as well as secretes hormones that stimulate the secretion of other hormones, it is known as the master gland. Page Ref: 755

5. d. Polydipsia or excessive thirst is found in both conditions but occurs for different reasons. Page Ref: 773,779

6. b. Also known as the water deprivation test, this evaluates the patient's ability to concentrate urine. Page Ref: 773

7. c. Radioactive sodium iodide is given to the patient for hyperthyroidism to destroy some thyroid cells to relieve the excessive secretion of thyroid hormones. Page Ref: 788

8. a. Hashimoto's thyroiditis is an autoimmune disease of the thyroid gland. Page Ref: 777

9. d. Obesity and heredity are precipitating factors for type 2 diabetes. Page Ref: 779

10. b. Although these words look similar, they have different functions.When blood glucose levels are low, glucagon, the hormone, breaks down glycogen (stored glucose) to form glucose Page Ref: 759

11. a. Epinephrine from the adrenal medulla is a neurotransmitter in the sympathetic nervous system. Page Ref: 761

12. c. Hypoglycemia or low blood sugar is associated with those symptoms because of the lack of sugar in the blood. Page Ref: 780

13. b. The parathyroid gland hormone releases calcium from the bone and raises calcium levels in the blood. Page Ref: 777

14. a. Goiter is a chronic enlargement of the thyroid gland. Page Ref: 774

15. d. Cortisol is secreted by the adrenal cortex, which is affected in Cushing's syndrome. Page Ref: 781

16. d. FSH, follicle stimulating hormone, from the pituitary gland stimulates hormone secretion from the ovaries and testes. Page Ref: 756

17. a. Seasonal affective disorder (SAD) is found in people living in northern climates. Page Ref: 774

18. a. Humulin is a form of insulin. Choices B and C are oral diabetic drugs that are not useful for a type 1 diabetic. Page Ref: 788

19. d. The pituitary gland is also called the hypophysis. This surgical approach to remove the pituitary is done through the sphenoid sinus. Page Ref: 787

20. c. This measures the average amount of glucose bound to RBCs. It is also called glycohemoglobin or glycosylated hemoglobin. Page Ref: 785

21. a. The diabetic cannot metabolize glucose so the body turns to fat for energy. The byproduct of this process creates ketones, acids that, when found in excess in the body, can cause coma or even death. Page Ref: 780

22. d. The production of thyroid hormone, T3, depends upon iodine. Page Ref: 774

23. c. Oxytocin from the posterior pituitary gland causes the pregnant uterus to contract. Page Ref: 755

24. a. Addison's disease is an autoimmune disease in which the body produces antibodies that destroy the adrenal cortex. Page Ref: 782

25. c. The pineal body, which is located posterior to the hypothalamus, secretes melatonin. Page Ref: 757

26. c. The parathyroid glands are beside the thyroid.The prefix para- means two parts of a pair beside. Page Ref: 758

27. b. Diabetes insipidus causes excessive amounts of water to be excreted in the urine (polyuria).Other symptoms include weakness, thirst (due to water loss and dehydration), and increased intake of fluids (polydipsia). Page Ref: 773

28. c. Cushing's syndrome is caused by an adenoma in the adrenal cortex that causes hypersecretion.The treatment is surgery to remove the adenoma in the adrenal cortex or pituitary gland. Page Ref: 781

29. c. Goiter is derived from a French word for throat. Mild-to-moderate thyroid gland enlargement is known as thyromegaly. Page Ref: 774

30. c. The symptoms of myxedema include swelling of the subcutaneous and connective tissue in various parts of the body, tingling in the hands and feet because of nerve compression, an enlarged heart, bradycardia, an enlarged tongue, slow speech, and mental impairment. Page Ref: 776

31. c. Synergism contains the combining form erg/o- which means work, and syn- means together. Page Ref: 763

32. d. Non-insulin-dependent diabetes mellitus is also called type 2 diabetes mellitus or adult-onset diabetes mellitus. Page Ref: 778

33. b. The pituitary gland, or master gland, is also called the hypophysis. Page Ref: 755

34. a. Hypophysis is a Greek word that means an undergrowth because the hypophysis grows below the hypothalamus. Page Ref: 755

35. d. The growth hormone stimulates cell growth and protein synthesis in all body cells. Page Ref: 756

36. b. Insulin is used to treat type 1 diabetes mellitus. It can be used to treat type 2 diabetes mellitus that cannot be controlled with oral antidiabetic drugs. Page Ref: 788

37. c. The pituitary gland is called the hypophysis. The anterior pituitary gland is called the adenohypophysis. The posterior pituitary gland is called the neurohypophysis. Page Ref: 755

38. a. A fasting blood sugar (FBS) is used to evaluate the function of the pancreas. Page Ref: 784

39. d. The combining form antagon/o- means fight against. Page Ref: 763

40. c. The prefix ad- means above. The combining form ren/o- means kidney. The suffix -al means pertaining to. The adrenal gland is located above the kidney. Page Ref: 760

41. d. In acromegaly, the face, hands, and feet enlarge. The treatment of acromegaly involves the use of drugs to suppress the production of the growth hormone. Page Ref: 772

42. d. The prefix hyper- means above. The combining form calc/o- means calcium. The suffix -emia means condition of the blood or substance in the blood. Page Ref: 777

43. b. Tetany occurs when the calcium level in the blood becomes very low. Page Ref: 777

44. d. Glycos/o- means glucose. Glycosuria is a symptom of diabetes. Excessive amounts of glucose in the blood are excreted in the urine. Page Ref: 779

45. b. Type 1 diabetes is caused by destruction of the beta cells of the islets of Langerhans in the pancreas. Type 1 diabetes mellitus is an autoimmune response that may be triggered by a viral infection or an inherited genetic predisposition. Page Ref: 779

46. a. Uterine inertia causes weak or uncoordinated contractions of the pregnant uterus during labor. Page Ref: 774

47. b. Hyp/o- means below or deficient. The treatment for dwarfism is to use a synthetic growth hormone drug. Page Ref: 776

48. a. Only some of the organs and glands of the endocrine system are influenced by the pituitary gland. Page Ref: 753,755

49. b. Only the pituitary gland secretes hormones that stimulate the ovary. Page Ref: 755

50. d. The pituitary gland is known as the master gland. Page Ref: 755

51. a. The parathyroid glands secrete a parathyroid hormone, which regulates the level of calcium in the blood. Page Ref: 758

52. d. The pancreas contains islets of Langerhans and is responsible for regulating blood glucose level. Page Ref: 759

53. a. This is the most abundant and biologically active of the mineralocorticoid hormones. This hormone regulates the balance of electrolytes, keeping sodium and water in the blood while excreting potassium in the urine. Page Ref: 760

54. b. Estradiol is the most abundant and biologically active female hormone. Page Ref: 761

55. d. The anterior pituitary gland, located in the brain, produces FSH (follicle stimulating hormone). Page Ref: 755

56. a. When hormones work together it is called synergism. When hormones work against each other, it is know as antagonism. Page Ref: 763

57. d. It contains the suffix -gen meaning that which produces because when broken down it releases sugar (glucose). Page Ref: 759

58. c. The pituitary gland, or hypophysis, is known as the master gland of the body. Page Ref: 755

59. a. Neurohypophysis (NYOOR-oh-hy-PAWF-ih-sis), neur/o- nerve, hypo- below; deficient, -physis state of growing. Neurohypophysis refers to the posterior pituitary gland that is below the hypothalamus. It does not make or secrete its own hormones but releases hormones produced by the hypothalamus when signaled to do so by nerves from the hypothalamus. Page Ref: 755

60. b. Gonadotropin (GOH-nah-doh-TROH-pin), gonad/o- gonads (ovaries and testes), trop/o- having an affinity for; stimulating; turning, -in a substance. Page Ref: 756

61. c. Pancreas. Glucagon (GLOO-kah-gawn), gluc/o- glucose (sugar), ag/o- to lead to, -on substance; structure. Glucagon is a hormone that breaks down stored glycogen. Insulin (IN-soo-lin), insul/o- island, -in a substance. Insulin is secreted by little "islands of cells," the islets of Langerhans in the pancreas. Somatostatin (SOH-mah-toh-STAT-in), somat/o- body, stat/o- standing still; staying in one place, -in a substance. Add words to make a correct and complete definition of somatostatin: A substance [that makes the] body [to be] standing still [without growth]. Somatostatin inhibits the release of growth hormone, glucagon, and insulin from the pancreas. Page Ref: 759

62. b. Graves' disease (GRAYVZ), named by Robert Graves (1796-1853), an Irish physician. The most common form of hyperthyroidism. This is an autoimmune disease in which the body produces antibodies that stimulate TSH receptors on the thyroid gland, increasing the production of thyroid hormones. Page Ref: 775

63. a. Cushing (KOOSH-ing), named by Harvey Cushing (1869-1939), an American surgeon. Syndrome (SIN-drohm), syn- together, -drome a running, A syndrome is many different symptoms and signs that make up one disease. Page Ref: 781

64. b. Blood glucose monitor—the patient pricks the fingertip and the drop of blood is placed on a test strip.It is inserted into the blood glucose monitor and the monitor displays the numerical value of the patient's blood glucose level. Page Ref: 784

65. a. Urine dipstick—urine test that measures glucose, ketones, and other substances in the urine.Rapid screening test used to evaluate diabetic patients. Page Ref: 785

66. c. Thyroidectomy (THY-roy-DEK-toh-mee), thyroid/o- thyroid, -ectomy surgical excision. Surgical procedure to remove the thyroid gland. All of the thyroid gland or just one part (one lobe) can be removed (subtotal thyroidectomy or thyroid lobectomy). Page Ref: 787

67. a. Stimulate (STIM-yoo-layt), stimul/o- exciting, strengthening, -ate composed of; pertaining to. Hormone (HOR-mohn), Hormone is derived from a Greek word meaning to set in motion. Page Ref: 756

68. b. Hypophys/o- is the Greek combining form that means pituitary gland. Page Ref: 790

69. d. Aden/o- means gland and -oma means tumor. Page Ref: 771

70. b. The blood level of growth hormone reflects the functioning of the anterior pituitary gland that secretes growth hormone. Page Ref: 755,784,785

71. d. Type 2 diabetes mellitus, or adult-onset diabetes mellitus, can be treated with weight loss, exercise, and diet.If those measures are not sufficient, oral antidiabetic drugs can be prescribed. Page Ref: 778,787

72. a. Follicle-stimulating hormone (FSH) from the anterior pituitary gland is needed to stimulate follicles in the ovary to produce eggs and in the testes to produce sperm. Page Ref: 783,789

73. c. NPH is a type of insulin given to treat diabetes mellitus. Page Ref: 788

74. b. Diabetes mellitus is treated with a diet that restricts the use of calories as per the guidelines of the American Diabetes Association (ADA). Page Ref: 786

75. c. Hypophys/o- refers to the pituitary gland, and -ectomy means surgical excision. The incision is made through the sphenoid bone. Page Ref: 787

76. a. The thyroid gland secretes the T3 and T4 thyroid hormones that regulate cellular metabolism. Page Ref: 758

77. c. After puberty, the ends of the long bones no longer grow, so excessive amounts of growth hormone cause facial and extremity enlargement (acromegaly). Page Ref: 772

78. b. Too little antidiuretic hormone (ADH) allows excessive amounts of water to be lost in the urine. This condition is diabetes insipidus. Page Ref: 773

79. d. Cretin is a French word that means mentally deficient person; a congenital lack of thyroid hormone causes mental retardation. Page Ref: 776

80. c. The thyroid gland is the only option given that has lobes. Page Ref: 757

81. c. Hemoglobin A1C measures the average amount of glucose carried in the red blood cells during their life span of three to four months. Page Ref: 785

82. d. During the time of pregnancy or gestation the pregnant woman can develop gestational diabetes mellitus. Page Ref: 779

83. c. Graves' disease is a type of hyperthyroidism in which too much thyroid hormone causes edema in the tissues behind the eye. Page Ref: 775

84. b. Insulin-dependent diabetes mellitus (IDDM) is also known as type 1 diabetes mellitus. Page Ref: 789

85. d. Antidiuretic hormone is produced by the hypothalamus but stored and released by the posterior pituitary gland. Its action is to bring water from the kidney tubules back into the blood. Page Ref: 754,755,773

86. b. Melatonin from the pineal gland is associated with the wake-sleep cycle. Page Ref: 757

87. d. TSH is the abbreviation for thyroid-stimulating hormone. Page Ref: 757

88. a. Parathyroid hormone from the parathyroid glands regulates the amount of calcium in the blood. Page Ref: 758

89. b. Low levels of glucose in the blood must be raised to normal levels, so the alpha cells of the pancreas produce the hormone glucagon that releases stored sugar from the liver. Page Ref: 759

90. d. The thyroid hormone affects body metabolism, insulin from the pancreas affects blood glucose, parathyroid hormone affects blood calcium, and aldosterone from the adrenal gland affects blood sodium. Page Ref: 757,759,760

91. b. The testes produce testosterone, the primary male hormone. The ovaries produce male-like hormones known as androgens. Page Ref: 761,762

92. c. Hormones are the chemical messengers of the endocrine system. Page Ref: 753

93. d. Hormones, the chemical messengers of the endocrine system, are released through ducts and travel through the blood to stimulate or inhibit other glands and organs. Page Ref: 753

94. c. Parathyroid hormone increases blood calcium levels in the blood and calcitonin decreases blood calcium levels in the blood. Page Ref: 753

95. b. The correct spelling is diabetes mellitus. Page Ref: 778

96. d. The suffix -ism is used frequently in endocrinology to discuss diseases caused by too much or too little of certain hormones. Page Ref: 771

Short Answer

97. glucose tolerance test. This is a test on blood or urine that measures the amount of glucose. Page Ref: 785

98. goiter. Thyr/o- means thyroid, and -megaly means enlargement. Page Ref: 774

99. dwarfism. Without growth hormone, the body does not grow during childhood and puberty. Page Ref: 773

100. myxedema. Characteristics are a mucus-like substance (myx/o-) and edema plus bradycardia and mental retardation. Page Ref: 776

101. hirsutism. Hirsut/o- means hairy. Page Ref: 782

102. acromegaly. Acr/o- means extremity; -megaly means enlargement. Page Ref: 772

103. polyuria. Poly- = many; -uria = condition of the urine. Page Ref: 773

104. Cushing's. Cushing's syndrome is caused by hypersecretion of cortisol. Page Ref: 781

105. medulla. This tumor causes severe hypertension because of hypersecretion of epinephrine from the adrenal medulla. Page Ref: 782

106. milk. Galact/o- is a Greek combining form and lact/o- is Latin. Page Ref: 790

107. hormones. The endocrine system uses substances known as hormones. Page Ref: 753

108. homeostasis. Homeostasis is maintained by the endocrine system. Page Ref: 753

109. cortex. The outermost part of the adrenal gland is the adrenal cortex, which produces and secretes three groups of hormones. Page Ref: 760

110. endocrine. This system is the endocrine system. Page Ref: 753

111. Acromegaly. The condition is called acromegaly and causes the face and extremities to widen rather than grow longer. Page Ref: 772

112. thyroid. The goiter is an enlargement of the thyroid gland resulting from thyromegaly. Page Ref: 774

113. Graves' disease. Graves' disease, the most common form of hyperthyroidism, is an autoimmune disease. The entire thyroid gland becomes enlarged and exophthalmos also occurs in Graves' disease. Page Ref: 775

114. Gestational. Gestational diabetes mellitus resolves once the pregnancy is delivered, although many patients develop type 2 diabetes later in life. The combining form gestat/o- means from conception to birth. Page Ref: 779

115. gynecomastia. Gynecomastia results from an imbalance of androgens and estrogens caused by puberty, aging, surgical removal of the testes or estrogen drug treatment for prostate cancer. Page Ref: 783

116. hormones. Hormone (HOR-mohn), Hormone is derived from a Greek word meaning to set in motion. Page Ref: 753

117. homeostasis. Homeostasis (HOH-mee-oh-STAY-sis), home/o- same, -stasis condition of standing still; staying in one place. Page Ref: 753

118. hypothalamus. Hypothalamus (HY-poh-THAL-ah-mus). Hypothalamic (HY-poh-thah-LAM-ik), hypo- below; deficient, thalam/o- thalamus, -ic pertaining to. Page Ref: 754

119. pituitary. Pituitary (pih-TOO-eh-TAIR-ee), pituit/o- pituitary gland, -ary pertaining to. Pituitary is derived from a Latin word meaning mucous secretions from the nose. The Romans thought that nasal mucus came from the pituitary gland. So pituitary originally meant pertaining to mucous secretions from the nose. Page Ref: 755

120. aldosterone. Aldosterone (al-DAWS-ter-ohn) is produced by the adrenal cortex. Page Ref: 760

121. progesterone. Progesterone (proh-JES-ter-ohn) is a combination of the prefix pro- (before), the combining form gest/o- (from conception to birth), the letters er from sterol (a category of chemicals), and the suffix -one (a chemical substance). Page Ref: 761

122. Testosterone. Testosterone (tes-TAWS-teh-rohn) is secreted by the testes. Page Ref: 762

123. inhibition. Inhibition (IN-hih-BISH-un), inhibit/o- block; hold back, -ion action; condition. Page Ref: 762

124. synergism. Synergism (SIN-er-jizm), syn- together, erg/o- activity; work, -ism process; disease from a specific cause. Page Ref: 763

125. hypersecretion. Hypersecretion (HY-per-seh-KREE-shun), hyper- above; more than, normal secret/o- produce; secrete, -ion action; condition. Page Ref: 771

126. Panhypopituitarism. Panhypopituitarism (pan-HY-poh-pih-TOO-eh-tah-rizm), pan- all, hypo- below; deficient, pituitar/o- pituitary gland, -ism process; disease from a specific cause. Page Ref: 771

127. Galactorrhea. Galactorrhea (gah-LAK-toh-REE-ah), galact/o- milk, -rrhea flow, discharge. Page Ref: 772

128. Acromegaly. Acromegaly (AK-roh-MEG-ah-lee), acr/o- extremity; highest, point, -megaly enlargement. Page Ref: 772

129. Postpartum. Postpartum (post-PAR-tum), post-after, behind, -partum childbirth. Page Ref: 773

130. Goiter. Goiter (GOY-ter), Goiter is derived from a French word for throat. A goiter can be a mild, subtle swelling in the neck, or it can enlarge enough to cause difficulty swallowing and breathing. Page Ref: 774

131. growth. Growth hormone is active during puberty as children grow into teenagers, but excessive amounts produce excessive growth. Page Ref: 772

132. Testosterone. Testosterone is the most abundant and biologically active of all the male hormones. Page Ref: 762

133. polyuria; polydipsia. Poly- means much, ur/o- means urine, and dips/o- means thirst. Page Ref: 773

134. thyroid storm. It is known as a storm because of the suddenness and severity. Page Ref: 776

135. diabetologists. Diabet/o- means diabetes, log/o- means the study of, and -ist means one who specializes in. Page Ref: 790

True/False

136. True. Testosterone is the primary male hormone. Page Ref: 762

137. False. Bulging eyes may be found in some patients with hyperthyroidism. Page Ref: 775

138. True. Gestational diabetes occurs only during pregnancy, but the same patient is at risk for type 2 diabetes later in life. Page Ref: 779

139. False. Gynec/o- = female; mast/o- = breast, -ia = condition.This condition is male breast enlargement from an imbalance of androgens and estrogens. Page Ref: 783

140. False. The correct word is cretinism. Page Ref: 776

141. False. The suffix -itis (inflammation) is inappropriate in this medical word. Mellitus with an ending of -us is derived from a word meaning honey or sweet. Page Ref: 778

142. True. It is associated with hypersecretion of prolactin. Page Ref: 772

143. False. Uterine inertia involves weak contractions during labor and is associated with hyposecretion of oxytocin. Page Ref: 774

144. False. The correct word is diabetic neuropathy. The combining forms, neur/o- = nerve and nephr/o- = kidney can be confused because of similar spelling. Page Ref: 780

145. False. The word is derived from word parts meaning innermost (endo-), secrete (crin/o-) and the study of (-logy). Page Ref: 752

146. True. The release of hormones is one of several ways in which the organs and glands are alike. Page Ref: 753

147. False. Only some of the organs and glands of the endocrine system are influenced by the secretions of the pituitary gland. Page Ref: 755

148. True. Both structures are located within the brain, but have very different functions. Page Ref: 754,755

149. False. The thyroid gland is composed of two lobes separated by a thin bridge of tissue called the isthmus. Page Ref: 757

150. True. The pancreas is part of the endocrine system because it secretes the hormones insulin, glucagons, and somatostatin, and is also part of the digestive system. Page Ref: 759

151. True. The cortex and the medulla of the adrenal gland function like different glands and secrete different hormones. Page Ref: 760

152. True. The function of the ovaries is controlled in part by the pituitary gland, but they also secrete their own hormones and are part of the female reproductive system. Page Ref: 761

153. True. Hormones have very different actions, some of which are inhibitory and some of which are stimulatory. Page Ref: 762

154. True. Hormones from the pituitary gland stimulate other glands, such as the thyroid gland, ovaries, and testes. Page Ref: 755

155. False. These antidiabetic drugs are given orally. Only insulin is given by subcutaneous injection. Page Ref: 787,788

156. True. It decreases in size and function after adolescence. Page Ref: 758

157. True. Insulin is always injected subcutaneously. Antidiabetic drugs are taken orally. Page Ref: 787,788

158. False. The glands of the endocrine system are located in the brain, neck, thoracic cavity, abdominopelvic cavity, and in the scrotum of the male. Page Ref: 752

159. False. The pituitary gland produces FSH in both females and males. In females FSH stimulates the follicles of the ovary to produce eggs, and in males FSH stimulates the seminiferous tubules of the testes to produce sperm. Page Ref: 755

160. False. Although gynec/o- means female, gynecomastia is actually an abnormal enlargement of the breasts in males. Page Ref: 783

Essay

161. Calcium in the blood is partially regulated by parathyroid hormone functioning. Since the parathyroid glands are located very close to the thyroid gland, some parathyroid tissue may have been inadvertently removed. This could cause hypocalcemia or low calcium levels in the blood. Page Ref: 777

162. Because of the possibility of decreased sensation in their feet (diabetic neuropathy), possible

poor eyesight (diabetic retinopathy), and sores that do not heal well, diabetics are advised to have foot care such as toenail trimming done by a professional such as a podiatrist and to avoid ill-fitting shoes. Complications with wound healing such as skin ulcers and gangrene can be prevented with these practices. Page Ref: 780

163. The pituitary gland in the brain is the master gland because it releases many hormones that direct and control other glands of the endocrine system and many organs as well. Page Ref: 753

164. The TFT is a blood test that measures the levels of T_3, T_4 and TSH. It is used to evaluate the function of the thyroid gland and the anterior pituitary gland. Page Ref: 785

165. These tests are nuclear medicine procedures that combine a radioactive iodine uptake and a thyroid scan. Two radioactive tracers are given, orally and intravenously. The thyroid gland takes up the radioactive substances and the rate of uptake determines how well the thyroid gland is functioning. Page Ref: 786

166. Endocrinology is the healthcare specialty that studies the anatomy and physiology of the endocrine system and uses diagnostic tests, medical and surgical procedures, and drugs to treat endocrine system diseases. Page Ref: 752

167. Stimulation involves acting on a gland or organ to release the hormones contained within. Inhibition involves acting on a gland or organ to prevent it from releasing its hormones. Page Ref: 762

CHAPTER 15

Multiple Choice

1. d. Anis/o- = unequal; cor/o- = pupil; -ia = condition. Page Ref: 823

2. a. Dilating the pupils allows better visualization of the structures of the eye for an internal exam. Page Ref: 838

3. d. The colored portion of the eye is the iris. Page Ref: 808

4. b. The sclera is opaque, therefore light rays cannot pass through it. It is a firm layer that shapes the eye and is where the extra ocular muscles attach. Page Ref: 808

5. c. Mi/o- means lessening, as the pupils contract in size. Page Ref: 809

6. d. This exam views the structures in the anterior chamber but not the posterior cavity Page Ref: 830

7. b. Antibiotic drugs are used to treat bacterial infections. Page Ref: 838

8. a. Concave lens are measured in minus diopters and are used to treat nearsightedness. Page Ref: 834

9. c. From the Latin for left eye: *Oculus Sinistra*. Page Ref: 834,839

10. d. The optic disk is not stimulated by light or color. It is located in the area of the retina where the optic nerve enters the eye. Page Ref: 812

11. c. Limbus is a Latin word for border. Page Ref: 808

12. b. Converg/o- means coming together. Page Ref: 831

13. d. This is a pus-filled swelling near the edge of an eyelid. Page Ref: 821

14. a. Of the selections above only the ophthalmologist, a physician, can perform eye surgery. An occultist is not a medical practitioner. Page Ref: 840

15. c. En- means inward, trop/o- means turning, and -ion means condition. Page Ref: 821

16. c. Herpes simplex is a viral infection and therefore is treated with an antiviral, not antibiotic medication. Page Ref: 838

17. d. Each of the above abbreviations involve the examination of some aspect of the eyes. Page Ref: 839

18. d. Inferior pertains to below. Page Ref: 813

19. b. A macule is a flat, pigmented spot on the skin. This word can be confused with macula, an area of the retina. Page Ref: 812

20. b. Pinkeye is a bacterial infection of the conjunctiva of the eye. Page Ref: 822

21. d. Ex- = outward; ophthalmos = eye. Page Ref: 823

22. a. Macular degeneration occurs in older patients. Page Ref: 825

23. d. Ex- = outward; trop/o- = turning; -ia = condition. Page Ref: 826

24. a. This surgery reshapes the curvature of the cornea to correct nearsightedness (myopia). Kerat/o- = cornea; -ectomy = excision. Page Ref: 837

25. c. Increased intraocular pressure from blocked aqueous humor causes glaucoma. Page Ref: 823

26. a. A hordeolum is also known as a stye. Page Ref: 821

27. a. Cataract is derived from a Greek word meaning waterfall. Page Ref: 824

28. a. The treatment of presbyopia is corrective eyeglasses. Page Ref: 825

29. c. Esotropia is also called crossed eyes. Page Ref: 826

30. c. Patients who have astigmatism experience blurry vision both near and at a distance. Page Ref: 827

31. a. Air-puff tonometry emits a short burst of air and measures the pressure of the air rebounding from the cornea without touching the eye. Page Ref: 830

32. c. The abbreviation OD means right eye. The abbreviation O.D. means doctor of optometry. Page Ref: 839

33. b. The lacrimal glands release tears that lubricate the anterior surface of the eye. Excess tears leave the eye through small openings and eventually drain into the nose. Page Ref: 809

34. b. In the medical word aqueous humor, the combining form aque/o- means watery substance and the suffix -ous means pertaining to. The word humor is derived from the Latin word meaning liquid. Page Ref: 811

35. b. Laser is an acronym for the words light amplification by stimulated emission of radiation. Photocoagulation means using light from a laser to coagulate bleeding. Page Ref: 836

36. d. The combining form accommod/o- means to adapt. The suffix -ation means a process, or being or having. The ciliary muscles must adapt to the changing distances. Page Ref: 831

37. d. Xerophthalmia is also known as dry eyes syndrome. Page Ref: 822

38. a. The abbreviation OS means oculus sinister or left eye. Page Ref: 839

39. c. The combining form pupill/o- means pupil of the eye. Page Ref: 808

40. d. The treatment for pinkeye is antibiotic eye drops or oral drugs for infection. Page Ref: 822

41. b. The combining form myop/o- means shortsighted. Page Ref: 827

42. a. The correction of exotropia involves repositioning of the extraocular muscles during early childhood. Ex/o- means outward. Page Ref: 826

43. a. The sebaceous glands are also called meibomian glands. Page Ref: 807

44. b. The orbit is a bony socket in the skull that surrounds all but the anterior part of the eyeball. Page Ref: 807

45. a. Scotoma is a temporary or permanent visual field defect in one or both eyes. Page Ref: 828

46. d. During gaze testing, the patient follows the physician's finger from side to side and up and down. Page Ref: 832

47. c. An intraocular lens can be implanted after removal of a cataract. Page Ref: 835

48. b. The combining form fund/o- means part farthest from the opening. Page Ref: 812

49. c. Diabetic retinopathy is a chronic progressive condition in which new, fragile retinal blood vessels are formed. Page Ref: 825

50. b. Ophthalm/o- means eye and -logy means the study of. Page Ref: 806

51. d. The small area between the cornea and the surface of the iris through which the aqueous humor circulates is called the anterior chamber. Page Ref: 811

52. d. The lacrimal gland produces and releases tears. Page Ref: 809

53. b. The organ of the eye responsible for the color of the eye is the iris. It is the colored ring of tissue whose muscles contract or relax to change the size of the pupil in the center of the iris. Page Ref: 808

54. d. The orbit is a bony socket in the skull that surrounds all but the anterior part of the eyeball. Page Ref: 807

55. c. Inflammation or infection of the eyelid with redness, crusts and scales at the bases of the eyelashes is called blepharitis. Page Ref: 821

56. a. Xerophthalmia is insufficient production of tears. Page Ref: 822

57. c. Exophthalmos is a condition which causes pronounced outward bulging of the anterior surface of the eye. Page Ref: 823

58. a. Diabetic retinopathy is a chronic, progressive condition which may eventually cause hemorrhage and blindness. Page Ref: 825

59. b. The medical term for farsightedness is hyperopia. In hyperopia light rays from a far object focus correctly on the retina, creating a sharp image. Page Ref: 827

60. a. Scleral (SKLEER-al), scler/o- hard; sclera (white of the eye), -al pertaining to. Icterus (IK-ter-us), Icterus is a Greek word meaning jaundice. Page Ref: 823

61. c. Cataract (KAT-ah-rakt), Cataract is derived from a Greek word meaning a waterfall. Looking through a cataract can be like looking through a water-fall or a piece of waxed paper. Page Ref: 824

62. d. Mydriatic (MIH-dree-AT-ik), mydr/o- widening, -iatic pertaining to a state or process. Page Ref: 838

63. d. Right eye (oculus dexter). Page Ref: 839

64. a. Optician (op-TISH-un), opt/o- eye; vision, -ician a skilled professional or expert. Page Ref: 840

65. d. See Figure 15-2. Page Ref: 808

66. a. Sebaceous (seh-BAY-shus), sebace/o- sebum (oil), -ous pertaining to. Meibomian (my-BOH-mee-an). Meibomian glands were named by Heinrich Meibom (1638-1700), a German anatomist. This is an example of an eponym: a person from whom something takes its name. Page Ref: 807

67. a. Lenses (LENZ), Lens is a Latin word meaning lentil. The two curved sides of a lentil seed resemble a lens, and the lentil plant itself is named Lens culinaris. Capsule (KAP-sool), Capsule is derived from a Latin word meaning little box. Page Ref: 810

68. d. See Figure 15-7. Page Ref: 813

69. c. Sclera is the tough, white outer covering of the eyeball. Page Ref: 808

70. a. The Snellen chart is a standardized chart used to measure distance vision. Page Ref: 831

71. b. Cones contain color pigments and provide color vision. Page Ref: 814

72. a. The optic disk is the circular area where the optic nerve enters the retina. Page Ref: 812

73. b. Tonometry or the air puff test measures the intraocular pressure of the eye and detects glaucoma. Page Ref: 830

74. d. The macule is the area of greatest visual acuity on the retina. Page Ref: 812

75. c. Phak/o- means lens. Page Ref: 835

76. c. Only an ophthalmologist is an M.D. An optometrist is a Doctor of Optometry (O.D.). Page Ref: 840

77. d. Presby/o- means old age. The lens becomes less flexible in older persons. Page Ref: 825

78. c. Vitreous humor fills the posterior cavity, not the anterior chamber. Page Ref: 812

79. d. The membrane is the retina, and surgically fixing it to reattach it is a retinopexy. Page Ref: 837

80. c. Nystagmus means a nodding. Page Ref: 826

81. d. Sagging skin on the eyelids is corrected with a blepharoplasty. Page Ref: 835

82. b. Fluorescein dye highlights damaged tissue. Page Ref: 830

83. a. The sebaceous or meibomian glands secrete oil on the eyelid. Page Ref: 807

84. c. Aqueous humor is produced by the ciliary body. Page Ref: 811

85. a. The ciliary body produces aqueous humor and has ligaments that hold the lens in place and muscles that change the shape of the lens. Page Ref: 810

86. d. Light rays are first focused by the cornea, and then by the lens. Page Ref: 808,810

87. c. The visual cortex that interprets visual impulses is in the occipital lobe of the cerebrum. Page Ref: 815

88. a. Fluorescein dye injected intravenously travels to the retina and glows bright green in areas of tissue damage and bleeding. Page Ref: 829

89. b. Amblyopia occurs when the brain ignores the visual image from one eye affected with strabismus. Page Ref: 828,832

90. d. The correct spelling is accommodation. Page Ref: 822

Short Answer

91. blepharitis. Blephar/o- = eyelid; -itis = inflammation. Page Ref: 821

92. presbyopia. Presby- = old age; -opia = vision. Page Ref: 825

93. lacrimal. Lacrim/o- means tears. Page Ref: 809

94. enucleation. Enucle/o- = remove the kernal or nucleus; -ation = a process. Page Ref: 835

95. dry eyes. Xer/o- = dry; ophthalm/o- = eyes; -ia = condition. Page Ref: 822

96. nystagmus. Nystagmus is a Greek word that means nodding. Page Ref: 826

97. Snellen. Normal visual acuity is 20/20. The numerator stands for 20 feet, the standard distance between the chart and the patient. The denominator stands for the distance at which a person with normal vision could see a particular line on the chart. Page Ref: 831

98. phacoemulsification. Phak/o- means lens. Page Ref: 835

99. corneas; corneas. A diseased or damaged cornea can be removed and a donor cornea sewn in its place. Page Ref: 835

100. half. Hemi- = half; an- = without; -opsia = condition of vision. Page Ref: 828

101. tonometry. A diagnostic procedure to detect increased intraocular pressure and glaucoma is called tonometry. Page Ref: 830

102. Ultrasonography. Ultrasonography is a radiologic procedure that uses high-frequency sound waves to create an image of the eye. Page Ref: 831

103. ophthalmoscope. An ophthalmoscope is a handheld instrument with a light and changeable lenses of different strengths used to examine the retina from all angles. Page Ref: 832

104. transplantation. Corneal transplantation is a surgical procedure to replace a damaged or diseased cornea. Page Ref: 835

105. enucleation. A surgical procedure to remove the eye from the orbit because of trauma or tumor is called enucleation. Page Ref: 835

106. mydriatic. A drug class called mydriatic drugs is used to dilate the pupil. Page Ref: 838

107. optometrist. A doctor who diagnoses and treats patients with vision problems, but who does not perform surgery and is not a physician, is called a/an optometrist. Page Ref: 840

108. sclera. The sclera is a tough, fibrous connective tissue that forms a continuous outer layer around the eyeball. Page Ref: 808

109. caruncle. A red, triangular tissue at the medial corner of the eye is called the caruncle. Page Ref: 807

110. conjunctiva. Conjunctiva (CON-junk-TY-vah), (con-JUNK-tih-vah). Page Ref: 807

111. cornea. Cornea (KOR-nee-ah). The cornea is a transparent layer. Page Ref: 808

112. pupil. Pupil (PYOO-pil), Pupil is derived from a Latin word meaning little girl or doll, because you can see a tiny reflection of yourself when you look closely at someone else's pupil. Page Ref: 808

113. miosis. Miosis (my-OH-sis), mi/o- lessening, -osis condition; abnormal condition; process. Some word parts have more than one definition. The best definition of miosis is a process of lessening [the size of the pupil]. Page Ref: 809

114. nasolacrimal. Nasolacrimal (NAY-soh-LAK-rih-mal), nas/o- nose, lacrim/o- tears, -al pertaining to. Page Ref: 809

115. anterior. Anterior (an-TEER-ee-or), anter/o- before; front part, -ior pertaining to. Page Ref: 811

116. optic. Optic (AWP-tik), opt/o- eye; vision, -ic pertaining to. Page Ref: 812

117. choroid. Choroid (KOH-royd), Choroid is derived from a Greek word meaning like a membrane. Page Ref: 810

118. lens. Lens (LENZ). The lens is a clear, hard disk with two curved sides. Page Ref: 810

119. Aqueous humor. Aqueous humor (AA-kwee-us HYOO-mor), aque/o- watery substance, -ous pertaining to Humor is derived from a Latin word meaning liquid. Page Ref: 811

120. posterior. Posterior (pohs-TEER-ee-or), poster/ o- back part, -ior pertaining to. Page Ref: 812

121. Rods. Rod (RAWD), Rods are so named because one end of each cell is shaped like a cylindrical rod. Page Ref: 814

122. thalamus. Thalamus (THAL-ah-mus). The thalamus is a structure in the brain. Page Ref: 815

123. Ectropion. Ectropion (ek-TROH-pee-on), ec- out, outward, trop/o- having an affinity for; stimulating; turning -ion action; condition. Page Ref: 821

124. conjunctivitis. Conjunctivitis (con-JUNK-tih-VY-tis), conjunctiv/o- conjunctiva -itis inflammation of. Page Ref: 822

125. II. The optic nerve is a cranial nerve for the sense of vision. Cranial nerves are written as Roman numerals. Page Ref: 812

126. 20. The numerator on a visual acuity measurement is always 20 because it represents the standard distance between the Snellen chart and the patient. Page Ref: 831

127. exotropia. Ex/o- means outward, and trop/o- means turning. Page Ref: 826

128. left eye; each eye or both eyes. OS means left eye (oculus sinister) and OU means each eye or both eyes (oculus uterque, oculus unitas). Page Ref: 838

129. 20/200. The numerator (20) on a visual acuity measurement represents the standard distance (in feet) between the Snellen chart and the patient. The denominator (200) represents the distance (in feet) at which a person with normal vision could see a particular line on the chart. Page Ref: 828

True/False

130. True. Tonometry tests for increased intraocular pressure, and gonioscopy examines the trabecular meshwork for blockage. Page Ref: 830

131. True. This is the pupil of the eye, the area that allows light rays to enter the eye. Page Ref: 808

132. False. It fills the posterior cavity of the eye. Page Ref: 812

133. True. Phac/o- is Greek for lens, and lenticul/o- is Latin. Page Ref: 840

134. False. It is called LASIK surgery. Lasix is a diuretic drug. Page Ref: 837

135. False. They are the cones. Page Ref: 814

136. True. Infants can become infected with conjunctivitis from a microorganism found in the mother's birth canal during birth. Page Ref: 822

137. True. Aphakia, or the absence of a lens, is acquired surgically Page Ref: 824

138. False. It is a malignancy of the eye in a child. Page Ref: 826

139. True. The lacrimal glands produce tears that flow through the lacrimal ducts. Page Ref: 809

140. False. Aqueous humor is a clear, watery fluid produced by the ciliary body of the eye. Page Ref: 811

141. True. The extraocular muscles control the movements of the eye in all directions. Page Ref: 813

142. False. A clear, hard disk in the internal eye is called the lens. Page Ref: 810

143. True. These are a type of oil gland. Page Ref: 807

144. False. The clear, gel-like substance that fills the posterior cavity of the eye is actually called vitreous humor. Page Ref: 812

145. True. Lenticul/o- is a combining form meaning lens. Page Ref: 810

146. False. Inflammation or infection of the eyelid is called blepharitis. Page Ref: 821

147. True. This is caused by weakening of connective tissue in the lower eyelid of older patients. Page Ref: 821

148. True. This is usually caused by a staphylococcus infection in a sebaceous gland. Page Ref: 821

149. False. Hyphema is blood in the anterior chamber of the eye. Page Ref: 824

150. False. These chambers are filled with aqueous humor. Page Ref: 811

151. False. Blephar/o- means eyelid. Page Ref: 821

152. False. Loss of transparency of the lens is a cataract. Page Ref: 824

153. True. Melanocytes are present with brown eye color. Page Ref: 809

154. True. Tears lubricate the eye and protect it from infection. Page Ref: 809

Essay

155. The heat from the laser coagulates and seals the retinal detachment to prevent further tearing, thus saving the eyesight. Page Ref: 836

156. The sclera would appear yellow rather than white. This condition, known as jaundice or scleral icterus, occurs when the liver is not functioning properly. Page Ref: 823

157. A young child is tested with a distance vision chart that uses pictures rather than alphabet letters. Page Ref: 831

158. Their irises lack melanin production. This begins with exposure to light. Page Ref: 809

159. The lacrimal gland continuously produces and releases tears through the lacrimal ducts to moisten the eye. Tears also contain an antibacterial enzyme to prevent bacterial infections. Page Ref: 809

160. The retina contains special light-sensitive cells known as rods and cones. Rods are sensitive to all levels of light, but not to color. They function in both daytime and nighttime vision. Rods can detect objects in very low light, although the image may be less than optimal in very low light. Cones, on the other hand, are sensitive only to color. The cones respond to red, green, and blue light. It is difficult to see colors in dim light because it takes many photons to activate a cone. Page Ref: 814

161. The conjunctiva is a delicate, transparent mucous membrane that covers the inside of the eyelids and the anterior surface of the eye. It produces a clear, watery mucus that helps lubricate the eye. Page Ref: 807

162. Blepharoptosis is the drooping of the upper eyelid from excessive fat or sagging of the tissues due to age or disease that affects the muscles or nerves. The treatment for blepharoptosis is a plastic surgery repair called blepharoplasty. Page Ref: 821

163. Fluorescein staining is a diagnostic procedure in which fluorescein, an orange fluorescent dye, is instilled in the eye to detect corneal abrasions and ulcers. A blue light is used to examine the eye where corneal abrasions and ulcers appear as fluorescent green. Page Ref: 829

CHAPTER 16

Multiple Choice

1. c. Bucc/o- means cheek. Page Ref: 861

2. a. This infection is caused by *Candida albicans,* a yeast-like fungus. Page Ref: 877

3. b. Epistaxis is Greek meaning blood falling from the nose. Page Ref: 875

4. d. These are examples of hearing tests. Page Ref: 880

5. b. Uvula is Latin for little grape. Page Ref: 861

6. d. Presby/o- = old age; -acusis = hearing. Page Ref: 872

7. c. Ménière's disease was named by Prosper Ménière, a French physician. Page Ref: 872

8. a. The pinna is the visible external ear. An otoplasty is the reshaping of the ear. Ot/o- = ear; -plasty = process of reshaping. Page Ref: 884

9. c. This surgery is done to remove the diseased footplate of the stapes, one of the small bones in the middle ear, with insertion of a prosthesis. Page Ref: 885

10. a. Tuss/o- is a combining form for cough. Some medication names have hints for the usage of the drug. Page Ref: 886

11. c. A part of the mastoid process was removed. Page Ref: 883

12. b. Because the tympanic membrane is nearly transparent, the first ossicle of the middle ear, the malleus, can be seen. Otoscopy is a procedure to visualize the structures of the ear. Ot/o- = ear; -scopy = using an instrument to visualize. Page Ref: 856,882

13. d. Rhin/o- means nose and -phyma means tumor or growth. Page Ref: 875

14. d. An upper respiratory infection occurs in the nose, throat, and/or ears. One example would be the common cold from a virus. Page Ref: 875

15. c. The temporomandibular joint, located in the lower jaw, is affected in this condition. Page Ref: 877

16. a. This child has a middle ear condition with fluid buildup. His surgery would involve making an incision into the eardrum with tube insertion for fluid drainage. Ot/o- = ear; -itis = inflammation; media = middle. Tympan/o- = eardrum; -ostomy = create an opening. Page Ref: 873,885

17. d. Allegra will block the effect of histamine, the substance released during an allergic reaction. Page Ref: 885

18. b. An auditory nerve tumor, such as an acoustic neuroma, will produce an abnormal brainstem auditory evoked response. Page Ref: 879

19. c. An- = without; -acusis = hearing. Page Ref: 872

20. d. Otitis media is a middle ear inflammation with fluid buildup. Page Ref: 873

21. b. Acute pharyngitis is a throat infection. A culture and sensitivity is a laboratory test done to identify the causative bacterium and the most appropriate antibiotic. Pharyng/o- = throat; -itis = inflammation of. Page Ref: 877

22. c. Thush is a yeast infection. Mycostatin is an anti-yeast medication. Page Ref: 866, 877

23. b. To treat head and neck cancer, the portions of anatomy usually removed are the mandible (jaw), tongue, lymph nodes, neck muscles, and sometimes the larynx. Page Ref: 884

24. a. The frontal sinuses are located in the frontal bone that forms the forehead. Page Ref: 860

25. c. Tinnitus is a Latin word that means a jingling or clinking sound. Page Ref: 874

26. c. The mentum is the most anterior part of the lower jaw bone or mandible. Mentum is a Latin word meaning chin. Page Ref: 858

27. c. Thrush is common in infants, but is also seen in the mouths of immunosuppressed patients with AIDS because their immune response cannot control the growth of *Candida albicans*. Page Ref: 877

28. b. The combining form ot/o- means ear. The suffix -rrhea means flow, discharge, or drainage. Page Ref: 874

29. b. Suppurative otitis media contains pus; whereas serous otitis media contains clear fluid. Page Ref: 873

30. a. Epistaxis is due to irritation or dryness of the nasal mucosa and the rupture of a small artery just beneath the mucous membrane. It can also be caused by trauma. Page Ref: 875

31. a. Vertigo is a Latin word meaning dizziness or turning. Vertigo is caused by upper respiratory infection, middle or inner ear infection, head trauma, or degenerative changes of the semi-circular canals. Page Ref: 874

32. a. Herpes simplex is a virus. Type 1 is found near the mouth. Type 2 causes genital herpes, a sexually transmitted disease. Page Ref: 877

33. a. The three tiny bones are called ossicles. In order of vibration, they are the malleus, incus, and stapes. Page Ref: 856

34. d. The external ear is called the auricle or pinna. Page Ref: 855

35. b. The turbinates are found in the nose. Page Ref: 859

36. a. An- means without, and osm/o- means sense of smell. Page Ref: 875

37. c. The abbreviation AS or avris sinsiter means left ear. Page Ref: 887

38. c. The combining form cheil/o- means lip. The suffix -plasty process of reshaping by surgery. Page Ref: 883

39. a. Cholesteatoma is caused by chronic otitis media. It can eventually destroy the bones of the middle ear and extend into the mastoid air cells. Page Ref: 871

40. d. Some of these drugs, like hydrocodone, contain a narcotic. The prefix anti- means against; the combining form tuss/o- means cough; the suffix -ive means pertaining to. Page Ref: 886

41. d. Decongestant drugs often are in the form of nasal sprays or oral drugs, such as Afrin, Dristan, Drixoral, and Sudafed. Page Ref: 886

42. d. T & A is a surgical procedure to remove the tonsils and adenoids in patients with chronic tonsillitis and hypertrophy of the tonsils and adenoids. Page Ref: 885

43. c. BAER stands for brainstem auditory evoked response. The patient listens as an audiometer produces a series of clicks. Electro-encephalography (EEG) is performed at the same time. A lesion or tumor in the auditory cortex of the brain or on the auditory cortex of the brain or on the auditory nerve will produce an abnormal BAER. Page Ref: 879

44. c. When the bacteria group A beta-hemolytic streptococcus causes the infection, it is known as strep throat. Page Ref: 877

45. b. Ossicle is derived from a Latin word meaning little bone. Page Ref: 856

46. d. The combining form tympan/o- means tympanic membrane or eardrum. The suffix -plasty means process of reshaping by surgery. Page Ref: 885

47. c. The patient stands with the feet together and the eyes closed. Swaying or falling to one side indicates a loss of balance and inner ear dysfunction. Page Ref: 883

48. a. Postnasal drip (PND) is related to the nose. Page Ref: 887

49. a. Otolaryngology is the proper word. The word parts ot/o- (ear), laryng/o- (larynx) and -logy (the study of) combine to make the complete word. Page Ref: 854

50. c. Malle/o- is a combining form that means hammer. Malleus is derived from Latin. Page Ref: 856

51. a. These are all part of the inner ear. Page Ref: 857

52. d. The paranasal sinuses contain the frontal, maxillary, ethmoid, and sphenoid sinuses. Page Ref: 860

53. c. The phrase buccal mucosa contains a word part that means cheek. The word part is bucc/o-. Page Ref: 861

54. c. The semicircular canals are oriented horizontally, vertically, and obliquely. Page Ref: 858

55. b. Dysequilibrium is also known as motion sickness, but is not associated with hearing loss. Page Ref: 872

56. d. Cervical lymphadenopathy is not a tumor of any sort but is enlargement of the lymph nodes in the neck. It can be caused by infection, cancer, or the spread of a cancerous tumor from another site. Page Ref: 876

57. a. A cochlear implant is done to correct hearing loss by surgically placing a small device behind the ear. Page Ref: 883

58. d. See Figure 16-9. Page Ref: 864

59. b. Presbyacusis (PREZ-bee-ah-KOO-sis), presby/o- old age, -acusis hearing. Page Ref: 872

60. b. Hemotympanum (HEE-moh-TIM-pah-num), Hemotympanum is a combination of hem/o-

(blood) and the Latin word tympanum (eardrum). Page Ref: 872

61. b. Otitis media (oh-TY-tis MEE-dee-ah). Media is a Latin word meaning middle. Page Ref: 873

62. a. Effusion (ee-FYOO-shun), effus/o- a pouring out, -ion action; condition. Page Ref: 873

63. a. Mastoiditis (MAS-toy-DY-tis), mastoid/o- mastoid process, -itis inflammation of. Page Ref: 873

64. c. Otosclerosis (OH-toh-skleh-ROH-sis), ot/o- ear, scler/o- hard; sclera (white of the eye), -osis condition; abnormal condition; process. Page Ref: 874

65. d. Vertigo (VER-tih-goh); The sensation of being off balance when the body is not moving. Vertigo is a Latin word meaning dizziness or turning. Page Ref: 874

66. a. Rhinophyma (RY-noh-FY-mah), rhin/o- nose, -phyma tumor, growth. Page Ref: 875

67. a. Otoplasty (OH-toh-PLAS-tee), ot/o- ear, -plasty process of reshaping by surgery. Page Ref: 884

68. c. Tympan/o- is Greek for eardrum; myring/o- is Latin. Page Ref: 888

69. d. Ot/o- means ear, laryng/o- means larynx, log/o- means the study of, and -ist means one who specializes in. Page Ref: 888

70. d. A myringotome is an instrument used to cut the tympanic membrane before a ventilating tube is inserted. Page Ref: 884

71. b. Cheil/o- means lip. Page Ref: 883

72. c. Audiometry is the process of measuring the sense of hearing. Page Ref: 879

73. c. Ot/o- means ear and -scope means instrument used to examine. Page Ref: 882

74. a. Ot/o- means ear, and -itis means infection. Media means middle. Page Ref: 873

75. a. Ossicul/o- means ossicle (little bone). Page Ref: 857

76. d. Impacted cerumen in the ear canal is removed with alligator forceps. Page Ref: 871

77. a. Temporomandibular joint (TMJ) refers to the joint of the mandible (jaw bone). Page Ref: 887

78. b. Ot/o- means ear, and -plasty means process of reshaping by surgery. Page Ref: 884

79. d. The tympanic membrane is where the tubes are inserted. Page Ref: 885

80. b. The maxillary sinuses are within the cheekbones. Page Ref: 875

81. b. The vestibular branch comes from the semicircular canals of the inner ear that help maintain balance. Page Ref: 858

82. c. The conchae or turbinates in the nose warm and moisturize incoming air. The sound-alike word cochlea is a bone in the inner ear. Page Ref: 858,859

83. b. Epistaxis is a Greek word that means blood falling from the nose. Page Ref: 875

84. d. Mentum is a Latin word that means chin. Page Ref: 860

85. a. The vermilion border is the pink-red border around the lips. Page Ref: 860

86. a. The adenoids are found along the roof and walls of the nasopharynx. Page Ref: 861

87. c. Epi- means above or upon. The epiglottis is above the glottis, the opening into the larynx. Page Ref: 863

88. c. The hard palate or roof of the mouth is formed by the maxilla, palatine bone, and vomer bone. Page Ref: 861

89. a. Neur/o- means nerve, and -oma means tumor. Page Ref: 871

90. d. Ménière's disease affects the inner ear and the semicircular canals. Page Ref: 872

91. c. The correct spelling is tonsillectomy. Page Ref: 885

92. c. The Rinne test uses a vibrating tuning fork placed on the mastoid process and then next to the ear to measure bone conduction and air conduction of sound. Page Ref: 880

93. d. The rapid strep test is to detect beta-hemolytic group A streptococcus in a patient with a sore throat. The results are available within an hour so that antibiotic drugs can be started immediately. Page Ref: 881

94. a. The helix is the rounded outer edge of the external ear. Page Ref: 855

95. c. He would have conductive hearing loss because the jellybean keeps sound waves from being conducted through to the inner ear. Page Ref: 872

96. c. A speculum does not have its own light source, so a penlight has to be used along with it. Page Ref: 882

97. b. Endo- means within, and -scope means instrument used to examine. It has a magnifying lens, fiberoptic light source, and can be used to take a biopsy. Page Ref: 883

98. a. A myringotomy or incision into the tympanic membrane is not performed during a radical neck dissection for cancer of the mouth and neck. Page Ref: 884

99. d. Tympan/o- means tympanic membrane, and -plasty means process of reshaping by surgery. Page Ref: 885

Short Answer

100. cold sores. Herpes simplex virus type 1 causes cold sores. Page Ref: 876

101. otorrhea. Ot/o- = ear; -rrhea = flow. Page Ref: 874

102. leukoplakia. Leuk/o- means white, plak/o- means plaque, and -ia means condition. Page Ref: 876

103. tongue. Gloss/o- is a Greek combining form and lingu/o- is a Latin combining form. Page Ref: 888

104. audiometry. Audi/o- means the sense of hearing, and -metry means process of measuring. Page Ref: 879

105. rhinoplasty. Rhin/o- = nose; -plasty = surgical reshaping. Page Ref: 885

106. AD. This abbreviation stands for auris dextra. Page Ref: 887

107. sinuses. Sinus is a Latin word meaning hollow cavity. Page Ref: 851

108. impaction. Impact/o- means wedged in. Page Ref: 871

109. auricle or pinna. The external ear is also known as the auricle or pinna. Page Ref: 855

110. malleus; incus; stapes. The middle ear contains three tiny bones called the malleus, incus and stapes. Page Ref: 856

111. turbinates. The turbinates are three long projections of the ethmoid bone that jut into the nasal cavity and function to break up the stream of air as it enters the nose. Conchae is another correct answer. Page Ref: 859

112. acoustic neuroma. An acoustic neuroma is a benign tumor of the nerve cells of the auditory nerve. Page Ref: 871

113. Tinnitus. Tinnitus is the sound of buzzing, ringing, hissing, or roaring heard constantly or intermittently in one or both ears, even in a quiet environment. Page Ref: 874

114. Ototoxity. Ototoxity is a drug effect in which certain drugs damage the cochlea. Page Ref: 886

115. Pansinusitis. Pansinusitis is sinusitis which involves all of the sinuses on one side of the face. Page Ref: 875

116. Pansinusitis. Pansinusitis is a medical procedure done to examine the external auditory canals and tympanic membranes. Page Ref: 882

117. Otolaryngology. Otolaryngology (OH-toh-LAIR-ing-GAWL-oh-jee), ot/o- ear, laryng/o- larynx (voice box), -logy the study of. Page Ref: 854

118. cerumen. Cerumen (seh-ROO-men), Cerumen is derived from a Latin word meaning wax. Page Ref: 855-856

119. tympanic. Tympanic (tim-PAN-ik), tympan/o- tympanic membrane, (eardrum), -ic pertaining to. Page Ref: 856

120. eustachian. Eustachian (yoo-STAY-shun), The eustachian tube was named by Bartolommeo Eustachio (1524-1574), an Italian anatomist. This is an example of an eponym:a person from whom something takes it name. Page Ref: 857

121. vestibule. Vestibule (VES-tih-byool), Vestibule is derived from a Latin word meaning small entrance chamber. Page Ref: 858

122. cochlea. Cochlear (KOHK-lee-ar), cochle/o-cochlea (of the inner ear), -ar pertaining to. Page Ref: 858

123. septum. Septum (SEP-tum). Septum is derived from a Latin word meaning a partition. Page Ref: 858

124. chonchae. Conchae (CON-kee). Concha is a Latin word meaning a shell. Another correct answer is turbinates. Page Ref: 859

125. sinus. Sinus (SY-nus), Sinus is a Latin word meaning hollow cavity. Page Ref: 860

126. nasolabial. Nasolabial (NAY-zoh-LAY-bee-al), nas/o- nose, labi/o- lip; labium, -al pertaining to. Page Ref: 860

127. vermilion. Vermilion (ver-MIL-yon). Vermilion is an English word meaning bright red. Page Ref: 858

128. temporomandibular. Temporomandibular (TEM-poh-roh-man-DIB-yoo-lar), tempor/o- temple (side of the head), mandibul/o- mandible. Page Ref: 861

129. palatine. Palatine (PAL-ah-teen), palat/o- palate, -ine pertaining to. Palatine and palatal are both adjective forms for palate. Page Ref: 862

130. larynx. Larynx (LAIR-ingks). The larynx is the voice box. Page Ref: 863

131. epiglottis. Epiglottis (EP-ih-GLAWT-is), epi-upon, above, glott/o- glottis (of the larynx), -ic pertaining to. Page Ref: 863

132. polypectomy. The suffix -ectomy means surgical excision. Page Ref: 883

133. Rhinorrhea. Commonly called a "runny" nose, rhinorrhea is often caused by allergens such as pollen, dust, or animal dander. Page Ref: 874

134. cerumen. Glands in the ear canal secrete cerumen, a waxy substance that traps dirt and has an antibacterial effect to prevent infection. Page Ref: 856

135. pharyngitis. Pharyng/o- means pharynx (throat) and -itis means inflammation of. Page Ref: 877

136. hertz; decibels. Hertz and decibel are units of measurement for sound waves. Page Ref: 879

137. dysequilibrium. Dys- means abnormal and the word equilibrium means evenly balanced. Page Ref: 872

138. myringotomy; myringotome. Myring/o- means tympanic membrane. The suffix -tomy means process of cutting or making an incision, and the suffix -tome means instrument used to cut. Page Ref: 884

True/False

139. False. This area of the upper lip is the philtrum. The mentum is the chin. Page Ref: 858

140. False. This mass is found in the middle ear. The cochlea is in the inner ear. Page Ref: 871

141. True. This is the removal of the palatine tonsils and adenoids or tonsillectomy and adenoidectomy. Page Ref: 885
142. True. The pharynx is the throat. Page Ref: 861
143. False. Audit/o- pertains to the sense of hearing but aur/i- pertains to the anatomic site, the ear. Page Ref: 888
144. False. Naris is singular; nares is plural. Page Ref: 858
145. False. The audiologist performs hearing tests and assesses hearing loss. The physician who specializes in conditions of the ear is an otorhinolaryngologist. Page Ref: 888
146. True. Tinnitus is a Latin word meaning a jingling sound. Page Ref: 874
147. True. An- = without; -osmia = sense of smell. Page Ref: 875
148. False. The correct spelling is tonsillitis. Page Ref: 878
149. False. Otosclerosis is the abnormal formation of bone between the stapes and oval window in the inner ear. Page Ref: 874
150. True. The nose and the throat are parts of the respiratory system and the digestive system respectively. Page Ref: 861
151. False. A rhinoplasty is plastic surgery of the nose. A ruptured tympanic membrane requires a surgical repair called tympanoplasty. Page Ref: 885
152. False. Otosclerosis is abnormal formation of bone in the middle ear and is not related to the vasculature. Page Ref: 874
153. True. The suffix -rrhea has the same meaning in both words it means flow or discharge. Page Ref: 874
154. True. Vertigo is the sensation of being off balance when the body is not moving. Page Ref: 874
155. True. The key to this word is the combining form gloss/o- which means tongue. Page Ref: 876
156. False. Audiometry measures hearing acuity and documents hearing loss. Brainstem auditory evoked response (BAER) analyzes the brain's response to sounds. Page Ref: 879
157. True. Swaying or falling to one side indicates a loss of balance and inner ear dysfunction. Page Ref: 883
158. False. A mastoidectomy is a surgical procedure to remove an infected part of the mastoid process of the temporal bone. Page Ref: 883
159. False. Decongestant drugs constrict the blood vessels, which limits the blood flow and reduces swelling in the mucous membranes. Page Ref: 886
160. False. The mandible is the lower jawbone. The nasal cavity is formed by the ethmoid bone and the maxilla or upper jawbone. Page Ref: 859

161. True. The tonsils and adenoids are collections of lymphoid tissue. Page Ref: 861-862
162. False. Exhaled air causes the vocal cords to vibrate. Page Ref: 863
163. False. A laryngectomy or removal of the larynx is done for cancer of the mouth and neck. Page Ref: 884
164. True. Audi/o- means the sense of hearing, and -metry means process of measuring. Page Ref: 879
165. False. The eustachian tube allows pressure in the middle ear to equalize with pressure in the throat and mouth and outside of the body. The eustachian tube goes between the pharynx and the middle ear. Page Ref: 857

Essay

166. The eustachian tube is shorter and more horizontal, making it easy for bacteria to travel from the nasopharynx to the middle ear. Page Ref: 873
167. Vocal cord polyps are benign growths that contain blood vessels. People who use their voice for a living such as newscasters or vocalists are predisposed to these growths that are related to vocal strain, cigarette smoking, and allergies. Page Ref: 878
168. Nasopharynx, oropharynx, and hypopharynx. The nasopharynx is the uppermost portion of the throat, the oropharynx is the middle portion of the throat, and the hypopharynx is the lowermost portion of the throat. Page Ref: 861-862
169. Malleus, incus, stapes. Malleus is Latin for hammer, incus is Latin for anvil, and stapes is Latin for stirrup. Page Ref: 856
170. During speech, the vocal cords close partially or entirely. Exhaled air from the lungs causes the vocal cords to vibrate. The surface layer of each vocal cord is looser than the layers beneath it, and this layer vibrates in a wavelike fashion at a frequency of up to 100 times per second. These vibrations produce sound waves. These sound waves travel through the vocal cords and past the soft palate, tongue, and lips, all of which shape the sound waves into the words as we speak. Page Ref: 863
171. The external ear captures sound waves which travel down the external auditory canal to the tympanic membrane. There the sound waves are converted to mechanical motion as they cause the tympanic membrane to move inward and outward. As it moves, the tympanic membranes move the malleus, incus, and stapes which in turn cause the oval window to move. This causes inner ear fluid on the other side of the oval window to begin to vibrate, which is in turn transmitted throughout the length of the cochlea. In the cochlea, tiny hairs detect different frequencies of sound, sending nerve im-

pulses to the auditory nerve to the brain. The brain interprets the mechanical movement as sound. Page Ref: 864

172. Conductive hearing loss prevents sound waves from reaching the inner ear. It may be caused by a foreign body or infection in the external auditory canal, perforation of the tympanic membrane, fluid behind the tympanic membrane, or degeneration of the ossicles of the middle ear. Sensorineural hearing loss prevents generation of nerve impulses to the auditory nerve and may be caused by otosclerosis, disease of the cochlea, damage to the inner ear from excessive noise, or aging. Mixed hearing loss is a combination of both conductive hearing loss and sensorineural hearing loss. Page Ref: 872

173. Thrush is an oral infection caused by the fungus *Candida albicans* which coats the tongue and oral mucosa. It is common in infants, but is also seen in immunocompromised patients with AIDS because they have a diminished immune response. It is also commonly seen when antibiotics kill normal bacteria in the mouth, allowing overgrowth of *Candida albicans*. Thrush is also known as oral candidiasis. It is treated with oral antiyeast drugs. Page Ref: 877

174. BAER analyzes the brain's response to sounds. The patient listens as an audiometer produces a series of clicks. Electroencephalography (EEG) is performed at the same time. A lesion or tumor in the auditory cortex of the brain or on the auditory nerve will produce an abnormal BAER. Page Ref: 879

CHAPTER 17

Multiple Choice

1. c. Obsess/o- means besieged by thoughts and compuls/o- means drive or compel. Page Ref: 908

2. a. The hippocampus controls long-term memory. Page Ref: 904,910

3. d. Ech/o- = to reflect back and -lalia = condition of speech. Page Ref: 911

4. b. This disorder was named for Karl Munchausen, a well-known liar. Page Ref: 913

5. c. Anti- means against and anxi/o- means fear or anxiety. Page Ref: 926

6. b. Liquor or alcoholic beverage, known as ethyl alcohol, is abbreviated as ETOH. Page Ref: 927

7. a. The psychiatrist is a physician and only physicians can prescribe drugs. Page Ref: 928

8. a. Narcissos was the character in Greek mythology who fell in love with his own image. Page Ref: 921

9. d. ECT is electroconvulsive therapy, also known as electroshock therapy. Page Ref: 924

10. d. Axis II contains personality disorders and mental retardation. Selections a,b, and c would be included in Axis I. Page Ref: 923

11. c. Epinephrine is a neurotransmitter for the sympathetic nervous system that is active in times of anger, danger, or fear. Page Ref: 905

12. b. Antipsychotic drugs are used to treat psychosis; anorexia nervosa is an eating disorder, not a psychosis. Page Ref: 927

13. b. Acr/o- = highest point or tip, phob/o- = fear and -ia = condition. Page Ref: 908

14. c. This disorder consists of distinct, different, personalities in one person. These personalities may not be aware that the others exist. Page Ref: 913

15. d. This disorder is characterized by pulling out one's hair. Trich/o- = hair; till/o- = pull out; -mania = condition of frenzy. Page Ref: 916

16. c. Cycl/o- = cycle, thym/o- = mind and -ia = condition. Page Ref: 918

17. c. Alcoholic beverages mixed with Antabuse will give a person headache, nausea, and dizziness. That is why Antabuse is useful in treating alcoholism. Page Ref: 927

18. a. The Rorschach or inkblot test was named by Herman Rorschach, a Swiss psychiatrist. Page Ref: 923

19. d. Norepinephrine is the neurotransmitter for the parasympathetic nervous system. Serotinin is a neurotransmitter in the brain and spinal cord. Page Ref: 904-905

20. b. Claustrophobia is the fear of closed-in spaces. In systematic desensitization, a patient is exposed to fear using different, progressive scenarios to relieve anxiety associated with the phobia. Page Ref: 908,926

21. c. Lithium inhibits excessive norepinephrine while increasing sensitivity to serotonin. Page Ref: 927

22. c. Voyeurism is secretly viewing others to obtain sexual arousal. Page Ref: 915

23. b. Thorazine is an antipsychotic drug. Page Ref: 927

24. a. Affect is used to describe external expressions of emotions. Page Ref: 905

25. c. Pyr/o- = fire and -mania = condition of frenzy. Page Ref: 916

26. c. The Thematic Apperception Test (TAT) involves 31 different pictures that the patient views, describing theme of each picture. Page Ref: 923

27. c. The abbreviation DT means delirium tremens. Delirium tremens is brought on by withdrawal after prolonged periods of heavy alcohol ingestion. Page Ref: 910

28. c. The combining form affect/o- means state of mind or mood. The suffix -ive means pertaining to. Page Ref: 905

29. d. Obsessive means pertaining to besieged by thoughts. Compulsive means pertaining to drive or compel. This disorder includes activities that consume a significant portion of each day. Page Ref: 908

30. a. Microphobia is a fear of germs. A phobia is an intense, unreasonable fear of a specific thing or situation or even the thought of it. Page Ref: 909

31. b. The BDI (Beck Depression Inventory) is a screening tool completed by the patient. Each item has four answers that show progressively more depressed emotions. The patient selects the statement that most closely matches his or her feelings. Page Ref: 922,927

32. a. Hallucinations are sensory perceptions; whereas delusions are false beliefs or thoughts. The combining form hallucin/o- means imagined perception. The suffix -ation means a process or being or having. Page Ref: 920

33. b. The combining form hebe/o- means youth. Page Ref: 920

34. c. Patients with major depression suffer from anhedonia. The prefix an- means without or not. The combining form hedon/o- means pleasure. The suffix -ia means a state of. Page Ref: 918

35. c. The Rorschach test contains cards with abstract shapes or inkblots on them. Patients are asked to describe what the shape of the inkblot represents to them. Page Ref: 922

36. d. Lithium (Lithobid) is an example of a drug used for mania. Page Ref: 927

37. d. Seasonal affective disorder is caused by hypersecretion of melatonin from the pineal gland in the brain. The treatment for SAD is exposure to sunlight or use of a light box for several hours each day. Page Ref: 919

38. b. Play therapy is used to treat social withdrawal, anxiety, depression, aggression, and ADHD. Page Ref: 925

39. a. Aversion therapy is a form of conditioning that creates an aversion to doing that behavior. It is used to treat drug and nicotine addiction and sexual identity issues. A- means away from, vers/o- means to turn. Page Ref: 924

40. d. Antianxiety drugs are used to treat anxiety and neurosis. This category is also known as anxiolytics and minor tranquilizers. Page Ref: 926

41. b. Bipolar disorder involves chronic mood swings between mania and depression. Patients with mania are hyperactive with limitless energy and euphoria. After an episode of mania, the patient swings abruptly into severe depression. Page Ref: 917

42. c. The combining form trich/o- means hair, the combining form till/o- means to pull out, and the suffix -mania means frenzy. Page Ref: 916

43. a. In malingering, patients are aware that they are lying and know exactly what they want. In Munchausen by proxy and Munchausen syndrome, patients are aware that they are lying, but are unaware that their motivation is the desire for assistance, attention, compassion, pity, and being excused from normal expectations of life. Page Ref: 913

44. d. Thanatophobia is a fear of death. A phobia is an intense, unreasonable fear of a specific thing or situation or even the thought of it. Page Ref: 909

45. a. The hypothalamus is located below the thalamus and forms the floor of the third ventricle. It controls emotions of pleasure, excitement, fear, anger, sexual arousal, and bodily responses to these emotions. Page Ref: 904

46. b. The combining form limb/o- means edge or border. The word limbic means pertaining to the edge or the border of the brain. The combining form amygdal/o- means almond shape. Page Ref: 903

47. d. Patients with anorexia nervosa are driven to decrease food intake to the point of starvation. They deny being too thin and they deny abnormal eating habits. Page Ref: 912

48. b. The person who practices sadism is known as a sadist. Sadism is named for Count Marquis de Sade, a French novelist in the late 1700s who experienced and wrote about these specific characteristics of sexual arousal. Page Ref: 915

49. b. The abbreviation ETOH means ethyl alcohol or liquor. Page Ref: 927

50. d. Thanatophobia is a fear of death. Page Ref: 909

51. d. The fornix is not part of the limbic system. Page Ref: 903

52. c. Injury to or degeneration of the hippocampi causes loss of all long-term memory. Page Ref: 904

53. a. When the level of dopamine decreases, schizophrenia may result. This chemical is also responsible for the "high" associated with narcotics and other substances. Page Ref: 920

54. d. An intense, unreasonable fear of a specific thing or situation is called a phobia. Page Ref: 908

55. c. Aversion therapy is a type of psychiatric therapy characterized by a patient thinking about a desired, but destructive behavior, coupled with a mild electrical shock or noxious smell. Page Ref: 924

56. a. Photophobia is NOT associated with a fear or mental disorder. Page Ref: 908

57. d. Cognitive disorders are characterized by a temporary or permanent impairment of thinking and memory. Page Ref: 910

58. c. Antianxiety drugs are also known as anxiolytic drugs. Page Ref: 926

59. d. Emotion (ee-MOH-shun), emot/o- moving, stirring up, -ion action; condition. Page Ref: 905

60. b. Dopamine (DOHP-ah-meen), Neurotransmitter in the brain. Page Ref: 906

61. d. Anxiety (ang-ZY-eh-tee), anxi/o- fear, worry, -ety condition, state. Page Ref: 908

62. c. Encopresis (EN-koh-PREE-sis), en- in, within, inward, copr/o- feces, stool, -esis condition of. Page Ref: 911

63. b. Tourette (TOOR-et), Tourette's syndrome was named by Georges Gilles de la Tourette (1857-1904), a French physician. This is an example of an eponym:a person from whom something takes its name. Page Ref: 911

64. b. Bulimia (byool-LIM-ee-ah), Bulimia is a combination of two Greek words meaning ox and hunge,r plus the suffix -ia (condition, state, thing). Page Ref: 912

65. a. Depersonalization (dee-PER-son-al-ih-ZAY-shun), Depersonalization is a combination of the prefix de- (reversal of, without), the word personal, and the suffix -ization, (the process of making, creating, or inserting). Page Ref: 912

66. d. PET scan, Radiologic procedure that shows areas of abnormal metabolism in the brain related to dementia and Alzheimer's disease. Page Ref: 922

67. c. Rorschach (ROHR-shahk), Rorschach test was named by Hermann Rorschach (1884-1922), a Swiss psychiatrist. Page Ref: 923

68. a. Hypnosis (hip-NOH-sis), hypn/o- sleep, -osis condition; abnormal, condition; process. Page Ref: 925

69. c. Phob/o- means fear, and -ia means condition. Page Ref: 908

70. a. Psychosis is characterized by a loss of touch with reality and disintegration of thought processes. Page Ref: 919

71. d. Hippocampus is a Latin word that means seahorse because of its enlongated structure. Page Ref: 904

72. a. Patient experiencing the manic phase of bipolar disorder show hyperactivity with limitless energy and extreme happiness (euphoria). Page Ref: 917

73. b. This area is most active when experiences are associated with the emotions of fear, anger, or rage. Page Ref: 904

74. d. Injury to the brain or changes in the levels of various neurotransmitters in the brain can produce abnormal emotional responses. Page Ref: 905

75. c. The hippocampus controls long-term memory and comparison with past and present events. Page Ref: 904-905

76. a. The frontal lobe of the brain is the site of all these things. Page Ref: 905

77. b. Hyperstimulation produces violent, aggressive behavior, and injury or degeneration of the amygdaloid bodies produces loss of emotions of fear and anger. Page Ref: 905

78. b. Dopamine is a neurotransmitter in the brain. Page Ref: 906

79. d. Posttraumatic stress disorder continues as a disabling reaction following an excessively traumatic event such as war, rape, etc. Page Ref: 901

80. a. Delirium is an acute condition that subsides as the toxic levels of drugs or alcohol decrease in the blood. Page Ref: 910

81. c. Narcissism is derived from the Greek myth about Narcissos, who fell in love with his own reflection. Page Ref: 921

82. b. No testing is done during a psychiatric interview. Interpreting inkblots is part of the Rorschach test. Page Ref: 923

83. d. De- means reversal of, toxic/o- means poison or toxin, and -ation means a process. Page Ref: 924

84. c. Ne/o- means new, log/o- means word, and -ism means process. Page Ref: 920

85. b. Glob/o- means comprehensive, and -al means pertaining to. Page Ref: 910

86. d. The pyromaniac's motive is the pleasure of seeing the fire and the people sent to fight the fire. Page Ref: 916

Short Answer

87. manic-depressive. Emotions swing between two poles:mania and depression. Page Ref: 917

88. dementia. De- means without, and ment/o- means mind. Page Ref: 910

89. transvestite. Trans- means across, vest/o- means to dress. Page Ref: 915

90. hypnosis (or hypnotherapy). Hypn/o- means sleep. Page Ref: 925

91. mind. Phren/o- and psych/o- are Greek, and ment/o- is Latin. Page Ref: 928

92. bulimia. Bulimia shows a characteristic pattern of binging and purging. Page Ref: 912

93. pedophile. Ped/o- = child and -phile = affinity for. Page Ref: 915

94. delirium. Delirium is disorientation and tremens refers to tremors of the hands. Page Ref: 910

95. schizophrenia. Hebe/o- means youth, and phren/o- means mind. Page Ref: 920

96. DSM-IV. DSM-IV stands for *Diagnostic and Statistical Manual of Mental Disorders,* 4th edition. Page Ref: 923

97. Affect. Affect is the outward display on the face of the inward emotions and thoughts. Page Ref: 905

98. Epinephrine. Epinephrine is a sympathetic nervous system neurotransmitter that prepares the body for "fight or flight." Page Ref: 905

99. limbic. Related structures in the brain that control emotion, mood, memory, motivation, and behavior are called the limbic system. Page Ref: 903

100. Mood. Mood is prevailing, predominant emotion affecting a person's state of mind. Page Ref: 905

101. amygdaloid. The amygdaloid bodies are almond-shaped areas within each temporal lobe that interpret facial expression and new social situations to identify danger. Page Ref: 904

102. fornix. The tract of nerves that joins all the parts of the limbic is called the fornix. Page Ref: 904

103. Obsessive-compulsive. Obsessive-compulsive disorder is a mental disorder characterized by constant, persistent, uncontrollable thoughts that occupy the mind, cause anxiety, and compel the patient to perform excessive, repetitive, meaningless activities. Page Ref: 908

104. panic. A panic disorder is a sudden attack of severe, overwhelming anxiety without an identifiable cause. Page Ref: 908

105. delirium. Acute confusion, disorientation and agitation due to toxic levels of drugs or alcohol in the brain is known as delirium. Page Ref: 910

106. Rorschach. The Rorschach test uses cards with abstract shapes on them to help determine a patient's mental state. Page Ref: 923

107. thalamus. Thalamus (THAL-ah-mus). The thalamus is a relay station in the brain. Page Ref: 904

108. hippocampus. Hippocampus (HIP-oh-KAM-pus), Hippocampus is a Latin word meaning seahorse. The structure of the hippocampus was thought to resemble the head and tail of a seahorse. Page Ref: 904

109. emotion. Emotion (ee-MOH-shun), emot/o- moving, stirring up, -ion action; condition. Page Ref: 905

110. affect. Affect (AF-fekt), Affect is derived from a Latin word meaning state of mind. Page Ref: 905

111. mood. Mood (MOOD). The prevailing emotion is known as the person's mood. Page Ref: 905

112. Neurotransmitters. Neurotransmitter (NYOOR-oh-trans-MIT-er), neur/o- nerve, trans- across, through, mitt/o- to send, -er person or thing that produces or does. Page Ref: 905

113. Epinephrine. Epinephrine (EP-ih-NEF-rin) is the nerve transmitter for the sympathetic nervous system. Page Ref: 905

114. Norepinephrine. Norepinephrine (NOR-ep-ih-NEF-rin) is the neurotransmitter for the parasympathetic nervous system. Page Ref: 905-906

115. Acrophobia. Acrophobia (AK-roh-FOH-bee-ah), acr/o- extremity; highest point, phob/o- fear, -ia condition, state, thing. Page Ref: 909

116. Claustrophobia. Claustrophobia (KLAW-stroh-FOH-bee-ah), claustr/o- enclosed space, phob/o- fear, -ia condition, state, thing. Page Ref: 909

117. Dementia. Dementia (dee-MEN-shee-ah), de- reversal of; without, ment/o- mind; chin, -ia condition, state, thing. Page Ref: 910

118. Malingering. Malingering (mah-LING-ger-ing). Malingering is derived from a French word meaning weak. Page Ref: 913

119. Hypochondriasis. Hypochondriasis (HY-poh-con-DRY-ah-sis), hypo- below; deficient, chondr/o- cartilage, -iasis state of; process of. Hypochondrium is a Greek word for the areas of the abdomen below the cartilage of the ribs. These areas contain the liver and spleen, which the ancient Greeks thought contained humors that caused moods. Page Ref: 914

120. antisocial. Antisocial (AN-tee-SOH-shal), anti- against, soci/o- human beings; community, -al pertaining to. Page Ref: 921

121. dopamine. Infatuation and the "high" produced from illegal drugs are both caused by increased levels of dopamine in the brain. Page Ref: 906

122. delusion. Delus/o- means false belief. Page Ref: 919

True/False

123. False. This condition is PTSD or posttraumatic stress disorder. PMDD is premenstrual dysphoric disorder. Page Ref: 910,919

124. False. This statement describes a conversion disorder, not psychosis. Page Ref: 914

125. False. This is the definition for kleptomania. Fetishism is obtaining sexual arousal from an object. Page Ref: 914,916

126. True. Xen/o- means foreign, phob/o- means fear, and -ia means condition. Page Ref: 909

127. False. Dependence is the need for the substance. Tolerance is the decreasing effect of the substance even with increasing amounts of it. Page Ref: 917

128. True. Psych/o- means mind, analy/o- means to separate, and -osis means process. Page Ref: 925

129. True. Treatment for this disorder is sunlight exposure because melatonin is produced in daylight hours. Page Ref: 919

130. True. The limbic system links the unconscious mind to the conscious mind. Page Ref: 903

131. True. ADHD is attention-deficit hyperactivity disorder. Page Ref: 911

132. False. The condition described is a fugue. Autism is an inability to form significant relationships and communicate with others. Page Ref: 911

133. False. Attention deficit hyperactivity disorder is characterized by distractability, short attention span, and inability to follow directions among other things. Page Ref: 911

134. True. Patients with autism have an inability to communicate or form significant relationships with others. Page Ref: 911

135. False. The inability to bond emotionally and form intimate relationships with others because of severe abuse or neglect of the patient's basic needs before age two is known as reactive attachment disorder. Page Ref: 911

136. False. Anorexia nervosa is an extreme eating disorder characterized by a decrease in food intake to the point of starvation. Page Ref: 912

137. True. Patients feel as if they are in a dream or watching a movie of themselves and things feel unreal and strange. Page Ref: 912

138. True. These patients are aware that they are lying and know exactly what they want. Page Ref: 913

139. True. In these types of patients diagnostic tests are negative but the patients have poor insight into their problem. Page Ref: 914

140. False. Bipolar disorder is characterized by chronic mood swings between mania and depression. Mania and euphoria may be considered to be the same. Page Ref: 917

141. True. Examples of common delusions are that other people are in love with the patient, one's spouse is unfaithful, or the patient has the powers of a god. Page Ref: 919

142. False. The PET scan is actually a radiologic procedure that shows areas of abnormal metabolism in the brain related to dementia and Alzheimer's disease. Page Ref: 922

143. False. This describes kleptomania. Klept/o- means to steal. Pyromania is deliberately setting fires. Page Ref: 916

144. False. The addict is aware but chooses to ignore this information and continue using the addicting substance. Page Ref: 917

145. True. The patient is in a sleeplike trance but still knows who they are and what is happening. Page Ref: 925

146. False. Triskaidekaphobia is a fear of the number 13. Page Ref: 908

Essay

147. The area located beneath the ribs (or the cartilage of the ribs) contains the liver and the spleen. Ancient Greeks thought that these organs were the source of humors that affected different moods or mental states. Page Ref: 914

148. mania and depression. Mania is a Greek word meaning frenzy. Depress/o- means to press down. Page Ref: 917-918

149. amygdaloid bodies. This area is most active when experiences are associated with the emotions of fear, anger, or rage. Page Ref: 904

150. hypothalamus. This area regulates sex drive and sexual behavior. Page Ref: 904

151. LSD, PCP. Hallucinogens are substances that produce hallucinations. Page Ref: 917

152. Posttraumatic stress disorder is a continued disabling reaction to an excessively traumatic situation or event, such as war, terrorist attacks, torture, rape, kidnapping, natural disasters, explosions, or fires. The patient feels helpless, has a numbed emotional response with disinterest in people and current events, and relives the trauma of the event over and over. Page Ref: 910

153. Amnesia is partial or total loss of long-term memory due to trauma or disease of the hippocampus. The patient is said to be amnestic. In retrograde amnesia, no events before the onset of the amnesia can be recalled. In anterograde amnesia, no events after the onset of the amnesia can be recalled. In global amnesia, all memories are lost. Page Ref: 910

154. Dementia is a gradual but progressive deterioration of cognitive function due to old age or a neurological disease process. Alzheimer's disease is the most common type of dementia. There is a gradual decline in mental abilities, with forgetfulness, inability to learn new things, inability to perform daily activities, and difficulty making decisions. Dementia can also include personality changes, anxiety, irritability, poor judgment, impulsiveness, hostility, combativeness, depression, and delusions. Page Ref: 910

155. Hypochondriasis is a mental disorder characterized by preoccupation with and misinterpretation of minor bodily sensations and fear that these indicate disease. Patients are convinced they have serious illness and make frequent trips to the doctor despite medical evidence and reassurance to the contrary. Page Ref: 914

156. The Beck Depression Inventory is a self-reported screening tool that assesses the degree of depression. The patient responds to several questions that are designed to show progressively more depressed emotions. The patient selects the statement that most closely resembles their own feelings. The responses are rated by the patient from 0 to 3, with 3 being the most sad. Page Ref: 922

CHAPTER 18

Multiple Choice

1. a. The gene p53 repairs DNA mutations and prevents the cell from dividing until damage can be repaired. If it cannot, the cell destroys it-

self (apoptosis) at the direction of p53. Page Ref: 947

2. b. Philadelphia chromosome is an abnormal chromosome with a translocation from chromosome 9 to 11. Page Ref: 964

3. d. Brachytherapy involves placement of radioactive elements close to the site of the cancer. Brach/y- = short; -therapy = treatment. Page Ref: 972

4. c. Many cancers spread through the lymphatic system. This biopsy would remove the sentinel lymph node, the one that would most likely be the first to receive cancerous cells spreading from the breast. Page Ref: 970

5. c. These catheters have access to circulation via the superior vena cava, thus providing a way to deliver chemotherapy to the entire body. Page Ref: 971

6. a. Debulking removes part of the tumor to make it smaller and therefore more receptive to chemotherapy or radiotherapy. Page Ref: 970

7. d. Tamoxifen produces a hormonal environment that does not promote the growth of certain tumors. Page Ref: 974

8. c. Retin/o- means retina and blast/o- means immature or embryonic. This tumor arises from the retina of the eye. Page Ref: 963

9. b. Hodgkin's lymphoma was named by Thomas Hodgkin, an English physician. Page Ref: 962

10. a. Aden/o- means gland. Adenocarcinomas arise from the epithelial cells that line the ducts of an endocrine gland like the pancreas whereas sarcomas arise from connective tissue. Page Ref: 957

11. b. Intra- = within; vesic/o- = bladder; -al = pertaining to. Page Ref: 969

12. b. This is a cancer of melanocytes or pigment cells of the skin. Page Ref: 958

13. a. Exfoliation means to shed. The Pap smear involves examination of cells that are shed from the cervix, lungs, or stomach. Page Ref: 963

14. d. The prostate-specific antigen is normally found in small amounts in the blood of a male. Elevated levels are seen in prostate cancer. Page Ref: 965

15. b. T = size of the tumor (T1-4); N = regional lymph nodes affected (N 1- 4); M = metastasis (M 0-1). Page Ref: 969

16. d. Cry/o- = cold; -surgery = an operative process. Page Ref: 968

17. c. This method uses the cerebrospinal fluid as a means to deliver chemotherapy to not only the spinal cord but also the brain. Page Ref: 968

18. b. Compazine is an antiemetic (against vomiting) drug. Page Ref: 974

19. a. PICC stands for peripherally inserted central catheter. Page Ref: 968

20. d. Ana- = excessive; plas/o- = growth. Page Ref: 955

21. b. This is a cancer of the deepest layer or base layer of the skin. Page Ref: 957

22. c. Tests for estrogen or progesterone receptors are done on cancer cells from the breast. Page Ref: 964

23. a. AFP is a hormone found in fetuses. When it is present in an adult, it can indicate liver, testicular, or ovarian cancer. Page Ref: 955

24. d. Lymph nodes represent the most likely site of spread or metastasis of certain tumors. Page Ref: 972

25. c. A benign tumor is encapsulated but a cancerous tumor is not. Page Ref: 950

26. d. A remission occurs after the successful treatment of cancer. Page Ref: 956

27. d. Sarcomas affect the cartilage, bone, tendon, ligament, aponeurosis, fascia, fat, and subcutaneous tissue. They grow rapidly and usually metastasize via the circulatory system. Page Ref: 959

28. a. The TNM staging system is used to describe the size of the tumor and whether the tumor has spread to lymph nodes and other sites. T = size of the primary tumor (T1 through T4) N = number of regional lymph nodes affected (N1 through N4) M = presence or absence of metastasis to other sites in the body (M0 or M1). Page Ref: 969

29. d. The combining form interstit/o- means spaces within tissue; the suffix -al means pertaining to. Page Ref: 974

30. b. The combining form stere/o- means three dimensions; the combining form tact/o- means touch; the suffix -ic means pertaining to. Page Ref: 970

31. a. A tumor marker is a blood test that detects antigens on the surface of cancer cells. Tumor markers are used to evaluate the extent of cancer and the effectiveness of the treatment being given. Page Ref: 965

32. d. Exenteration is used to treat widely metastatic cancer in the abdominoplevic cavity. Page Ref: 970

33. a. The combining form cry/o- means cold; the combining form surg/o- means operative procedure; the suffix -ery means process of. Page Ref: 968

34. d. A plasma cell is a B lymphocyte that has been activated by a pathogen so it secretes antibodies. Multiple myeloma is a malignant tumor of a plasma cell. Page Ref: 962

35. a. Areas of increased uptake during a scintigraphy are abnormal and can be infection, cancer, or metastasis. Page Ref: 967

36. a. Examples of environmental substances (called carcinogens) include radiation, chemi-

cals, fumes, foreign particles, some chemotherapy drugs, and some hormone drugs. Page Ref: 948

37. c. Ewing's sarcoma was named by James Ewing, an American pathologist. Page Ref: 959

38. d. The abbreviation PICC means peripherally inserted central catheter. The combining form peripher/o- means outer aspects; the suffix -al means pertaining to. Page Ref: 976

39. d. The prefix ana- means apart from or excessive; the combining form plas/o- means growth or formation; the suffix -ia means condition, state, or thing. Page Ref: 955

40. a. During electrosurgery, the electrical current passes through the electrode and evaporates the intracellular contents of the cancerous cell. Page Ref: 968

41. c. Normal cells appear well differentiated and characteristic of that tissue type. Poorly differentiated or undifferentiated cells lack evidence of specialization and appear immature and embryonic. The greater the number of undifferentiated cells, the poorer the prognosis. Page Ref: 968

42. a. The prefix meta- means after, subsequent to, transition, or change; the suffix -stasis means condition of standing still or staying in one place. Page Ref: 950

43. d. Basal cell carcinoma is cancer of the deepest layer of the epidermis of the skin. Page Ref: 957

44. c. Oste/o- means bone. Osteosarcoma is also known as osteogenic sarcoma. Page Ref: 961

45. b. CEA stands for carcinoembryonic antigen. The higher the level of CEA, the more advanced the cancer is. Page Ref: 965

46. a. In addition to the Bethesda system, the CIN classification is used to detect cervical cancer. Page Ref: 969

47. b. Intra- means within, and visic/o- means bladder. Page Ref: 969

48. d. Radioresistant tumors are those are not adversely affected by radiation therapy; whereas radiosensitive tumors are those that are readily destroyed by radiation therapy. Page Ref: 973

49. c. Programmed cell death rate is known as apoptosis. This helps keeps the normal cell from mutating. Page Ref: 947

50. a. While heredity may be a factor in whether or not a person inherits an oncogene from a parent, it is not a direct cause of cancer and therefore not a carcinogen. Page Ref: 948

51. b. This process is known as angiogenesis. In angiogenesis, the tumor grows rapidly but often has a central core of tissue that is necrotic because the blood supply was inadequate. Page Ref: 950

52. d. During the process of metastasis, cancer cells break off and move to other sites within the body. Even though the cells move to other sites within the body, they maintain the tissue characteristics of the original site. Page Ref: 950

53. b. The process of *differentiation* allows tissues and organs to assume their intended shape and purpose. Page Ref: 949

54. b. Dysplasia is a result of chronic irritation and inflammation. Page Ref: 955

55. a. The correct answer is cholangiocarcinoma. The word part cholangi/o stands for bile duct, which is a part of the gallbladder. Page Ref: 958

56. d. The high alpha fetoprotein level indicates that the cancer may be advanced. AFP can also be elevated in noncancerous conditions like cirrhosis and hepatitis. Page Ref: 965

57. a. A core needle biopsy is inserted into the tumor to obtain several long pieces (or cores) of tissue. Page Ref: 969

58. c. Lysosomes (LY-soh-sohm), lys/o- break down or dissolve, -some a body. Add words to make a correct and complete definition of lysosome: a body [that contains enzymes that] break down or dissolve [a bacterium or virus]. Page Ref: 946

59. d. Cytoplasm (SY-toh-plazm), cyt/o- cell, -plasm growth; formed substance. The cytoplasm is the substance in which cell organelles float. Page Ref: 946

60. b. Nucleus (NYOO-klee-us), Nuclei (NYOO-klee-eye), Nucleus is a Latin singular masculine noun meaning kernel. Form the plural by changing -us to -i. Page Ref: 947

61. a. The p53 gene recognizes DNA damage and activates proteins to repair the damage. While the DNA is being repaired, the p53 gene inhibits mitosis to decrease the chance of producing more defective cells. Page Ref: 947

62. b. See Figure 18-3. Page Ref: 948-949

63. b. Metastasize (meh-TAS-tah-size), meta- after, subsequent to; transition; change, stas/o- standing still; staying in one place, -ize affecting in a particular way. Page Ref: 950

64. c. Ca is a brief form for carcinoma or cancer. Page Ref: 976

65. b. PICC; peripherally inserted central catheter. Page Ref: 976

66. a. Combining chemotherapy drugs increases their effectiveness against cancerous cells while minimizing the side effects caused by large doses of just one drug. Page Ref: 975

67. a. Radiation treatment uses one of several types of radiation to disrupt the atoms in the DNA in cancer cells to keep them from dividing. Page Ref: 973

68. c. Ana- means apart from, plas/o- means formation, and -ia means condition. Page Ref: 955

69. d. Carcinomatosis is formed from the plural of carcinoma, which is carcinomata, meaning

more than one cancerous tumor site. Page Ref: 955

70. d. Terat/o- means bizarre form and -oma means tumor or mass. Page Ref: 963

71. b. Bone marrow aspiration is used to diagnose leukemia or lymphoma. Bone marrow transplantation is used to treat leukemia or lymphoma. Page Ref: 963

72. a. The Pap smear is not a blood test. It uses exfoliative cytology to detect early cervical cancer. Page Ref: 963, 965

73. a. Fractionation divides the total dose of external beam radiation to be given into smaller doses that can be given daily. Page Ref: 972

74. d. Adjuv/o- means giving help or assistance, and -ant means pertaining to. Page Ref: 975

75. c. CTR stands for certified tumor registrar. Page Ref: 976

76. b. Lys/o- means break down or dissolve, and -some means a body. Page Ref: 946

77. c. A cell has a cell membrane. A bacterium has a cell wall. Page Ref: 945

Short Answer

78. Oncology. Onc/o- = tumor; -logy = study of. Page Ref: 944

79. metastasis. Meta- = change; -stasis = staying in one place. Page Ref: 950

80. Carcinomatosis. Carcin/o- means cancer. Page Ref: 955

81. liposarcoma. Lip/o- = fat; sarc/o- = connective tissue; -oma = tumor. A lipoma is a benign tumor of fatty tissue. Page Ref: 960

82. Mammography. Mamm/o-= breast; -graphy = process of recording. Page Ref: 966

83. excision. Excis/o- means to cut out. Page Ref: 970

84. biopsy. Bi/o- means living tissue, and -opsy means process of viewing. Page Ref: 969

85. brain. Astr/o- = star; cyt/o- = cell; -oma = tumor. Astrocytes are cells that support neurons in the brain. Page Ref: 959

86. Lymphangiography. Lymph/o- = lymph; angi/o- = vessel; -graphy = process of recording. Page Ref: 966

87. radical. Radic/o- means all parts including the root. Page Ref: 972

88. cervical. The human papillomavirus causes genital warts and chronic inflammation that can lead to cervical cancer in women. Page Ref: 948

89. tumor necrosis. Lymph nodes release a substance called tumor necrosis factor which causes cancer cells to become necrotic and die. Page Ref: 949

90. Anaplasia. Anaplasia is a process by which cells that were once mature and differentiated become undifferentiated and immature in appearance and behavior. Page Ref: 955

91. relapse. A relapse is the return of symptoms or signs of cancer after a period of improvement or even remission. Page Ref: 956

92. Bronchogenic. Bronchogenic carcinoma is cancer of the mucous membranes lining the bronchi of the lungs. Page Ref: 958

93. hepatoma. Hepatocellular carcinoma is cancer of the liver and is also known as a hepatoma. Page Ref: 958

94. lymphoma. Hodgkin's disease is a type of lymphoma. Page Ref: 962

95. Exfoliative. Exfoliative cytology is a cytology test that examines cells from secretions or from cells scraped or washed from a body surface. Page Ref: 963

96. hormone. A tumor with increased numbers of estrogen receptors or progesterone receptors is considered to be hormone dependent. Page Ref: 964

97. cell. Cell (sell), Cell is derived from a Latin word meaning a storeroom or chamber. Page Ref: 945

98. cytoplasm. Cytoplasm (SY-toh-plazm), cyt/o- cell, -plasm growth; formed substance. Page Ref: 945

99. RNA [or Ribonucleic Acid]. Ribonucleic acid (RY-boh-nyoo-KLEE-ik AS-id). Page Ref: 946

100. Mitosis. Mitosis (my-TOH-ss), mit/o- thread like structure, -osis condition; abnormal condition; process. Add words to make a correct and complete definition of mitosis: a condition of cell division during which the chromosomes align along thread-like structures In the nucleus. Page Ref: 947

101. Angiogenesis. Angi/o- blood vessel; lymphatic vessel; gen/o- arising from; produced by. Page Ref: 951

102. Dysplasia. Dysplasia (dis-PLAY-zee-ah) (dis-PLAY-zha), dys- painful, difficult, abnormal, plas/o- growth, formation, -ia condition, state, thing. Page Ref: 955

103. Neoplasm. Neoplasm (NEE-oh-plazm), ne/o- new, -plasm growth; formed substance. Page Ref: 956

104. Basal. Basal (BAY-sal), bas/o- base of a structure, al pertaining to. Page Ref: 957

105. Angiosarcoma. Angiosarcoma (AN-je-oh-sar-koh-mah), angi/o- blood vessel; lymphatic vessel, sarc/o- connective tissue, -oma tumor, mass. Page Ref: 959

106. Kaposi's. Kaposi (KAH-poh-see). Kaposi's sarcoma was named by Moritz Kaposi Khan (1837-1902), an Austrian dermatologist. See Figure 18-8. Page Ref: 960

107. Osteosarcoma. Osteosarcoma (AWS-tee-oh-sar-KOH-mah), also known as osteogenic sarcoma, oste/o- bone, sarc/o- connective tissue, -oma tumor, mass. Page Ref: 961

108. leukemia. Leukemia (loo-KEE-mee-ah), leuk/o- white, -emia condition of the blood; substance in the blood. Page Ref: 961

109. nephroblastoma. Nephroblastoma (NEF-roh-blas-TOH-mah), nephr/o- kidney; nephron, blast/o- immature; embryonic, -oma tumor, mass. Page Ref: 963

110. Ultrasonography. Ultrasonography (UL-trah-soh-NAWG-rah-fee), ultra- beyond, higher, son/o- sound, -graphy process of recording. Page Ref: 967

111. change in bowel or bladder habits. A change in bowel or bladder habits can be a sign of cancer in the lower gastrointestinal tract. Page Ref: 956

112. orange. The dimpling of the skin resembles the dimpling on the skin of an orange. Peau d' orange means peel of the orange. Page Ref: 957

113. lymphangiography. Lymph/o- means lymph or lymphatic system, angi/o- means lymphatic vessel, and -graphy means process of recording. Page Ref: 966

114. ovary. FIGO is used to stage ovarian cancer. Page Ref: 969

115. prostate gland. The Gleason Score is used to stage prostate cancer. Page Ref: 969

116. protocol. A protocol tells which chemotherapy drugs should be given and in what dosages. Page Ref: 975

117. oncology. Onc/o- means tumor or mass, and -logy means the study of. Page Ref: 944

True/False

118. True. A Pap smear can be perfromed to detect abnormal cells that could become cervical cancer. Page Ref: 948

119. False. It is angiogenesis. Angi/o- means blood vessel; gen/o- means arising from; -esis means condition. Page Ref: 950

120. False. This is the description for an in situ malignancy. Dysplasia is not yet a malignancy. Page Ref: 955

121. False. This is relapse. A remission is a period of no symptoms or signs of cancer. Page Ref: 956

122. False. It is a chondrosarcoma. Sarcomas occur in connective tissue such as cartilage. Page Ref: 959

123. True. This is a cancer of skeletal or voluntary muscle. The biceps muscle is skeletal muscle. Page Ref: 961

124. False. Chori/o- = fetal membrane; carcin/o- = cancer; -oma = tumor. Choriocarcinoma arises from the chorion, the fetal membrane that later becomes the placenta. Page Ref: 962

125. False. In situ means the tumor is still contained in the spot where the cancer started. Page Ref: 956

126. False. This is Kaposi's sarcoma. Ewing's sarcoma is cancer of the growth plate at the end of an arm or leg bone. Page Ref: 959

127. False. The process described above is an excisional biopsy. Page Ref: 969

128. True. The procedure helps the physician pinpoint the location of the mass with great accuracy. Page Ref: 970

129. False. The implantable wafer is implanted in an area where a tumor has already been removed. Page Ref: 971

130. True. This helps make the patient more comfortable or leaves a smaller tumor that can be more successfully treated with chemotherapy or radiation therapy. Page Ref: 970

131. True. This is a very invasive surgery and is used to treat widely metastatic cancer in the abdominopelvic cavity. Page Ref: 970

132. True. These drugs work by substituting an alkyl group for a hydrogen molecule in the DNA. Page Ref: 974

133. False. Antiemetic drugs treat nausea and vomiting, but they are not chemotherapy drugs. They treat the side effects of chemotherapy. Page Ref: 974

134. True. It is within the cell that all cancerous aberrations first begin. Page Ref: 945

135. False. Suppressor genes *inhibit* mitosis and keep each cell from dividing excessively. Page Ref: 947

136. True. In situ tumors have a high cure rate because they have not metastasized. Page Ref: 956

137. False. Suppressor genes suppress mitosis and keep cells from dividing excessively. Page Ref: 947

138. False. A neoplasm is any new growth or tumor, benign or malignant. Page Ref: 956

139. True. This acronym is a memory aid created by the American Cancer Society. Page Ref: 956

140. False. Aden/o- means gland. An adenocarcinoma forms from the epithelial cells that line the ducts of glands found in the breast, gallbladder, pancreas, prostate, or salivary glands. Page Ref: 957

141. False. Chemotherapy antibiotics are a special class of antibiotic drugs that affect normal and cancerous human cells, not bacteria. Page Ref: 974

Essay

142. 1. Lymphocytes known as natural killers (NK) will destroy the cancer cell.

    2. A cancer cell will enter a lymph node where it is destroyed by macrophages.

    3. Lymph nodes release tumor necrosis factor that destroys a cancer cell. Page Ref: 949

143. This test done on the cancer cells detects a gene that points to an aggressive type of breast, ovary, or bladder cancer. If the tumor is Her 2/neu positive, the tumor may be resistant to certain drug therapies. Page Ref: 964

144. Adenocarcinoma is cancer of the epithelial cells that line the ducts of glands of the breast, gallbladder, and pancreas, prostate gland, or salivary gland. The word part aden/o- means gland. Carcinoma is cancer of the epithelial cells of the skin and mucous membranes of various organs. Page Ref: 957

145. Sarcoma is cancer of connective tissues such as cartilage, bone, tendon, ligament, aponeurosis, fascia, fat, or subcutaneous tissue; muscles; or nerves. Sarcomas grow rapidly and most often show anaplasia of their cells. Sarcomas usually metastasize via the circulatory system. Page Ref: 959

146. A blood smear is a manual blood test done to examine the characteristics of erythrocytes and leukocytes under the microscope when an abnormal automated complete blood count (CBC) suggests that the patient has leukemia. Page Ref: 965

147. Grading is a medical procedure that classifies how well differentiated the cells appear under the microscope. Normal cells appear well-differentiated and characteristic of the tissue type from where they originate. Poorly differentiated cells lack evidence of specialization and appear immature and embryonic. The greater the number of undifferentiated cells, the poorer the prognosis. Page Ref: 968

148. The TNM system is a classification system for cancer. It is used to describe the size of tumor and whether the tumor has spread to lymph nodes and other sites. T stands for tumor size, N stands for node-the number of regional lymph nodes affected, and M stands for the presence or absence of metastases to other sites in the body. Page Ref: 969

CHAPTER 19

Multiple Choice

1. d. The examination would be called a barium enema. Page Ref: 998

2. c. Xer/o- = dry; mamm/o- breast; -gram = picture. Xeromammography uses a special plate processed with dry chemicals with the image printed on paper. Page Ref: 1001

3. b. MRI uses a magnetic field to align protons. High-frequency radiowaves are sent through the body. The protons absorb the radiowaves and send signals converted to images. Page Ref: 1003

4. d. In positron emission tomography, a positron is a positively charged particle used to produce images. Page Ref: 1011

5. a. AP means anteroposterior. Page Ref: 995

6. c. During an MRI the patient's body is inserted into a hollow tube. If a person is claustrophobic, or has the fear of being in closed spaces, the modified MRI scanner, which is open on some sides rather than being totally enclosed, is used. Page Ref: 1003

7. a. The x-ray beams enter the patient's upper back and exit through the anterior chest to enter the x-ray plate. Page Ref: 995

8. b. Although a crown and a joint prosthesis have metal parts, they may cause artifacts on the image but will not become dislodged. Page Ref: 1004

9. c. Trac/o- = visible path; -er = thing that performs. Page Ref: 1007

10. d. These substances are used in MUGA scans and scintigraphy. Radioactive substances emit positrons. Page Ref: 1007,1011

11. c. This tomography uses a beam of electrons to do a full body scan from shoulders to upper legs. These scans are marketed to the public and do not need to be ordered by a physician. Page Ref: 1004

12. a. KUB stands for kidneys, ureters, and bladder. Page Ref: 995,1020

13. b. It produces a two-dimensional image in various shades of gray. Page Ref: 1005

14. c. Dos/i- means dose and -meter means instrument used to measure. As a protection, all health care professionals who work in radiology or nuclear medicine wear a clear, unexposed piece of x-ray film that changes with increased exposure to radiation. Page Ref: 996

15. d. The Doppler effect in physics relates to the change in the pitch of sound depending where the observer is hearing the sound. This principle was used to develop Doppler ultrasonography. Page Ref: 1006

16. a. Both are inhaled gases used to detect lung cancer. Page Ref: 1008-1009

17. c. The x-ray is called a scout, or preliminary film. Page Ref: 996

18. c. Cho/o- = bile or gall; angi/o- = vessel; -graphy = process of recording. Page Ref: 998

19. d. The MUGA detects how well the heart wall moves during contraction and how much blood it can eject from the ventricle. Page Ref: 1009

20. b. Later/o- = side; -al = pertaining to. Decubitus = lying down. Page Ref: 995

21. b. Pyel/o- means renal pelvis, and -graphy means process of recording. Page Ref: 999

22. d. This is a test for bone density to see if demineralization from osteoporosis has occurred. Page Ref: 1001

23. c. An abdominal aneurysm occurs in the aorta, the body part visualized on an aortogram. Page Ref: 997

24. a. Air (in a body cavity or the lungs) has a low density, and x-rays pass through it, creating a nearly black area on the x-ray plate. Page Ref: 994

25. b. AP stands for anteroposterior. The x-ray beam first enters the anterior chest. This position is used for portable chest x-rays taken at the patient's bedside. Page Ref: 995

26. b. A scout film provides an initial view of an area before the patient receives the contrast dye. Page Ref: 996

27. a. Xeromammography uses a special plate processed with dry chemicals, and its image is printed on paper. Page Ref: 1001

28. c. The patient lies on a narrow bed inside the CT scanner. CT stands for computed tomography. Page Ref: 1001

29. a. MRI stands for magnetic resonance imaging. Page Ref: 1003

30. c. EBT stands for electron beam tomography. Page Ref: 1004

31. a. Another name for sonography is ultrasonography. Page Ref: 1005

32. c. TEE stands for transesophageal echocardiography. Page Ref: 1005

33. b. Tests that use x-rays expose the patient to radiation, but ultrasonography uses sound waves. Page Ref: 1005

34. a. Every radioactive substance is in a constant state of decay (changing from being unstable to being stable), as measured by the half-life. Page Ref: 1007

35. c. Radiopharmaceuticals are called tracers because their presence in a particular area of the body can be traced by the gamma rays they produce. Page Ref: 1007

36. b. The thyroid gland takes up iodine to make thyroid hormones. When it takes up iodine-123, the radioactivity produces an image of the thyroid gland. Page Ref: 1010

37. d. Only krypton-81m and xenon-133 are in the form of gases that can be inhaled. Page Ref: 1008

38. a. Areas of increased uptake are called hot spots and areas of decreased uptake are called cold spots. Page Ref: 1010

39. c. Gadolinium is a metallic element that responds to a magnetic field. Page Ref: 1003

40. b. A lead apron is also used to shield parts of the patient's body that are not being x-rayed. Page Ref: 996

41. c. The image is known as a myelogram. Page Ref: 999

42. a. The abbreviation rem stands for roentgen-equivalent man. Page Ref: 996

43. a. This nuclear medicine procedure uses scintigraphy and the inhaled radiopharmaceutical to create an image of the lungs. Page Ref: 1010

44. a. A KUB is an x-ray of the kidneys, ureters, and the bladder. Page Ref: 995

45. c. Sonography is a radiologic procedure that uses sound waves. Page Ref: 1005

46. a. Arthrography is a radiologic study that uses contrast dye to examine a joint. In this study, contrast dye is injected directly into the joint. Page Ref: 998

47. d. MRI is a test that uses magnetic fields to examine the body. MRI stands for magnetic resonance imaging. Page Ref: 1003

48. a. Hearing aids, insulin pumps,and earrings contain are metal and should not be used in an MRI study. Page Ref: 1004

49. b. Three-dimensional ultrasonography produces images that are colorized in shades of brown. Page Ref: 1005

50. d. The body uses iodine to produce thyroid hormones. Radioactive iodine-123 concentrates in the thyroid gland where it can be easily measured by a nuclear medicine camera. Page Ref: 1008

51. b. The word that contains a word part that means point of light is scintigraphy. Page Ref: 1009

52. d. The incorrect statement is that the x-ray emitter moves in a triangle around the patient. The x-ray emitter in CAT scans actually moves in a circle around the patient. Page Ref: 1001

53. b. Gastrointestinal (GAS-troh-in-TES-tin-al), gastr/o- stomach, intestin/o- intestine, -al pertaining to. Page Ref: 1000

54. b. Computerized axial tomography (CAT), also known as computerized tomography (CT) Tomography (toh-MAWG-rah-fee), tom/o- a cut, slice, or layer, -graphy process of recording. Page Ref: 1001

55. d. Magnetic (mag-NET-ik), magnet/o- magnet, -ic pertaining to. Magnetic resonance imaging uses a magnetic field. Page Ref: 1003

56. b. Barium (BAIR-ee-um), an insoluble metallic element found in the earth. A liquid suspension of barium particles creates a white and chalky contrast dye that is radiopaque. Page Ref: 1019

57. a. Permanent metal dental work, such as a crown, will not detach, although it may cause artifacts on the MRI image. Page Ref: 1004

58. a. Half-life measures how long substances stay radioactive. Page Ref: 1007

59. a. Electron beam tomography (EBT) uses a beam of electrons to create an image. This is known as a full body scan, although only the

area from the shoulders to the upper legs is actually scanned. Page Ref: 1004

60. a. Spiral (SPY-ral), spir/o- a coil, -al pertaining to. Helical (HEL-ih-kal), helic/o- a coil, -al pertaining to. Spir/o- is derived from a Latin word meaning a coil and helic/o- is derived from a Greek word meaning a coil. Page Ref: 1002

61. d. Myelography (MY-eh-LOG-rah-fee), myel/o- bone marrow; spinal, cord; myelin, -graphy process of recording. Page Ref: 999

62. c. Lateral (LAT-er-al), later/o- side, -al pertaining to. Page Ref: 995

63. a. Magnetic resonance imaging uses a strong magnetic field inside the scanner to align protons in the atoms of the patient's body. Page Ref: 1003

64. c. PET stands for positron emission tomography. Page Ref: 1011

65. d. It is a screening test, but it does not need to be ordered by a physician. Page Ref: 1004

66. d. Cin/e- means movement. Fluoroscopy involves a monitor that shows a continuously changing image of the movement of the internal organs. However, only a few select individual x-rays are taken to preserve the images. With cineradiography, the entire fluoroscopy is preserved. Page Ref: 1000

67. d. The transducer is held against the skin over the organ or structure to be visualized. The probe is placed inside a body cavity. Page Ref: 1005

68. a. The monoclonal antibodies combine with the cancerous cells and the radiopharmaceutical emits radioactivity that shows up on a scan. Page Ref: 1019

69. d. A chest x-ray (CXR) is the most common radiologic procedure. Page Ref: 1020

70. d. An intravenous pyelography (IVP) uses contrast dye to create an image of the urinary tract, beginning with the pelves of the kidneys. Page Ref: 1020

71. b. An upper gastrointestinal (UGI) series uses barium to outline the upper gastrointestinal tract, including the esophagus, stomach, and small intestine. Page Ref: 1000, 1020

72. b. Nuclear medicine uses radioactive substances. Page Ref: 1007

73. c. Fluoroscopy uses a fluorescent screen that transforms x-rays into wavelengths of light that can be displayed on a TV monitor. Page Ref: 1000

74. d. Increased uptake produces an area of the image that shows more vividly on the image. Page Ref: 1009

75. c. Marie Curie discovered radium in 1898 while working with uranium. Page Ref: 1010

76. d. A PET scan can detect abnormal brain activity caused by many diseases. Page Ref: 1015

Short Answer

77. radioactive. Radioactive substances produce gamma rays or positrons and are used for nuclear medicine imaging. Page Ref: 1007

78. sonogram. Son/o- = sound; -gram = picture. Page Ref: 1005

79. lead apron. Lead will not allow x-rays to pass through it. Page Ref: 996

80. lung. This scan detects areas of "cold spots" that could indicate poor air flow in the lungs. Page Ref: 1010

81. CXR. The chest x-ray (CXR) is the most common radiologic procedure. Page Ref: 1020

82. Rems. Rem stands for Roentgen-equivalent man. Page Ref: 1020

83. fluoroscopy. Fluoroscopy follows the movement of internal organs in real time. Page Ref: 1000

84. MRI. MRI stands for magnetic resonance imaging. Page Ref: 1003

85. joint. Arthr/o- = joint; -graphy = process of recording. Page Ref: 998

86. Barium. Barium is a radiopaque contrast medium made of small, chalky particles suspended in a liquid and used for radiologic procedures of the digestive tract. It is normally swallowed or instilled in the rectum and colon. Page Ref: 998, 1000

87. decubitus. The decubitus position is a lying-down or on the back position used for radiologic imaging. Page Ref: 995

88. trans-. In the phrase transesophageal echocardiography, the word part that means across is trans-. Page Ref: 1005

89. dosimeter. A dosimeter measures the cumulative exposure of a health care worker to radiation. Page Ref: 996

90. portable. A portable film is a radiograph taken at the patient's bedside or in the emergency department when the patient cannot be transported to the radiology department. Page Ref: 996

91. cholangiography. An imaging study that uses injected contrast dye to visualize the gallbladder is called cholangiography. Page Ref: 998

92. Fluoroscopy. Fluoroscopy uses a continuous x-ray beam to capture motion of the internal organs as it occurs. Page Ref: 1000

93. radiolucent. Radiolucent (RAY-dee-oh-LOO-sent), radi/o- radius (forearm bone); x-rays; radiation, luc/o- clear and shining, -ent pertaining to. Page Ref: 994

94. radiopaque. Radiopaque (RAY-dee-oh-PAYK), Radiopaque is a combination of the combining form radi/o- and the word opaque (not transparent). Page Ref: 994

95. posteroanterior. Posteroanterior (POHS-ter-oh-an-TEER-ee-or), poster/o- back part, anter/o- before; front part, -ior pertaining to. Page Ref: 995

96. Dosimetry. Dosimetry (doh-SIM-eh-tree), dos/i- dose, -metry process of measuring. Page Ref: 996

97. arteriography. Arteriography (ar-TEER-ee-AWG-rah-fee), arteri/o- artery, -graphy process of recording. Page Ref: 997

98. cholangiography. Cholangiography (KOH-lan-jee-AWG-rah-fee), chol/o- bile, gall, angi/o- blood vessel; lymphatic vessel, -graphy process of recording. Page Ref: 998

99. Mammography. Mammography (mah-MAWG-rah-fee), mamm/o- breast, -graphy process of recording. Page Ref: 1001

100. densitometry. Densitometry (DEN-sih-TAWM-eh-tree), densit/o- density, -metry process of measuring. Page Ref: 1001

101. Echocardiography. Echocardiography (EK-oh-KAR-dee-AWG-rah-fee), ech/o- echo (sound wave), cardi/o- heart, -graphy process of recording. Page Ref: 1005

102. Nuclear. Nuclear (NYOO-klee-er), nucle/o- nucleus, -ar pertaining to. Page Ref: 1007

103. Radiopharmaceuticals. Radiopharmaceutical (RAY-dee-oh-FAR-mah-SOO-tik-al), radi/o- radius (forearm bone); x-rays; radiation, pharmaceutic/o- medicine, drug, -al pertaining to. Page Ref: 1007

104. positron. Positron (PAWZ-ih-trawn), Positron is a shortened form of positive plus a shortened form of electron. Page Ref: 1011

105. radiation. Radiation (RAY-dee-AA-shun), radi/o- radius (forearm bone); x-rays; radiation, -ation a process; being or having. Some word parts have more than one definition. The best definition of radiation is being or having x-rays. Page Ref: 993

106. roentgenogram; radiograph. Roentgenogram, radiograph. Roentgenogram (RENT-gen-oh-gram), roentgen/o- x-ray; radiation, -gram a record or picture. Roentgen is the unit of measurement for x-rays or gamma rays. It was named for Wilhelm Roentgen. Radiograph (RAY-dee-oh-graf), radi/o- radius (forearm bone); x-rays; radiation, graph instrument used to record. As commonly used in medicine, the word radiograph is a misnomer because it refers to the x-ray image, which does not follow the traditional meaning of the suffix-graph (instrument used to record). Page Ref: 993

107. projections. Projection (proh-JEK-shun), project/o- throw forward, -ion action; condition. Page Ref: 994

108. cyclotron. Cycl/o- means circle, and -tron means instrument. A magnetic field keeps particles going in a circle to near the speed of light. Page Ref: 1011

109. radiology. Radi/o- means radiation, and -logy means the study of. Page Ref: 992

110. venography. Ven/o- means vein and -grapy means process of recording. Page Ref: 997

111. sound. Sonography uses sound waves to create an image. Page Ref: 1005

True/False

112. True. Both refer to x-ray images. Page Ref: 993

113. True. The sound waves bounce off the heart (cardi/o-) and the echo is captured to create an image. Page Ref: 1005

114. False. Bone has a high density but is radiopaque, creating a white image on the film. Page Ref: 994

115. True. Radi/o- means radiation, and pharmaceutic/o- means medicine or drug. Page Ref: 1007

116. False. Thallium-201 is the radionuclide that is given. Page Ref: 1007

117. True. Interventional radiology uses ultrasound, CT scans, or MRI scans as a guide for other procedures such as biopsies or needle insertions. Page Ref: 1002

118. False. X-rays, fluoroscopy, and CT scanning expose patients to radiation but the MRI uses a magnetic field. Page Ref: 1003

119. False. It is called a barium swallow. Page Ref: 1000

120. True. The computer can then combine these slices into three-dimensional images. Page Ref: 1001,1003

121. False. The x-ray described in this question is the AP x-ray. Page Ref: 995

122. True. Angiography is made of the parts angi/o-, which means blood vessel, and -graphy, which is a process of recording. Page Ref: 997

123. True. It is absorbed in the small intestine and then processed by the liver and excreted into the gallbladder. Page Ref: 998

124. False. A mammogram is used to create an image of the breast. The combining form mamm/o- means breast. Page Ref: 1001

125. True. The bone density tests determine if demineralization from osteoporosis is present. Page Ref: 1001

126. True. MRI uses strong magnetic fields instead of radiation to create diagnostic images. Page Ref: 1003

127. True. The radioactive substances are given intravenously or by inhalation but have short half-lives and do not cause any radiation damage to the patient. Page Ref: 1008

128. False. PET scans use positively charged particles called positrons, not magnetic fields. Page Ref: 1011

129. True. In this type of study, fluoroscopy and individual radiographs are used to document the results. Page Ref: 998

130. True. It is also known as a full body scan. Page Ref: 1004

131. False. It does expose the patient to radiation because it is performed in conjunction with a CT scan to create an image and that involves x-rays. Page Ref: 1004

132. False. All types of ultrasonography use sound waves and not radiation to create an image, so the patient is not exposed to any radiation. Page Ref: 1006

133. False. Magnetic resonance imaging uses a strong magnetic field to align protons in the atoms. Page Ref: 1003

Essay

134. PET scans require a cyclotron which is a very large, expensive piece of equipment that emits positrons. Page Ref: 1011

135. The radiologist dictates the findings to be transcribed into a radiology report that is incorporated into the patient's medical record. Page Ref: 994

136. The suffix -graphy indicates a process of recording a procedure while the suffix -gram indicates the record or picture that is produced. Page Ref: 997

137. Color flow duplex ultrasonography combines a two-dimensional ultrasound image and Doppler technology to create an ultrasound image that shows anatomy, as well as colors, according to the velocity, direction, and turbulence of the blood flow in that area. It is used to image the coronary arteries, carotid arteries, or arteries of the legs. Page Ref: 1006

138. Echocardiography is an imaging test that uses ultra high-frequency sound waves emitted by an ultrasound transducer placed on the chest or swallowed and positioned in the esophagus. The sound waves bounce off the heart, creating echoes that are changed into an image by a computer. This procedure shows the heart contracting and relaxing. The resulting image is called an echocardiogram. Page Ref: 1005

139. X-rays are a type of invisible ionizing radiation. They have a very short wavelength and contain so much energy that they are able to pass through the body. Page Ref: 993

140. The images in an x-ray appear in various shades of black, white, and gray that correspond to the density of various tissues. Areas of low density are said to be radiolucent. An example is an air-filled space which shows up black on an image. Areas of high density are said to be radiopaque. An example of this is bone, which shows up white on the image. Page Ref: 994

141. A film badge is worn by all health care professionals who work in the radiology and nuclear medicine departments. The badge contains a clear, unexposed piece of x-ray film that becomes progressively more opaque with cumulative exposure to radiation (x-rays and gamma rays from radioactive substances). Radiation exposure is measured in rems. Dosimetry is the process of measuring the amount of radiation exposure as detected by a film badge and measured by a dosimeter. Page Ref: 996